Pregnancy is a "Real Mother!"

Our Multitasking Modern-Day "Real Mother"

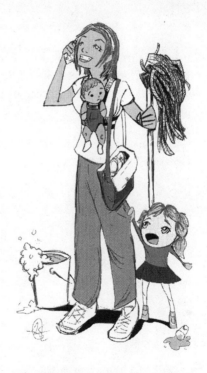

Jeffrey L. Zweig, MD

Figure 0-1 Pregnancy real mother mascot

Copyright © 2015 by Jeffrey L. Zweig, MD.

Library of Congress Control Number:		2015901622
ISBN:	Hardcover	978-1-5035-1973-2
	Softcover	978-1-5035-1974-9
	eBook	978-1-5035-1972-5

All rights reserved. No part of this book may be reproduced or transmitted in any form or by any means, electronic or mechanical, including photocopying, recording, or by any information storage and retrieval system, without permission in writing from the copyright owner.

Any people depicted in stock imagery provided by Thinkstock are models, and such images are being used for illustrative purposes only.
Certain stock imagery © Thinkstock.

Print information available on the last page.

Rev. date: 05/16/2015

To order additional copies of this book, contact:
Xlibris
1-888-795-4274
www.Xlibris.com
Orders@Xlibris.com

PREGNANCY IS A "REAL MOTHER!"

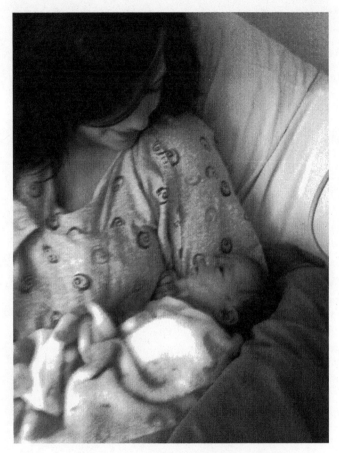

Figure 0-2 Mother and Baby Bonding

The very best job I ever had in this world was being a Mom
--Naomi Judd, RN, Mother of Wynonna,
Judd's Farewell Concert 1989

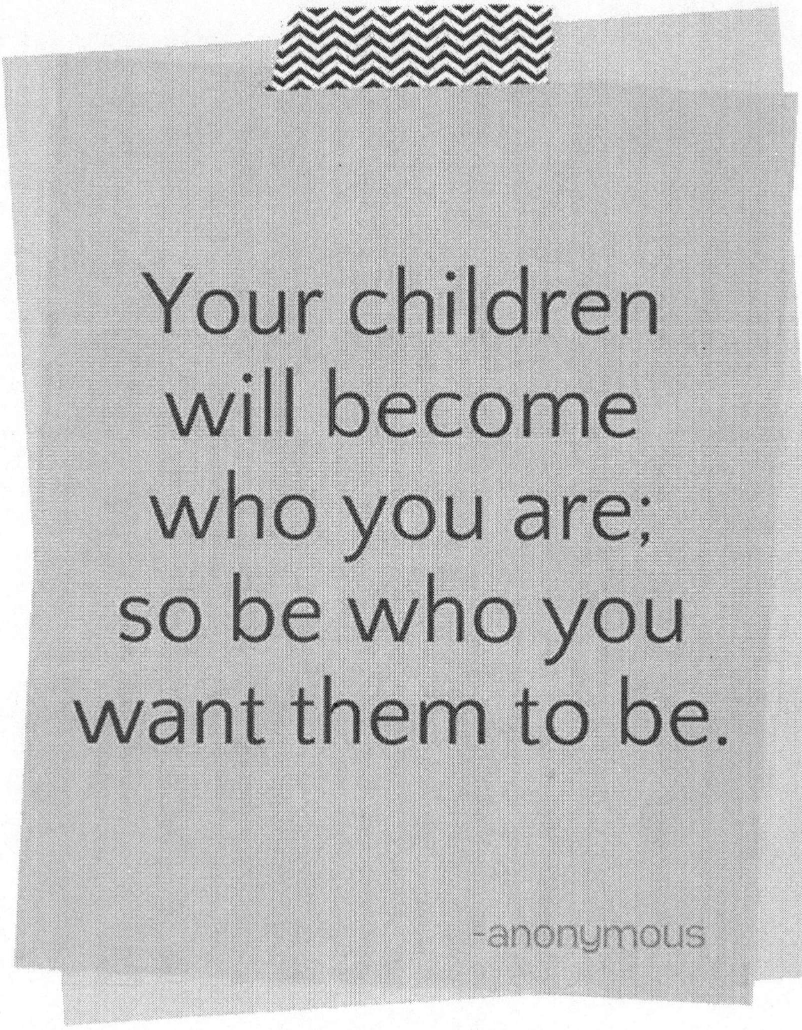

> Your children will become who you are; so be who you want them to be.
>
> -anonymous

Figure 0-3 Anonymous Quote about Children

ABOUT THE AUTHOR

Jeffrey L. Zweig, MD, was born in Los Angeles and grew up in Santa Ana, California. He has the following credentials:

> BA Johns Hopkins University, Baltimore, Maryland
> MD University of California, San Francisco, California (UCSF)
>
> Residency, Chief, Department of Obstetrics and Gynecology, UCLA Medical Center, Los Angeles, California
>
> Chief, Department of Obstetrics and Gynecology, Southwestern Medical Center, Lawton, Oklahoma.
>
> Board Certified, American College of Obstetrics and Gynecology (ACOG)
>
> Fellow, American College of Obstetrics and Gynecology

Dr. Zweig serves on the active Medical Staff of the following hospitals in Lawton, Oklahoma

> Comanche County Memorial Hospital and Southwestern Medical Center

He has the following specialty skills:

> Obstetrics with experience in Ultrasound and High Risk Pregnancies

Gynecological Surgery including Advanced Laparoscopic and Hysteroscopic Surgery

Infertility including Ovulation Induction and Insemination (no IVF)

Office Gynecology with treatment of menstrual disorders, infections and ovarian disorders

Dr. Zweig lives with his wife and family in Lawton, Oklahoma. He played tennis and was on the varsity tennis teams in high school and college. Dr. Zweig was a "runner" and was usually doing 15 miles per week. Currently his workout routine is with the elliptical for about 50 minutes per day followed by crunches with the Healthrider (I believe my knee and hip joints are being spared). He may get into light jogging soon but walking also works right now.

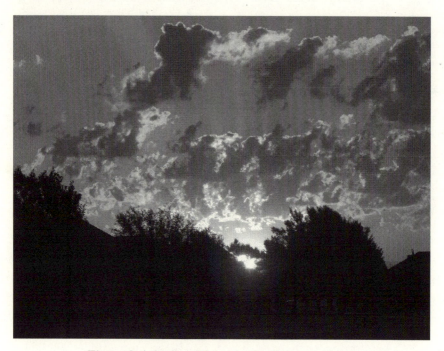

Figure 0-4 the Sun Rising in the Heavens Above

And the secret to life (on earth) is ....to reproduce!

This quote has "haunted" the author for many years because surely there must be more to life (on earth) than just to reproduce. The "survival of the species," preserving and recreating life itself seems to be the critical mission on this unpredictable planet. It is "wired in" as the basic instinct throughout all animal and plant life. This drive that is powered by the pleasure of sex: it is such a controlling and ingrained force. Is that all there is to life on this planet?

Curly, (in the movie *City Slickers*) states that secret to life is "about just one thing." When Billy Crystal asked what that "one thing'" was, Curly shot back and said, "Well, that's what you have to figure out."

States Julie Ann Williams, the "secret to life" is having trust and faith in God.

Scott Peck, in his book *The Road Less Traveled*, states that the purpose of life is for the individual is to constantly develop and improve oneself as a person.

Albert Schweitzer said, *"*The purpose of *life* is to serve and to show compassion and the will to help others."

However, Groucho Marx, the famed 1950's comedian, hit the nail on the head when he reflected and expounded, "The Secret to Life is honesty and fair-dealing. If you can fake that, then you got it made!"

Finally, Mae West stated, "You only live once, but if you do it right, once is enough."

"A BABY is born with a need to be LOVED and never outgrows it"--Frank A. Clark

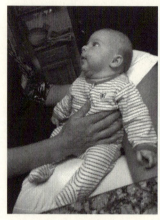 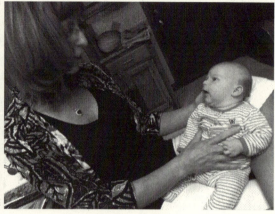

Figure 0-5 Judianna gazing at her mom

Figure 0-6 Julie and Judianna and the Secret

PREFACE

This book fulfills a need for all expecting parents wanting to know what pregnancy and having a baby is really "all about." Because many couples do not have the time or the inclination to read, I have attempted to create a book that was informative yet was a humorous and "an easy read." Entertaining you and making you laugh are some key ways of keeping you, the reader, captivated. The reader will be yearning to read the very "next page." This book guides the reader vicariously "down the road" of pregnancy with the destination of having a baby in their arms at the end. It portends to be, in a true sense, a pregnancy "reality book." The author is hopeful that this book may accomplish in presenting information on pregnancy in a way similar to that Dr. Benjamin Spock achieved with his classic book, *Baby and Child Care*.

The information in this book will provide the expectant couple the knowledge they need to know about pregnancy and childbirth. The main difference in this book compared to others is that I want reader to actually *enjoy* reading this book. The stories, the anecdotes, and the very <u>silly</u> humor punctuate the didactic information that is being conveyed. The premise behind this book's writing style and presentation is that it will more likely be read if:

    a. the reader sees pictures of real patients, nurses and hospital scenes
    b. the reader is presented with anecdotes of pregnancy situations that actually transpired
    c. the reader enjoys comicalness of natural human behavior

All of the above ingredients are interjected between the educational materials being presented. I want this book to be easily readable for every expectant couple. People will spend many hours in researching specifications and equipment on a vehicle prior to any purchase, but they tend to spend less time reading about the baby that is about to come into their lives.

No book on pregnancy for expecting parents can be "completely comprehensive." This book seeks "the middle ground:" not too brief but not too drawn out and technical. The reader should look to other specific books and articles for those detailed topics on which further information is desired, such as breastfeeding, caring for the newborn, etc. Though extensive in page numbers, the pictures and illustrations take up much of the manuscript.

The book starts out with a "Quick Start" section (the first two chapters). The reader can immediately obtain the "Cliff Notes" information about diet, physical activities, and other topics that they need to know through all of the phases of pregnancy. These two chapters comprise of the 200 or so most frequently asked questions (FAQs) of pregnancy.

The third part of the book comprises the essential but more detailed information that most couples might want to know about childbirth:

> Nutrition
> Labor and delivery
> Pain relief and anesthesia
> Cesarean section
> Postpartum Instructions
> Breastfeeding
> The Newborn

The last section is called the "Tales:" "Old wives" tales and, yes, "Old Obstetrician Tales" (real pregnancy stories *but* with some author editorial latitude taken to make the narratives more interesting). There are about 27 real-life stories that have transpired during the author's career. These stories entertain while educating the reader about an important aspect of obstetrics. Simultaneously the stories provide comic relief and laughter as well as thought-provoking reality.

Couples will become very familiar with the everyday workings of the labor and delivery rooms, the dedicated and compassionate nurses, and the anesthesia "miracle workers." After reading this book couples will be completely prepared for their pregnancy and delivery experience.

This book is not a "pregnancy manual" which is typically dry and boring. It is not a book on Pregnancy: Week by Week (like the other popular books on pregnancy: the reader is referred to those books if a pictorial growth guide of their baby is desired). This book follows the typical road a patient will usually travel down during her pregnancy.

This book is both informational and a little bit of a "novel" at the same time. As one of author's patients stated to him, the book has its own "personality" and is "a living saga." Even if you are not pregnant, the "Old Obstetrician's Tall Tales" in the last section will amuse and amaze you yet be very spiritual and insightful. The reader will never forget this book because the reader will identify themselves with the same pregnant folks that are highlighted throughout the book. The book reveals much about an Obstetrician's life and the patients that he cares for. If you enjoyed the books (and movies), *The Help, The Blind Side or National Treasure (semi-documentaries-dramas),* you will definitely delight in reading this book.

Teaching and education have been an integral part of the author's career. Early in his career he taught medical students as an assistant clinical professor at Stanford University School of Medicine. Since 2006 the author has been teaching the Specialty of Obstetrics and Gynecology to the Family Practice Residents at the University Of Oklahoma School Of Medicine. In 2008 he was awarded the "Best Teacher of the Year" award – an achievement he personally cherishes as a milestone in his career.

"Education is the most powerful weapon which you can use to change the world."

---Nelson Mandela

Expounding on the life of a writer, Tom Stoppard, the English playwright, once stated,

"You spend your whole life putting words together. Every once in a while you put them together in just the right order and it gives the world *"a nudge."*

As Charles Krauthammer remarked (and the author concurs), "That is what I live for."

--Chris Wallace Show, October 27, 2013.

ACKNOWLEDGMENTS

The author would like to give his gratitude to all of those people who have helped and encouraged him with the creation this book. First, he would like to thank all of his patients from the past 40 years who have inspired as well as educated him to the point that he would be able to pen this book. He would especially like to thank all of those patients who have allowed the author to use their pictures and stories in the book.

I would like to thank Dr. Janice Lepp for taking her valuable time to read, review and correct didactic information in the book. Her critical recommendations were indeed very significant.

The author asked many professionals in his community to review and constructively make suggestions to improve the book as follows:

Dr. Minda Roan, Pediatrician at Southwestern Medical Center, for her review and corrections and input to the chapter on the Newborn.

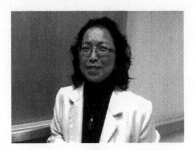

Figure 0-7 Minda Roan, MD

Deana Price, RN, Women's Services at Southwestern Medical Center, Newborn Nursery, for her contribution to the chapter on Breastfeeding

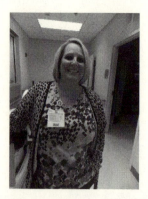

Figure 0-8 Deanna Price, RN

Mrs. Paige Holder, Dietician at Southwestern Medical Center (SWMC) for reviewing and editing the chapter on Nutrition.

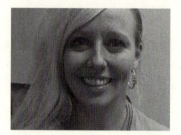

Figure 0-9 Paige Holder, RDA

Albert Arrendondo, CRNA, Chief of Anesthesia Services, Southwestern Medical Center for his patient information hand-out that is contained in the chapter on Anesthesia.

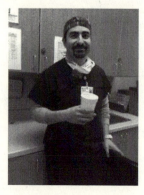

Figure 0-10 Albert Arrendondo, CRNA

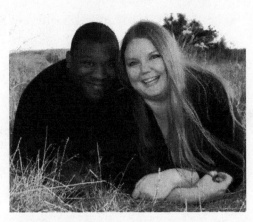

Figure 0-11 Warren and Audra Stewart

I would like to thank Artist, Mr. Warren Stewart and Mrs. Audra Stewart, RN for helping to further sketch out the mascot- of "The Real Mother" that adorns the cover plus other illustrations for the book and to his wife, Audra, for reviewing the book while she was pregnant with her first baby.

I would like to thank Mrs. Susan Pokorny, one of my patients, who helped re-draw and touch up many of the illustrations and photographs in the book.

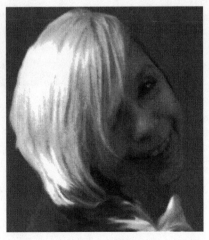

Figure 0-12 Susan Pokorny, Artist

I would like to thank all nurses of Women's Health at Southwestern Medical Center in Lawton who not only were pictured in this book but also helped me in so many ways: especially Angie, Courtney, Tammy, Lindsey, Becky, Caitlin, Jodi, Jessica, Marianne, Stacy, Kasmira, Rayanna, Emily, Diana and Judy.

I would like to thank my office staff, Donna Cunningham, Angela Gardner, Ramona Garcia, and April Bluford, for their support, obtaining the permissions for the book, and feedback on the content of the book.

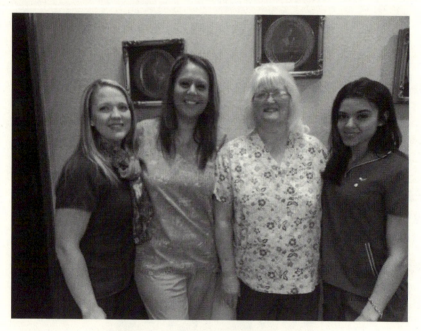

Figure 0-13 Dr. Zweig's Office Staff
Left to right: Angela Garner, Ramona Garcia,
Donna Cunningham and April Bluford

I would like to thank my family for their patience with the project and allowing me the time to pursue the writing and completion of this book. I would like to especially thank Julie Williams, my life partner, for reading the manuscripts and offering her thoughts and advice on the topics covered in the book. She was so gracious and kind to pose for some of the illustrations in many of the chapters in the book.

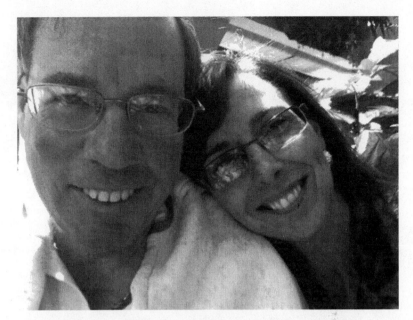

Figure 0-14 Author and Julie

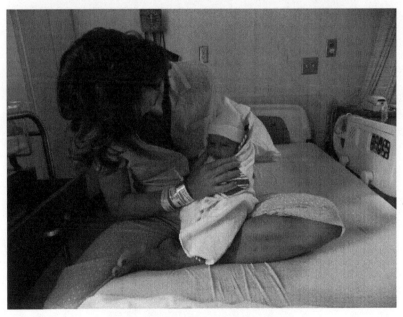

Figure 0-15 Julie and Judianna

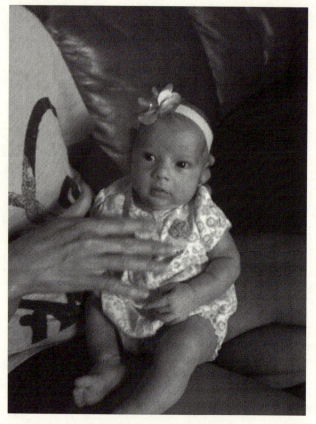

Figure 0-16 Baby Judianna

"If you live to be a hundred, I want to live to be a hundred minus one day so I never have to live without you."

"Some people care too much. I think it's called love
—A.A. Milne, Winnie-the-Pooh

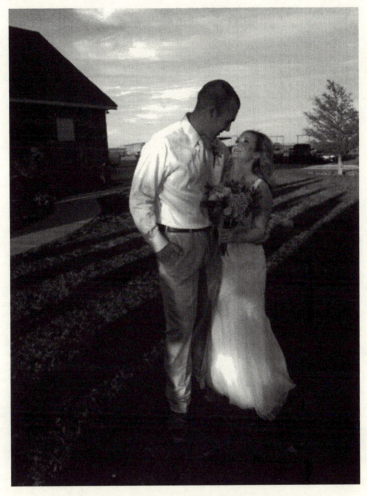

Figure 0-17 Wedding Day of CJ and Katie

Photographer's Note: They did not pose for this picture. It was caught on camera spontaneously!

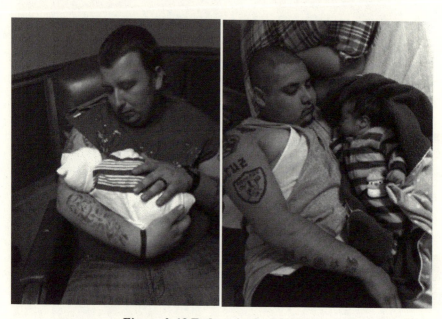

Figure 0-18 Fathers in the Moment

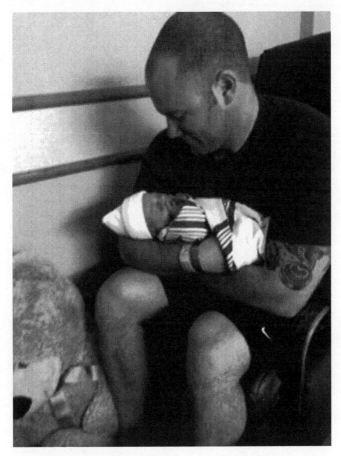

Figure 0-19 Moments those take your breath away.

CONTENTS

About the Author.. vii
Preface.. xi
Acknowledgments xv

Chapter 1   Quick-Start Section..1
   Everything I Ever Needed to Know about Pregnancy
   I Learned from the 20 Rules of Advice 2
   Introduction to Being Pregnant...6
     1. Positive pregnancy test 6
     2. Diet: What you should be eating 9
     3. "Morning Sickness" 12
     4. My Body is Changing Already! 16
     5. Exercise and Physical Activities......................17
     6. Due Dates 18
     7. Appointments. 19
     8. Your Email, telephone numbers
         and addresses, please! 24
     9. Smoking and other Substance Use 25
    10. Medications and Drugs 25
    11. Prenatal Vitamins and Iron: 28
    12. Weight Gain Guidelines 31
    13. How long is my pregnancy? It can't be that long!...35
    14. Laboratory Testing...37
    15. When can I know the sex of my baby?............41
    16. Vaccinations: FLU Vaccine and dTap..............45
    17. What was one of the original purposes
         of Obstetrical Care?...47

18. Why pregnancy is a "Real Mother?"..................................48
19. Sex and Pregnancy: A frequent question
    asked during Pregnancy..49
20. People Giving You Advice and Stories:
    "You need to ignore them!"..52
21. Get out and Enjoy Life (because,
    Life as you know it now is coming to an end!).............54
22. Relationship Changes and Challenges 54
23. Traveling during Pregnancy 59
24. Bathing, Showering, Clothing and Shoes......................60
25. "Quickening" (Feeling the baby's movements).............61
26. Hospitals and Delivery..61
27. Prenatal Classes and Hospital Tours..............................63
28. Insurance Coverage and Billing 63
29. Telephone Calls and Problems..67
30. How much does my baby weigh
    and how long is my baby?..70
31. Obstetrical Adverse Events and Malpractice.................71
32. Missing fingers and toes 73

Chapter 2 Medical Conditions and their
          Treatment during your Pregnancy...............................75

1. Colds and flu:...75
2. Stomach and bowel symptoms
   (GI symptoms) explained..76
3. Anemia 80
4. Headaches..82
5. Seasonal Allergies:...82
6. Dizziness, Lightheadedness and Fainting: 83
7. Leg swelling (edema) and Varicose Veins: 83
8. Strange cravings
   (ice, ice cream, vinegar and pickles)................................86
9. Hair coloring, Permanents and Manicures 87
10. Swelling of your hands: now how
    do I get my wedding ring off?..87

11. "Baby Brain" 88
12. "Dreams" during Pregnancy. 88
13. The "Black Line," Tan nipples and other Color Changes on your body during Pregnancy......................89
14. Sunbathing, Saunas, Tanning beds and Creams 89
15. How do I prevent from getting "stretch marks"? 90
16. Colostrum and Leakage of your nipples late in pregnancy 92
17. Carpal Tunnel Syndrome (Why are my fingers numb?) 92
18. Pregnancy-Related Abdominal and Pelvic Pains...........92
19. Low Back Pain 94
20. Sciatica and Round Ligament Syndrome (your baby is "getting on your nerves") 95
21. Insomnia: It means I cannot fall or stay asleep!.............99
22. Can I sleep on my back or lay down on my back during exercise class?..100
23. Yeast and other vaginal Infections...............................102
24. Urinary Tract Infections (UTI's)..................................103
25. Other Noticeable Skin "Things" (Red Palms and Spider Angiomas)...............................103
26. "My Face is breaking out!" 104
27. "I'm tired of being pregnant and I want my baby out!"—the most common complaint OB's hear daily 105
28. Sexually Transmitted Diseases (STD's) 106
29. Leakage of urine during Pregnancy (Urinary Incontinence) 112
30. Obesity 112
31. Cramping and Braxton-Hicks contractions 114
32. Gender Reveal Parties 115
33. Pregnancy Q&A's 118
34. Getting use to the "Bumpy" Road. 119
35. The Natural "Pelvic Exam Reflex" 121

36. It seems like everything "bleeds" when I am pregnant!...................................122
37. Abnormal Pap Smears during Pregnancy....................123
38. Smoking Cessation...124

Chapter 3 Labor and Delivery:
          The Short and Pithy Version................127
1. When will I deliver my Baby?...............................127
2. How do I know if I am in Labor?..........................129
3. I lost my mucus plug, now what do I do?
    The most common phone call to the OB
    suite as reported by the nurses!............................129
4. When do I call the office or go to the hospital?............130
5. What do I need to bring to the hospital?....................130
6. Introduction to the Labor and Delivery Suite.............131
7. How many people can be in the Birthing Room?........132
8. How long will I be in Labor?...............................137
9. When do I need to see my doctor after delivery?...........150
10. Inductions of Labor and C-Sections........................150
11. Baby Care and Pediatricians.................................150
12. Breastfeeding..151

Chapter 4 Pictorial Tour of Labor and Delivery....................153

Chapter 5 Prenatal Care:
          "The Good, the Bad, and the Details".....................169
1. High Expectations, But 170
2. The Ten Important Steps you can take
    to stay healthy when pregnant...............................171
3. Dental Health and Care during Pregnancy...............173
4. Eye Care and Changes..178
5. Seat Belts..179
6. What about Sex during Pregnancy?........................180
7. Incompetent Cervix and Early Second
    Trimester Loss...181

Chapter 6   Mostly Third Trimester Pregnancy Issues or
            "The Final Stretch"...184

1. "Baby-Moon" 185
2. Preparing in advance for your Hospital Stay.................187
3. Pre-eclampsia or Toxemia of Pregnancy 191
4. Pre-term Labor 196
5. Premature Rupture of Membranes 198
6. Twin and Multiple Pregnancy, Just a few
    important comments ("Double Trouble")....................199
7. Abruption of the Placenta..202
8. Placenta Praevia 204
9. Fetal Kick Counts and Fetal Movements......................206
10. GBS Testing ("The Swab Test") 207
11. Vertex position in the 3rd trimester...............................208
12. Fetal Surveillance testing
    (Baby "health checkups" while pregnant)..................210
13. 3D Ultrasound 213
14. How long after my due date will my OB
    allow me to stay pregnant? 216
15. When can I stop working?...216
16. Cord Blood Banking..217
17. 3rd Trimester Testing 217
18. "Nesting" Instincts 219
19. Birthing Plans..219
20. Other 3rd trimester Experiences and Feelings. 222
21. Pregnancy Portraits..224

Chapter 7   Labor and delivery:
            How you can be "Birthing with the Stars" 226

1. Preliminary Remarks..226
2. When does Labor Occur?...227
3. But How Do I Know When I'm in Labor? 228
4. Definition of Labor 232
5. What is the Purpose of Labor?
    Your baby wants to Head Out! 232

6.	What Does a Turtle-Neck Sweater Have To Do with Childbirth?	233
7.	"Engagement?" Doesn't that occur before marriage?	237
8.	The "Mechanism of Labor"	237
9.	Other Medical Definitions and Terminology	241
10.	True Labor: Sometimes may be difficult to diagnose!	244
11.	The Amniotic Sac	245
12.	The Bishop's Score	247
13.	Leaking Amniotic Fluid	248
14.	What do I do when Labor Starts?	249
15.	The Trip to the Hospital	251
16.	Video camera or other recordings of the baby's birth	255
17.	How many people can I have in my Labor and Delivery Room? Can we have Cameras and Videos?	256
18.	What if my doctor is not there?	258
19.	Eating during Labor? I don't think so!	259
20.	The Umbilical Cord	260
21.	The Emergency C-section and the prevention of Aspiration	261
22.	The Process of Labor	262
23.	The Typical Scenario of Childbirth	264
24.	The First Stage of Labor	268
25.	Delivery	277
24.	The Immediate Care of the Newborn in the Delivery Suite	283
25.	Third Stage of Labor	283
27.	Causes of Uterine Atony (TMI section)	287
28.	The Delivery Room "Shivers and Shakes"	288

Chapter 8   Analgesics during Labor and Delivery:
            Medications available for Pain Relief 292
    1.   What Are the Most Commonly Used Medications? 292

Chapter 9   Obstetrical Anesthesia 301
    Epidural Anesthesia 302
    Technique of Epidural Anesthesia 304
    Spinal Anesthesia 318
    General Anesthesia 319

Chapter 10   Operative or Assisted Vaginal Delivery 321
    1.   Vacuum Extractor 321
    2.   Obstetrical Forceps 327

Chapter 11   Fetal Monitoring 332

Chapter 12   Induction of Labor 347

Chapter 13   Cesarean Delivery:
            Babies born that are "A Cut Above!" 354
    Abdominal Incisions: 357
    Other types of Uterine Incisions 358
    Closure of the Incision: the Skin Layer 359
    Medical Indications for a C-Section 360
    Obstetrical Legal Indications. 360
    Author Observation of Patients with Polycystic
            Ovarian Syndrome (PCOS) –His Special Concern 362
    The Uterine Incision 364
    The Risks of a C-Section 364
    C-Section Complications 368
    The Cascade of Events for a C-Section 368
    Visual Tour of a C-section 374
    Questions Most Frequently Asked
            After C-Section Surgery 383
    VBAC: Vaginal Birth after C-Section 386
    VBAC Protocol 389

    Risks of: Repeat C-Section and VBAC 389
    Benefits: VBAC 389
    Breech Babies 391
    External Cephalic Version (ECV) 392

Chapter 14 Exercise and Physical Fitness in Pregnancy 395
    Exercise Don'ts: 395
    Exercise Do's: 396
    Cardinal Principles of Exercise during Pregnancy: 397
    Exercise Cautions: 397
    Water or Snow Skiing 399
    Scuba Diving 399
    Weight Lifting Programs 399

Chapter 15 Other Questions most asked about
                during Pregnancy 400
    Saunas And Hot Tubs . . . Can I Use Them? 400
    Electric Blankets 401
    Can I Sunbathe or Tan?
        No, unless you use Sunscreens! 401
    Can I Smoke? 402
    Can I Travel During Pregnancy? 403
    Any Wardrobe Changes? 405

Chapter 16 Foods And Nutrition 406
    Nutrition during Pregnancy 406
    Consumer Reports recommends that pregnant women
        avoid eating tuna altogether. 408
    Caloric Requirements 408
    Weight Gain 409
    Nutrients 410
    Red Meats 413
    Milk and Dairy Products 419
    Fiber 422
    What Is In A Food Label? 435

    Food Preparation 442
    Store Food Properly 447

Chapter 17 Potential Hazards During Pregnancy 450
    Imaging studies during Pregnancy: X-Rays 452
    Other Diagnostic Imaging Technology 453
    Occupational Safety and Environmental Exposures 454
    Special Concern for Medical and Dental Fields 457

Chapter 18 Medications During Pregnancy
               And Breastfeeding 462
    General Principles 462
    Food Additives 466
    Specific Harmful Drugs 466
    Commonly Prescribed Safe Medications 467
    Vaccinations during Pregnancy 470
    Substance Abuse 473
    Caffeine Use 474

Chapter 19 Pre-existing Medical Conditions
               and Infectious Diseases during Pregnancy 477
    1. Pregnancy and Diabetes 477
    2. The Rh Negative Factor 480
    3. Herpes and Pregnancy 487
    4. HIV, Hepatitis and Pregnancy 498
    5.   Infectious Diseases during Pregnancy That Cause
         Serious Birth Defects: 501
    6.   Medical Diseases during Pregnancy that cause
         serious Birth Defects: 501

Chapter 20 Obstetrical Tragedies 502
    Ectopic Pregnancies 509
    Stillborn 509

Chapter 21 Postpartum Instructions 510
   How long will I stay in the hospital? 511
   Baby Identification and Security bracelet 511
   Bathing and Showering 512
   Bleeding, discharge and Infection after Delivery 512
   Warning Signs: 514
   Physician Rounds and Hospital Visits after Delivery 514
   "New Father Sleeping Sickness" 517
   Perineal Care after Delivery 519
   After-pains 520
   If you had an episiotomy 520
   Treatment Of Sore Episiotomies 522
   Constipation 522
   Hemorrhoids 523
   Bladder problems 524
   Leg Swelling and Pain 524
   Back and pelvic pain after delivery 525
   Eye Changes 525
   Nutrition and Dieting 525
   General Physical Activity 526
   Exercise 527
   C-section Deliveries 527
   Postpartum Depression 532
   Birth Control 532
   Other Special Postpartum Situations
      you want to know about after delivery 535
   Rh factor 536
   Rubella Vaccine 536
   Smoking 536
   Breast Feeding Postpartum 538
   Lactation Suppression 539
   The 6 Week Check-up Appointment 544
   Breasts and Breastfeeding 544
   Discharge Medications 545

    Supply Checklist for Baby 545
    Losing weight after your birth 551

Chapter 22 Breast And Bottle Feeding 553

    Breastfeeding 554
    Advantages of Breastfeeding 555
    Disadvantages of Breastfeeding 556
    Preparation for Breastfeeding 557
    Technique of Breastfeeding 558
    Breast feeding Key Points 562
    Initiation of Breastfeeding 563
    Sustaining Milk Production 564
    Breast Engorgement 565
    The Actual Nursing Process 566
    Lactation Specialist Deanna Price, RN,
        Has Some Special Advice 569
    Breast Infection (Mastitis) 573
    Clogged Ducts 574
    Swollen Glands under your Arms 574
    Embarrassing Let-Down 575
    Inverted Nipples 575
    Previous Breast Surgery 575
    Baby Favoring Only One Breast 576
    Nutrition for Breastfeeding 576
    Can I start a weight loss diet when breastfeeding? 576
    How do I know when there is enough milk? 578
    How often should I feed? 578
    Milk Expression 578
    Facilitating Milk Expression 579
    How to Express 579
    Milk Supply 580
    When to Express 581
    Breast Pumps 581
    Storing Breast Milk 581

Thawing Breast Milk 582
Breastfeeding Sequence in Brief 582
Bottle-feeding 583
Lactation Suppression: 586
Weight Loss and getting back into Shape 587
Weight Management Discussion 587

Chapter 23 The Newborn 589
Prenatal Visit with Your Pediatrician 589
The Newborn 591
Concept of Parenting 591
The importance of giving your baby a proper name............592
Newborn Health Screening and Testing................................594
Preparing for your baby's arrival at home.............................595
Newborn Physical Examination 596
The Baby's Skin 597
The Baby's Genitalia ("Sexual anatomy")...........................600
The Babies Digestive System 602
Breastfeeding 602
Your Temperature Settings at home 605
Diapers...607
Circumcision...610
A Little Historical and Religious Perspective......................611
Newborn Monitoring Systems..616
Crying Babies 617
Sudden Infant Death Syndrome (SIDS) 619
Keeping Your Marriage Alive After the Baby Arrives 622
Getting your baby to go to sleep..625
Author's Experiences with his young children 627
Author's Advice to his own Children...................................631

Chapter 24 Old Wives Tales..634
More Old Wives Tales that try to predict
    the sex of your baby 642

Drano Test-Revised 643
"Old Mayan Wives' Tale: Even and Odd numbers 643
The Key Test 643
The Acne Test 644
The Ring Test.. 644
The Linea Nigra Test 645
Mayan" Numbers Variation"... 646
Cold Feet Tale 646
Pillow Test... 646
How are you sleeping in your bed?....................................... 647
Urine Color Test... 647
Hair Growth Theory... 648
Shape of Your Belly Test 648
Nose Shape and Growth 649
Facial Changes 649
Demeanor and Agility.. 649
Show me your Hands 649
Do you smell Garlic?.. 649
Saving the best for Last? Skip this one if you are smart! 650
More Myths about Pregnancy... 650

Chapter 25 "Old Husband's Tales" 651

Chapter 26 Old Obstetrician Tales
 (Yes, there are such Tales!)................................... 652
The DaSilva Family 652
The Garabaldi Family 653
Melanie, the Hairdresser Athlete 654
The City Councilman's Wife 655
Zweig's Laws of Obstetrics... 656
How to be sure your teen uses birth control
 (especially my teenager).. 657
The Story of Jennifer's Birth 658
Four babies in 26 minutes... 662
The Isuzu Baby (Isuzu Trooper SUV) 664

April fool's Days 666
The Camper on Interstate 680 668
Remembering Rita 669
The Tennessee Trucker Woman 671
Mr. Juan Garcia of Alviso, CA but it is a not a
    pregnancy story 673
My Hispanic Newlywed 674
The Red Hair Girl from Santa Maria, CA 676
Hamrell's line 680
Buying "Protection" for my Ultrasound Probe 680
Runaway Teen travels down a hard road with
    metamorphosis into a Respected Physician 683
The Biggest Baby I ever delivered 694
Little Patient in San Ramon, CA 697
Dr. Karen Branch and the Male Medical Students 701
Future Lawton Nurse says "Castor Oil does not work!" 703
The Breech delivery with Dr. Bill Dignam 706
The Pregnant Teenager who was lost and Hurt 708
Dr. Gandhi and his Breech Girl 713
The Koerber Story 715
Typhoon Yaling/Typhoon Patsy 719
"I want a Pepsi" 723
Pregnant 16 year old single Tennessee Teenager 725
The Pyrimidalis Muscles 729
Cassandra, a Pregnant Runner
    who saved her Doctor's Life 730
Match.com 741
The Linda Castro Story 753
Women make all the RULES 756

Chapter 27 Concluding Words: Footprints in the Sand
                    and Winnie-the-Pooh 761

Appendix A: Other questions asked
by my pregnant patients. 765

Why did the Author write this Book? 765
Why did you choose Obstetrics as a medical specialty? 766
Dedication 770
Jude Lyons Legacy Raisin Bran Muffin Recipe 772
"Toast" of the Town 773
Dr. Zweig 2013 Commencement Speech to the
graduating OU Medical Family Practice
Residents in Lawton, OK. 774

Appendix B: Additional Resources
Prenatal Non-Invasive Testing
(NIPS) Diagnosis 782

Harmony Blood Test 783
Materni21 784
Panorama Test 785
About Panorama™ 785
New sunscreen labels 786
The Obstetrical Forceps 789
A "Doctors Note" 790

Appendix C: How did I become Pregnant? 791
Yes, it was a girl in a red sundress 791

Appendix D: Vaccination Guidelines
for Pregnant Women 801

List of disorders included in newborn
screening programs 811
What should parents know to protect the safety
and security of their Baby? 817
Common Questions About Newborn
Hearing Screens/Tests 819

Appendix E: VBAC Protocol at Southwestern
              Medical Center, Lawton, OK 821
    VBAC Consent Form 828

Appendix F: References and Sources of Information 830

Appendix G: Sample of a Birth Plan 831
    Procedures Prior To Or During Early Labor 832
    Procedures For Delivery 833
    Postpartum 834
    Newborn Care 835

Appendix H: Baby Weight and Length for each week of
              Pregnancy 836
Index 839

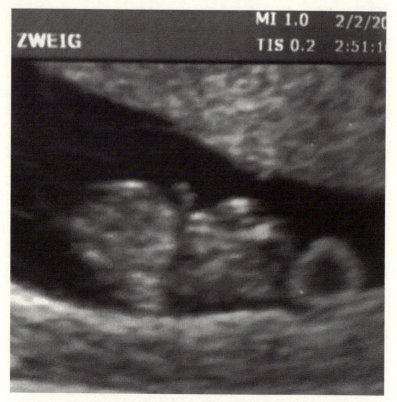

Figure 0-20 Halo is still being worn by embryo on ultrasound

Garth Brooks sings the 'Mom' Song

You'll never have a better friend
Or a warmer touch to tuck you in
She'll kiss your bruises, your bumps and scrapes
And anytime you hurt, her heart's gonna break

www.**garthbrooks**.com/news/**garth**-sings-on-gma-2/

"Mom" was written by Don Sampson and Wynn Varble

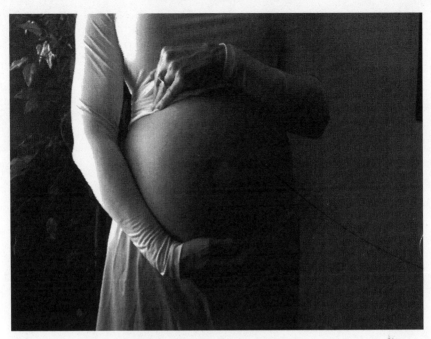

Figure 0-21 Circle of Life Photo

"The Circle of Life"

**From the day we arrive on this planet, and blinking, step into the sun
There's more to see than can ever be seen, more to do than can ever be done
There is far too much to take in here, more to find than can ever be found
It's the circle of life, and it moves us all**

The song lyrics of Tim Rice as sung by Sir Elton John present a suitable "poem" at this *"The Beginning"* of the book. Similarly this is *the beginning* of your pregnancy and your new life to arrive.

(The author urges the reader to look up **all** the lyrics for their philosophical insight about humans and their destiny on this planet)

CHAPTER 1

Quick-Start Section

Most women will suspect that they may be pregnant when they are late for their cycle. Their breasts become even more sensitive than usual. Loss of appetite, some nausea, and being more sleepy than usual are some of the other suspicious symptoms. But, it is not until you have purchased a pregnancy test and find a "positive" result (or your pregnancy test is done at your physician's office, the laboratory, or hospital) that you know "it is for sure."

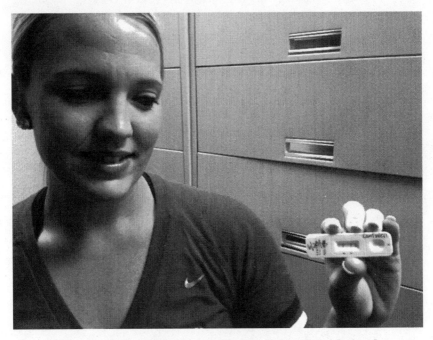

Figure 1-1 Pregnancy Test is "Positive." Angela is obviously "glowing" with her positive pregnancy test results.

Everything I Ever Needed to Know about Pregnancy I Learned from the 20 Rules of Advice

1. LIFE SYLE ABUSE AND BABY ABUSE DURING PREGNANCY: *QUIT* SMOKING, *QUIT* DRINKING, AND *QUIT* TAKING DRUGS, MEDICATIONS AND OTHER HARMFUL SUBSTANCES.

2. EAT HEALTHY: Whatever you eat is what your baby's tissues and organs will be made from.
Quality protein (80 grams per day) can build a strong baby and help reduce pregnancy complications.

3. IRON AND FOLIC ACID ARE THE MOST IMPORTANT MINERAL/VITAMIN SUPPLEMENTS YOU CAN TAKE DURING PREGNANCY. Almost every pregnant woman is anemic: decreased red blood cells that carry and circulate oxygen to your baby. Just taking one iron pill with Vitamin C per day can avoid this most common condition during pregnancy. Extra folic acid is also very effective in building a better baby: you can purchase folic acid OTC (over the counter) in 0.8 mg tablets and take up to 4 mg per day.

4. SEE YOUR OB PHYSICIAN EARLY IN PREGNANCY AND KEEP YOUR APPOINTMENTS! Pregnancy complications can be diagnosed earlier and can thereby be addressed to decrease your and your baby's health risks and assure better outcomes. "Life Happens!" so make an appointment with your OB in the very first few weeks of pregnancy.

5. LABOR AND DELIVERY TAKES ABOUT 12 HOURS ON AVERAGE. Fortunately an Epidural can eliminate most of these hours of pain. 25% of patients will have a Cesarean delivery for a good reason.

6. PREGNANCY IS THE MOST IMPORTANT LIFECYCLE EVENT YOU WILL EXPERIENCE IN YOUR LIFETIME. The emotional and physical rollercoaster has just begun: from

the horrible morning sickness in the beginning to the tears that will be streaming down your face when you hold your baby in your arms for the first time.

7. BREASTFEEDING YOUR BABY HELPS GIVE YOUR BABY THE BEST "HEAD START" (I'M TALKING BRAINS!) IN HIS/HER LIFE. Breast milk has the proper composition of protein, carbohydrate and fat designed naturally for a human baby. Further, breast milk contains and passes on immune protection antibodies from your breast milk to your baby. Antibodies protect your baby from viruses and bacteria. Your baby may not suffer the same number or severity of colds and diarrhea that other babies may experience. It is your baby's first "fast food."

8. PREGNANCY IS NOT "A DISEASE:" YOU CAN AND SHOULD CONTINUE TO GO TO SCHOOL AND WORK. Continue with school and your education. You are still able to do most physical activities and work as much as your body and mind can bear.

9. TAKING CARE OF A BABY IS THE MOST DIFFICULT (AND THE MOST RESPONSIBLE) JOB YOU WILL EVER HAVE IN YOUR LIFETIME. You will never believe how a little baby can consume all of your time, energy and emotional strength. Mentally you need to prepare for the crying, the poopy diapers and the lack of sleep. You will be rewarded when your baby smiles back at you: it is their way of telling you, "Thank you, Mommy and Daddy. I love you!"

10. PRACTICE SAFE SEX (please!). It is a different world now and STD's are more common than they ever were. Keep up your personal hygiene (that means a shower or a bath!) and brush your teeth after meals.

11. AVOID DANGEROUS ACTIVITIES AND SITUATIONS. Drive carefully and do not text while driving. Stay away from physical activities that increase your risk of body injury or falls. Being protective of yourself, protects your unborn baby.

12. BUY AT LEAST 4 RECEIVING BLANKETS AND 4 BABY BLANKETS FOR YOUR BABY. Your baby cannot leave home or sleep without them! You and your baby will lose one or two of them along the way. Similarly, buy 4 stuffed animals for your baby.

13. HAVING MORE THAN 8 CONTRACTIONS PER HOUR IS A SIGN OF PRETERM LABOR: If you are feeling these contractions more than 4 weeks prior to your due date, please contact your OB or go to your hospital.

14. DO DAILY FETAL KICK COUNTS: it is the only way a pregnant mother can monitor her baby's health on her own.

15. LEARN WHAT a "CATEGORY 3" FETAL HEART STRIP LOOKS LIKE (see Crash Course on Fetal Monitoring).

16. IF POSSIBLE, A PRE-CONCEPTUAL PREGNANCY PLANNING APPOINTMENT MAY BE VERY CRITICAL TO YOUR BABY'S DEVELOPMENT:

    a. CONTROL YOUR BLOOD PRESSURE AND SWITCH OUT MEDICATIONS THAT MAY BEDANGEROUS TO YOUR BABY

    b. TAKE CONTROL OF YOUR DIABETES (BLOOD SUGAR): IT CAN *SIGNIFICANTLY* LOWER THE RISK OF BIRTH DEFECTS IN THE VERY FIRST FEW WEEKS OF PREGNANCY

    c. TAKE CONTROL OF ANY OTHER MEDICAL CONDITIONS AND THEIR TREATMENT: Depression, Rheumatoid Arthritis, Lupus, Heart disease, Crohn's and Ulcerative colitis, Psoriasis, Acne, Substance abuse, etc.

17. IF YOU THINK YOU ARE IN LABOR, ESPECIALLY IF YOU THINK YOU ARE IN *ADVANCED* LABOR AND READY TO DELIVER, CALL (OR HAVE SOMEONE

ELSE CALL) THE OB SUITE AND LET THEM KNOW YOU ARE COMING!

The OB nursing staff must prepare for your delivery. If other patients are in labor, they may have to "call in" extra nurses for your delivery. The OB nursing and hospital staff will have to notify your OB and anesthesia staff if you want an epidural, and give them and a Nursery nurse time to travel to the hospital and get ready for your delivery and baby.

18. PREPARE IN ADVANCE FOR YOUR TRIP TO THE HOSPITAL AND MAKE CHILDCARE ARRANGEMENTS FOR YOUR OTHER CHILDREN.

In the last month of pregnancy patients should get together items they will need during their stay at the hospital (see Third Trimester Issues chapter). Patients should also make arrangements for the care of their other children (if other children are present in the home). Not a day goes by that the OB staff sees parents schlepping their other children to the hospital when they think they may be in labor (even at four o'clock in the morning!).

19. Pregnancy is *not* a comfortable physical condition: particularly in the last few months. Most patients will experience abdominal pain, pelvic and pubic pain. You will feel upper abdominal pain from the expanding uterus and rib pain as the pregnancy pushes your liver and spleen into your chest. There will be times when you cannot walk, turn over, get up or pick up your other child. Your may walk or even wobble like an old woman with arthritis.

If your baby is moving and there is no bleeding from your vagina, probably all of your discomfort is related to your enlarging baby, uterus and placenta. The physical weight and location of your pregnant uterus is putting pressure on a bone, a nerve or a muscle. As Coach Lou Holtz told his football players, "It's not the load that breaks you down, it's the way you carry it. "Having a 30 pound uterus and an 8 pound "creature" moving around inside your abdomen is painful.

20. Read the rest of this book!--Thank you, Robert Fulgrum, (Author of *Everything I ever needed to know I learned in Kindergarten*)

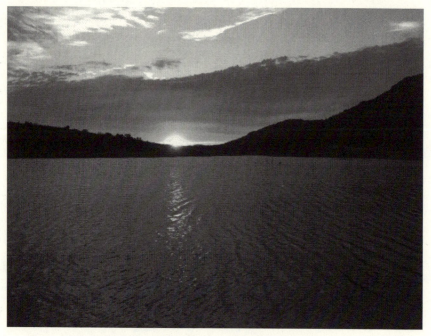

Figure 1-2 Sunset at Lake Elmer Thomas

Introduction to Being Pregnant

1. Positive pregnancy test

At this instant moment you realize that you have an important responsibility: the healthy development of your child. There are some changes you may have to make to your lifestyle now: no more beer or alcohol on weekends, smoking must be stopped and you have to be conscientious about your diet and any medications that you are taking.

Pharmacies and many supermarkets (Wal-Mart, Target, etc.) sell pregnancy tests. Name brands such as EPT, ClearBlue Easy, etc. are very reliable. Generic brands sold at national and local pharmacies also provide accurate results.

The first problems that you will typically report during your first OB appointment will include your early pregnancy symptoms: nausea, frequency of urination, etc. Of all your pregnancy symptoms, breast tenderness could be your very first physical sign of pregnancy: your nipples or your breasts themselves are noticeably tenderer. Just turning slightly over in bed at night will be difficult without groaning. The breasts become larger and fuller: the husbands start complaining, "And I cannot even touch them!" You can no longer even be hugged!

Author note: The author always tells patients that your breasts will be your first clue to pregnancy. Your breasts become sensitive prior to your period but when you are pregnant, they just become even tenderer. Nipple tingling is a sure sign of pregnancy!

Your sense of smell will become heightened: suddenly perfumes, food smells, etc. will become noxious. One patient stated, "I can even smell my husband eating Fritos and he is all the way downstairs in the kitchen!"

Lastly, you have become very sleepy all day long: patients go to bed or fall asleep on the couch at 7:30 (so called pregnancy sleeping sickness).

Some foods and meals that sound good will just no longer seem appetizing or desirable.

As one pregnant patient said, "you know you are pregnant when you throw up one minute and then, during the very next minute you are looking for something to eat!"

The LBD Pregnancy Test

The author has recently heard of this pregnancy test that was developed by Hollywood reporters, i.e., the celebrity paparazzi. Apparently they have developed the technique of detecting an *unannounced* pregnancy of celebrities by observing the small bump protuberance in their lower abdomen. The early pregnancy bump is best observed when these stars wear their little black dress.

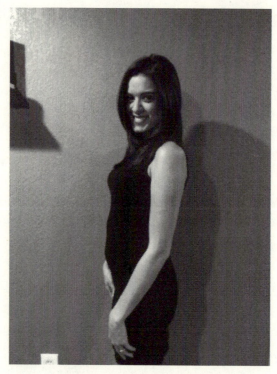

Figure 1-3 Little Black Dress

Common Symptoms of Pregnancy

Breast tenderness and Nipple Sensitivity/Tingling Sensations
Loss of appetite, nausea, and vomiting
Sleepiness, fatigue ("I can sleep all day!") and exhaustion
Frequent Urination
Emotional swings and other psychological feelings
Smell sensations are changed and accentuated
Appetite and Taste changes and aversions (suddenly new cravings and dislikes)

Author Note: Sometimes the breast sensitivity is so intensified that patients have difficulty just turning over in bed at nights. Author sometimes asks, "Can you still be hugged?" Patients usually respond, "Very, very gently!"

2. Diet: What you should be eating

Since you are reading this information, you are newly pregnant and most likely in the first trimester (first 13 weeks) of your pregnancy. You are quite nauseated and have no desire to eat at all! Even the smell of food makes you sick! In fact, all odors including perfumes, smoke, and the smell of cooking food are making you ill right now. However, you will feel better and you will start feeling hungry during some parts of your day. Stick with liquids first. Take small sips of liquids so you will not get dehydrated. Do not worry about calories as there are sufficient fat and carbohydrates stored in your body to nourish you and your baby. Liquids such as Gatorade, soups and broths, bananas, and natural teas will usually stay down and then you can advance your diet to soft foods as you see fit(read more about "morning sickness" later in this chapter in section 3. When you start to get your appetite back for more solid foods, it is important to eat a well-balanced diet (e.g. *the classic food pyrami*d) during your pregnancy. The following foods are recommended for a well-balanced diet:

- fruits and vegetables
- protein such as beef, chicken, fish, lean pork, bean products, energy bars, tofu, etc.
- dairy products such as milk, eggs, cottage cheese, and yogurt
- carbohydrates such as beans, whole grain cereals, rice, potatoes, etc.

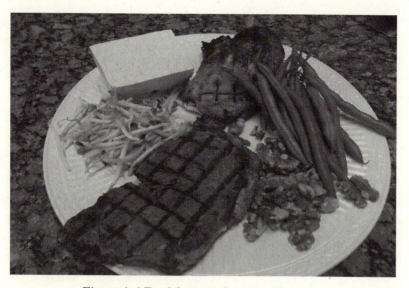

Figure 1-4 Food Sources for a healthy baby

A high protein diet, about 80 grams, is extremely important in building quality bones, muscles, and organs in your baby. Consuming a high protein diet has been shown to help prevent a very serious pregnancy condition called pre-eclampsia (Toxemia).

The author tells his patients on the first OB visit, *"Whatever you eat may become what your baby will be made of (for the most part)!"* Of course, your own body proteins (as well as vitamins and minerals) are undergoing constantly being turned over, re-circulated, recycled or otherwise transported from your tissues to be integrated into your baby's body (as well as your body).

Though this advice is not completely true (because the mother's body will supply necessary proteins, etc.), it highlights to patients the need to eat *right*.

As an example, a 6-ounce container of yogurt contains as much as 8 grams of protein. Therefore, we recommend a high protein, low carbohydrate diet such as the Atkins or South Beach diets. These diets and other similar diets can be found at your bookstore or on-line. More detailed information regarding diet, nutrition, and meal plans is found in the chapter on Nutrition later in this book.

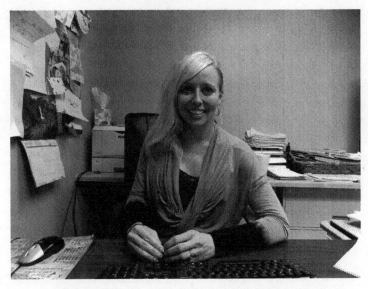

Figure 1-5 Nutritionist: Worlds' Most Interesting

Quoting the *Most Interesting Nutritionist in the World*, "I may not drink milk very often, but when I do, I prefer the taste of *Great Plains* milk. Stay nourished my friends." Further, as the milk industry has long advocated and advertised, *"Milk does a body good"* (reference, www.gotmilk.com).

Author's Note: This author can see the *real* results of proper nutrition when he is performing surgery: some patients will have strong thick ligaments and muscles while other patients have tissues that seem to fall apart easily. For the most part, your baby will be manufactured from both "whatever you eat" as well as from the quality and quantity of proteins, etc. now present in your body that become absorbed into your baby. The author tells the mothers of his patients, "I can tell you ate quality protein when you were pregnant with your daughter: your daughter's tissues were very hard to cut during her C-section ("built tough").

Further, the food choices you make during pregnancy become incorporated into tissues and organs of your baby: the muscles, bones, organs and all other supporting tissues of your future child is dependent on the quality and amount of protein in your diet. One caveat, although heredity plays a significant factor in the construction of your baby, nutrition is just as significant.

Most foods are *combinations* of protein, carbohydrate and fat: rarely *pure* protein or fat. However, some foods are predominately protein or carbohydrate and just mostly fat as listed below:

Examples of the Main Food Groups

Mostly Protein	**Mostly Carbohydrates**	**Mostly Fat**
Grilled 90% Hamburger	Pasta	Butter
Protein Bars	Rice	Bacon
Beef Jerky	Potato	Chips
Lean Pork	Fruit	Fried foods
Lean Turkey	Beans	
Fish and Tofu		

Remember that vegetables, (e.g. salads) consist mainly of fiber and water but it is the salad *dressing* that can be loaded with mostly fat calories: 60 calories per tablespoon for *light* dressings and up to 230 calories for others. Also check the labels for all preservatives and other chemicals in your dressings, canned goods, and other *processed* foods (avoid *processed* foods as much as possible).

3. "Morning Sickness"

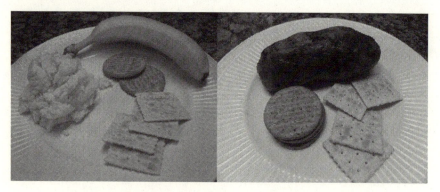

Figure 1-6 Morning Sickness Diet: Saltine crackers and instant mashed potatoes soothe your queasy stomach

In order to avoid becoming dehydrated, just sip liquids: carry around a sports bottle and try sipping small amounts through a straw every so often. Try to keep you stomach coated with instant mashed potatoes, saltine crackers, slices of baked potatoes, etc.

Sea-bands® (or copper bracelets), even acupuncture or hypnosis, may be tried but most patients have not reported significant symptom improvement.

Usually when your stomach is completely empty your nausea ensues. Until 1999 the most commonly prescribed medication for nausea was Bendectin.® Bendectin® contained doxylamine and Vitamin B6. This medication was voluntarily withdrawn from the market because of the cost of on-going costly medical liability. In *recent* large clinical trials this medication was found to be *safe and efficacious* in ameliorating nausea and vomiting during early pregnancy. Isolated instances of any cause-effect on the unborn baby were completely unsubstantiated. Because of the safety profile of this drug combination, the medication was approved by the FDA Panel re-released as Diglegis.®

> On April 9, 2013 the U.S. Food and Drug Administration approved new drug, Diclegis for use in women with morning sickness. It is the only FDA-approved drug to treat *specifically* pregnancy-related symptoms of nausea and vomiting.

Diclegis® costs about $5 per pill. However, you can find OTC (over-the-counter) Vitamin B6 and doxylamine at your local (or chain store) pharmacy or grocery store.

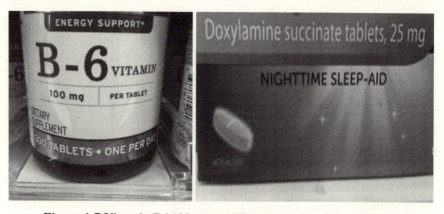

Figure 1-7 Vitamin B6 100 mg and Doxylamine succinate 25 mg

Generic Doxylamine 25 mg and Vitamin B6 100 mg every 6 hours can ease your nausea.

At your pharmacy you can find that the combination of generic OTC (over-the-counter) Vitamin B6 (Pyridoxine) 50 mg and Doxylamine.

There are also name brands such as Unisom SleepTabs® that contain doxylamine. If one were take 50 mgs of Vitamin B6 plus *one half (1/2)* tablet of the sleep aid Unisom©, you would recreate the same formulation that exists today in Diglegis. It would be very similar to the decades used medication Bendectin. The dose of the medication is 25 mg of doxylamine® and 50 mg of Vitamin B6 as needed every 6 hours. Most patients can testify that this combination works well and is very effective in counteracting nausea. Unisom® contains 25 mg of doxylamine.

Author money tip: Using generic or brand name doxylamine and Vitamin B6 OTC could be 10 times *less* expensive than prescription Diglegis® (when you compare costs of generic versus brand name). There are *two* forms of Unisom© sold in stores: so you have to be careful to read the ingredient labels.

Unisom SleepTabs®: containing 25 mg of doxylamine (also sold as Bentyl®)

Unisom Gel caps®: containing 25 mg of diphenhydramine (also known as OTC Benadryl®)

The Unisom pills may make you sleepier than the gel caps. However, if you also have insomnia, the traditional Unisom pills will help your nausea but also help you get a better night's sleep!

If these measures are not helpful, then the medications listed below may be necessary and can be prescribed to you:

Phenergan 25 mg either orally, by cream application or rectally every 6 hours

Compazine 10 mg and 25 mg (oral and rectal suppositories every 6 hours as needed)

Zofran 4 mg either orally or sublingual (under the tongue) every 4 hours

    Zofran is classified as a Category B drug in pregnancy. There are reports of its use in early pregnancy with an increase association of certain malformations such as cleft palate or lip defects as well as septal defects in the heart. However, after all other therapy fails to alleviate symptoms, most OBs will prescribe Zofran because of its effectiveness compared to the rare possibility of associated birth defect.

Morning Sickness usually improves after the first trimester of pregnancy. However, in a few patients it can last throughout the entire pregnancy. Occasionally it can come back just for a few weeks in the last trimester: the point is that these symptoms *vary* with each patient and with each pregnancy that you may have.

<u>Another point</u>: Prescription prenatal vitamins can make the nausea worse in many patients. In such cases, I recommend that patients hold off taking their Prenatal Vitamins and try using chewable Prenatal or Children's Vitamins until their morning sickness subside after the 1st trimester (although nausea at any time of day can last throughout the pregnancy is some patients). If possible, try to continue taking OTC folic acid 0.8 milligrams (mg) and Iron OTC per day until you are feeling better.

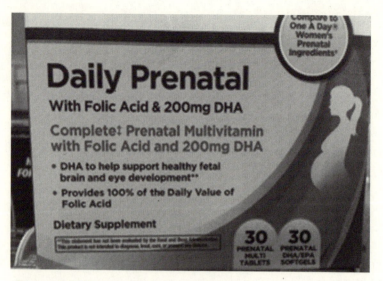

Figure 1-8 Vitamin Substitutes. Children's chewable Vitamins

Author's Note: Severe "morning sickness," also known as *Hyperemesis Gravidarum,* affects less than 5% of pregnancies. Occasionally patients must be hospitalized for intravenous fluids and medications to prevent dehydration and metabolic disturbances. To give patient's some reassurance, a UCLA Medical Center study found that morning sickness was correlated positively with having healthier babies!

The chief objection to prenatal vitamins by patients is the size of the pills. Some pharmaceutical companies have tried to make them smaller, chewable and even divided them in half (making you take one twice a day. If you are eating a healthy well balanced diet, particularly fresh vegetables, fruits, dairy products, etc. you will be taking a sufficient amount of vitamins to sustain your growing baby.

Bottom-line, OTC folic acid (.8 mg twice daily) and Iron supplementation (325 mg twice daily) along with a healthy diet can replace your need for a prenatal vitamins.

4. My Body is Changing Already!

Unbelievably, your body is changing in just a few weeks after you miss your period.

Your breasts are fuller and larger. They are more sensitive if not tender. It is hard to turn in bed or even be hugged.

Your abdomen seems to be a little bigger or "pouchie." Clothes are snugger. You are going to the bathroom to empty your bladder more frequently (and not just during the day but now in the middle of the night!)

FYI, asking a pregnant woman "if she has to go to the bathroom" is a very stupid question!--Author

Smells and odors now even more pronounced. Your appetite has changed: you lose your taste for your morning coffee and spicy foods. Most people who smoke quit because of the smell. Your personality may change: there are times when you become emotional: some patients get short with their partners and even start getting annoyed with them!

5. Exercise and Physical Activities

You can continue to do your normal physical activities and exercises as you have prior to your pregnancy. Exercise should be moderated if you get short of breath or "get winded." You should slow down if you cannot talk while working out. Pulse rates should not exceed 140 beats per minute.

We do not recommend *bouncy* activities such as jumping jacks, horseback riding, skiing or intense running because such up and down jerky motions can potentially disrupt the attachment of the placenta. Biking, swimming, elliptical, walking on a treadmill, step climber and working out with weights are permissible.

Note: Sex is fine during pregnancy: it can be challenging in certain positions late in pregnancy. Yes, I know you are too tired to even think about it!

6. Due Dates

"What is my baby's due date" and "How Far along am I," and "How much does my baby weigh?"

Your OB will tell you your "due date" or estimated date of confinement (EDC) on your first OB visit. To calculate your due date is a simple matter (Naegele's Rule): Subtract 3 months from your last menstrual period (LMP) and add 1 week (add a year if your LMP was March 25th or later).

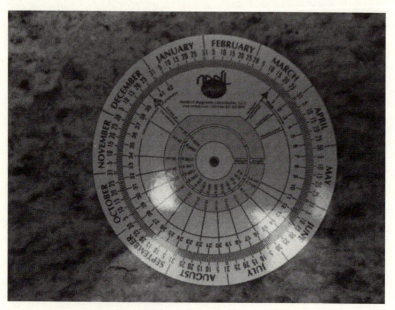

Figure 1-9 Pregnancy Wheel Calculator

The Pregnancy Wheel shows that LMP is March 15th with conception on March 29th and an EDC on December 22nd see dark arrows on Pregnancy Wheel

For example: Your LMP is June 6, 2014 then your due date would be March 13, 2015.

In another way of figuring: 6/6/2014 minus 3 months equals 3/6/2014 plus one week makes 3/13/2014 then add one year equals 3/13/2015

The calculations go as follows:

06/06/2014

    Minus 3 months

03/06/2014

    Add one year

03/06/2015

    Add one week

03/13/2015

"Due dates" rarely change. Due dates are the most reliable when calculated in the first trimester. If you want to monitor your baby, "there is an App for that!" The "Pregnancy Wheel" and other similar Apps (baby developmental steps, what is my baby doing now, etc.) are available for download for Smartphones and on your computer. The Apps will also tell you all the information you desire on a weekly basis. In the illustration provided, there is a Pregnancy Wheel that is helpful when the LMP is not certain: just input the weeks calculated by ultrasound (or fundal height) on the wheel and the date of conception and EDC is shown.

7. Appointments.

Your OB will see you every 4 weeks during the first and second trimesters (a trimester equals 13 weeks) of pregnancy. In the last trimester (the last 13 weeks) he will see you every two weeks and in the last month he will see you every week. Of course, you can be seen and evaluated for any problems that occur between office visits. High Risk Pregnancies complicated by diabetes, hypertension etc. will be seen more frequently as dictated by your specific medical and obstetrical needs.

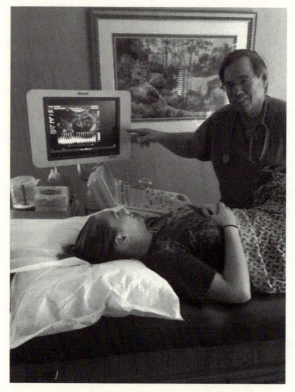

Figure 1-10 Ultrasound in 1st Trimester

Your *first OB visit* is very important. It is best to make that appointment 6-8 weeks after the first day of your last menstrual period (LMP). During this first appointment the office will enter your demographic and insurance information as well as input your complete medical history into the computer. The patient will undress and undergo a complete physical exam with attention paid to your thyroid gland, lungs, heart, and abdominal areas. A pelvic exam will be performed: a test for cervical cancer (HPV) and a test for STD's will be done. An important feature will be the determination of your pregnancy size and your "due date." Significant "high risk" factors will be highlighted by your OB.

Laboratory testing will be performed as detailed below. Your *first OB visit* in the first 8 weeks of pregnancy is a critical moment for "dating" your pregnancy:

It is the most accurate point in time for calculating your correct "due date."

<u>Author Note</u>: The author usually meets and greets his "New OB" patients in the exam room. It is only after the medical and previous OB history is completely taken down that the author asks the patient to undress for the physical and pelvic exams. After doing the preceding and documenting her medical history, I asked one my recent *New OB* patients that now it was time to do her physical and pelvic exam and she needed "to take her clothes off." She promptly responded, "You mean I do not even get dinner first!"

Your *return OB* visits will be focused on weight gain, urine testing and growth of the baby. The uterine fundal height will be ascertained each visit: each centimeter (cm) of fundal height corresponds to each week of pregnancy. You will be able to hear the baby's heart beat after 13 weeks of pregnancy. It is very moving to the author to observe the faces of the patient and her husband when they first hear the heart beat sounds coming loudly from the baby with the Doppler.

While you are listening to your baby's heartbeat, the author might even say, "They make a lot more noise after they are born! That is when you need to stock up on the duct tape! (Seriously, I am just kidding!)

Other Questions and problems can be addressed at these visits.

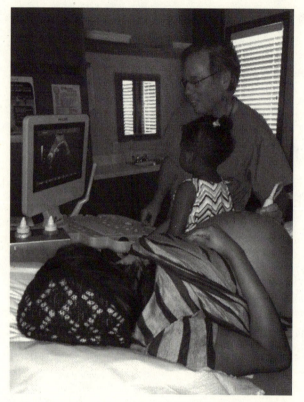

Figure 1-11 First Ultrasound Picture for mom and sibling.

The above first ultrasound in which the sibling is seeing their future sibling ("the enemy") for the first time, i.e. you are no longer "an only child!"

High risk factors and concurrent medical conditions can be re-evaluated. Depending on your OB's routine, ultrasound exams will be performed usually in the first trimester to validate the "due date" and, in some cases, document the number of babies you are carrying! An "anatomy screening" ultrasound is usually done between 18 to 22 weeks of pregnancy. The sex of the baby can usually be determined at this time.

Author Note: When looking at the ultrasound of her baby, one patient noted "that my baby looks fat! But, then I remind them of the well-known fact, "You always look 5 lbs. heavier when you are on the TV screen!"

It is very important to alert the office if you cannot make your appointment *as far in advance as* you can. Further, alert the office if you are going to be late. If you miss more than 2 return OB visits without adequate reason or notice, most OB's will discharge you (As Donald Trump says, "You're fired!") from their professional care.

Many times when the author sees an OB for her appointments, he will enter the room and ask her, "So, what is the Baby Report today?" The following comments are just a small sample of what I hear on an everyday basis when I see a "return OB" patient:

"Just want to get it over with" "just want *it* out!" "I'm ready, done!"

"Awesome so far" and "I'm sick of being sick" "I'm beyond tired"

"I can't even sleep 2 hours before I start snoring: it is the *fatness* that makes me snore!"

"Hot flashes 1-2 times per day" "I feel like I'm in a perpetual hangover state"

"Groin Pain" "Kidney Pain" "Pain going down my butt and leg"

"Miserable, can't sleep" "My hips and pubic bone hurts: I cannot get up or walk!"

"Feet are swollen" "Hands are swelling" "Pressure in my pelvis"

"It is too hot outside to be pregnant"

"Are you sure I am not due now?

"No one told me I would be sneezing and leaking!"

"Heartburn"—my baby is going to have a lot of hair!"

"Just ready" "Tired of being pregnant" "Just tired" "Don't sleep much until 3 am"

"Moving around a lot and the baby is resting his foot on my ribs"—this latter quote from a Fitness Instructor

A husband stated, "If I touch her abdomen, the baby stops moving. I guess the baby doesn't like me!"

The baby is not moving as much now (close to term), I guess the baby is running out of room!

The hardest thing to do in the morning is to getting up out of bed after sleeping all night.

A pelvic exam to check for cervical effacement and dilatation is done in the last few weeks of pregnancy. If I find that the cervix is not thinned out or dilated, I may comment to the patient (analogous to the cards in the Monopoly board game), "Not dilated, you may not "pass Go and you do not collect $200!'"

I might also quip to the patient as she is leaving the room, "I will see you back in one week unless you *"de-pregnate"* sooner!"

8. Your Email, telephone numbers and addresses, please!

It is extremely important that you keep your physician's office up-to-date with your *current mobile* and/or your home phone number. Further, we need your email address and recommend that you keep checking your email for any notifications from our office. There are many instances when the office or hospital needs to talk to you about important test results or alert you to an impending medical problem with your pregnancy. Set up your voicemail service if you have not already done so and keep it clear for more messages. Provide the office with the contact information of family members, co-workers, and friends who we can reach if we cannot for some reason get you! Due to technological advances in computers and the Internet, many communications to your OB's office can be made through the "Patient Portal." Through this connection you can leave messages, check your lab results, etc. The office web site and patient portal are HIPPA compliant and secure: like other sites you will need a username and with your own password to log on.

9. Smoking and other Substance Use

Smoking is very much discouraged during pregnancy. Nicotine causes decreased blood flow to the uterus and baby. Thus, smoking is directly associated with smaller babies (and lung cancer in you!). There are many resources and drug therapies to help you quit smoking. Please feel free to discuss these options with your OB's office.

Marijuana is likewise discouraged during pregnancy. Many States require a DHS (Department of Human Services) investigation if marijuana is discovered in your system during the pregnancy.

Alcohol intake should be discontinued. Many patients have consumed alcohol just prior to missing their period and did not know they were pregnant: such early use does not have a significant on the embryo. Recent studies have also shown that an occasional drink may not be harmful as previously thought. However, it is best advice is to avoid altogether.

Lastly, all other unlawful drugs (methamphetamine, narcotics, PCP, benzodiazepines, ecstasy, etc.) must be stopped. Use of these drugs will prompt a child protection (DHS) investigation and possible removal of the baby (and any other children in the home) from your custody.

10. Medications and Drugs

It is important to avoid all drugs during pregnancy unless absolutely necessary.

If you have been prescribed medications for medical conditions such as hypertension (high blood pressure) diabetes, etc., please continue these medications until you are able to check with the office for their safety during your pregnancy.

Most OTC (over-the-counter) medicines are safe *for limited use* during pregnancy. Please see the enclosed medication table below. There is also a chapter on Medications later in this book. Further the reader is also referred to the textbook, *Drugs in Pregnancy and Lactation."* The website, *www.Pregnancycenter.org* provides another source on the safety of most medications in use today. Lastly, readers can "Google" the particular medication if further information is desired.

Even acetaminophen (Tylenol) has recently been reported (2014) to be linked to ADHD in childhood if used frequently and for long durations during pregnancy: no drugs are absolutely safe during pregnancy.

Your OB will electronically send your prescriptions to your pharmacy, whether that pharmacy is local, regional or mail order. Most pharmacies are *connected* electronically. If your pharmacy is not connected, a paper prescription can be written out for you to carry to your pharmacy. Your OB's office may also fax prescriptions to your pharmacy.

Figure 1-16 Medications for common symptoms

SYMPTOM/ AILMENT	MEDICATION/REMEDY
Common Cold Allergies: Claritan	Sudafed 30 mg: 1–2 every 6 hours; Robitussin DM or Novahistine DMS for cough; Sucrets; Chloraseptic lozenges; nasal spray such as Neosynephrine or Afrin; steam shower clears passageways
Indigestion	Tums, Digel; Mylanta II (chewable or liquid); Maalox Plus; Mylicon Chewable
Headaches	Tylenol, Extra Strength Tylenol Advil*(Ibuprofen)*, Aspirin*;
Discomfort	Extra Strength Tylenol Aspirin*; Advil), Tylenol,
Backache	Tylenol, Extra Strength Tylenol (apply heat, heating pad, massage)

Constipation	Milk of Magnesia; Dialose Plus; Pericolace: Surfak; Miralax
Nausea	Hot tea; Pepsi or Coke; crackers; small meals; vitamin B–6 50mg (morning and night); Emetrol (if cannot be controlled with diet)
Growing Pains	Avoid heavy lifting; elevate feet when sitting; relax
Swelling	Decrease salt intake; elevate feet when possible; eat

Notes:

All Drug names above are brand names with trademark and copyright protection: used for information purposes only

* Aspirin, Ibuprofen (Nuprin, Advil, Motrin i.e., NSAIDs) should not be used in the last 4 weeks of pregnancy (see Medications chapter)

Please inform your OB of all the prescription and Over-the-Counter (OTC) medications that you are taking and not being a patient with the story below.

<u>Author Note</u>: As I was saying "good-bye" to a new OB patient at 6 weeks pregnancy, she pulled out a sheet of paper with the medications that she was taking:

Strattera 80 mg	Citalopram 20 mg
Mirtazapine 30 mg	Lisinopril-HCTZ 20/12.5 ng
Acyclovir 400 mg	Clonidine .1 mg
Topiramate 200 mg	Telmisartan 80 mg
Metformin 500 mg	Proctozone-HC cream

In the List above, there are 2 medications for hypertension, 3 drugs for psychiatric indications, one for diabetes and one for herpes.

Except for the last 2 drugs all the rest are *not* recommended to be taken in pregnancy. I asked her if she had planned to be pregnant and she stated, "No." Fortunately, with her prompt stopping of 7 of these medications her baby was not compromised.

This story illustrates the extremely important point to plan and consult with your OB PRIOR to pregnancy if you have current medical and psychological conditions. More importantly, the patient should discuss the medications used for current treatment.

Unless for a specific condition and a limited time, controlled drugs are not recommended during pregnancy. Xanax, Klonopin, etc. are controlled drugs. Controlled or scheduled drugs require a written prescription by your physician: they cannot be phoned or faxed into your pharmacy by law.

Please notify the office staff if there a change occurs to your pharmacy of choice.

Most insurance and Medicaid plans cover generic brand of medications with low or no co-pays. Brand names medications may require more out-of-pocket expense.

11. Prenatal Vitamins and Iron:

Physicians routinely prescribe a prenatal vitamin with folic acid/iron for your pregnancy. However, vitamin deficiencies, by themselves, are rare during pregnancy (also when you are not pregnant). However, *anemi*a, (i.e. low red blood cell count), is one of the most common conditions during pregnancy. One third (1/3) of all American women are anemic. It is caused by *Iron* deficiency: only 5% of the iron a woman consumes in her diet is absorbed into her intestines. Therefore, *iron* is the most important *mineral* that you can take during your pregnancy.

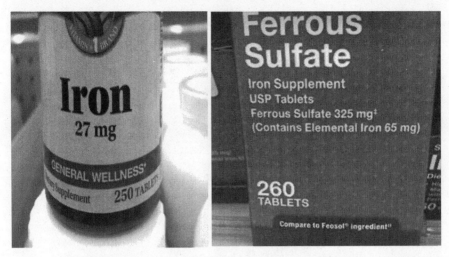

Figure 1-12 Iron supplements 27 mg and 65 mg

Iron Supplements come in many different doses and with other ingredients: 27 to 65 mg of *elemental* iron. Patients should take an extra iron in addition to their prenatal vitamins to prevent anemia. Check with your pharmacist, consumer magazines and your physicians for the most cost effective formulations.

The following is a list of "brand name" and generic medications commonly used during pregnancy:

Leading Rx Prenatal Vitamin[1,3-7]	DHA Source	DHA	Vitamin D3	Docusate Stool Softener
Nexa® Plus		350 mg	800 IU	✓
CitraNatal Harmony®		265 mg	400 IU	✓

PreferaOB ONE®	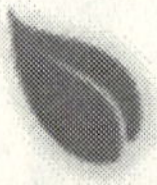 🍃	200 mg	400 IU
Prenate Essential®	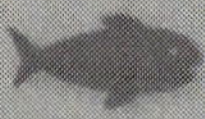 🐟	300 mg	220 IU
Vitafol®-One		200 mg	1000 IU
vitaMedMD™ One Rx	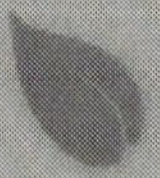 🍃	200 mg	400 IU

Figure 1-13 Prenatal Vitamins: Brand Names

There are a multitude of brand names of Prenatal Vitamins available: each company tries to extol the virtues (i.e. better or more ingredients in their brand such as DHA, etc.). The main difference between prescription prenatal vitamins and over-the counter (OTC) brands is usually an extra 0.2 mg of folic acid. It is just as acceptable to take generic (Walgreens, CVS or Wal-Mart) brands of prenatal vitamins and add both generic folic acid 0.8 mg and Iron (please see Appendix for the list of prenatal vitamins covered by most Medicaid programs—your pharmacist will know!)..

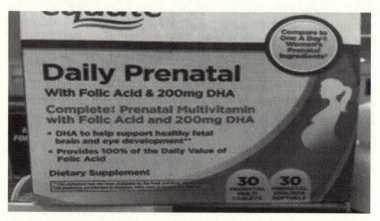

Figure 1-14 Vitamins: Prenatal Vitamin Generics

Further, some prescription prenatal vitamin capsules/pills are so large that many patients gag or get sick just from taking them. If you are experiencing morning sickness or cannot tolerate the large prenatal vitamins, you can substitute Gummy Bears, Flintstones or other smaller or chewable children's vitamins!

Folic acid supplement is probably the most important *co-factor* necessary to prevent serious birth defects such as *spina bifida*. One study showed that as the amount of folic acid in milligrams is increased (up to 4 mgs per day) there is a corresponding decrease in the incidence of birth defects.

Vitamin C helps the absorption of iron. Therefore, taking iron such as ferrous gluconate or ferrous sulfate (elemental iron) with Vitamin C 500 mg twice a day is an excellent way of avoiding pregnancy-related anemia. You can use stool softeners or extra fiber to avoid the constipating effect that iron has on your intestines.

Fluoride supplementation after the 1st trimester has been shown to effectively reduce the likelihood of your child to have cavities (i.e. caries) in his/her future.

**Take Home Point: Iron (and extra folic acid) is the most important mineral supplement you can take during your pregnancy.

12. Weight Gain Guidelines

ACOG (American College of Obstetrics and Gynecology, the professional association of Ob-Gyns in the United States) recommends a total weight gain of 24 lbs. during pregnancy. Most of your weight gain should be achieved in the last part of pregnancy, that is, 11 lbs.

PREGNANCY WEIGHT GAIN BY TRIMESTER	
First Trimester Weight Gain (the 1st 13 weeks)	5 lbs
Second Trimester Weight Gain (14 to 27 weeks)	9 lbs
Third Trimester Weight Gain (27 to 40 weeks)	10 lbs
Total Recommended Weight Gain for Pregnancy	24 lbs

Figure 1-14 Weight Gain by Trimester

Weight Gain is a balancing act between food consumption (calories in) and food burned (calories out). Gaining more than the recommended 24 lbs. means that you will hold on to that weight after your delivery, i.e. net weight gain. If you are gaining more weight than recommended, then you need to do one or both of the following actions:

Eat less

Exercise more

Exercise and physical activity help burn calories. Also the composition of your diet can influence weight gain: try to reduce fats and eat more protein. My advice is to focus on protein foods: fat has **twice** as many calories as protein and carbohydrates. Further, protein does not cause the higher level of insulin release from your pancreas as do carbohydrates ("sugars"). The moment your blood sugar (or glucose) bottoms out, your body's "hunger center" becomes activated. Consequently, high carbohydrate diets cause "rebound hunger" in about 2 hours: you experience the up and down cycles of hunger and eating with resultant unwanted weight gain (particularly during the morning sickness of the first trimester.

Fat: 9 calories/gram (you need to burn 9 calories to use up one gram of fat)

Protein and Carbohydrates: 4.7 calories/gram

Eat less fat by avoiding fried foods. Decrease your amount of carbohydrates by eating less breads, pasta, and desserts. Excess weight gain makes you feel more uncomfortable and just makes weight loss more difficult postpartum. Most food establishments fry or add a lot of fat and butter to their food (because fat tastes so good! Like French fries and pizza!). Avoid eating out: dining at fast food restaurants will make you consume more fat and sugar calories (and you can save a lot of money and waiting time simultaneously!).

Where does the weight gain come from?

Placenta	1.0
Amniotic fluid	1.5
Breast Growth	1.0
Blood Volume	3.0
Fat on mother	4.0
Extra Fluid on mother	4.0
Baby	7.5
Total	24.0

Figure 1-15 Weight Gain Components

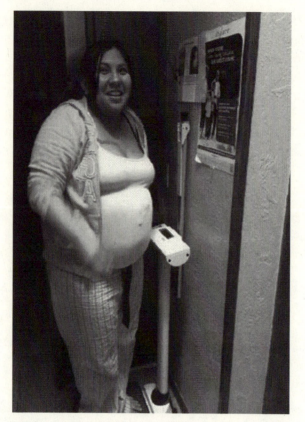

Figure 1-16 Weighing in: "Can't weigh that much!"

Another patient also stated, "According to my BMI calculator, I am too short!"

If you are gaining more than a pound per week in the first 28 weeks of pregnancy, then you are gaining too much weight. As above, avoid fats (butter, fried foods) and decrease your "carbos": ice cream, cake, candy, deserts, breads, pasta, etc.)

Weight gain or loss is based on a simple formula:

Calories IN – Calories Burned = Net Calories

Simply, that means that the amount of calories you consume minus calories you burn up equal <u>net</u> weight gain or loss.

So if you are gaining too much weight, just eat a little less and exercise more.

> *Author's Note*: Miracle Grow© Not Recommended as "Growth Nourishment" for Your Baby!

Other helpful ways to watch your weight:

Drink more water, such as 6 to 8 full glasses of water per day (it fills you up!)

If you are not hungry, do not eat! Just because it happens to be lunch time does not mean that you have to eat.

Conversely, when you are no longer hungry: stop eating! You do not have to finish your plate: better in the waste than on your waist! Further, you do not have to finish your child's plate: throw it out or store it up for leftovers for another time.

Eat more vegetables such as carrots, celery and cucumbers: they tend to fill you up and eliminate your appetite.

Eat and chew your food very slowly. Chew gum when you feel like snacking.

Exercise or be more physically active: go outside for walks or if the weather is not conducive, walk on a treadmill or use other equipment. If you watch any TV shows, put your treadmill in front of the TV and walk when you ordinarily just sit on your butt!

13. How long is my pregnancy? It can't be that long!

Most people hear that pregnancy is "9 months." Well, not exactly: there are two ways of measuring the average length of pregnancy (264 days):

Menstrual weeks: 40 weeks from the first day of your last menstrual period (LMP)

Conceptual weeks: 38 weeks from the day of conception

Most physicians use the conventional "40 weeks" of measurement when they talk to their patients about "how far along" they are.

Further, the length of your pregnancy is divided into thirds (1/3's) or trimesters of 13 1/3 weeks as shown below:

First Trimester	0 weeks to 13 1/3 weeks
Second Trimester	13 1/3 weeks to 26 2/3 weeks
Third Trimester	26 2/3 weeks to 40 weeks

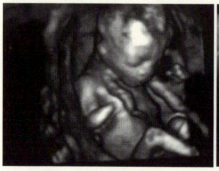
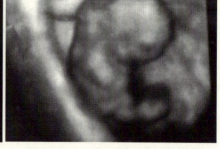

Figure 1-17 First Baby Picture   **Figure 1-18 Baby Picture in 3D**

During your appointments or at the hospital Ultrasound Unit, you may receive your "first" baby pictures: Do the pictures look like anyone on your side of the family?

A full term pregnancy is 40 weeks from the last menstrual period. Your baby, not you, should determine when it is the right time to be born.

There is approximately a 16% chance of a miscarriage with any given pregnancy (higher percentages dependent on methodology of specific studies).

Once you see the fetal heart beat on your first trimester ultrasound, your chance of a miscarriage drops drastically to less than 3%! See the "first baby pictures" in Illustrations.

14. Laboratory Testing

Your OB's office will refer you to a regional or hospital laboratory for your pregnancy laboratory work. There many national and local laboratories such as the following laboratories available in the author's area:

Quest laboratory nationally

LabCorp

SmithKline

Your local hospital laboratory

There are a series of *Standard* laboratory testing during your pregnancy as follows per ACOG guidelines:

Table 1-1 of Standard Pregnancy Laboratory Testing

Weeks 1-13

> CBC, RPR, Blood type and Rh, Antibody Screen, TSH with or without reflex T4, Rubella immunity, HIV, Hepatitis B, Sickle Cell (if Afro-American heritage), Cystic Fibrosis, Chlamydia, Gonorrhea, Pap and reflex HPV, and Drug testing, Maternal Genetic Testing (as indicated)

Week 16-20

> Multiple Marker screen for neural tube defects, GI defects and Down's syndrome

NIPS (Non-invasive prenatal screening: Harmony®, Materna 21® and Panorama

Week 28-32

Anemia and 1 hour 50 grams Glucose (Gestational Diabetes test)

Week 36

Group B Strep Testing (GBS, not GPS!) and Repeat Hemoglobin (anemia check)

Table 1-2 Table of Extended Genetic and Physical Testing

Test	Detecting	Timing (weeks)	Patient	Risks
PAPP–A, beta HCG with nuchal translucency	Trisomies*	11–14	All	None
Fetal Blood DNA	Trisomies*	10+	All	None
Chorionic Villus Sampling (CVS)	Genetic**	11–15	Age 35+	1% loss
Multiple Marker Screen	Trisomies*	15–22	All	None
Amniocentesis	Genetic**	15+	Age 35+	0.5% loss
Anatomy Ultrasound	Physical***	16+	All	None

Notes:

*Trisomies (Trisomy 21, 18, 13) but can also tell sex

**Genetic Testing: Trisomies, specific metabolic disorders, sex

***Physical Abnormalities such as cleft lip/palate, as well as cardiac, renal, neuro and skeletal etc. abnormalities

Laboratory and Pregnancy Surveillance Testing TIME LINE					
Prenatal Panel**	Quad screen	1 hr. Glucose*		1 hr. GTT	GBS test
Pap GC, Chlamydia	NIPS	Harmony/Panorama		Hgb/Hct**	NST's
		Penta Screen			BPP
Urinanalysis		Anatomy U/Sound			BPP
SureSwab	Nuchal Fold	Amniocentesis			S/D Doppler
Drug Screen		Dating U/sound			
	PAPP-A	NIPS			
Weeks 6-12	Weeks 11-14	Week 16-18		Week 28	Week 36 -42

* 3 hour Glucose Tolerance Test performed if 1 hour glucose>130 mg%
** Anemia studies and Glucose Tolerance are done at any time during pregnancy as indicated

In 2013, Laboratory Services and other Laboratories have introduced new antenatal blood tests, NIPS or Non-invasive Prenatal Screening (commercially branded as *MaterniT21Plus, Harmony, Panorama*, etc.) that can screen for Trisomy 21 (Down's syndrome), Trisomy 13, and Trisomy 18 starting around *11 weeks of pregnancy*. Further these tests can reveal the sex of your baby. Your blood is drawn (maternal blood) and the laboratory checks your blood for the *baby's* blood *hemoglobin* that has crossed into your circulation. This blood test can be done as early as the 10th week of pregnancy. Because this test can make an extremely early diagnosis of some chromosomal defects, parents can be made aware of the baby's condition and decide earlier in the pregnancy on the various options and treatments that are available to them.

One important caveat: if there is less than 3.5% of fetal hemoglobin in the patient's blood sample, these tests may not be able to produce any results. Further, if you weigh over 160 lbs. this type of testing may return showing "not enough fetal Hemoglobin extraction for testing. The testing may have to be postponed until the time window between 16 to 20 weeks.

These tests may take up to 2 weeks before a report is available. Accordingly, other screening tests and anatomy ultrasounds will continue to have a place in the antenatal diagnosis of fetal abnormalities.

During these times of rapid technological advances OB's will continue to perform "Anatomy Ultrasounds" for physical defects that are not genetically related.

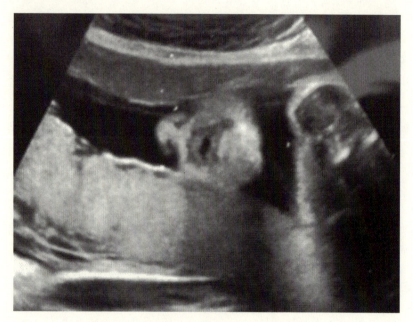

Figure 1-19 Baby's Mouth on Ultrasound

Ultrasound in itself can be helpful in diagnosing cleft lip and palate as seen in the ultrasound picture above.

Multiple Marker screening on maternal blood is performed at 18 to 20 weeks to help diagnose chromosomal abnormalities. Also, during this window of time in pregnancy ultrasound can screen for physical defects as well as the sex of the baby. If an abnormality is found on these latter two tests (ultrasound and Multiple Markers) then maternal blood sampling for Fetal DNA (NIPS testing) can be performed to make a more clear diagnosis. Most OB's are moving away from the more invasive testing, i.e., amniocentesis and CVS, particularly if the targeted ultrasound study is normal. Obviously, invasive testing carries increased risks to the pregnancy such as rupture of the amniotic sac, infection, bleeding, etc. Very rarely, the pregnancy can be lost due to complications of these more invasive procedures (1:350 approximately).

15. When can I know the sex of my baby?

Between 15-18 weeks of pregnancy an ultrasound can reveal the sex of your baby. As mentioned above, a NIPS blood test can reveal the sex of the baby at 10 weeks gestation. Early diagnosis of the sex is particularly important when screening for serious sex-linked genetic defects (Hemophilia, etc.) Similarly, at 18 to 20 weeks of pregnancy an "anatomy scan" can be performed to make sure all the baby's major organs are developing normally. When you see your baby on the ultrasound screen, do not be upset if your baby looks like "Achmed, the terrorist" (reference, Jeffrey Dunham video on YouTube). The baby has just not yet developed much tissue and muscle over the skeleton.

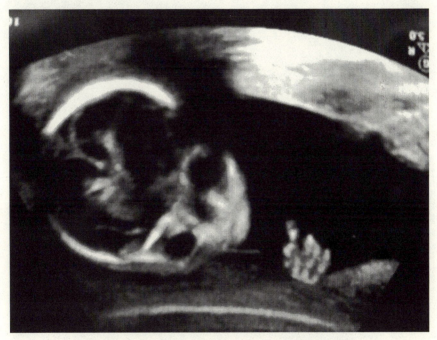

Figure 1-20 Ultrasound of baby's head. Your baby looks like *Achmed* the Terrorist

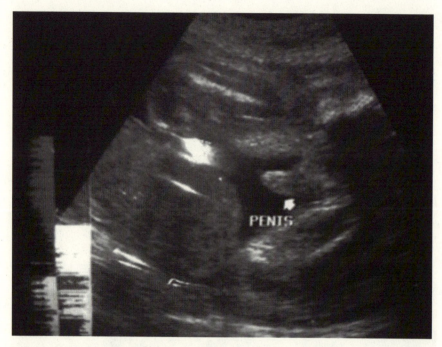

Figure 1-21 Sex of baby boy on ultrasound

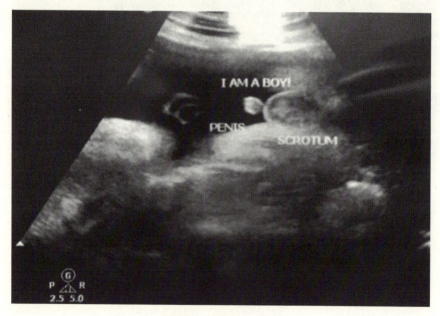

Figure 1-22 Boy Sex

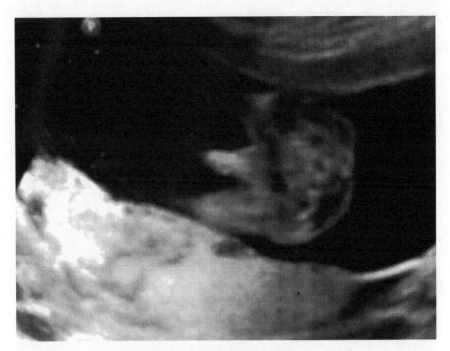

Figure 1-23 Baby Boy above

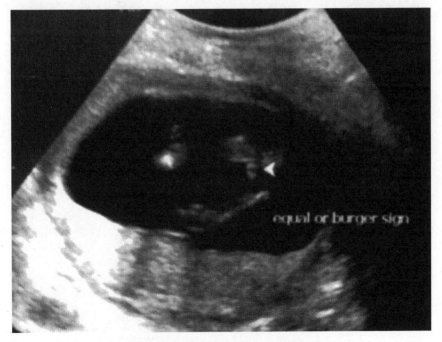

Figure 1-24 Sex of female baby on ultrasound above

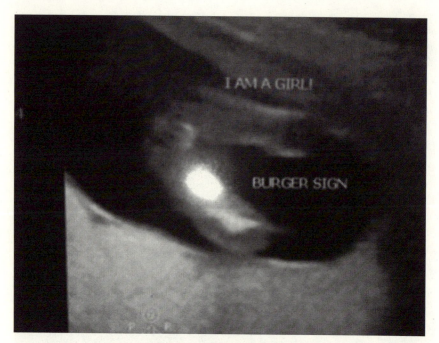

Figure 1-25 Baby Girl

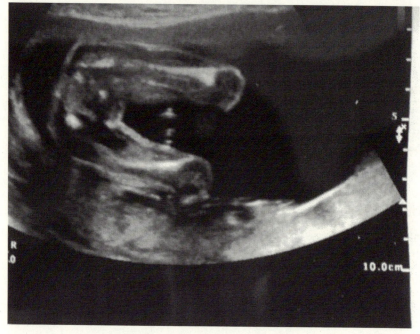

Figure 1-26 Sex of baby girl on ultrasound above

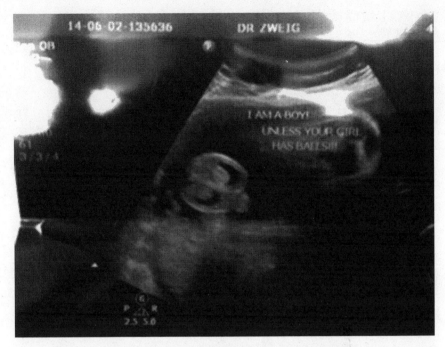

Figure 1-27 Sex of baby boy on Ultrasound

Ultrasound pictures demonstrating the sex of your baby are shown in the figures 1-21 to 1-27 above.

The sex of the baby is more easily diagnosed correctly at 16 weeks of pregnancy (maternal obesity can delay proper detection until 22 weeks). If the baby is properly positioned (getting the right "angle on the dangle"), an ultrasound can visualize the sex as early as 12th week. The typical sign for a baby girl is the "Hamburger sign/ Burger sign/Equal sign "representing the two labia together giving the appearance of burger buns. For boys, the "hot dog" sign is pretty self-explanatory!

16. Vaccinations: FLU Vaccine and dTap

The ACOG (American College of Obstetrics and Gynecology) and the Centers for Disease Control and Prevention (CDC) recommend that all pregnant patients obtain the flu vaccine as soon as it becomes available in the months of September and October. There is at least a two week interval of time before your body starts producing antibodies against the flu virus. Each year the flu vaccine (inactivated virus) is formulated for the most common strains likely to be prevalent the upcoming flu season: influenza A (H1N1—Swine type and H3N2)), and variations of influenza B).

Note: Some Health professionals in high risk environments will actually obtain 2 separate vaccinations during the 5 month flu season in order to cover during these months: in September and another booster injection in January.

Chickenpox and measles (e.g., the 2015 Disneyland measles outbreak) is also making a new come back in the United States today. If you are uncertain about whether you were vaccinated in childhood or whether your vaccination is still effective, a varicella or measles immune titer can be done at the Laboratory. Chickenpox during pregnancy can be very serious: if Chickenpox is contracted during pregnancy, there a 20% risk of pneumonia requiring hospitalization and intensive care.

DTap is a diphtheria and pertussis vaccination (inactivated viruses) that is being recommended now by the CDC for pregnant women in the 3rd trimester. The vaccination is given at this time when viral antibodies can be stimulated and peak for transmission to the newborn through the maternal blood and breast milk. Hence, the baby is *passively* protected with antibodies in the first few months of life.

Check to be sure your standard vaccinations are all up to date: polio, measles, mumps and rubella (MMR), tetanus, etc. Other vaccinations (pneumococcal, meningococcal) can be delayed until after pregnancy. The CDC Guidelines for Vaccination in Pregnant Women is reproduced in Appendix D. Check with *www.cdc.gov* website for additional information.

TB skin testing and other diagnostic skin tests are permissible during pregnancy as needed.

17. What was one of the original purposes of Obstetrical Care?

It has something to do with Pre-eclampsia: it is the main disease that helped create the medical specialty of Obstetrics. More than 100 years ago, most women delivered their babies at home with perhaps a midwife or some other person experienced in delivering babies. However, many serious complications and many deaths occurred.

Your office visits are timed at specified intervals of time so your OB can discover whether or not you are developing toxemia of pregnancy.

Authors Note: The New England Journal of Medicine is one of the oldest and most respected medical journals in the United States today. When the author was in medical school, the front cover of the NEJM always carried the weekly *Report of Maternal Mortality* and Morbidity from the Massachusetts General Hospital (MGH): it would report on a monthly basis the number and causes of death of pregnant women. Very unfortunately, complications and even death can occur when you become pregnant.

One of the main complications of pregnancy is *pre-eclampsia* which is also commonly known as *toxemia*.

Pre-eclampsia:

1. High blood pressure (Hypertension)
2. Protein (Proteinuria) leaking from kidney filtration into your urine
3. Swelling (edema) of legs, hands face, etc. and sudden weight gain (2 lbs. in 1 week)

Eclampsia:

All of the above with the addition of seizures or generalized convulsions

Significant blood pressure elevations can cause strokes, heart attacks and damage to your kidneys. Accordingly, in order to avoid these tragic complications, physicians in the early 1900's started monitoring pregnancies with routine checks *before the end of pregnancy rather than waiting until the commencement of labor.* The main assessments were weight gain (edema), blood pressure checks, and looking for protein in the urine. Since pre-eclampsia is a ***pregnancy-induced*** disease that occurs in the last trimester of pregnancy (the last 13 weeks), office visits are scheduled at more frequent interval of time: every 2 weeks and then every week during the last month of pregnancy.

Nowadays, prenatal care has evolved into many other aspects of attention:

- Surveillance and protection of baby's health status during the pregnancy (NST, Biophysical Profile, etc.)
- Nutrition and Vitamin supplementation (i.e., protein intake focus and folic acid)
- Fitness and avoidance of excess weight gain
- Smoking cessation and other substance abuse treatment
- Prenatal diagnosis (physical and genetic abnormalities)
- Medical care of patients with pre-pregnancy conditions such as diabetes, asthma, hypertension, etc. In the past these patients were advised not to ever become pregnant.
- Assessment of the emotional/family support of the mother and the home environment to which the baby will be living.

18. Why pregnancy is a "Real Mother?"

Welcome to all of the "fine" changes you will be experiencing during your pregnancy:

- Morning Sickness, sometimes "all day sickness" in the first trimester (which some patients may experience throughout the entire pregnancy!)
- Extreme sleepiness and fatigue
- Sensitivity to odors, smoke, perfumes and colognes, foods, etc.
- Breast tenderness and swelling as well as enlargement
- Weight gain and swelling
- Leg swelling
- Stretch marks
- Hemorrhoid swelling

- Heartburn
- Feet swelling and the need to wear flip flops

19. Sex and Pregnancy: A frequent question asked during Pregnancy.

Sex is "safe" during pregnancy. Actually, "safe sex" is even safer during pregnancy! Are there any more questions?

Sex is different during pregnancy depending on what stage of pregnancy you are at. At any time in pregnancy it is hard to get in the mood when you are nauseated and vomiting. In the first trimester most women, if not too queasy, are too tired and fatigued to think about sex. Somehow there are times of wellness when sex is desired. Sex is probably best enjoyed in the 2nd trimester when the morning sickness and sleepiness has worn off. In addition, your energy levels have improved. The enlarging abdomen and discomfort in all positions in the 3rd trimester makes sex difficult for the pregnant patient. The best advice: whatever the couple decides that is best for them works! Pregnancy has a variable effect on sexual desire in both women and men:

Some women may have an increased desire for sex. In general, most women experience an overall decrease interest in sex.

Men may continue to have their usual desire for sex but at the same time they definitely are worried about harming their unborn child. Consequently they may completely avoid their wife's desires. Further, no matter how much the wife may coax him, there is an innate feeling in men that a woman with child is "taboo" and, therefore, it is improper to have sex with her.

Lastly, there are certain <u>absolute</u> conditions in pregnancy when sex should be discontinued:

- Placenta praevia (an OB complication in which the placenta overlies the cervix and can bleed during intercourse)

- Premature Labor (in which intercourse could stimulate contractions and preterm labor)
- Cervical Incompetence (weakness of the cervical support tissues) with or without cerclage placement.

<u>The Bushman Reaction (anecdote)</u>: The author has been awakened two nights in a row at 1 am due to contractions induced by Evelyn Bushman having sex in the 3rd trimester. Yes, sex can start contractions. The physical orgasm coupled with the release of semen (containing prostaglandins and other fluids) can stimulate contractions but not necessarily labor itself. In the Bushman the expectant couple typically expresses their physical and emotional love for each other at 10 PM each night. In the next hour or so, uterine contractions become more frequent. When they do not subside quickly, the couple usually rushes to the OB suite at 1 am. The author is then awakened by MaryAnn, "Ms. Bushman is here again with contractions but her cervix is not dilated. The contractions are irregular. "Is it okay to send her home with the recommendation of "vaginal rest" for the remainder of her pregnancy?" "Yes," I replied, as I quickly put the phone down and try to go back to sleep!

Hint: The guy should wear a condom if the consequence of sex, i.e. significant uterine activity, occurs regularly after sex. Then, her OB can get some needed sleep!

Table 1-3 Key OB Instructions and Questions Frequently Asked

If your water breaks or you think you may be in labor, CALL THE OFFICE during office hours or after hours go the hospital

If your baby is not moving or there are decreased fetal movements, call your OB's office or the OB unit.

If you are bleeding during your pregnancy, call your OB's office or the OB unit. Bleeding after sex can occur but it is usually a very minimal amount.

If you have any questions or concerns regarding symptoms (fever, uncontrollable nausea, severe abdominal pain, headache, etc., call your OB's office first. If so directed or after office hours, then go to the hospital if necessary.

Do not get into hot tubs with a temperature greater than 104 degrees: you will get burned!

Hair permanents and hair colorings may "not take" as well during pregnancy and have not been shown to be absorbed to cause any significant effect on the baby. The vapors in the salon that are not ventilated well have been investigated but, to date, no harmful effect has been shown to exist. The same holds true in nail salons.

With regard to Dental Exams, your dentist may call your OB's office for guidance in prescribing medications

> Dental X-rays are permitted with proper apron shield protection

> Local anesthetics are permissible but not gas.

20. People Giving You Advice and Stories: "You need to ignore them!"

People, family, friends and even "strangers" are going to say things to you that are totally outrageous. The author's advice to deal with such encounters: "just let it go in one ear and out the other!" Much of the information is just plain incorrect. It is almost guaranteed that 90% of what they say will be *negative* and will make you feel insecure and bad.

It is unknown why people love to makes comments about your pregnancy or about how you look. These people are either jealous of you being pregnant or just feel so impulsive to unthoughtfully "flap their jaws." In the case they do say something despicable about your pregnancy or try to tell you some "horror story that happened to them or another person, just ask her "Where he/she got their Medical Degree?" or "Where they went to Medical School?". They will say stupid stuff like, "your belly is so big that you must be having twins." Conversely, they might say something worse like, "you're so small, I hope your baby is growing properly." We live in a "negative" culture world. People just like to talk! Inherently they seem compelled to make some comment about your pregnancy.

People are going to tell you "stuff!"

Author's Note: So many people will come up to you, even if you are in a supermarket, etc. and try to tell you the sex of your baby by "the way you are carrying" or the shape of your abdomen. Such predictions of sex based on the contour of your "baby bump" are totally erroneous and lack scientific fact (see "Old Wives' Tales Section of this book). If someone asks if you are carrying twins because they think your abdomen is so large, just tell them straight out "that I am **not** pregnant and that you have *really* hurt my feelings!" Then, you can start crying in front of them!

If people are going to try to mess with your brain and feelings (probably un-intentionally?), you might want to turn it back around and start to mess with theirs!

Also, according to the author's wonderful patient, Gabrielle Barnett, "do not believe some of the information you read on the internet!" That is another one of the reasons the author has written this book: so that you will get accurate straight talk from an experienced OB.

Author's True Anecdote: To illustrate the part about "OB horror stories" I can tell the story about two labor patients that I delivered on the same day. One patient had a long and difficult labor. She labored close to 14 hours and had to push for over 2 hours before she delivered. We used almost maximum doses of Pitocin to get her contractions strong enough to fully dilate her cervix. She did have an epidural. She had been up all night long in labor. By the time she delivered, she was totally exhausted.

The other patient was having her third baby. She, too, had an epidural. Her labor was short: about 6 hours. She pushed the baby out relatively easily.

The next day I was making rounds on both patients whose rooms were right next to each other. As I was outside their doors, I could hear both women talking to others about their labor experience. The one patient that had the long and difficult labor stated, "Oh, it wasn't that bad. It was really no problem." The author thought to himself, *what are you talking about? You had one of the most difficult labors any woman could have.* Then I heard the other patient talking, *the labor was horrible. I was in so much pain. I was miserable during the entire time!* I said to myself again, *Girl, you had a short and easy labor. You do not know how lucky you were.*

My point: In less than 24 hours after a patient delivers, her own perception of what she experienced is completely different than what actually happened. That perception will actually change even more as time goes by. So, you cannot really believe anything that a person tells you about her labor and delivery! Author Note: I presume that women talk about their pregnancy and childbirth just like guys talk about their fishing and hunting stories!

21. Get out and Enjoy Life (because, Life as you know it now is coming to an end!)

It is truly how incredible a baby can completely take over your life. Taking care of a baby in the first few weeks completely occupies most of your time (and sleep!). I advise patients to "enjoy life now" by going out to your favorite movies, restaurants, museums, concerts, and weekend getaways, it is still "before baby" time. "After baby" you will need a babysitter just to get a few hours off. You still will be thinking of your baby at all times ("I bet he/she is crying, wet, etc.).

22. Relationship Changes and Challenges

The high level of hormones being secreted from the placenta into your circulation can have profound effects on your feelings and moods. Husbands (or SO's or FOB's) report that their "wives change into some other psychotic weird crazy person when they are pregnant." I tell them that they expect that "that beautiful, kind and sexy woman you fell in love with will return back to them within weeks after their delivery (It is just a temporary episode when pregnant *Girls Gone Wild*)." Nevertheless, pregnant women will experience immense emotional swings, get moody and hateful to their spouses and members of their family. Some of these hateful reach extremes may become manifest when she goes into labor. I heard a lot of statements from women in labor as follows:

"You're never going to have sex with me ever again" "Don't look my way or look at me that way!"

"Don't expect any more children after this one!"

"Get away from me. I hate you. You did this to me!"

My own wife at the time (now she is my "ex-wife," also known as "Plaintiff" by my attorney) grabbed me by the b...s when she was in labor. I am sure she didn't mean to?

<u>Author anecdote</u>: I tell some people that "I always try to *drown* my problems, but I can't get my ex-wife to go swimming!" "No, I don't think I still harbor *any* ill feelings toward her!

I always tell the expectant fathers that they should *never* (*never, ever* per Taylor Swift or you may never be back together!*) argue or contradict the future mother of your child.

"It is better to be happy than to be right!"

"You might have another opinion, but it is best to keep it to yourself"

*"You should never, ever insult or call her any names. Never use swear words or criticize her because those words will never (never, ever) be forgotten (you'll be hearing them again and again in every subsequent argument and maybe in a court room, for years) and it does not **ever** lead to a solution to the conflict at hand.*

(If you do not follow this sage advice, then you will be paying child support like the author did!")

Remember: Marriage is "Grand," but divorce is $50 Grand!

Author Anecdotes:

There was a new sociological study recently completed from California: the study showed that the main cause of divorce in California was…….. Marriage!

I am always surprised when I see a California divorce lawyer getting married for the first time: perhaps "hope does triumph over experience!"

Pregnancy and newborn babies completely change the concept of your relationship. From being "lovers and best friends" you become mothers, fathers, and a family. Your roles to each other and to society have changed. It is very important to recognize and acknowledge the change. It occurs so suddenly and unexpected as you are holding your baby in your arms for the first time. Accordingly, there are a few recommendations I have for you.

Inform your partner that you have less or occasionally no control over your moods and emotions. He needs to know that your pregnancy has "gotten hold of you" for 9 months and that he just needs to be patient. I say to the guys, "You may have a different thought or answer, but please, just keep to yourself." Remember, "A happy wife means a happy life."

According to John Gray (author of Men are from Mars, Women are from Venus), women talk out (externalize) their problems and conflicts. Women get together in groups in order to think out their problems and solve them. Men try to solve their problems inwardly (internalize) by being alone while working on the car or constructing or fixing something in the garage. Men are hard-wired to "fix things." But, they cannot fix what is happening to their wives. It is best for the men to just respond to their partner's feelings, such as the following:

I feel your frustration.

You have a right to feel angry.

You are such a good person, a good friend, a good daughter, a good student, etc.

When their wife comes home after being cut off in traffic by another vehicle, most men would respond, "I am getting my gun, just tell me what kind of car he was driving and which direction he was headed." By reflex, men are going "to fix" the problem but what he should do is the following:

Solution: Go over and put your arms around her, give her a kiss, and say, "I feel your frustration and honey, and you are such a good driver." Men need to respond to all statements by acknowledging their feelings: frustration, depression, loss, etc.

According to Dr. Phil (from his book, *Relationship Rescue*), "the best relationships" equal "being best friends" and "meeting each other's needs." I like to extend the part "being best friends" to also mean "being best roommates." It is important for each partner to communicate their most important "needs." Think about what really matters to you and what makes you happy. "Don't sweat the small stuff." "Being best friends" means respecting and honoring each other. Being critical or worse, calling each other a name or belittling each other is the surest road to relationship death.

<u>Author Anecdote</u>: After the author's divorce he began researching more information about relationships in order to try to understand what had happened. He wanted to avoid such a disaster in the future. The author read, "Men are from Mars and Women are from Venus." The author admitted to himself that, despite being an Ob-Gyn, he really had been completely ignorant of how women think and act. It was as if a bright light had been turned on in a dark room of information on how women "tick." The next day he went into the OR and asked the anesthesiologist, Henry Nesis, MD, if he had ever read the book. He replied, "Wasn't that book written by John Gray? The author replied, "Yes. It was written by him." Henry then asked, "Wasn't he married to Barbara DeAngelo, the other renowned relationship expert?" I replied, "Yes, he was married to her!" Henry then said, "Well, if those two "Relationship Experts" could not make it, how do they expect *us* to?"

The bottom line to all you fathers out there, as sung by Queen Latifa in the musical, *Chicago* (with modification by author):

Get a little motto that will always see you through -
When you're good to Mama, Mama's good to you!
Spice it up for Mama, She'll get hot for you!

Read more: <u>Chicago The Musical - When You're Good To Mama Lyrics | MetroLyrics</u> From *Chicago The Musical*

The Marriage Box (or the Relationship Box)

The following is a quotation that the author hopes the reader will appreciate: its wisdom applies not just to marriage but to *all* relationships. The information in this book is not just inclusive of "pregnancy facts." It would not be perfectly fine to know all the didactic information regarding pregnancy, but that information would pale if the couple could not get along or have a successful and happy relationship after the birth of the baby.

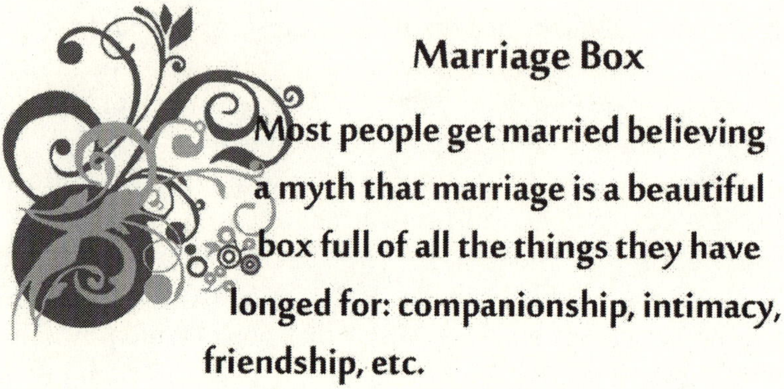

Marriage Box

Most people get married believing a myth that marriage is a beautiful box full of all the things they have longed for: companionship, intimacy, friendship, etc.

Figure 1-28 The Marriage Box

*Unknown (but has been attributed to **J. Allen Petersen**)*

However, as another had surmised after being married, "Marriage is like a deck of cards. In the beginning all you need are two hearts and a diamond. By the end, you wish you had a club and a spade!" Lastly, as Groucho Marx stated, "Marriage is a wonderful institution as long as you don't mind being in "an institution" the rest of your life.

A successful Marriage is the act of two people having great mutual respect and admiration for each other as well as trying to "overserve" each other.

23. Traveling during Pregnancy

It is usually safe to travel during most of your pregnancy with some precautions. However, the safest time to travel is in the second trimester (13–27 weeks) as your pregnancy is well established and your delivery is remote. Most physicians caution against travel in the last four weeks of pregnancy because of the increased probability of labor starting.

<u>Author's Note and True Story</u>: One of my patients traveled from Lawton, OK, to Killeen, TX, five days prior to her scheduled C-section. Of course, she experienced a problem: she ruptured her membranes while visiting her fiancé at Fort Hood. She had to be delivered there by a physician she never met until just prior to surgery.

Please do not travel during the last few days or weeks of pregnancy unless you have notified your physician and a true family emergency exists. The patient should obtain a copy of her OB records if she must leave town at this time.

Travel in the first trimester can be difficult: motion may cause increased nausea. Further, you may not travel far without resorting to frequent pit stops to empty your bladder!

<u>Another Authors Note and True Story</u>: When I was a younger doctor, I traveled to an Obstetrics Conference in Maui, Hawaii. A group of us decided to take the 25 mile "Road to Hana." Dr. Branch's wife, Martha, was early pregnant at the time: because of all the twists and turns in the road, we had to stop frequently for her to get out of the car and "hurl" in the bushes by the roadside. It was not a very pleasant road trip and by the time we got to Hana, the water falls had already closed. It was now 5:30 PM and we were getting pretty hungry (except Martha!). We entered the only restaurant in town which was open. As we walked into the foyer, we saw that the place was completely empty: there were no other diners sitting in the restaurant at all! We asked for a table but the host turned us down: apparently there was a "dress code" and a group of doctors in Hawaiian shirts and shorts was not appropriate for their eating establishment!

It is important, whether traveling by car or plane, that you move your legs frequently and flex your muscles so that you can avoid leg/feet swelling and worse yet, possible blood clots forming in your legs.

If you are traveling to other countries, it is best to check with your OB or your family physician regarding appropriate vaccinations and other protective injections that you may need. The CDC and other health organizations may have recommended guidelines prior to your entry into the specific country.

24. Bathing, Showering, Clothing and Shoes

Daily bathing and/or showering during pregnancy is recommended. There is no harm to taking a bath at any point in pregnancy. Clothing should be clean and be loose fitting and comfortable. The photo above shows how resourceful OB patients can be when they want to keep wearing their favorite jeans

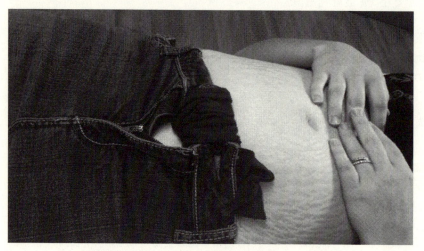

Figure 1-29 Waist Expanders for your pants to fit into your favorite pair of jeans ()

Wear flat and comfortable supporting shoes, like tennis or running shoes, and avoid high heels to avoid imbalance and falling. The further along in pregnancy you are, the more you have to balance out the weight of the baby growing in the front of you. Be careful getting in and out of the bathtub, walking outside in adverse weather conditions (snow, ice and rain), etc. because of the risk of falling and significant injury.

Author's Note: There is always one of my patients wearing a cast on her arm or her foot because of a fall from the natural imbalance caused by the growing baby in the front of you!

25. "Quickening" (Feeling the baby's movements)

You will feel the baby move for the first time between 16–20 weeks of pregnancy. First time moms will feel the baby move later at 18 to 20 weeks whereas second and other babies can be felt sooner. The very day that the expectant mother first feels her baby move is a significant milestone in her pregnancy: please notify your OB of the date and mark that date in your Baby Diary. Each baby's frequency and force of movements is different, but the baby usually moves at least 10 times per hour. It does have "sleep" periods of time that can last 30 minutes or so. It is important to get to know your baby's movement pattern and report any sudden decrease in fetal movements to the office. Most times, drinking orange juice or eating some yogurt or fruit will cause the baby to be more active.

26. Hospitals and Delivery

There are thousands of excellent hospitals throughout the United States and the world. The author lists the two hospitals in his city as examples of the obstetric facilities that have dedicated and compassionate nursing staffs

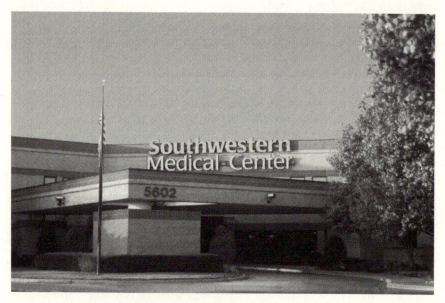

Figure 1-30 Southwestern Medical Center, Lawton, OK.

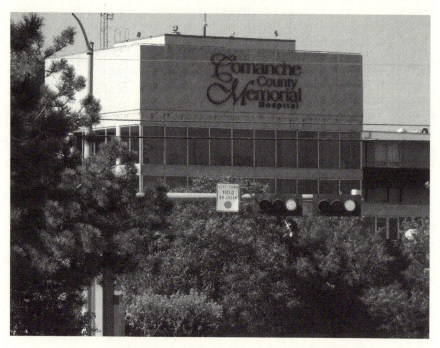

Figure 1-31 Comanche County Memorial Hospital Pic

For example, there are two outstanding hospitals in the author's city. The patient should check with their insurance plan to see if the hospital where they want to deliver is "contracted" or "preferred." It is important to pre-register at the hospital during your pregnancy. The receptionists in your OB's front office will gladly print out a copy of your demographic and insurance information from the computer to bring to the Admitting Office so that you do not have to fill out the same paperwork again (Many OBs are employed or are connected electronically to the hospital so that medical, personal and insurance data can be shared or transmitted).

27. Prenatal Classes and Hospital Tours

Because so many patients are requesting and desiring epidurals for pain relief during labor, many hospitals are no longer offering Lamaze or Bradley classes. Check with your hospital (call the OB suite or the Education Office) to see if and when classes are being held. If you are planning on a natural birth without anesthesia then I recommend you obtain Lamaze or Bradley instruction via a DVD from their internet site or from Amazon.com.

The reader should call Labor and Delivery at the hospital (or check their website) for the schedule of tours of the obstetric suite and the postpartum floor.

28. Insurance Coverage and Billing

The Office will verify that your insurance coverage is active for your pregnancy. It is recommended that you obtain a copy of your insurance benefits from your job/work and bring them to the office during your first appointment. Important insurance telephone numbers, coverage of procedures, etc. are detailed in your booklet. Put your insurance plan "800" number in your smartphone Contacts for easy access. Your pregnancy will be billed as a "global" procedure meaning that your total OB care is billed as a "package deal," i.e. includes all of your OB visits, your delivery and your 6 week Postpartum visit are all inclusive. Your laboratory testing, medications, vitamins and ultrasound examinations are *not* included and will be billed separately by the laboratory, pharmacy, hospital, and the office. Insurance is explained below. The reader can skip to the next section if you desire.

Table 1-4 Insurance Crash Course 1A

Insurance 1A Crash Course

Some definitions:

Deductible: annual amount of money you must pay "out of pocket" i.e. your wallet.

Allowable charges: a service that is allowed to be charged by the insurance company. Some health care costs/services are not covered or allowed under the plan.

Commercial 80/20 plan: insurance plan covers 80 percent of charges and you pay the other 20 percent out of pocket.

Out-of-Network: usually a 70/30 Plan with 30 percent cost to you.

Co-pay: defined amount of money to be paid to physician, pharmacy, ER, etc. approximately $20

There is an annual deductible amount and there is an annual maximum out-of-pocket amount. Further, some health plans do and do not allow you to "carry over" to the next calendar year.

Deductibles are usually applied or credited to the "maximum out of pocket" amount if you reach it.

Example: Health Maximus Plan A (plans vary—check your plan out)

$750 annual deductive with a Maximum $3000 out of pocket plan

Obstetrical Physician total cost:	$5000.
Laboratory fees and cost:	$2000.
Hospital Total cost including Epidural:	$10,000.
Pharmacy Costs	$300.
Total Cost:	$17,300.

The patient will be responsible for the maximum out of pocket of $3000 for this pregnancy. However, if your policy runs on a "Calendar Year" basis or plan, and your pregnancy carries over to the next calendar year, you have to start all over with paying your deductible and the new Maximum out of pocket gets zeroed out and begins all over again.

If you get pregnant in September 2013 and deliver in June of 2014, then you will be paying in two calendar years.

Let's say for example, your 2013 costs of pregnancy to date (office visit, ultrasound, pharmacy, and lab) is $2000 on December 31, 2013.

80/20 Plan: Normally you will pay $400 (20% of $2000) and your Plan will pay $1600, but you must meet your deductible of $750. Therefore, you will pay a total of $750 in 2013 and your plan will pay $1250.

Your Total Bill still stays at $17,300 so in 2014 you have a balance of $15,300.

You must subtract another $750 deductible, but your Total Cost is over you maximum allowable out-of-pocket of $3000. Your deductible is applied to the $3000. You will pay $750 in the beginning of 2014 and then another $2250 for the remainder of your cost after you deliver.

	Two Calendar Year Physician cost	One Calendar Year Physician cost
2013 Out of pocket cost:	$1250.	
2014 Out of pocket cost:	$2250	
Total Cost:	$3500	$3000.

One other point: Your Insurance Plan may have a total "contracted" amount that they will pay with each of the service entities (Hospital, Lab, Pharmacy and OB). That is total amount allowed by the insurance company and agreed upon by contract with the service entities. There will be "no balance billings" for any billing above the "allowable." These "billings" above the "contracted amount" must be "written off" by the same service entities: you will probably pay less out of pocket (also known as "co-insurance).

*HMO, *PPO and *MCO type health plans work with or contract with the healthcare entities. If your insurance is through Tricare, Medicare and Medicaid there may be little or no out of pocket costs to your pregnancy.

Tricare Prime: Referral is necessary but no co-pay or deductible

Tricare Standard: Deductible $50-$500, Co-pays at initial office visit, with Out-of-pocket varies per Plan

HMO: BlueLinks in Oklahoma requires Referral from your primary care MD (with a reference number) for OB care.

*HMO is a Health Maintenance Organization (the largest is Kaiser Foundation Health Plan in CA)

*PPO is a Preferred Provider Organization (most Blue Cross/Blue Shield Plans)

*MCO is a Managed Care Organization

*Capitated Health Care is a Health Plan in which part of your monthly premiums go to your Primary Care Physician

For in-depth information see *www.healthcare-information-guide. com/insurance-policy-terms.html*

Any deductibles and out of pocket expense determined by your insurance should be paid by the 7th month of your pregnancy. This can be estimated, and paid a little each month at your return OB visits. Please speak with the office manager or front office staff on or before your second visit to make arrangements for the costs and your payment schedule.

29. Telephone Calls and Problems

Please call the office if any problems or have any questions that come up *between* the Ob visits Call the office during regular office hours and *do not wait* until the evening to try and address your problems. If you are having problems during regular office hours, call to determine if you should be seen in office. *OBs prefer that you do not go to the Emergency room or Obstetrics Suite during office hours unless the problem you are experiencing cannot be handled at your physician's office. Questions about possible labor can be fielded by the office.*

Please stay off your phone so that we may return your call. Our office staff will usually get to your messages between patients or at the end of the day. Accordingly, do not "screen" your calls from the office and then call back 2 to 5 minutes later when office staff is taking care of other patients (you cannot believe how often patients do this! Pick up your phone!).

Prescription Refills: Please remember that most physicians will refill prescriptions *during office hours only and NOT after hours or on weekends*: please pay attention and note when your medication bottles are getting low! When there are just a few days left of pills left in your container, call your physician's office for refills (most physicians fill prescriptions for a year so that you can obtain refills at your pharmacy. Please check with your pharmacy on how many refills you have left.

Stupid Phone Calls the author has received after Office hours

    a. Memorial Day Special at 3 a.m.

Hello, Dr. Zweig. This is Dr. Smith at the ER. Your patient, Lisa Morrell is here for dental pain due to a tooth abscess. She has not taken her diabetes or high blood pressure medications. Her blood sugar is 259 and her blood pressure is "through the roof" at 210/110. Is it okay if I give her an antibiotic for dental infection?

I cannot remind patients enough to keep up their dental care (cleanings, cavities filled, etc.) during and between pregnancies. Toothaches and gingivitis seem to become more painful after going to bed. In fact, all pain and body aches become accentuated after bedtime: you are not bothered by other daily activities and the patient focuses solely on her body pains.

    b. The Bar closes at 2 AM.

Hello, Dr. Zweig? Yes? This is Mary Anne at Labor and Delivery. Your patient, Yessica Gonzalez is here after getting into a fight with her boyfriend at the bar (she was "talking" and dancing with another guy!). She is 28 weeks pregnant. She says she was punched in the face and hit in the stomach. She has had no bleeding or leakage of fluid. Her baby's fetal heart strip is otherwise normal. Is it okay if we send her back down to the ER for an evaluation of her black eye and bruises?

I really wondered why a 7 months pregnant woman was at the bar at 2 AM. I am sure she was not drinking any alcohol!

    c. Hello, Dr. Zweig? Yes? This is Jody at Labor and Delivery. Your patient, Sara Sakorski, just came up from the ER with back pain. She is 26 weeks pregnant. The ER thought she might be in labor. She is not having any contractions. She is just having back pain! She is 292 lbs. She has not tried any Tylenol or even a heating pad! Is it okay if we tell her to avoid heavy lifting, try Tylenol, hot shower, back massage and a heating pad? Yes, of course: standard treatment recommendation. Good night!

d. Hello, this is Stacy in Labor and Delivery. Your patient Kimberly Smith just arrived at 12:30 am. While she was going down her stairs at home her dog got in her way and she fell down. She has had no bleeding or loss of fluid. She has no bruises or other injuries. The baby's fetal heart strip is normal for 22 weeks. Is it okay for us to let her go home? I just wonder why a pregnant woman is up at midnight in the first place: I would expect her to be fast asleep by 9 PM!

e. Hello, Dr. Zweig, this is Dr. John at Comanche County Hospital ER. Your patient, Mrs. Jones went to take out the trash tonight and slipped and fell on the ice outside her garage. She is a little sore on her left side but there is no bruise. There has been no bleeding or loss of fluids. Baby appears well on our portable ultrasound. Do you have any advice for her? Yes, tell her, she should wait to take the trash out until the ice has melted tomorrow!" I guess she must have missed the weather reports blazing all over the News that we had 5 inches of snow and that there will be ice as the temperatures outside will be in the low 20's.

f. Hello, Dr. Zweig, this Katie from labor and delivery at Comanche County. Your patient Tammy Pisani who is 37 weeks pregnant came in because she thinks she has the flu. The ER sent her up here for "baby check" prior to her being seen down there.

g. Hello, Dr. Zweig, this is Janell from Women's Services. Your patient, Mrs. West, has "indigestion." The author replied, "I guess she was eating the hospital food again! Please give her a tablespoon of antacid every 2 to 4 hours until her stomach recovers.

h. Lastly, one from early afternoon during office hours: "Hello," Dr. Zweig, we have your patient here Ms. Wells." She said, "She has an appointment scheduled with you in 30 minutes in the office." "Well, she was pulled over by the Lawton Police. She was found to have an outstanding warrant. She was arrested. However, she started having contractions (suddenly!) and they brought her here. She is 37 weeks pregnant. She has had a previous C-section. Baby's heart rate strip is "equivocal." The baby had just 10 accelerations in 10 seconds. What do you want us to do?" I said, get a biophysical profile because she had significant oligohydramnios last pregnancy and that was a factor in performing her first C-section. We will make a decision thereafter." "OK, Dr. Zweig, and by the way the Police have released her from custody now!"

Please see author's Chapter 2, Medical Conditions during Pregnancy: that section details the difference between the flu and a cold. In this case, there was a low grade fever, nasal congestion, post nasal drip and a slight cough. Most trips to the hospital can be avoided for both flu and a cold unless there is high fever, shaking chills, extreme prostration or respiratory distress. Fluids, decongestants, cough medications; rest and chicken soup are helpful for most symptoms.

30. How much does my baby weigh and how long is my baby?

There is not a day that goes by that a patient will ask these questions during her OB visit. Many "pregnancy apps" are available for your smartphone that will give you the approximate weight and length/height of your baby at any given day or week of your pregnancy.

For any given week of pregnancy, the reader is referred to The BabyCenter/Expert Advice at *http://www.babycenter.com/average-fetal-length-weight-chart*

A copy of their chart is placed in Appendix H at the back of the book so that the reader can reference the weight and height of their baby at any particular week of their pregnancy.

So please, do not ask your OB the same question <u>every</u> visit, "How much does my baby weigh or how long does he measure?" at your next appointment! Get the App! Or go to the web address above!

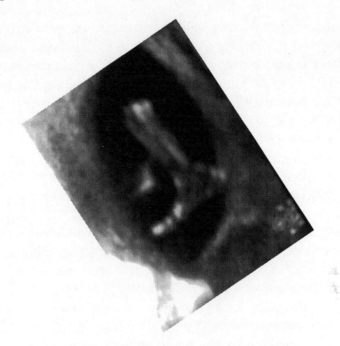

Figure 1-32 Baby's Foot on ultrasound

The reader can see clearly that the baby is wearing Nike tennis shoes! The above foot is similar to the "winged foot "in the Goodyear Tire Logo (originating from Greek God, Hermes or the Roman God, Mercury) The Lawton Goodyear Plant is one of the largest tire production facilities in the United States.

31. Obstetrical Adverse Events and Malpractice

The OB team strives to provide the most compassionate and State-of-the Art medical care that is possible. Physicians and nurses are "human" and are not perfect. Patients are human and are not perfect. When imperfects professionals care for imperfect patients, imperfect results are bound to happen. Physicians and the hospital staff do not "know everything" or have "seen everything" so that all situations can be handled with a satisfactory outcome.

Our nation and society have "high expectations," particularly when it comes to pregnancy and a baby. When something goes wrong or is not anticipated, patients are just too eager to file a lawsuit. The author remembers a story about a female OB-GYN physician who had written a Letter to the Editor of the OB-GYN News. She had finished an excellent university OB-Gyn training program and was one of the new "bright stars" of physicians on staff at one of the prestigious and reliable University Medical Centers. She stated in her Letter, "that she was quitting the practice of Obstetrics because the "standard of care" was "perfection." If patients expect "perfect results" that they should have God take direct personal care of their pregnancy."

Another story: The Women's Group located in Georgia was a much respected OB-GYN group of physicians, nurse practitioners and office staff. The President of the Southeast Section of ACOG (American College of OB-GYN) was the leading member of the Group. She was sued for an "adverse outcome" for which she was not directly responsible or could have otherwise made different. The Group settled the lawsuit for an undisclosed amount of money. In the coming few months the Group received a letter from their malpractice carrier that their insurance was going up to $117,000 per physician. With such a large malpractice premium, each physician would have to work 7-8 months before he could draw any salary. The Group immediately disbanded and disintegrated: two physicians left the city to practice elsewhere, one physician stopped practicing Obstetrics and practiced just Gynecology, and the esteemed highly respected female Ob-Gyn physician who was sued stopped Ob-Gyn and hospital practice altogether.

As sure as the sun will rise in the morning, tragically miscarriages, infections, premature birth, postpartum hemorrhage, stillborn, and birth abnormalities will continue to occur.

All patients should remember that, as medical professionals, we all do the best that we can to ensure safe and satisfactory outcomes. But, we are not perfect and no physician or nurse can guarantee or warrant that all medical care will be perfect.

32. Missing fingers and toes

It is a "classic question" from many generations of mothers in all OB's offices around the world, "Does my baby have all its fingers and toes?" The author replies, "In my career, I have mostly seen extra fingers and toes. In fact, one of my patients in Georgia had 12 fingers and 12 toes! However, she told me that other family members also had babies with extra digits. However, not every baby that is born is perfect: about 5% of babies have some minor "birth defect."

It is truly miraculous how many babies are born with no anatomical defects: the Creator has his hand in every birth.

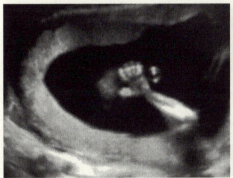
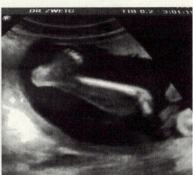

Figure 1-33 Baby's Hand Waving; All Fingers are present.

Figure 1-34 Foot with all toes

There is a *very uncommon* pregnancy condition, called "Amniotic Band Syndrome," in which a band of scar tissue forms and traverses the amniotic fluid. Like a spider web, it can wrap around body part and put pressure on fingers, toes and even the arm or leg itself (tourniquet effect). Accordingly, amniotic bands can cut off of circulation to the affected baby part.

Occasionally there is no explanation for a particular birth defect as is seen below:

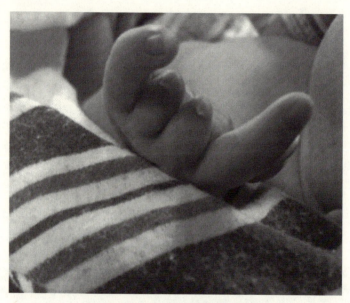

**Figure 1-35 Finger abnormality.
Above picture: Short middle fingers,**

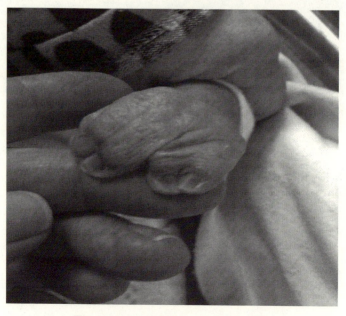

Figure 1-36 Webbing of the fingers

CHAPTER 2

Medical Conditions and their Treatment during your Pregnancy

1. Colds and flu:

It is extremely important to know the difference between a "cold" and "the flu."

"Cold"

> Cause: several different viruses: adenovirus, RSV virus, etc.
> Symptoms: nasal congestion, low grade fever, sore throat, and later a cough with minimally colored mucus

"Flu"

> Caused by the Influenza viruses: A, B
> Symptoms: fever greater than 101 degrees, chills, muscle aching and extreme prostration (weakness to the point of dizziness and the lack of energy to even stand up), headache, stuffy nose

Both conditions are caused by ***viruses*** and cannot be treated with antibiotics (Most antibiotics treat ***bacterial*** infections only). ACOG recommends the "flu" vaccine as a safe and an effective first step in the overall prevention of influenza A and B.

a. "Colds" can be treated with Tylenol for headache; lozenges and gargle mouthwashes for sore throat, and medicines such as Tavist D, Mucinex and Robitussin for cough and nasal sprays (Afrin, Neo-Synephrine) for decongestion.

b. "Flu" can be similarly treated as is a cold. The prescription drug, Tamiflu®, has been shown to be safe and effective in shortening the duration and symptoms of flu.

Ibuprofen, Aleve (naproxen) and aspirin can be taken for occasional and limited use during pregnancy but should *not* be taken during the last 2 months of pregnancy.

2. Stomach and bowel symptoms (GI symptoms) explained

A. *nausea and vomiting*

Usually in the first trimester, nausea and vomiting can continue throughout your pregnancy. These upsetting symptoms and their treatment are covered in the previous section of the book.

B. *Diarrhea/Stomach flu:*

Go on a Liquid diet: water, Gatorade®, bananas, tea and broth. Avoid solid foods, eggs and fried foods.

C. *Constipation:*

Try eating more fruits and vegetables. Drink more water. Do a little more walking. If these measures are not helping you, you can try stool softeners such a Colace, Surfak© or generic DSS (decosate sodium).

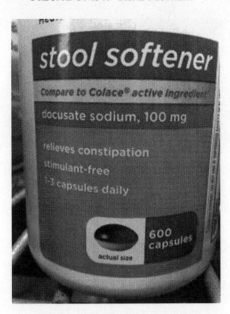

Figure 2-2 Stool Softener

Laxatives such Miralax®, Dulcolax® and milk of magnesia are safe. There is a natural "slow down" in your regular bowel movement due to the pregnancy: the pregnancy hormone *progesterone* relaxes smooth muscle activity in your intestinal walls such that intestinal contractility is slowed down. Again, eating plenty of fiber (vegetables and fruit plus fluids) will help counteract this tendency.

D. *Heartburn:*

Heartburn is a very common problem during pregnancy. It makes its appearance in the 2nd trimester just as the nausea of pregnancy is leaving. Many patients claim they "live on antacids and Tums." The muscle that prevents food from "refluxing" back from the stomach into the esophagus becomes relaxed during the mid-trimester. There are a number of suggestions for help:

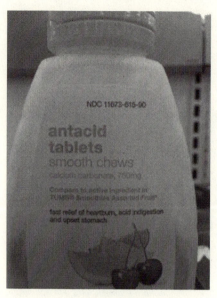

Figure 2-3 Antacid Medications
Sample Antacid medication

1. Do not eat late in the evening or go to bed shortly after the evening meal.

2. Avoid spicy foods (cayenne and other peppers) and other foods that you find cause "your heartburn."

3. Antacids such as Maalox®, Tums® and Mylanta® are soothing. Try to reserve Zantac®, Pepcid AC® and Prevacid® when antacids are not totally effective.

E. "Gas"

"Gas" (flatulence) in the intestines is seldom the only symptom a pregnant patient may experience. Most gas is related to diet: bean products, cabbages, etc. Digestion of these types of vegetables causes the production of various gases as by-products. Gas expands the intestinal tract. Bloating and an uncomfortable fullness may be felt by the already pregnant patient. OTC products with simethicone (Gas-X,© Mylicon©) can provide some relief.

Bowel Disorders during Pregnancy Are Common but these Moms are taking these disorders in Stride

Summary of Article Posted by Carolyn Buchanan May 22, 2013

SUMMARY:

a. About 72 percent of women in their first trimester experience constipation, diarrhea bloating, or irritable bowel syndrome.

b. The majority of women will experience some type of elimination irregularity.

c. Only 4.4 percent of women stated that constipation interfered with their lives. Bloating was a quality of life changer for another 4 percent. Not bad, when you consider how ubiquitous the symptoms are.

Underlying Causes: Increased progesterone levels produced by the placenta relax smooth muscles in the intestines. As a result, peristalsis is inhibited and food by-products take longer to travel through the intestinal tract. Prenatal Vitamins, calcium, and iron supplements taken during pregnancy further aggravate constipation.

Practical solutions to *constipation* are as follows:

- Increase your fiber intake. Most pregnant women consume only 16 to 17 grams of fiber per day. It is recommended that pregnant women increase their fiber consumption up to 25 to 30 grams per day.

- Eat more frequently with smaller amounts of food at one time.

- Increase fluid intake.

- Try to have regular bowel movements at given time of day.

- Be active! — Physical activity has a reflex stimulation.

- Consume Probiotics such as Culturelle, active yeast yogurts, etc.

3. Anemia

Anemia is the most common preventable problem during pregnancy. Anemia is, by definition, a lower amount of circulating *normal* red blood cells. Basically, if you take whole blood and let it settle in a test tube, 45% of the bottom half of the tube should be red blood cells (RBCs) and 55% will be plasma. Most men have a RBC *percentage* of 45% i.e., the *hematocrit*, and most women run at best 40%. The most common cause is iron deficiency. 33% of American woman are currently anemic due to iron deficiency regardless of their pregnancy status. There a few facts the reader must know:

a. Iron is poorly absorbed from your intestinal tract: Only 5% of the iron in your diet is actually absorbed from your intestines into your bloodstream.

b. Most "American diets" do not incorporate the necessary food groups that are rich in iron into their daily nutrition: meat, liver, cast iron cooking, etc.

c. Most women are anemic because they lose most of their blood (and iron) during their menstrual periods: iron may not be replenished by the usual dietary sources.

d. Most Prenatal vitamins do not contain sufficient amounts of iron to provide for the needs of both the baby's and mother's red blood cells. By themselves Prenatal vitamins alone cannot usually replenish the mother's iron stores.

e. An Iron supplement, such as ferrous sulfate or ferrous gluconate (available OTC), is a simple way to prevent iron deficiency anemia.

f. Some specific bowel disorders and previous intestinal surgeries (Bariatric surgery in particular) will further aggravate the absorption of iron into their bone marrow: the red blood cell "factory."

Author Anecdote: It is just heartbreaking and totally unnecessary for an expectant mother to be iron deficient: too many expectant mothers have a Hemacrit <30% when they are admitted in labor. This totally *preventable* condition is very frustrating for most OBs. Many patients just find it too hard to remember to take their prenatal vitamins. The Author has a helpful suggestion: keep your prenatal vitamin and Iron next to your toothbrush and take them both after you brush your teeth just before going to bed!

PICA

Pica is "craving" for a non-food item during pregnancy. Many OB patients will crave "ice" during pregnancy. Ice, in itself" does not cause anemia but it can be a symptom of anemia. In the Southeast OB patient crave "clay" or white dirt. It is such a common craving that many convenience stores stock the "white dirt" and sell it to their pregnant customers. Clay binds iron and therefore the small amount of iron in an OB's patient diet is NOT absorbed in the intestinal tract: iron deficiency can be made dramatically worse.

TMI (too much information) Added information if you are interested further or you can skip to the next section!)

There are other less common anemias (<10%) that occur during pregnancy:

a. Folic Acid deficiency. Despite a very poor diet, it still takes 3 months to develop this type of anemia. Folic acid is a constant component of all prenatal vitamins.

b. Vitamin B12 anemia. This type of anemia is very rare and is usually related to specific GI disorders that prevent absorption of this fat soluble vitamin. Pernicious Anemia, stomach surgeries including Gastric Bypass, etc. are some examples of some of these predisposing conditions.

c. Sickle cell anemia. Many patients with Black ancestry may carry the sickle cell *trait*. There is a 25% chance of the baby having Sickle Cell *disease* when both parents carry the trait.

Sickle cell status is checked routinely on the prenatal panel of blood work if the status unknown. If the father of the baby also carries the trait or the disease, then genetic counseling and testing would be advised.

d. Thalassemia. This type of anemia is caused by an inherited type of gene abnormality that affects the structural formation of hemoglobin, the protein in the red blood cell that carries oxygen. It is common in patients with Mediterranean ancestry, but can occur in all ethnic groups and all races due to intermarriage.

4. Headaches

Most headaches during pregnancy are "Tension Type" headaches. They are caused by muscle spasms of the neck muscles due to your change in posture (your back and neck curvatures) during the pregnancy. Neck massage, hot shower, heating pad and Tylenol are the safest remedies.

Patients with pre-existing migraine headaches may experience an attack during pregnancy. Migraine Headaches frequency is not changed by pregnancy. The usual treatment is bed rest in a dark room. If a patient experiences an "aura" prior to their headache, caffeine products (such as Coke, No-doze™ etc.) may be taken to abort the headache altogether. Imitrex™ (sumatryptans class), verapamil™ (calcium channel blockers or beta blockers) can be used for intractable pain or severe attacks during pregnancy.

5. Seasonal Allergies:

Most antihistamines are safe during pregnancy. Benadryl, Chlor-Trimeton, Zyrtec™, Claritan and other antihistamines can be used to treat your symptoms.

6. Dizziness, Lightheadedness and Fainting:

Most patients begin to notice some lightheadedness in the last part of pregnancy: especially when they may stand up from a sitting or lying down position. Due to the effects of progesterone from the placenta, a pregnant woman's blood pressure will drop during pregnancy (during the 2nd trimester with a slow rise in the 3rd trimester). Drinking plenty of fluids can help alleviate some (but not all) of these symptoms.

If dizziness occurs just before meal times, then hypoglycemia is the usual cause. The placenta siphons off the blood sugar out of a pregnant woman's blood stream in order to transport it over to the baby. The best way to avoid these symptoms is to have a healthy snack in-between meal snacks.

Fainting is a classic symptom of pregnancy: many older motion pictures portrayed young women fainting or swooning to the ground. At that point the other characters would classically blurt out, "She must be pregnant!" Fainting is caused by a loss of your blood pressure when standing still (or standing up) for a period of time. A significant portion of your blood volumes "pools" into the distended deep veins in your legs (caused by the combined effects of gravity keeping the blood volume down in the relaxed dilated walls of the veins). It is recommended "to keep moving" especially when standing, sitting when traveling by car or plane, or quickly getting up from a horizontal position. Keep flexing your leg muscles and, when getting up, hold on to some support so that if you feel faint you can brace your possible fall.

7. Leg swelling (edema) and Varicose Veins:

Leg swelling is quite common during pregnancy: it is usually worse at the end of day when you have been standing upright for prolonged periods of time. Gravity in conjunction with lowered venous tone prevent blood flow back to your heart (i.e. venous stasis in which relaxed concentric muscles in the vein walls do not contract and push the blood upward). In some patients the valves that keep blood from flowing back downward into your legs "leak." Such edema may be occur more frequently during the hot summer months: people sweat, lose salt and drink more fluids, thus creating blood less capable of holding fluid in the vessel walls with diffusion into the skin spaces. Prolonged periods on your feet standing can increase the gravitational effect to slow the return of venous blood flow back to your heart. Later in pregnancy the enlarged uterus compresses the vena cava to a small degree and can still aggravates the problem.

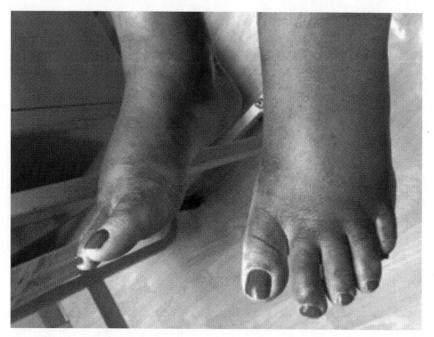

Figure 2-4 Swelling of the feet in pregnancy

It is important not to sit for prolonged periods of time (airplane and car travel or sitting at your computer).

There is a normal "flow of water" in the 3rd trimester of pregnancy (particularly in warm climates). It is quite common to awake in the morning with *hand* swelling. Upon arising and being on your feet all day, gravity moves the water from your hands to your legs. Hence, you have *swollen legs and feet* at the end of the day. The pregnant mother drinks fluids and salt during the day: hence, she has to get up during the night to eliminate the extra fluid load. After lying down flat all night, her hands become swollen again and "the water cycle" repeats itself.

Author's Note: Many of our patients who have to be on their feet all day (restaurant, hospital and nursing home and hospitality employees) are especially troubled by leg and feet swelling. Most of this swelling usually occurs in the last 1-2 months of pregnancy. Support hose and stockings may be useful in these situations.

All of the above factors (upright standing positions, the "progesterone effect" on concentric smooth muscles and valves in vessel walls, gravity and compression of the pregnant uterus on the vena cava) also predispose to vein swelling (varicose veins or varices) in your legs. Vein swelling can also occur in the pelvis and vulvar areas as well as around the rectum, i.e. hemorrhoids.

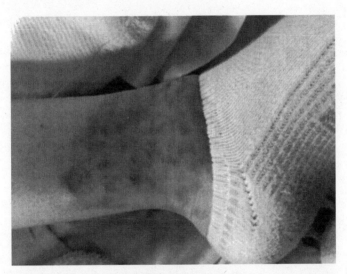

Figure 2-5 Varicose Veins

Warning Signs:

If your feet as well as *your face and hands* swell suddenly with excess weight gain of 8 or more pounds in a few days along with a constant headache, then contact the office or hospital to be evaluated for a special condition of pregnancy: pre-eclampsia or toxemia of pregnancy.

What can you do about the leg swelling and varicose veins?

1. Avoid prolonged standing or sitting. Lay down on your left side with your feet elevated for 20 minutes 3-4 times per day.

2. Wear support hose (such as TEDS, Jobst, etc.)

3. Correct any anemia with iron and eat a high protein diet: both of which can increase the "oncotic pressure "in your bloodstream to keep fluids from leaking out. Be careful of excess salt in your diet and in your foods (particularly some canned foods).

4. Vitamin B6 50 mg (OTC) may be helpful. It can be taken up to 4 times per days and.

8. Strange cravings (ice, ice cream, vinegar and pickles)

Many patients experience various cravings during pregnancy. Pickles and ice cream together has always been a stereotypical classic combination for an expecting woman.

<u>Salty food</u> cravings include pickles, chips, and even heavily vinegar covered salads.

<u>Sweets</u> such as cookies, ice cream, and chocolate can be very much desired by patients. It may also be a reason for the extra pounds that she may gain.

<u>Other</u>: watermelon

<u>Ice</u>: Some of my patients have also reported cravings for "ice." Ice in itself should not be a problem unless excessive.

<u>Clay</u>: The most alarming craving is for "white dirt," or clay (medical term, *"pica"*). It is most common craving experienced in the Southeast by patients of African-American Heritage. Unfortunately, many stores in the South "sell" white dirt to pregnant patients. White

dirt, or clay, absorbs much of the iron in a pregnant woman's diet. Accordingly, severe anemia can occur.

9. Hair coloring, Permanents and Manicures

It is permissible to use continue to color your hair and get a permanent during pregnancy. The only caution is making sure that the salon is well ventilated. There are many chemicals that are used in your hairdo: without adequate air flow and air conditioning these chemical vapors can be inhaled and *theoretically* be exposed to your baby (but in miniscule amounts). To be absolutely safe, do the following:

Avoid hair coloring and permanents in the first trimester (1st 13 weeks)

Avoid bleach and ask your hairdresser to use "organic" solutions

Manicuring the nails in your hands and feet is also permissible but again, as above, most of the salons should be ventilated to prevent excess inhalation. The chemical used on your nails are not absorbed by your body and cannot affect your baby.

10. Swelling of your hands: now how do I get my wedding ring off?

Along with swelling of your feet, the fingers in your hand can experience swelling. Occasionally the swelling prevents you from removing your rings. In such a case it is best to attempt removal of your rings in the late afternoon. Usually your hands are swollen in the morning and then, as you are on your feet all day, the swelling leaves your hands and face and goes to your feet by gravitational force.

    a. Put cooking oil or liquid KY lubricant under the ring and over your finger.
    b. Put your hands over your head or just above your hand so that the veins and lymph channels can drain
    c. Try slipping the ring off gently: don't use force or otherwise more swelling may ensue

d. Worst case scenario: you may have to go to the Jeweler and have the ring cut off
   e. Even worst case scenario: do not put them back on your finger later! Put your wedding or other rings on a necklace to be worn.

11. "Baby Brain"

Many OB patients may notice that their memory may come somewhat impaired during pregnancy. Such "lapses" have been excused by patients by simply stating that it is caused by their "Baby Brain." Difficulty in concentration, forgetfulness, sleepiness and fatigue, learning abilities etc. can be experienced.

12. "Dreams" during Pregnancy.

Your dreams during pregnancy can be more dramatic and occasionally frightening. Dreams about your baby and other people in your life become accentuated.

For example, the author was listening to the heart rate of a baby on a typical OB checkup appointment. The author then said to the patient, "the rhythm sounds like my washing machine at home." The next appointment, the patient told me that I needed to be careful of what I say and "that night after her OB visit she had a terrible nightmare. She dreamt that she was in a horrible long painful labor and when it was finally all over, she had delivered a washing machine!"

All OB patients should be reassured that such disturbing dreams will go away after pregnancy: they will just be changed out for the disturbing reality that parenthood brings you after your baby is born!

Such exotic dreaming is normal: just expect them to be more vivid and accentuated.

13. The "Black Line," Tan nipples and other Color Changes on your body during Pregnancy

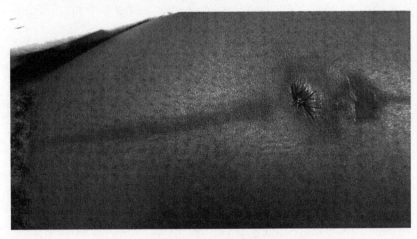

Figure 2-6 Linea Nigra

There is a higher concentration of pigment producing cells (melanocytes) in the very middle of your abdomen as well as your nipples and areola. Toward the end of pregnancy a "black line," or the "linea nigra, the medical term for the line that forms vertically down from your rib cage to your pubic area will be formed. Similarly the areola and nipples of your breasts will darken as your pregnancy progresses. The darkness of your nipples and the "black line" will fade in time only to come back again with future pregnancies. No treatment is necessary. The reader is also referred to the Old Wives Tales section of the book regarding the significance of this line in common gossip.

14. Sunbathing, Saunas, Tanning beds and Creams

Sunbathing during pregnancy is not too different than when you are not pregnant. When sun-tanning, you need to limit your times of exposure: a finite amount of time in direct sunlight (less than 30 minutes) on a daily basis. The use of a high level SPF lotion protection is recommended (25-50 SPF). People burn more easily in the covered areas of your body where there has been little exposure to the sun: feet, ear lobes, bottom areas, and chest.

Tanning beds are overall safer than direct sunlight as much of the damaging- UV type B radiation is filtered out in a tanning bed. Again, follow the recommended guidelines as far as length of time of exposure and the settings.

Suntan coloring (spray tans) are probably the safest route for a bronze body. The baby cannot absorb sunlight, tanning bed rays or the tanning colors you apply. For the latest information regarding sunscreen products and the new FDA labels, please go to Appendix B.

Saunas and hot tubs can be used by a pregnant patient. The safely guidelines are adjusted and are applied more strictly. Time of use should be limited: ACOG states that women might "reasonably be advised to remain in saunas for no more than 15 minutes and in hot tubs for no more than 10 minutes" to avoid increasing one's core temperature. Also, one should not submerge your head (unless you want to drown!), arms, shoulders and upper chest in a hot tub. Dehydration and overheating are important concerns: keep a water bottle is handy and drink fluids as much as possible.

15. How do I prevent from getting "stretch marks"?

Stretch marks are due to tearing of the elastic fibers in your skin. Your skin's ability to stretch over your enlarging uterus is due to genetic, hormonal and constitutional factors: meaning that you are really born with the factors that cause (or avoid) stretch marks. The following advice may help decrease the severity of stretch marks:

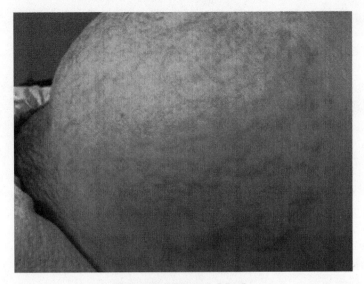

Figure 2-7 Stretch Marks

- Avoid sudden jumps in weight gain in pregnancy: let your skin stretch *very slowly* each day

- Use of skin creams to improve the softness and resilience of your skin (cocoa butter, Neutrogena, Lubriderm, Vaseline Intensive Care, etc.)

- Avoid any steroid creams medications: the high levels of cortisone from your placenta is a main factor that works on the elasticity of your skin

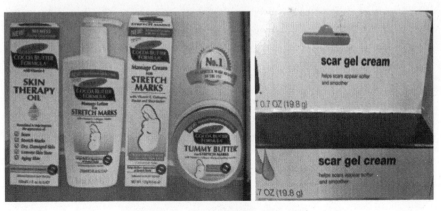

Figure 2-8 Stretch Mark Creams

16. Colostrum and Leakage of your nipples late in pregnancy

In the last month of pregnancy you will notice some leakage of liquid from your nipples. The liquid is called colostrum. It is a natural process and signals the beginning growth and preparation of your breasts and nipples for future lactation.

17. Carpal Tunnel Syndrome (Why are my fingers numb?)

Usually in late pregnancy, as happen with swelling of your feet noted above, you can experience numbness in your fingers due to accumulation of fluid in the "carpal tunnel," the small bony tunnel through which the median nerve travels and supplies feeling to your fingers. It is usually worse in the mornings but can last in some cases until you deliver. Again, pregnant women should decrease their consumption of salt and salty foods: Vitamin B6 50 mg every 8 hours can help alleviate some of the numbness.

18. Pregnancy-Related Abdominal and Pelvic Pains

Pregnancy is NOT a comfortable state of affairs: you have another "creature" inside of you and it can be unbearable.

The enlarging uterus or womb can cause painful discomfort in the abdomen. The growing uterus pushes out and stretches the abdominal muscles and tissues. The uterus can twist from side to side during its growth and pull on the Round Ligaments. These Round Ligaments attach to the sides of the pregnant uterus: they stabilize and "tether" the uterus and keep it in place (see below).

Further, as the pregnancy advances, the uterus pushes the liver and spleen into the chest area: rib and chest pain as well as shortness of breath ensue.

VERY COMMON PREGNANCY RELATED SYMPTOMS

Pelvic and uterine cramping as well as pain (Sharp pains in lower pelvic areas)
Backache
Pubic bone and hip pain
Tailbone pain
Flank discomfort (pain in the side)
Sciatica (pain going down your buttock into your legs with some numbness
Chest pains and Shortness of Breath (uterus or baby's leg pushing liver and spleen into your chest with sore ribs
Pains radiating into vagina and pelvis

Author's Note:

There is not a day that goes by that we do not have a patient call, come to the office, or go to the Obstetrics suite with abdominal pain. Please, do not panic when you are feeling very uncomfortable. You need to know how you can tell if this pain is normal or abnormal:

ABNORMAL PAIN

Table 2-1 Abnormal Abdominal Pain

The pain is accompanied by nausea and vomiting
The pain is associated with fever, chills and sweating
There is pain as well as blood, mucus or other fluid coming out the vagina
The uterus is "rock" hard and/or you are having contractions.
The baby is not moving or there is a significant decrease in the baby's movements.

There are going to be painful areas of your "stomach" that are due to the "growing pains" of your enlarging uterus and baby. If slowing down your activities or lying down for a while eases the pain, then the pain is probably related to your pregnancy and is just probably a "muscle spasm."

19. Low Back Pain

Low back pain results from the increased weight and related changes to your spinal curvature during pregnancy. If you already have had a back injury or other disc disease, it can be aggravated by a superimposed pregnancy. The American College of Obstetrics and Gynecology (ACOG**) suggest the following measures to prevent and treat low-back pain in pregnancy:

- Wear low-heeled (not flat) shoes with good arch support (and avoid high heels)
- Get help from family and co-workers when lifting heavy objects
- Place one foot on a stool or box when standing for long periods of time
- Place a board between your mattress and box springs if the bed is too soft (check out Tempur Pedic or other space-age technologies at your local mattress store (Mattress Firm, Sears, etc.)
- Squat down, bend knees, and keep back straight when lifting
- Sit in chairs with good back support or use a small pillow to provide support
- Sleep on side with pillows between knees for support
- Apply heat, cold or massage to the painful area

** Reference OBG Management, January2014 per ACOG Patient Information Booklet with web reference to http://www.acog.org//media/For%20Patients/faq115.pdf?dmc=1&ts=20130118T1434071958

Bottom Line: Avoid heavy lifting and wearing shoes with high heels. Back massage, heating pad and Tylenol should help with the discomfort.

20. Sciatica and Round Ligament Syndrome (your baby is "getting on your nerves")

Just about half way through your pregnancy the expectant patient may feel pain in her right or left groin. The "baby bump" is now more protuberant and the uterus itself can now "twist" or rotate in the abdomen. The Round Ligament is responsible for keeping the uterus straight: the Round ligaments are inserted on the top side portion or the uterus and basically, "tether" the uterus so it does not rotate.

> **Round Ligament Syndrome** is abdominal/pelvic pain usually on one side that comes from stretching of the Round ligament that radiates from the top of the uterus into the groin).

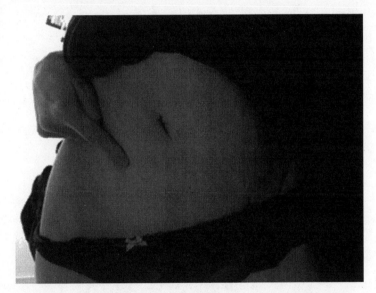

Figure 2-9 Round ligament from top of uterus to groin

However, the baby may move to one side or the expectant mother may position herself in such a way that the uterus twists: such twists stretch out the Round ligament and cause pain the respective groin areas. Round ligament pain does not endanger the baby but just makes you uncomfortable. Rotating or lying on the side of the pain may alleviate the pain. Round ligament pain usually resolves later in pregnancy when the pregnancy is more advanced and the uterus is more stable from rotational forces.

Sciatica is a nerve pain syndrome in which the sciatica nerve is compressed in the lumbar vertebral area of the back. Pain is felt down the buttocks into the lower leg just on one side of the body. Vertebral injuries, heavy lifting, constitutional factors play major roles in this condition. From the mid-portion of pregnancy the "baby bump" causes the expectant mom to lean back and increase the curvature of her lower back: it is very similar to the same positional change that everyone unconsciously does when lifting and carrying a heavy bag of groceries to their car.

Everyone would experience a backache if they had to carrying 25 lbs. of groceries for 7 months.—Author Note

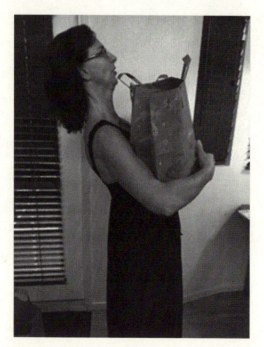

Figure 2-10 Low back pain due to increased sway and curvature

The combined changes of the "baby bump" and the increased "lean back" of the lumbar-sacral curve combined with the increased weight of the pregnancy itself put compression forces on the sciatica nerve.

The most common kinds of *pregnancy-aggravated* pain in the back and abdomen are summarized as follows:

Low back pain that is focused in the middle of the lower back is a result from increased weight-bearing and the increasing greater curvature of your lower spine as the baby grows.

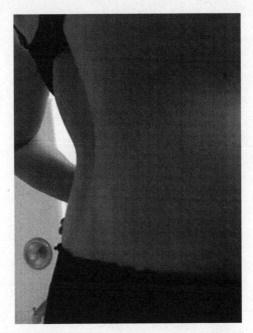

Figure 2-11 Low back pain due to the "lean back" of pregnancy

Round ligament pain in focused in the groin and upper pelvic area on one side or the other.

Sciatica pain ensues from nerve root compression due to disc protrusion in your lumbar-sacral (L5-S1). The pain radiates down your buttock cheek into the back of your leg on one side.

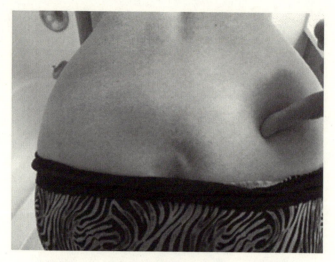

Figure 2-12 Sacra-iliac joint pain location

Sacroiliac pain is focused in the pelvic joint space about 2 inches to the right or left of the mid-spine. The pelvic joint space separates to enlarge the *pelvic circumference* and, thus make more room for the passage of the baby through the birth canal. This separation of the sacra-iliac joint space carries its own attendant discomfort.

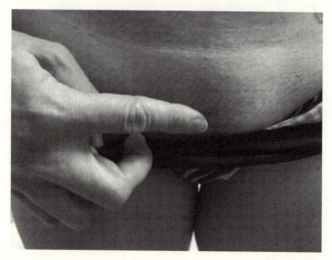

Figure 2-13 Pubic bone pain from symphysis separation

The pubic bone in front, anatomically the *pubis symphysis*, is composed of two wing bones of the pelvic girdle. The joint space between these two bones separates as the ligaments that hold them together relax and stretch as a result of the pregnancy hormone, *relaxin*. As a result of this separation and expansion of the pelvic ring, the patient may feel discomfort similar to the sacroiliac joint space noted above.

21. Insomnia: It means I cannot fall or stay asleep!

Having difficulty falling asleep is a common problem during pregnancy. There are many recommendations to help with this very common difficulty:

   a. Avoid *stimulating* activities prior to bedtime. Turn off the TV or your music. Physical activities such as your work outs may activate your alertness.

   b. Avoid having emotional conversations or phone calls.

   c. Avoid eating close to bedtime which may also cause heartburn or acid reflux.

   d. Reading tires your eyes and may help many people become sleepy.

   e. Light housework or a warm bath/hot shower may help you fall asleep. Your partner may volunteer to give you a very relaxing body massage but beware that other body parts may be touched leading to other activities. Sexual intercourse with a fulfilling climax can help you fall into a relaxed state and tranquility due to the release of endorphins from such pleasurable activities.

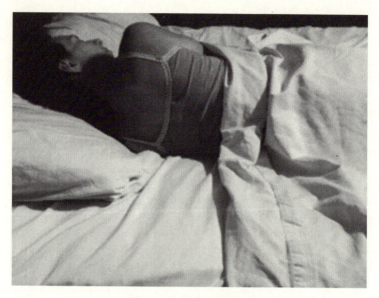

Figure 2-14 Insomnia

Insomnia usually occurs in late pregnancy whereas "always falling asleep" is common in the first part of pregnancy. Frequently, the need to empty your bladder and your baby's active movements in the middle of the night can keep you from falling back to sleep. Unisom, Benadryl and Melatonin® may be helpful at these times.

22. Can I sleep on my back or lay down on my back during exercise class?

You can relax and go to sleep at night and not worry about inadvertently sleeping on your back. Patients tell the author frequently that they "wake up in the middle of the night and find that they have been sleeping on their back. They ask, have I hurt my baby?" The answer is NO! Sleep studies show that a person at sleep is constantly moving, at least every 15 minutes, during the nighttime. Basically, you are constantly moving even though you may not know it. No medical studies have been published to show that unintentionally sleeping on your back has led to any adverse effects, or even stillborn, in your baby. The author's advice, "You have no control over what position you sleep in. You are always moving around. So do not even think about it. Just go to sleep and enjoy the rest you deserve!"

"Caval Syndrome." Later in pregnancy, in the 3rd trimester, patients will feel faint and dizzy if they are lying straight on their back while doing their exercises on the gym floor. It is called "Caval Syndrome:" the weight of the baby compresses the vena cava and obstructs the blood flow coming back from your legs back to your heart. When doing exercises flat on your mat in the gym floor, if dizziness is noticed, it is best to lean onto your left side floor. If you still experience light- headedness or visual changes, you may have to forgo all such "on your back" activities altogether.

Author's Note: It is not uncommon that patient's will start to feel lightheaded or feel like they are going to faint if they are lying down straight on their back during an OB exam (especially during a longer OB ultrasound evaluation). In these situations, the patient should lean over onto their left side and take some deep breaths: such respiratory efforts will "physically pull" more blood back from their legs into their heart and chest.

It is standard policy for patients in labor or patients who are undergoing a C-section to be positioned on their left side (or "Left Lateral Tilt") in order to avoid placing the full weight of the baby directly on and compressing the vena cava or blood flow coming from the lower portion of the body.

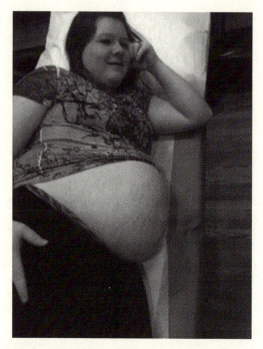

Figure 2-15 Lateral tilt during an office exam.

23. Yeast and other vaginal Infections

Yeast infections occur quite frequently during pregnancy. Burning, itching and a vaginal discharge are the common symptoms. OTC vaginal medications such a Monistat® or generic miconazole creams can treat the condition.

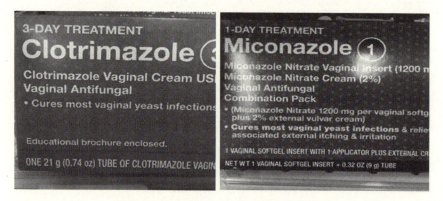

Figure 2-16 Yeast Medications (OTC)

If your discharge has an odor (or if the burning does not improve with yeast creams), then contact the office for an appointment for proper diagnosis and treatment.

You can avoid yeast infections by the following:

a. Wipe from front to back when using the bathroom
b. Wear cotton underwear to improve aeration and decrease moisture in the area
c. Watch your intake of "sweets," i.e. carbohydrates
d. Blow dry the vaginal area after showering

24. Urinary Tract Infections (UTI's)

Urinary tract infections are very common during pregnancy. Symptoms include the following:

a. urgency (need to rush to bathroom) and burning while voiding,
b. frequency to the point of going every 5-10 minutes and,
c. bloody urine

Call your OB's office for a urinalysis and treatment. There are a number of ways to help prevent UTI's:

a. Void right after sex
b. Do not hold your urine for long periods of time: void when you start to feel your bladder full
c. Wipe front to back
d. Take Vitamin C 500 mg twice (2) per day
e. Drink cranberry juice daily or take cranberry granules (available at Health Food Stores)

25. Other Noticeable Skin "Things" (Red Palms and Spider Angiomas)

In the last part of pregnancy patients may notice redness of the palms of their hand, i.e. also called "Liver Palms" because it is seen in patients with cirrhosis due to the inability to metabolize "estrogens." In pregnancy, however, there is a natural high elevation of estrogen which induces the redness of the palms.

Patients may also notice "spider angiomas," i.e. red capillary "spots" that form on the chest and face. Worse yet, some patients may actually form a "spider" right on the very tip of the nose! A spider in this very prominent location is embarrassing to any individual: make-up usually hides this "spot." After delivery these spiders will regress and disappear but may also re-appear to "haunt you" in a future pregnancy.

26. "My Face is breaking out!"

Due to increased levels of placental hormones, particularly testosterone, many patients will experience "teenage acne" again. The usual care of acne is recommended: frequent washing of your face or the areas of the specific outbreaks. Drying solutions such as Benzoyl Peroxidase can be helpful. Occasionally topical antibiotics may need to be prescribed.

Other Topical Acne Treatments and Pregnancy

Some experts recommend topical prescription products containing either erythromycin or salicylic acid. Other options include over-the-counter products that contain either benzoyl peroxide or glycolic acid. Only about 5% of the active medication applied to the skin is absorbed into the body. So it's believed that such medications would not pose an increased risk of birth defects.

Treatments for Pregnancy Acne

Pregnancy acne is a natural condition that usually resolves after delivery. What can you do about pregnancy-related acne? Limit washing to two times per day and after heavy sweating.

- Wash you face with a non-course, oil-free, alcohol-free cleanser.
- Cleanse gently with your fingertip of your hand or be careful with washcloths and sponges as they can irritate sensitive skin and increase acne breakouts.
- After washing, rinse your skin with lukewarm water. Then gently pat dry and apply moisturizer.
- Do not wash too often as it may re-stimulate your oil gland.
- Shampoo daily.

Most important point: never squeeze or pop your pimples as this may lead to acne scarring.

---Reference credit to Louise Chang, MD on June 02, 2011, WebMD

27. "I'm tired of being pregnant and I want my baby out!"—the most common complaint OB's hear daily

Doctors and nurses hear this complaint <u>every day</u>. Your baby needs to come out when it is ready *naturally*. Your health professionals understand all the discomforts you are experiencing but the baby's welfare comes first. ACOG and health leaders are all agreed on *the strict guidelines* that the baby is "best born" and healthiest when the baby delivers after 39 completed weeks of pregnancy. As I say to my patients, "you do the crime; you got to do the time!" TTBP Syndrome(Too Tired of Being Pregnant) is too common a condition that OB nurses see often.

Table 2-2 Danger Signals when pregnant

> **DANGER SIGNALS**
>
> 1. Bleeding during pregnancy (some spotting after sex is normal)
> 2. Loss of fluid or continued loss/leakage of fluid through the vagina that requires a pad
> 3. Decreased fetal movements
> 4. Severe constant headache accompanied by visual side effects (blurring), nausea and/or vomiting
> 5. Swelling all over your body (face, eyelids, hands and feet)
>
> If any of the above symptoms are experienced, call the office or go to the hospital immediately for evaluation.

28. Sexually Transmitted Diseases (STD's)

In the 1970's, when the author was young, STD's were an uncommon occurrence during pregnancy. Yes, the 1970's were a decade of "Free Love, bra-less women, marijuana and many other clothing and hair style changes. It was a generational rebellion against the rigid conforming life so drilled into "traditional" American life: school, job or college, career, marriage, and babies.

In fact, at the beginning of his practice, the author rarely checked for gonorrhea or chlamydia in his pregnant patients. Of course, I did check if there were other factors going on in the patient's life: single mom in whom the father of the baby had "gone missing," patients with a vaginitis such as bacterial vaginosis or trichomoniasis, etc.

It was the author's assumption at that time that couples who become pregnant were married or at least had a very stable committed relationship. These couples were very much "in love," were best friends and wanted to express their union of hearts and minds by having and raising a baby together.

The 21st century is very much different: most babies are born out of wedlock and worse, to just a single mom.

It is a fact that the cost of care for 80% of the babies born in the US today are paid by Medicaid, a welfare* program funded by the State and Federal Governments (i.e. the taxpaying citizens).

*   The author does not consider *welfare as an "entitlement"* program as so euphemized by that word but a pragmatic government program. It is a necessity of our American culture to protect the lives of women and their unborn babies.

Accordingly, the majority of babies born in the US are born into poverty. Further, in the case of military families or relationships many of our soldiers are deployed out of the country or to other training facilities far from their homes and loved ones. Being away for extended months of time along with the natural desire for sex and love together make the perfect ingredients for infidelity both at home as well as away from home. Unfortunately, it is on a patient's first OB exam that many STD's may be detected. Of course, the relationship is severely affected. The most common STD's seen are the following order:

HPV infection. This *viral* infection is the most common cause of sexually transmitted diseases diagnosed in pregnancy and is the main cause of genital warts both externally and internally. The cervical infections are almost always asymptomatic because of the lack of visibility. Most abnormal Pap smears are caused HPV. The Pap smear detects the HPV virus by concomitantly using DNA testing probes when the Pap smear is processed. There are more than 13 "high HPV types" but type 16 is responsible for 40 per cent of the pre-cancerous changes in the cervix. HPV type 6 and 11 are the cause of most genital warts. Vaccination (now covering 9 HPV subtypes) helps prevent infection in both women and men. These viruses attach and infect human cells in the genital area.

OB's usually reserve treatment until after the baby is delivered. By 6 weeks postpartum, the woman's immune system is no longer compromised by the pregnancy itself: warts and cervical disease caused by HPV notably regress and can, but not necessarily, be eliminated by the immune defense system.

Chlamydia Trachomata. This STD is a *bacterial* infection that is easily treated with an antibiotic. The CDC currently recommends that both partners take Azithromycin 500 mg: each partner will take 2 pills for treatment. A "test of cure" re-culture test will be done at the next OB checkup. This infection is "silent" and does NOT produce any noticeable symptoms in 80% of women. Unfortunately, it is because of the standard pregnancy testing done at the first OB visit that the diagnosis is usually first made. It is very agonizing for the OB office staff to have to inform the patient of this infection.

Trichomoniasis. Trichomoniasis is a common STD in pregnancy: it may be the cause of a urinary tract or a vaginal infection.

Trichomoniasis is frequently a cause of bleeding in pregnancy. It produces a severe cervicitis, vaginitis and cystitis (cervical, vaginal and bladder infection). It is easily transmissible from person to person by sexual relations.

This *parasitic* infection does produce symptoms: a copious amount of discharge with odor. It can cause bleeding during pregnancy as well as some bladder symptoms: urgency, painful urination, etc. Trichomoniasis is treated with metronidazole 500 mg. Both partners must take 4 tablets at one time for cure. Follow up examination is necessary to assure "test of cure." (TOC).

Bacterial Vaginosis. This is a poly-microbial infection: several bacteria are present when this diagnosis is made. This disease is not an infection but truly an infestation. The bacteria can be transmitted sexually. However, It is *not* considered a STD in the classic definition of an infection. However, because this infection is associated with adverse outcomes in obstetrics (such as Premature Rupture of Membranes, Preterm Labor, etc.), it is prudent to treat this infection when diagnosed. Local or systemic therapy with Clindamycin or metronidazole is available.

Herpes Type I (simplex) and Type II (genitalis). These viruses can re-surface during pregnancy, i.e. "cold sores on the lips for Type 1 and blisters on the genital areas (Type 2). A more in-depth discussion has been presented in this book and can be found in the section on infectious diseases during pregnancy. Herpes virus is very contagious. It is estimated that at least 5% of pregnant women have been infected with Herpes II. Acyclovir (Zovirax®, Valtrex®, Femvir®, etc.) can be used safely during pregnancy to treat primary and recurrent attacks. These medications can be used in the last 4 weeks of pregnancy to prevent a recurrence or viral shedding. Such prophylactic use can avoid an outbreak during labor and prevent the need for a C-section. Acyclovir does not become incorporated into human DNA and therefore is completely safe for the pregnant patient and her baby.

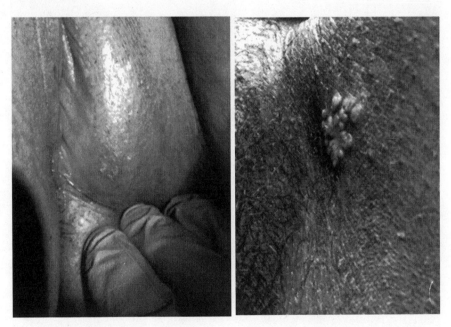

Figure 2-17 Herpes Ulcers   Figure 2-18 Herpes Blisters

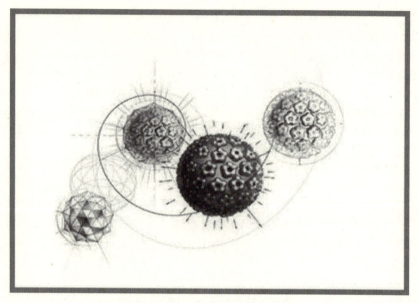

Figure 2-19 Herpes Viral Particles

<u>Gonorrhea</u>. Unfortunately, this infection is diagnosed all too frequently during pregnancy. This *bacterium* is treated with Ceftriaxone 250 mg injection plus Zithromax 500 mg orally. Both partners should be treated at the same time. Again, a "TOC" will be done at your next Ob visit.

It is may be quite surprising to know but this infection is also usually "silent" but may cause some extra vaginal discharge in the affected patient.

There are a number of other sexually transmitted diseases that can infect an expectant mother but are not seen very often:

- <u>Venereal Warts or Condyloma Accuminata.</u> These warts are caused by the HPV virus (an STD) and can be present on the outside or vulvar skin area. They can be present in the vagina and cervix. These warts can be spread to your sexual partner. They can be stimulated to grow and spread during pregnancy. They rarely can affect or infect the baby during vaginal birth. Local treatment is available to clear them or hold them in check. Surprisingly, these warts can completely disappear without treatment during the 6 weeks after delivery: when the pregnancy –associated immune suppression state is no longer existent.

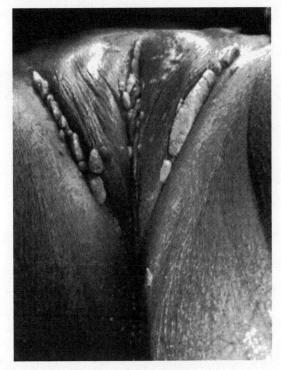

Figure 2-20 Condylomata Accuminata. Condylomata Accuminata during pregnancy

<u>Molluscum contagiosum</u>: warty looking lesions that look like little "JuJu Bees" or small volcanos.

These infections are usually not treated during pregnancy unless other factors are present. Most OBs will treat them in the postpartum period.

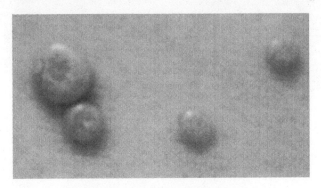

Figure 2-21 Molluscum Contagiosum

Syphilis: initially a single ulcer that manifests itself as a generalized skin rash in 2 months. Most cases are diagnosed during the normal prenatal blood work that is obtained in early pregnancy. Active disease during pregnancy must be treated. The "stage" of the disease should be evaluated as treatment is dependent on staging. Bicillin given intramuscularly over 4 to 6 weeks may be necessaryduring pregnancy.

Lymphogranuloma virus and chancroid diseases occur mostly in the tropical area (or infected people from those areas) and are rarely seen in clinical practice.

29. Leakage of urine during Pregnancy (Urinary Incontinence)

It is quite normal for the pregnant patient to become incontinent during pregnancy. In the 3rd trimester the baby can kick your full bladder and, due to gravitational forces and other mechanical factors, the pregnant patient my leak urine into her underwear. There is already an increased amount of vaginal secretions and mucus during the latter part of pregnancy: many patients may need to wear a pantiliner on a regular basis.

30. Obesity

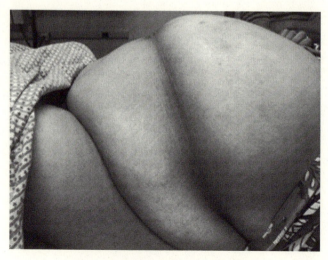

Figure 2-22 Obesity in Pregnancy

Obesity affects at least 33% of American women. Overweight women are encouraged to gain *less* weight during the pregnancy: approximately 18-20 lbs. Obesity is defined as a BMI (Body Mass Index) greater than 33%. Obesity puts patients in the "Higher Risk" category during pregnancy. The heart already has to "work" 50% more during pregnancy in woman with normal body weights. Obesity by itself strains the heart even further because of the increased circulatory needs of the mother along with the added challenge of circulation to the baby and placenta. Obesity in Pregnancy is associated with the following:

    a. Increased incidence of pre-eclampsia and hypertension
    b. Increased incidence of Gestational Diabetes
    c. Greater difficulty visualizing baby by ultrasound to detects abnormalities and position by physical exam
    d. Increased risk of a C-section
    e. Greater difficulty and time in placing epidural and spinal anesthesia
    f. Increased risk of wound infection if a C-section is needed (as well as other post-operative problems)
    g. Increased risk of Deep Venous Thrombosis (DVT)
    h. Increased risk of Heart Failure
    i. Increased risk of larger babies with concomitant risk of shoulder dystocia

Consultation with a Registered Dietician as well as gradually increased physical activities may help avoid these problems during labor and delivery. Optimally, patients should try to "get in shape" and get back as far as they can to their "ideal body weight" prior to getting pregnant.

<u>Author's Anecdote</u>: When I first started practice, I purchased the best examination tables available. The Hamilton Image power table (shown below) has been used for patient care since 1987. Katherine came in for her 6 week postpartum checkup. She lay down on the table. I pushed the power button so the table would go up. The table rose up 6 inches and then, to my complete astonishment and surprise, the table dropped to the ground! The hydraulics could not hold her up. You do not want to be the next patient to achieve this feat!

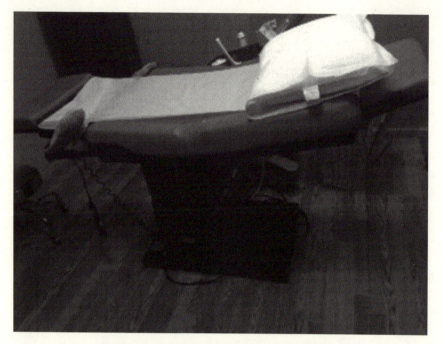

Figure 2-23 Exam Table Power Hydraulics

31. Cramping and Braxton-Hicks contractions

The uterus is a "muscle" and it can contract months before the onset of labor. It is a "smooth muscle" and the OB patient has no control over it (involuntary muscle). In the first trimester cramping can be quite pronounced as the uterus starts to expand ("Growing pains").

The uterus is basically "exercising." Muscles are always contracting (or fasciculation). Frequently these contractions can be painful: they can become an alarming cause of concern for the OB patient. These contractions become more frequent the closer the OB patient gets to her due date. Further, these Braxton Hicks contractions seem to come earlier and more noticeable with each subsequent pregnancy.

Though the contractions or cramps are painful, the best remedy for these "pains" is getting off your feet, laying on your left side and increasing your fluid intake. As long as there is no bleeding or significant mucus discharge (usually pink or blood tinged), there is no cause for concern.

"If there are children in the home, you can bet that pencils, scissors and socks will all go missing at some time."

32. Gender Reveal Parties

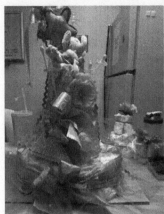
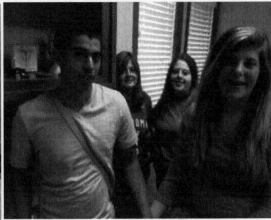

Figure 2-24 Gender Reveal Party: On the left, it a pink "cake" and on the right, partiers wearing blue and pink shirts to show their "vote" for the sex of the baby

Perhaps because of economic times many couples are sharing their excitement by celebrating the time they find out the sex of their child. These "Gender Reveal Parties" are very much like a traditional birthday party in which the usual blue and pink colors decorate the home.

Your OB usually will write down the sex of the baby on a piece of paper. He may point out the sex of the baby on an ultrasound photo in which the area between the baby's legs is so exposed. Your guests might then be able to guess at the sex of the baby. Some have a wrapped box containing either pink or blue balloons that will be opened up at a certain time. Another may make a large decorated cake with blue or pink colored filling, etc. Lastly, there are the "riddles" in which your OB may give you so that you can know the sex of the baby as follows:

Words of Riddle by Dr. Zweig (concept by Miss Clopton)

The Riddle for a Boy

In mommy's womb I love to grow,
The strongest hands and my beautiful toes,
Secret is what sex I am going to be,
Already on ultrasound you might be able to see
Be careful and look at the way each letter begins each line
Only the first letter is the key to my sex and kind
You will solve the identity of my sex by viewing these sentences of verse and how all together they align

The Riddle for the Girl:

In this riddle my gender you are trying to find
The first letter is important to each line
She, or I could even be a He?
All the "Old Wives Tales" cannot truly predict the sex I be
Girls are pink and boys are blue but both colors can look good on me
It really matters that all the lines you will need
Read vertically rather than horizontally will be the key
Love me not because I am a boy or girl but as a special baby that you will soon see!

Hint: The first letter of each sentence going downward: It's a boy and it's a girl in bold type face.

It's
A
B
O
Y

It's
A
G
I
R
L

And can you feel the Love Tonight?

It is where we **are.** ----Song written and sung by Sir Elton John, from the Disney movie, *The Lion King*

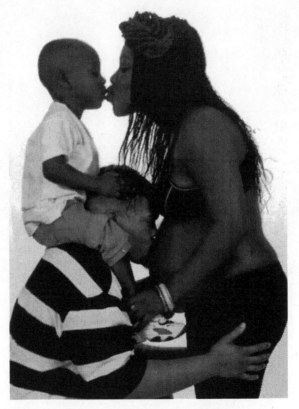

Figure 2-25 Love, Can you feel it

33. Pregnancy Q&A's

PREGNANCY Q & A'S

Q. Should I have a baby after 35?

A. *No. 35 children are enough*

Q. I am 2 months pregnant now. When will my baby move?

A. *With any luck right after he finishes college.*

Q. What is the most reliable method to determine a baby's sex?

A. *Childbirth*

Q. My wife is 5 months pregnant and is so moody that she is borderline irrational.

A. *So what is your Question?*

Q. My childbirth instructor says it is not pain that I will feel during labor but pressure. Is that right?

A. *Yes, in the same way a tornado might be called an air current.*

Q. When is the best time to have an epidural?

A. *Right after you find out you are pregnant.*

Q. Is there any reason I have to be in the delivery room while my wife is in labor?

A. *Not unless the word "alimony" means anything to you.*

> **Q. Is there anything I should avoid while recovering from childbirth?**
>
> **A.** *Yes, Pregnancy*
>
> **Q. Do I have to have a baby shower?**
>
> **A.** *Not if you change the baby's diaper very quickly*
>
> **Q. Our baby was born last week. When will my wife begin to feel and act normal again?**
>
> **A.** *When the kids are in college*

34. Getting use to the "Bumpy" Road.

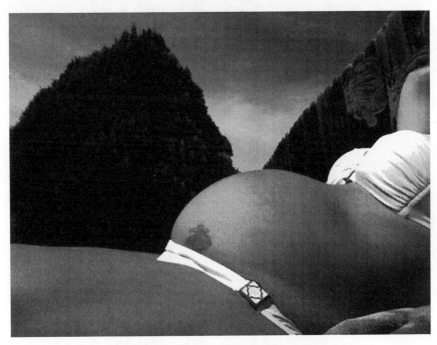

Figure 2-26 Baby Bump Beauty

As your pregnancy progresses, you will find it more difficult to do even the most routine tasks in life. Your baby "bump" is cramping your style.

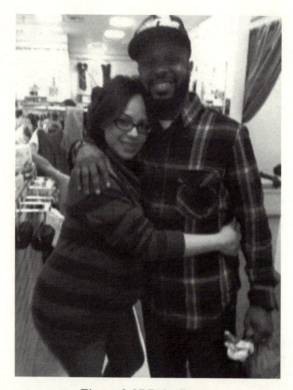

Figure 2-27 Baby Bump

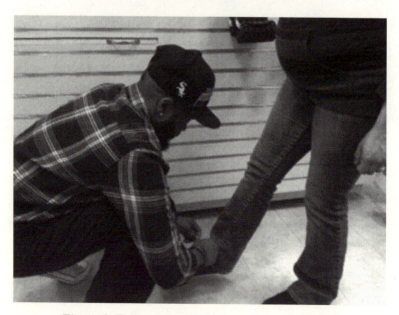

Figure 2-28 Baby Bump in the way of tying shoes

They were shopping in the Maternity Store in the mall. She tried on several pieces of clothing and was ready to check out. After leaving the dressing room, she realized that she could no longer reach her shoes to tie the laces. She said, "Honey, can you tie my shoe laces?" Without hesitation he dropped down on his knees and tied them for her ("true love" and the author was there to catch this precious act of devotion).

The following are some of the usual routines you no longer will be able to do:

1. Tie your shoelaces or put on your boots.
2. Shave your legs and other places.
3. Pick up things off the floor
4. Paint your toenails

35. The Natural "Pelvic Exam Reflex"

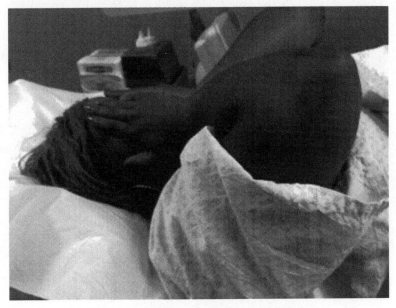

Figure 2-29 Pelvic Exam's Natural Reflex

The above picture illustrates a very common reflex a woman will automatically do when a pelvic examination is performed. This natural reflex appears to be "hard-wired" into the neurologic reactions of a woman: most of the patients do not realize that they are doing it. They did not learn or see this type of automatic movement from other family members. This reaction is most common in patients of Hispanic descent, but as you can see from the above picture, can be seen in patients of all races and ethnic groups.

36. It seems like everything "bleeds" when I am pregnant!

It is not uncommon to experience bleeding from areas in your body that have not bled previously. There is a tremendous amount of increased "vascularity" or blood vessel formation and filling when you are pregnant. The most troublesome question that the OB office hears: I am spotting, bleeding or having a brown discharge after sex. The cervix, the opening to the uterus, is quite delicate and fragile during pregnancy. With penetration and sexual contact with the cervix some blood vessels will break and bleed. As long as there is not excessive bleeding, i.e. heavier than a normal period, or pain, sex should be okay.

It is quite common to experience bleeding during pregnancy in the following situations:

a. Gums bleeding while brushing your teeth
b. Hemorrhoids or other rectal bleeding after a bowel movement
c. Nosebleeds after blowing hard or blowing frequently as you would when you have a cold
d. Blood or brown mucus when vomiting excessively in the first or other trimesters of pregnancy
e. "Blood shot" eyes from rubbing them too hard
f. Bleeding more excessively from minor cuts and injuries
g. Bleeding can occur after sexual intercourse but is usually light and stops within 30 minutes.

Vaginal bleeding ("bright red bleeding") at any time during pregnancy is not normal. Call your OB or the hospital for medical guidance.

Author Anecdote: "Hello, Dr. Zweig. This is April at Comanche Memorial OB unit. Your patient came to the hospital with vaginal bleeding after having intercourse *2 days ago*! Her speculum exam is negative for any blood or fluids. She is 20 weeks pregnant." Author responds to the OB nurse, "I am sure glad she sought prompt attention to this problem!"

37. Abnormal Pap Smears during Pregnancy

About 10-15% of Pap smears performed during pregnancy return abnormal. The most common cause is infection: bacterial vaginosis (BV), yeast, trichomoniasis and HPV. HPV is the most cause of cytological abnormalities of the cervical cells seen on Pap. Current recommendations for cervical cancer screening are Pap smears (cytology) with HPV testing or just HPV testing alone. If a Pap smear cytology returns show an abnormality, i.e. squamous intraepithelial lesion (Low grade=LGSIL or High grade=HGSIL), then your OB may perform a *colposcopy* exam during your pregnancy. *Colposcopy* is a procedure in which your OB looks at your cervix with "binoculars." By magnifying the skin surface of the cervix with the colposcope, your OB can determine if there is a significant abnormality or pre-cancerous change of the cervix. Rarely, there is such a very significant lesion that a "cervical skin biopsy" would need to be performed. Undergoing a colposcopy does not in any way harm your baby. However, it is NOT uncommon to spot after such an examination: just expect some red to brown discharge afterwards.

80% of HPV infections can be destroyed by your body's immune system such that viral infection can be eliminated within 12 months (similar to how a viral cold can be eradicated by your body within weeks). Gardasil is a vaccination that is available for teens and young women that helps prevent HPV infection and, thus help avoid abnormal Pap smears in your future. Gardisil® and other vaccinations help immunize patients against just a limited number of the "high risk" HPV types. Occasionally patients vaccinated with HPV may still become infected with other high risk, medium risk and low risk viruses that can cause Pap smears to become abnormal (there are greater than 82 subtypes of the HPV virus).

Many abnormal Pap smears and HPV tests will return to normal at your 6 week postpartum check-up.

Other causes of abnormal Pap smears, such as yeast or STD infections, can be readily diagnosed and treated with antibiotics.

38. Smoking Cessation

Smoking Cessation is a goal every smoker who becomes pregnant should strive to achieve. Frequently, just the smell of tobacco is so abhorrent that many pregnant women will quit smoking immediately. There are many treatment options that are available as follows:

1. "Cold Turkey" quitting. After making a decision for the health of their baby and themselves, the patient tosses her cigarettes out. It is extremely helpful that the father of the baby be supportive. If he is a smoker as well, then the two of them should make a "pact" and quit together. With the cost of cigarettes being over $4 per pack, a pack per day smoker can save $120 per month (equals $1440 per year: double that amount, $2880, if they both smoke). The author tells patients that this amount of money translates to two cruises per year!

2. Nicotine Gum and Skin Patches. Nicotine gum and skin patches have been available to the past decade to help smokers kick the habit.

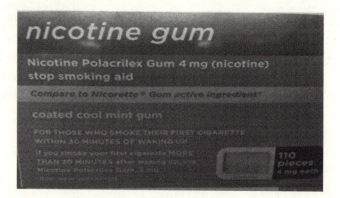

Figure 2-30 Nicotine Gum

3. Zyban or Wellbutrin©medication. These medications have assisted smokers lose their desire for smoking over several months.

4. Chantrix. Chantrix is the newest and most consistent therapy available that has a proven track record is helping smokers lose their addiction to tobacco. Most motivated patients can stop smoking within 1-2 months.

5. Smoke-Enders and other community based Smoking Cessation Programs. For additional help, the reader should google national and local smoking cessation programs and support groups located in their community. Most hospitals sponsor smoking cessation programs throughout the year.

Figure 2-31 Oklahoma Rising

Sunrise in Oklahoma and the birth of a new day. It is the rising of many new "Okies."

And, adding more Oklahoma flavor to this book:
Oklahoma Rising Lyrics
Artist and Songwriter: Vince Gill Lyrics

Say hello to the future, gonna shake the future's hand
And build a better world, upon this sacred ancient land
Well, I choke back the emotion, I'm an Okie and I'm proud
So when you call me Okie, Man, you better say it loud

Author recommends read entire lyrics at http://www.leoslyrics.com/vince-gill/oklahoma-risinglyrics/#Maw73lWsmpY1r2qP.99

CHAPTER 3

Labor and Delivery: The Short and Pithy Version

Because of all the pelvic exams being performed during your pregnancy and especially during labor and delivery, all the privacy and modesty you formerly possessed regarding your body and particularly your intimate parts will be lost forever.—from" every woman who has given birth"

1. When will I deliver my Baby?

Most (70%) patients will deliver within seven (7) days of their due date (EDC). Eighty percent (80%) will deliver within two (2) weeks of their due date.

A simple way to calculate your due date is as follows (see detailed discussion in Chapter 1):

Subtract 3 months from your last menstrual period (LMP) and then add 1 week (Naegele's Rule)

Example: June 6, 2014 minus 3 months equal March 6, 2014 plus 1 week = March 13, 2015

<u>"39 weeks and Later" Rule and the 2013 ACOG definitions of pregnancy lengths</u>

Most people commonly believe that a baby is "ready" and can be born without any problems anytime in the last month of pregnancy. Unfortunately, this belief is false and is further given credence by the public because of the great success medicine has had in treating and saving "premature" babies. In 2012 the "39 weeks or later" rule was instituted so that patients would not be requesting their OB's to deliver them because of all the discomforts and inconveniences of pregnancy.

The American College of Obstetricians and Gynecologists (ACOG) and the Society for Maternal-Fetal Medicine (SMFM) are discouraging use of the general label 'term pregnancy' and replacing it with a series of more specific labels: 'early term,' 'full term,' 'late term,' and 'post-term.'

The following represent the four new definitions of 'term' deliveries:

    Early Term: Between 37 weeks 0 days and 38 weeks 6 days

    Full Term: Between 39 weeks 0 days and 40 weeks 6 days

    Late Term: Between 41 weeks 0 days and 41 weeks 6 days

    Post-term: Between 42 weeks 0 days and beyond

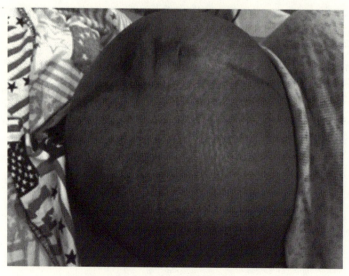

Figure 3-1 Belly Button changes

Just because your belly button popped out does not mean you are "ready" to deliver. Your baby is not a "turkey!"

The pregnant mother was talking to her husband (or "the baby daddy"),

"We better get this straight; the deal was that if I was going to have your baby, you promised to change all the poopy diapers!"

2. How do I know if I am in Labor?

You are experiencing already the hardening of the uterus in the last trimester: these are the so-called *Braxton-Hicks contractions*. These *practice contractions* is the process by which the uterus goes in-training for real labor. Braxton-Hicks contractions can become more frequent and more uncomfortable the closer you get to your due date. Labor contractions usually start out at regular or even irregular intervals: the uterus hardens and can be felt all the way around into the back like someone hugging you. True labor pains become more frequent, more regular and stronger. A bloody discharge or blood tinged mucus are the hallmark signs that usually signify that you are in *true labor*. If your amniotic sac ruptures, you will feel a steady stream of fluid coming out of your vagina ("almost like you are peeing on yourself"). It continues to leak and you will be grabbing a pad or washcloth almost immediately. Only about 10% of patients will have loss of amniotic fluid as their first sign of labor.

3. I lost my mucus plug, now what do I do? The most common phone call to the OB suite as reported by the nurses!

Losing your mucus plug does not necessarily mean you will be starting labor: as the cervix thins and dilates late in pregnancy, some of the mucus in your cervix can be discharged. Patients can pass a glob of mucus and it may be *days or some weeks* before you go into labor. If you are not having regular contractions or any bloody show, you do not have to call the OB suite or your physician to report it. Just *wait* and see if the other signs of labor such as more painful and more regular contractions develop or if your amniotic sac starts leaking continuous amounts of water.

4. When do I call the office or go to the hospital?

Prior to calling your OB's office or your hospital's OB unit, wait until the contractions are at least 4-5 minutes apart for one hour. If you are leaking amniotic fluid and having bleeding more than a menstrual flow, you should report to the hospital right away.

> It is a longstanding tradition at the author's hospital for the family to bring Chick-Fil-A to the nurses after your baby is born! It would be even better to have the Chick-Fil-A and the baby to arrive at the very same time!
>
> You will be amazed how much more nursing care you will receive when your nurses are given tasty treats!
>
> Yes, it is okay to substitute Pizza Hut, Papa John's, etc.

5. What do I need to bring to the hospital?

You should pack basically the same toiletries and clothes that you would take on a weekend trip away from home. Bring your hair dryer, brushes, combs, curling iron, shampoos and other toiletries. Pack yours and the baby's "Going Home" outfit. Do not forget to bring your camera (with charged batteries and extra SD memory cards, recharging cords) to the Delivery Suite. You can also bring a cooler containing popsicles to suck on while in labor. Further, pack some food for the "new dad to be" (see Postpartum Instructions Chapter).

Author Anecdote: Hardly a week goes by in the birthing room that someone is having a "media catastrophe." Many patients buy a new camera or a new phone and do not know how to use them. It seems like someone, usually the patient's mother, sister, or friend is fumbling with the camera and no one told her how to use it! Folks, a pregnancy is approximately 40 weeks long: you have plenty of time to read the directions and practice with your new camera prior to coming to the hospital. Designate and educate the "official photographer," whether that person is a parent or good friend, how to use the equipment!

6. Introduction to the Labor and Delivery Suite

After passing through the Labor and Delivery doors, you will be brought to the scale for the official weigh in and then to your Birthing Room. You will change into your hospital gown that is loose fitting. The nurse will put the fetal monitoring straps around your abdomen to evaluate the baby's heart rate and your contractions.

"The Last to Know Syndrome"

Hello, Dr. Zweig? Yes, this is Dr. Zweig. This is Jennifer from Labor and Delivery. Your patient, Barbara Green, just arrived and she is completely dilated. We need you NOW!

When I arrived 12 minutes later in the Labor room, the patient was pushing during a contraction. In making a quick visual survey around the room I saw the father of the baby, Barbara's mother and two cousins. The nurses had not even had time to start an IV or take down important medical information. Further to add to the nurses' consternation, her OB records had been sent to the other hospital in town.

This story is presented to remind patients to call the hospital before you leave home. It is just plain considerate to give "a head's up" to the hospital staff and your OB so that they can anticipate and prepare without a slow panic for your labor and delivery care. If labor starts in the middle of the night, your OB needs enough time to get dressed and travel to the hospital. Contrary to common beliefs, your OB does not live at the hospital 365 day per year or 24 hours per day.

Unfortunately, the above story plays out every day in hospitals all across the nation.

Eating before your ride to the hospital

It is very important that the OB patient NOT EAT or take a large amount of fluids before going to the hospital. Contractions can initiate a "reflex reaction" in which you can become quickly nauseated and vomit. So, if you do not want to see your food again, please be so advised!

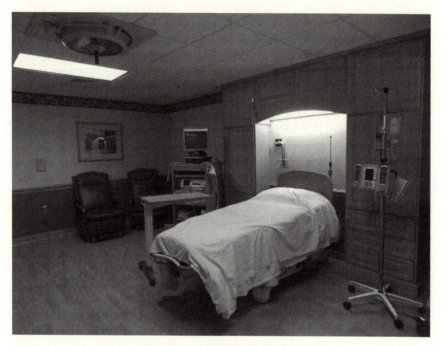

Figure 3-2 Birthing Room

7. How many people can be in the Birthing Room?

Every OB doctor has his own rules and regulations. The author usually allows as many people as the patient desires as long as they do not get in his way or in the way of the nurses. Yes, having a baby is a lifecycle momentous occasion and you want to share that experience with loved ones and others. Delivering a baby is also the most stressful event a woman will experience. It is not the occasion for people who just want to see a baby born ("Looky-Loos"). As Eldridge Cleaver had stated, "if they are not there to be part of the solution, then they are there to be part of the problem."

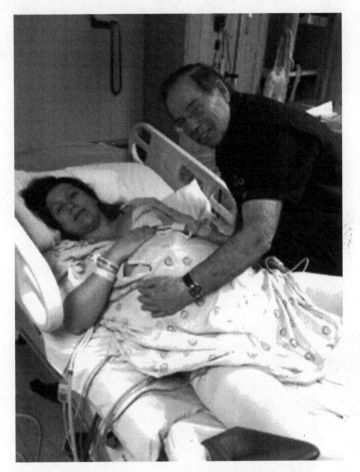

Figure 3-3 Leopold's maneuvers: baby's position with baby weight estimation

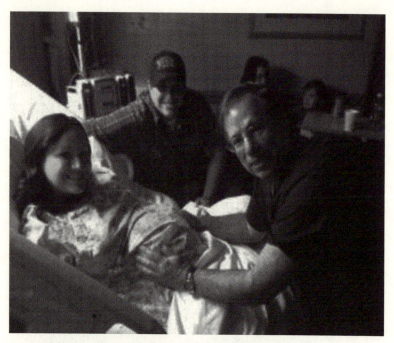

Figure 3-4 Baby's Weight: "Yes, I think the nurse is right. Your baby probably does weight about 11 lbs.!

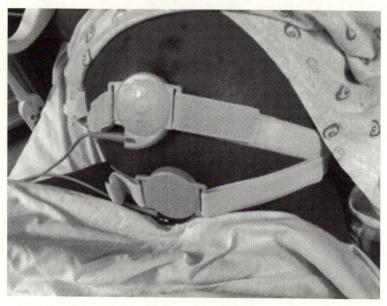

Figure 3-5 Fetal heart monitor: External and internal Uterine Contraction Monitor on abdomen of a patient in labor

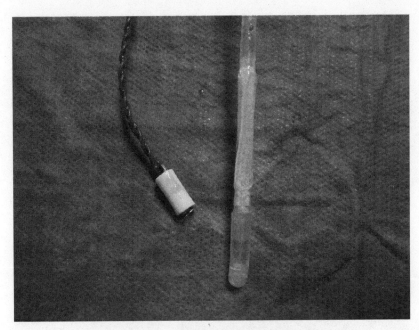

Figure 3-6 Internal Fetal Heart Electrode and Intrauterine Pressure Catheter

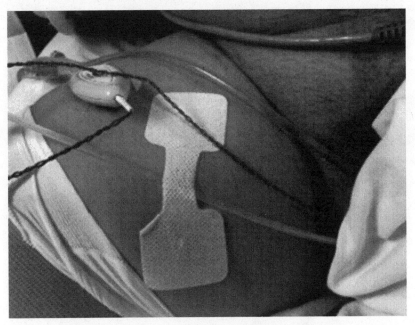

Figure 3-7 Internal uterine catheter (IUPC) and Fetal Scalp Electrode monitoring (FSE)

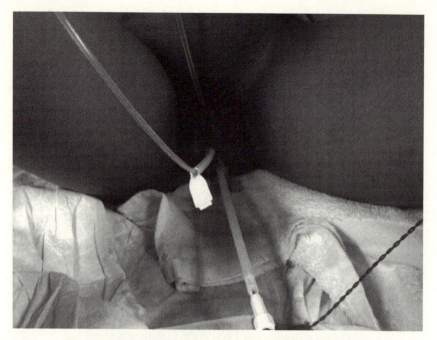

Figure 3-8 Uterine pressure catheter, FSE and Urinary catheter demonstrated on this patient in labor

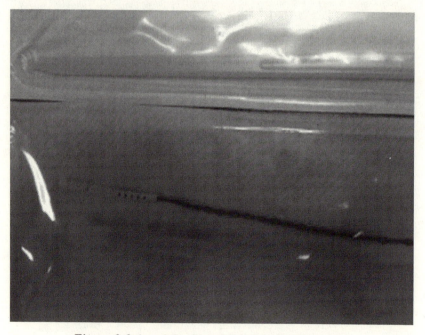

Figure 3-9 Amniohook and Fetal Scalp Electrode

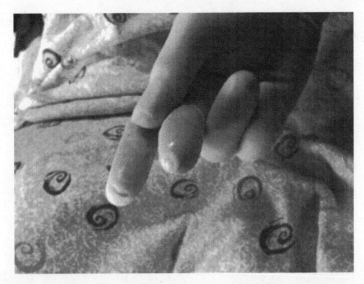

Figure 3-10 Finger cot on middle finger "hook" used to "break the water."

Author's Note: When external monitoring of the baby is not producing an adequate tracing, I will usually tell the patient that I need to place the monitors inside the uterus. The Internal monitors produce a more accurate "quantitative" recording of the contractions and a direct reading of the fetal heart beat off the baby. However, during the process that the author is placing "internal monitors," i.e., the intrauterine pressure catheter (IUPC) into the uterus and the fetal heart electrode on the baby's scalp, the family members or husband will ask what I am really doing. I usually chime in and say, "This is a "Dr. Dre Beats" electrode that goes into the baby's ear so the baby can rock out listening to KLAW, Oklahoma's best country music station. The catheter tubing is a computer cable so the baby can access the internet and Wi-Fi so he can get connected!"

8. How long will I be in Labor?

Most labors are approximately 12 hours from start to finish. Each labor and delivery is *very different* for each patient. Second time mothers labor approximately 8 hours. The third or higher order pregnancies are usually even quicker!

In the very early days of Obstetrics it was said that "a laboring mother should not see the sunrise more than once."

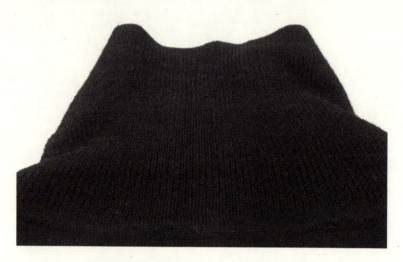

Figure 3-11 Neck of a turtle neck sweater

The Turtle neck sweater

The best analogy in order to understand the "process of labor" is as follows: imagine putting a turtle neck sweater over your head. The neck portion is initially long and about 3-4 inches in length. The cervical "neck" becomes stretched out (medical term, "effacement") until there is a small opening in the opening at the top of the turtle neck portion of the sweater. As you push your head through the neck portion, it stretches open until the neck is dilated far enough to push your head through it.

Basically the time it takes to stretch out the neck portion of the turtle neck until your head can fit through is called the First (1st) Stage of Labor. The 2nd Stage of Labor is the time from when neck opening can fit your head until the time it goes over your head to rest on your neck. The 3rd Stage of Labor is the time from when the baby is delivered until the placenta comes out. The 4th Stage of Labor is the most difficult: it is from the time the placenta is out until your child goes off to college!

Table 3-1 the Stages of Labor

1st Stage of Labor	Onset of contractions until the cervix is completely dilated
Latent Phase, 1st Stage: start of contractions until the cervix is 3-4 cm dilated	
Active Phase, 1st Stage: 3-4 cm of cervical dilatation until 10 cm	
2nd Stage of Labor	Time from cervix completely dilated until baby is born
3rd Stage of labor	Time from birth of baby until placenta is delivered
4th Stage of Labor	Time from placenta is delivered until your child goes off to college

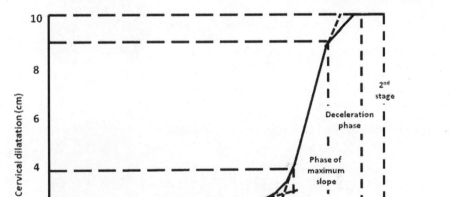

Phases of labor in primigravida. (From Friedman EA: Obstet Gynecol 6:567, 1955.)

Figure 3-12 Labor Curve This Labor Curve illustrates slow progress to 4 cm with "take off" slope of active phase of labor

(Reprinted with permission from Friedman EA: *Obstet Gynecol* 6: 567, 1955)

Baby is "Jumping through two Hoops" or Navigating the Birth Passageway

In order to be born the baby must negotiate "two hoops:" the female pelvic bone structure is constructed such that there is a "wide" elliptical shape at the opening of the upper pelvis. The shape of the pelvis changes in its mid-portion: the wide elliptical shape at the top of the-pelvis rotates 90 degrees and is therefore, is wider front to back a narrower and deeper ellipse as seen below in the changing shapes).

Inlet Shape of Pelvis (average)

Mid-pelvis Cavity Shape (ellipse rotates 90 degrees)

--Typical mid-pelvis shape

Accordingly, the baby comes into the pelvis facing one side or another. But, when the baby's head descends to the mid-pelvis, the baby's head must turn 90 degrees and face your back (or front—"posterior baby."). When the baby's head turns facing your back in the mid-pelvis, the shoulders are able to come through the inlet side to side. When the baby's head is born, the turning of the shoulders in the mid-pelvis causes the face to turn sideways after it is born. It is a good thing that the human neck is not too long or otherwise, we would never be born!

TABLE 3-2 THE CARDINAL MOVEMENTS OF LABOR

Descent of head into the pelvis	
Flexion of the baby's head	decreases diameter of head to better fit the bony pelvis
Internal Rotation of baby's head	baby's face turns to the backside (OA) to midpelvic elliptical shape, but shoulders now able to enter inlet
Extension	baby's head extends and de-flexes to get under pubic bone
External Rotation	Shoulders coming down side to side hit midpelvis and thus rotate to front-back direction but causes baby's head to rotate after it is born to one side or another

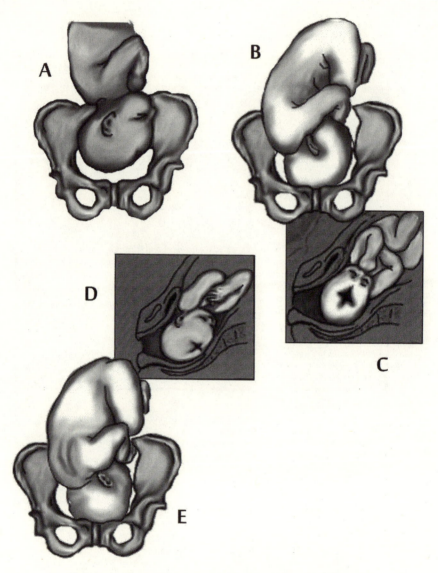

Figure 3-13 Pelvic Journey of baby during childbirth.
The Mechanism of Labor demonstrated: Flexion, descent,
internal rotation, extension and external rotation

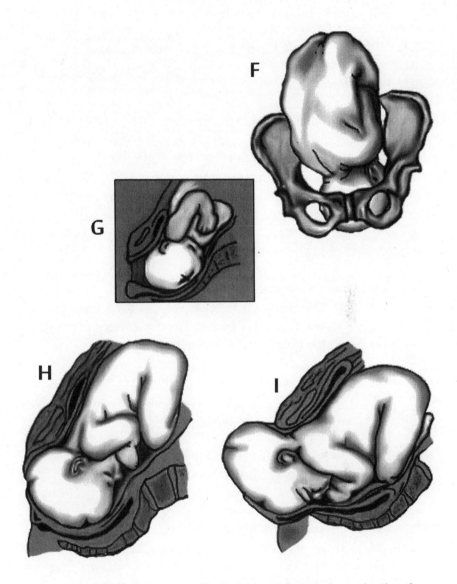

Figure 3-14 Birthing Process The baby is progressively navigating the pelvic curvatures and geometric changes (Adapted with permission from Elsevier, from Willson, *Obstetics and Gynecology*)

"It is not the size of the donut, but the size of the donut hole" is the important factor in calculating whether a baby will fit through the bony pelvis of the woman. Many women with wide hips may have very thick bone structure and, therefore, a small pelvis (small donut hole) which is, in fact, may be too small to deliver an average size baby.

Author's Anecdote

Just prior to Halloween one year the author's office staff had made a decision to get dressed up for Halloween. Everyone would wear their Halloween's outfits at the office. The author was required to participate and likewise got dressed into an outfit. He chose a Hobo's clowns attire. He wore it in the office and saw patients in it. No one was in labor and he did not have anyone in the hospital to make rounds on. So he was "safe." He thought, "No one other than his patients would see him so dressed."

But, as you would have guessed, he received a call from Labor and Delivery from Washington Hospital across the street. One of his patients just got checked in and she was completely dilated. He needed to come to the hospital *immediately*!

The author ran across the street in his outfit, went up the stairs hurriedly and blasted into the patient's labor room. The patient looked up and was astonished: like, who is this character in the room?

I had to deliver the baby in my Halloween outfit under a sterile gown. To this very day the patient tells everyone, "I was completely dilated and pushing when this *'clown'* showed up and delivered my baby!"

To decrease the discomforts of labor during the First Stage of Labor (1 to 4 cm), medications are available and can be given (as an injection in your skin or in your IV). The two (2) most common medications given during labor are Stadol® and Nubain®: they provide some pain relief and "take the edge" off your labor pain. They may make you somewhat sleepy. These medications will last 1-2 hours and occasionally they can be given again. However when most patients reach 4 cm, they usually opt for epidural anesthesia at this point.

Epidurals will provide the most satisfactory comfort from 4 cm to delivery time and thereafter.

The majority of patients will deliver their baby within 12 hours of *true active* labor. Most Primigravida (1st pregnancies) patients will dilate at 1 cm per hour. Multipara (2nd or more pregnancies) patients will dilate at 1.5 to 2 cm per hour. Most patients will be admitted to the OB suite at 2 centimeters. An IV will be started and the fetal monitor will be used to follow your contractions and baby's heart beat. When contractions are coming every 2 to 3 minutes, most patients will want "something for pain.' Usually Nubain or Stadol is given in your IV. When these medications wear off in about 2 hours, the cervix will have dilated to 4-5 centimeters. Your membranes may rupture or be ruptured by your OB at this point in labor. If it is difficult to obtain a good tracing of your contractions and the baby's heart rate, internal monitors may be placed at this time in order to obtain an adequate tracing of the baby's heart beat.

At home most families will "break bread" together, but in Labor and Delivery we "break water!"

Breaking the water or rupturing the amniotic sac is commonly performed to shorten the duration of labor: the uterine muscle can contract more efficiently due to the decrease volume of the uterus. Furthermore, rupture of the membranes causes other chemical reactions and hormone releases to increase the contractility of the uterus and the softening of the cervix.

Reasons Not to perform amniotomy (artificial rupture of the membrances, i.e. AROM)

1. GBS colonization of the Genital tract. Despite the universal use of antibiotic prophylaxis for GBS positivity in the OB patient, the OB and the patient may want to keep this barrier intact for a longer period of time.

2. Patients who want "natural childbirth." As noted above, the patient may be tolerating her labor pains without medication,

but rupture of the membranes may produce stronger contractions that she may not be able tolerate. Accordingly, such patients may desire a longer but less intense labor.

3. The amniotic sac provides a "cushion" or "water bag" to protect the baby's head as it travels through the pelvis.

4. The rare occurrences of cord prolapse and intrauterine infection can be avoided.

These above issues can be discussed with your OB and the advantages/disadvantages deliberated at any given point during labor.

If your cervix is dilated 4 centimeters or more, most patients will opt for their epidural anesthesia at this point. If the cervix is 4 cms, the first time mother should be completely dilated in approximately 6 or more hours (1 cm/hr).

The author will tell his patients, "when you are flying 'Epidural Airlines,' you can lay back, relax and go to sleep. We will tell you when your baby is at the gate and you are ready to "de-pregnate. "Labor takes a long time. It is like flying from Oklahoma City to San Francisco, you just have to lay back and watch the movie.

Most patients will push for about an hour before the baby is born.

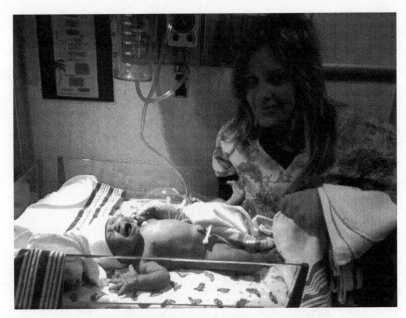

Figure 3-15 Newborn in baby warmer being tended to by one of our "Ace" nurses

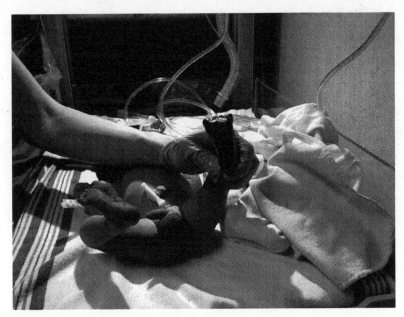

Figure 3-16 Baby Footprints Making Footprints after birth. In Oklahoma (the Native America State) the nurses say, "The baby is now an official member of the *Blackfoot* tribe!

Unfortunately there may be "drug pushers" in the community, but the OB staff really appreciates the "Baby Pushers!"

On average, 18% of first time Moms will need a C-section: baby is too big, positioned in the wrong direction or the baby does not tolerate labor, etc.

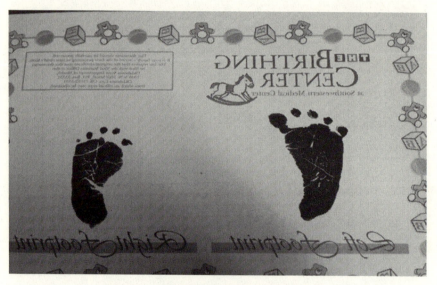

Figure 3-17 Birth Certificate Footprints

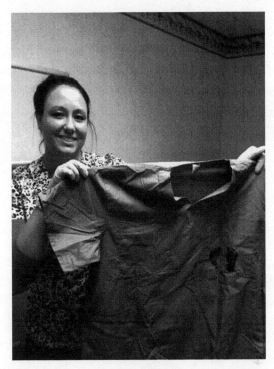

Figure 3-19 Footprints on Dad's Scrub Lindsey, RN has also put the Baby footprints on a Scrub top for parents to take home to frame

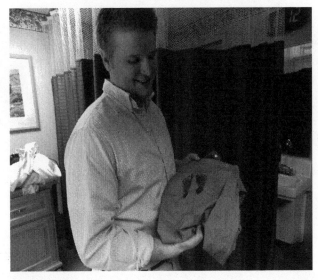

Figure 3-18 Footprints on the new Father's Scrub Shirt

9. When do I need to see my doctor after delivery?

You will need to make a 6 week checkup appointment after you leave the hospital. You may need to be seen sooner if you have high risk conditions such as hypertension, diabetes, C-section, anemia, etc.

Postpartum Instructions is further detailed in its own separate chapter later in this book.

10. Inductions of Labor and C-Sections

C-Sections are scheduled in the last week of pregnancy, i.e. after 39 weeks of pregnancy.

Elective (meaning for patient convenience without a medical reason) Inductions of labor for vaginal deliveries can be performed after 39 completed weeks with the added requirement of the cervix being "ripe" or conducive to the induction of labor. To try and naturally induce your labor you just need to remember the following "Old Wives Tale: What got you into this mess in the first place, may help you get out of it!"

Inductions of labor can be started with oxytocin alone if your cervix is "ripe," and has a satisfactory Bishop's score (see Chapter on Labor and Delivery for Bishop's scoring). If the cervix is not dilated or not satisfactorily effaced, then your OB may choose to "soften" your cervix with Cytotec or Cervidil. Frequently patients will go into labor with just the softening process alone.

11. Baby Care and Pediatricians

There are many fine Pediatricians and Family Physicians in your community. They are available to provide newborn care to your baby. If you do not already have a physician for your baby, the office will be happy to refer you to one. Of course, not all physicians may be on your health insurance plan: you may have to contact your health insurance company for a physician's referral.

Do not forget to bring your car seat and a newborn outfit for your baby to go home in.

12. Breastfeeding

Breastfeeding is recommended by all health professionals as the best nutrition for your newborn. Breast feeding has the following advantages:

1. It is Natures' original "fast food." It is totally "organic" and specially formulated only for human babies.

2. Breast milk contains maternal antibodies. Antibodies are produced by the immune system. Antibodies are produced in response to all of the previous infectious diseases that she has contracted and fought. These antibodies in her body will be transferred to the baby by passive diffusion from the mother's bloodstream through the placenta to the baby. They will protect the baby from infections during the first 3 months after birth. Consequently breastfed babies have less colds and diarrhea than bottle-fed babies.

3. Breast milk is at the right temperature, is located on your body and is cheap: not only a "fast food" but the first "convenience food" for your baby.

In essence, your breasts will naturally fill with milk within about three (3) days after birth. Prior to that time, the breast will produce colostrum, a high protein concentrate that will nourish your baby. By putting the baby to breast when the baby cries and allowing the baby to suck on the nipple, the milk will be stimulated to come.

Most hospitals have lactation specialists available for you in the event you need help and consultation.

There are many excellent breastfeeding materials that can help you master the art of breastfeeding. These instructional resources are available from:

Le Leche League

Medela Corporation (manufacturers of breast pumps and nursing supplies)

International Society of Breast feeding mothers

Google search sites

> *Everything you do is based on the choices you make.*
> *It's not your parents, your past relationships,*
> *Your job, the economy, the weather, an*
> *argument or your age that is to blame*
> *You and only you are responsible for every decision and*
> *Choice you make. Period.*
> *--Anonymous*

Patient said to the author, "I don't know why anyone would want to do this (have a baby) twice!"

Author replied--"Because of the beautiful baby you are now holding in your arms! And, at just that moment, you will forget instantly all the misery of your pregnancy and the pain and exhaustion of your childbirth

CHAPTER 4

Pictorial Tour of Labor and Delivery

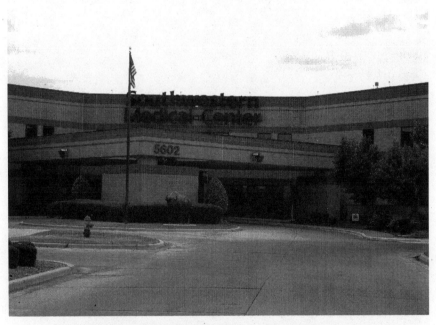

Figure 4-1 Hospital Entrance. Driving into the
Hospital Entrance or Emergency Room

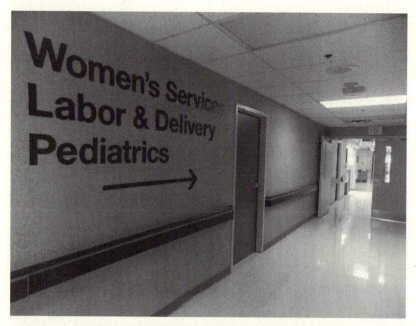

Figure 4-2 Hallway to OB Suite Hallway leading to the OB suite and postpartum floor.

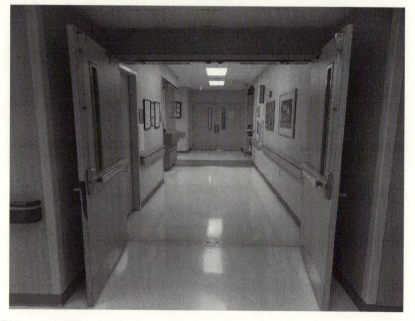

Figure 4-3 OB Suite. Doors open to welcome you to the OB Suite Entrance

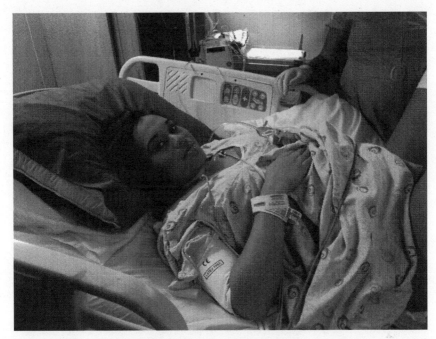

Figure 4-4 Patient in Labor.

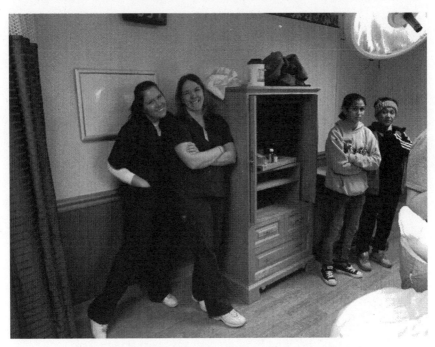

Figure 4-5 Family and Nursing Student support

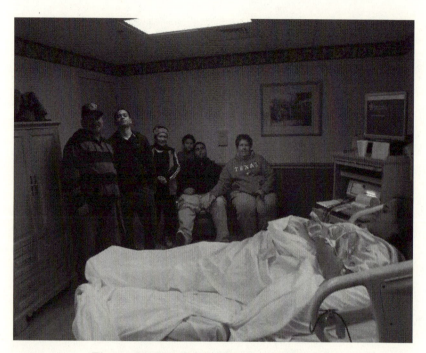

Figure 4-6 Family members to support you

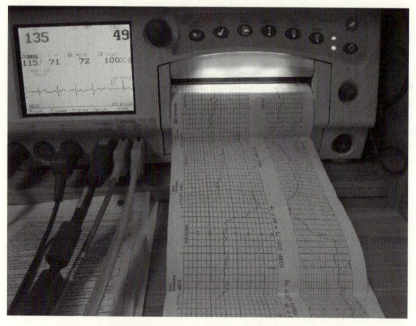

Figure 4-7 Fetal monitor traces your contractions and FHT (yes, that is a variable deceleration, 2nd stage.)

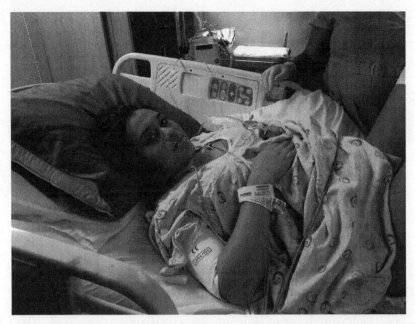

Figure 4-8 Patient with epidural getting close to being completely dilated

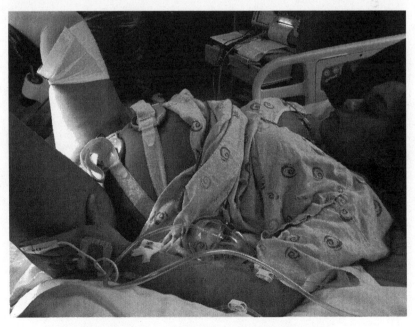

Figure 4-9 Patient in 2nd Stage of Labor with her legs up as she pushes the baby with each contraction.

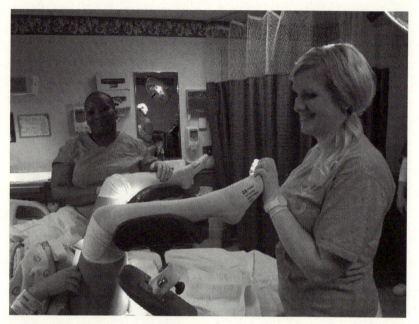

Figure 4-10 OB Nurses "coaching" the patient in her pushing efforts.

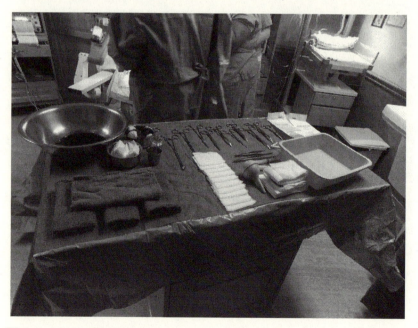

Figure 4-11 OB Table with warm water, anti-septic solutions and towels.

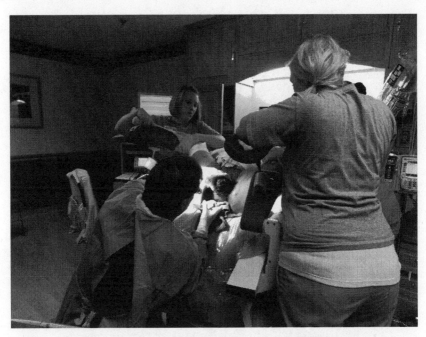

Figure 4-12 Baby's head is crowning on the perineum.

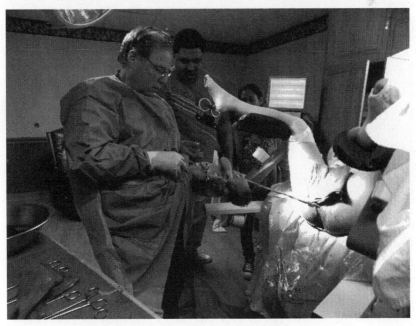

4-13 Husband Cutting the Cord the husband is in the "traditional act" of cutting the baby's umbilical cord

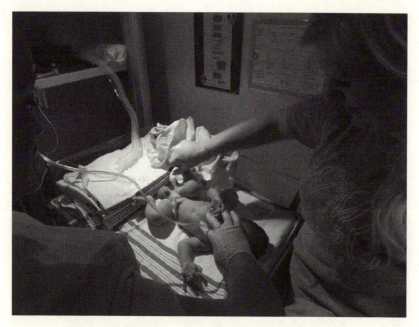

Figure 4-14 Baby in Warmer is given some oxygen blow by to help pink up this baby boy

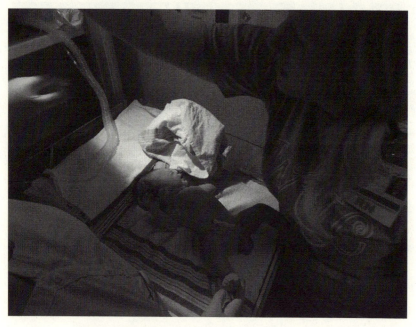

Figure 4-15 Newborn in Warmer Baby being attended to in the Baby warmer

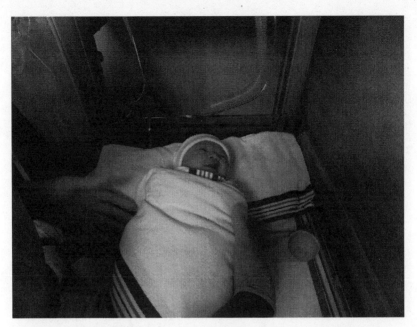

Figure 4-0-16 Baby "mummy-wrapped up in warm "blankie.""

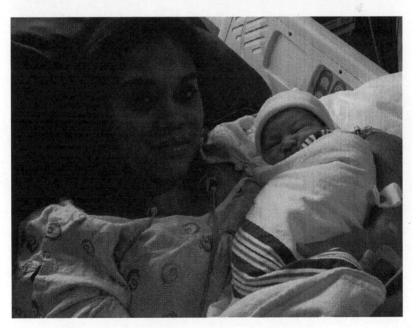

Figure 4-17 New Mother holding her baby for first time

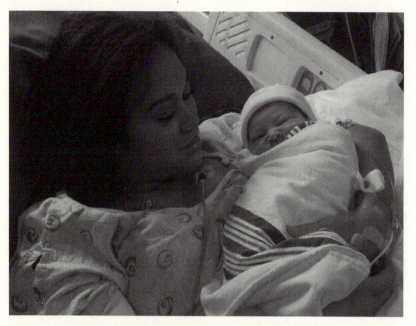

Figure 4-18 Mother bonding with her newborn

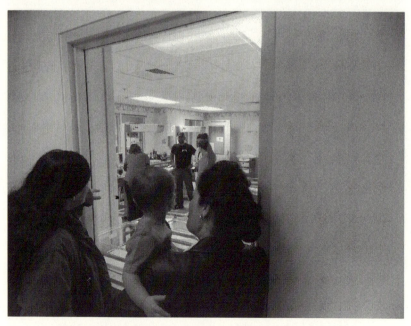

Figure 4-19 Relatives and friends looking through the nursery window at the "new family edition"

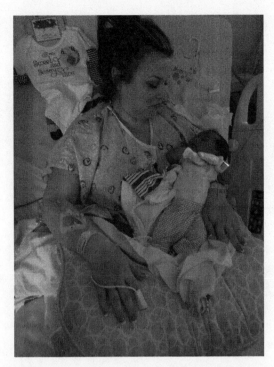

Figure 4-20 Postpartum mother completely outfitting her "new arrival"

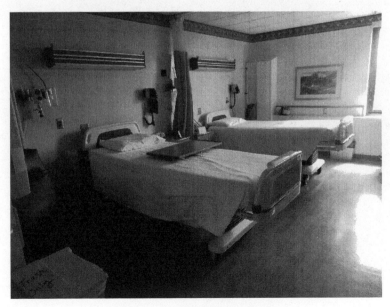

Figure 4-21 Postpartum Room

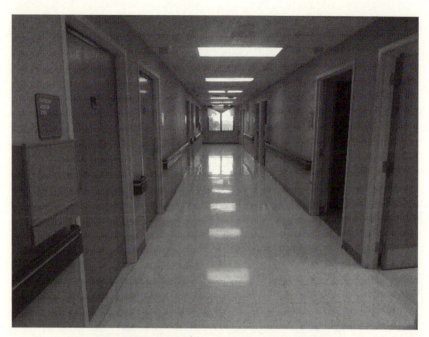

Figure 4-22 Postpartum Floor with private single beds.

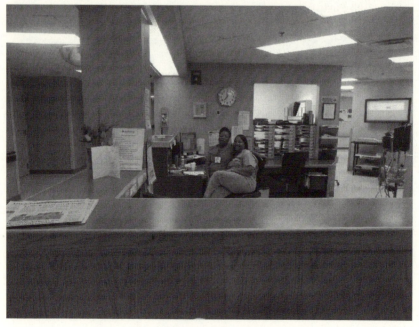

Figure 4-23 Postpartum Nursing Station.

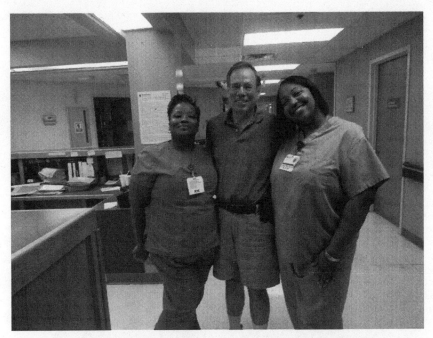

Figure 4-24 Your OB Physician-Nurse Team "at your service."

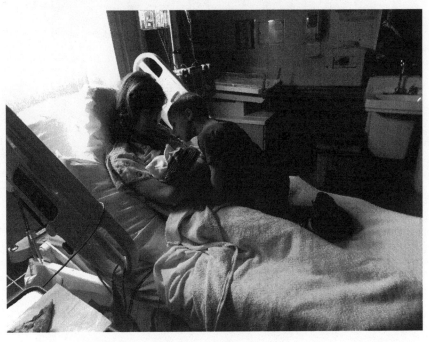

Figure 2-25 The wonder of a child gazing at his newborn sister

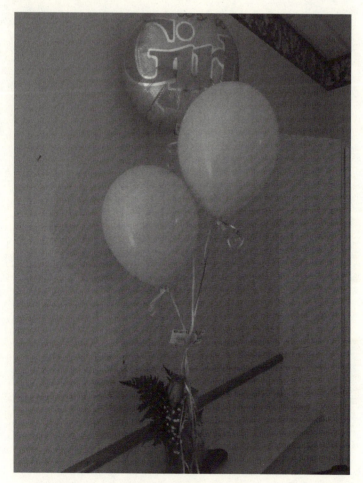

Figure 2-26 Traditional Roses for the new mom.

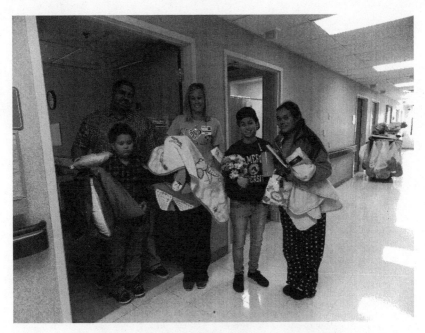

Figure 4-27 Family departing for home

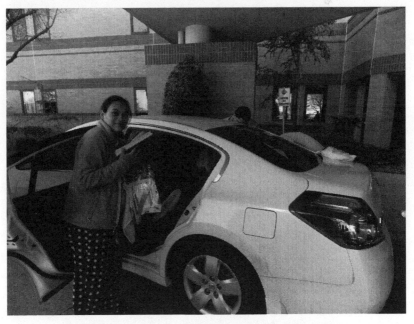

Figure 4-28 Mom placing baby in car seat New Mom getting ready to drive home after Dad figures out how to set up baby seat on the other side of the car

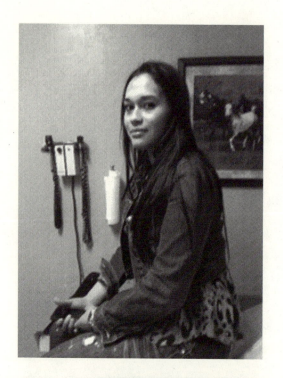

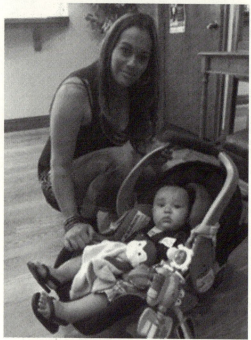

Figure 4-29 Graciela at her Checkups

CHAPTER 5

Prenatal Care:
"The Good, the Bad, and the Details"

The goals of prenatal care are:

1. To assure the healthy physical and mental development of the unborn baby;

2. To support and promote the health of the pregnant mother herself; and,

3. To develop a relationship with a physician in whom she can trust and confide.

Accordingly, it is the physician's responsibility to continue to supervise and monitor the health of the pregnant mother and her unborn child. Such surveillance is accomplished by proper instruction in nutrition and education about hygienic procedures and habits. The obstetrician teaches the expectant mother a proper way of living, exercising, and caring for herself, her husband, and their children. The physician will constantly search out any factors that may be detrimental to the development of the unborn child and any factors that may contribute to an unhealthy situation for the mother. The pregnant mother should be able to have great trust in her obstetrician throughout the pregnancy and especially during the labor and delivery. The mother may be fearful of labor and delivery. She is quite anxious about being in pain as well as suffering harm in the delivery process. She desperately needs her obstetrician, husband, relatives and friends to support her during this stressful period of time.

1. High Expectations, But . . .

No physician can guarantee a perfect pregnancy, labor, delivery, and, most of all, a healthy baby. Approximately five to ten percent of all babies have some abnormality or defect, whether it is an insignificant birthmark or a serious heart problem.

Statistically however, the chances are that you will have a normal pregnancy and a healthy baby. By going to a physician experienced in obstetrics (family physician with OB, an OB-GYN Generalist, OB Hospitalist, Perinatologist, i.e. a maternal-fetal health subspecialist), you are insuring yourself and your baby against preventable health risks.

Important Information

Congratulations! You are pregnant! Whether this is the first time or the tenth, you have made a conscious decision to learn more about pregnancy, childbirth and your newborn baby. (That is why you're reading this book!) First things are first. As soon as possible, write down or place the following information in your smartphone or near your home phone as well as your work phone. Further ; keep a copy in your wallet or your purse:

OBSTETRICIAN'S PHONE NUMBER: _____

HOSPITAL PHONE NUMBER: _____

NEIGHBOR'S PHONE NUMBER: _____

AMBULANCE COMPANY'S PHONE NUMBER: _____

BABYSITTER'S PHONE NUMBER: _____

PARAMEDIC EMERGENCY PHONE NUMBER: _____

(Fire or Police Department numbers should be used if there are no Paramedics in your area)

AREA EMERGENCY PHONE NUMBER: _____

POISON CONTROL CENTER: _____

DEAF INFORMED COMMUNICATION ORGANIZATION

EMERGENCY VOICE AND TTY: _____

2. **The Ten Important Steps you can take to stay healthy when pregnant.**

One of the most important aspects of your pregnancy for which you alone are responsible is personal hygiene. A good personal health routine is not just important medically, but it also can make a big difference in your self-esteem and mood. At times during pregnancy, it is not unusual to feel awkward and unattractive. Taking the time to be knowledgeable about good health routines can make you feel better about yourself. Make the following commitments a part of your personal hygiene. Many of these suggestions will be elaborated upon later in this book.

Ten Important Hygienic Measures to do when Pregnant

I.   Your hands come in contact with, and pass along, more germs than any other part of your body. Wash your hands with soap and water before eating or drinking, after they become dirty, after going to the bathroom, and after blowing your nose. Purel™ or other sanitary solutions/wipes should be purchased and kept in your possession when you are out and about.

Avoid people who are sick! Do not visit or get close to people that have colds, flu and diarrhea. If you are going to be or you are always exposed to the public, wear surgical masks (it is more socially acceptable now).

II. It used to be believed that you lost at least one tooth for every pregnancy. This foregoing "old wives' tale" is nonsense. There are some dental problems that are aggravated by pregnancy (such as gum problems), but your teeth should not suffer permanent problems from pregnancy. Brush your teeth after every meal and before going to bed. Now, as always, it is important to use dental floss regularly.

III. Wear properly fitted and comfortable shoes. The damage caused by ill-fitting bargain shoes is not worth the extra money saved. Avoid extreme high heels. They are neither good for your back nor your safety. Flat shoes during pregnancy help alleviate the strain on your lower back.

IV. Bathe and wash your hair regularly. Feeling clean and feminine is great for your morale!

V. Dress properly for the weather conditions. Anticipate weather changes by watching the Weather Stations.

VI. Do not re-use your pantyhose, stockings or underwear without washing them. Change your clothes daily.

VII. It is very important to properly cleanse yourself after going to the bathroom. After urinating, dab (do not rub) using a backward or downward motion. Likewise, after a bowel movement, gently wipe yourself from front to back. NEVER WIPE FROM THE ANAL AREA TOWARDS THE VAGINA: yeast and bacteria around the rectum contaminate the vagina and urethra (and may cause bladder and yeast infections). If you have any doubt that you have cleansed yourself completely, use soap and water on toilet paper or a washcloth. NOTE: during love making, couples should be careful not to stroke the rectal or anal area towards the vagina.

VIII. Do not smoke. Even if you usually smoke, think of your baby and sacrifice cigarettes for nine months.

IX. Do not drink alcoholic beverages. A small amount on special occasions, such as New Year's, is not harmful.

X. Control your emotions. Do not become violent or combative. Don't throw things. Find outlets for your anger that are not dangerous to you and your baby (or anyone else!). Hit a tennis ball around or go bowling with your anger. Don't forget those old standbys for emotional release – crying and screaming. They work wonders!

These are the Ten Healthy Measures for good personal hygiene and emotional stability, not only during pregnancy, but for the rest of your life as well.

3. Dental Health and Care during Pregnancy

It is especially important for women who are planning to become pregnant or who are in early stages of pregnancy, to have a comprehensive dental examination. Potential problems that could lead to infection, dental abscess, or pain should be treated and corrected at once. Dental abscesses can potentially "seed" the maternal bloodstream with bacteria which could lead to severe infection in both mother and baby at any time during pregnancy (poor dental hygiene has been linked to an increased incidence of premature labor).

It is recommended to maintain your annual dental checkups and cleanings even if you are pregnant. It is important to keep scheduled appointments with your dentist and dental hygienist for any dental treatments that are recommended. It is safe to have regular dental cleanings, cavities filled, whitening and fluoride treatments and teeth pulled as needed.

It is very important to continue to brush your teeth after each meal. Floss and use mouthwash regularly.

Mouthwash with fluoride or other whitening additives are not harmful during pregnancy. Whitening treatments are safe during pregnancy.

Because of the effects of various placental hormones, the gums enlarge, swell and bleed easily. Dental check-ups should be made, not postponed, during pregnancy.

It is NOT true "that you lose a tooth for every baby you have" (an old wives' tale). This old wives tale should be laid to rest.

Dental X-rays are safe to take during pregnancy. Be sure that the dental assistant covers your abdomen (i.e. the baby!) with the lead apron which shields and repels any radiation.

Calcium supplements may be helpful if sufficient amounts are not being consumed in your diet (or if not adequately supplied in your prenatal vitamin pill). No more than 1.5 grams (1500 milligrams or mgs) of calcium is necessary on a daily basis during pregnancy. Be sure to add up all the amounts from all the foods, liquids, vitamin pills, etc. that you take.

Dental caries ("cavities") can be treated and filled during pregnancy. Gold, silver, plastic and other metal fillings are safe. Swallowed dental pastes, metals, plasters, etc., do not affect the baby.

Use of nitrous gas is permissible after the first trimester.

Use of Novacaine® or other local anesthetics can be safely utilized to provide numbness prior to dental work. These agents are not toxic or in any way affect the baby.

Braces and other orthodontic appliances are also permissible and safe during pregnancy.

Oral surgery for root canal, dental abscess and extractions should be performed if considered necessary by your dental specialist. If any questions arise, both your dentist and your obstetrician can consult with each other about the particular problem. If surgery or involved dental work can be postponed until after delivery without incurring serious adverse effects to the teeth, then any such procedures can be delayed until after the baby is born.

Sodium fluoride supplements during pregnancy are available. They may have significant beneficial effects on your *baby's* developing teeth (see below). Ask your dentist and obstetrician for their advice.

Battery tooth brushes (for example, Spin-brush®, Phillips Sonic®, etc.) can be used and are recommended as being superior brushing techniques during pregnancy.

Use of analgesics, i.e. "pain pills," for pain before and after dental procedures is permissible. Codeine, Percocet®, Lortab® 5 mg, Esgic®, Tylenol #3®, etc., are safe to use.

Pregnant patients with heart conditions should be placed on antibiotic coverage before and after treatment prior to undergoing any dental procedures or treatment. The following heart conditions need such antibiotic coverage:

a) Rheumatic heart disease

b) Mitral valve prolapse (selected patients)

c) Valve replacements

d) Other specific medical conditions as directed by your physician. The point is that bacteria around the gums and teeth enter the abundant blood vessels in the mouth during dental manipulations. Such "showers of bacteria" enter the bloodstream and travel to your heart and the placenta. Theoretically, there is a risk of infecting an already damaged heart. Likewise, the placenta (and baby) can become infected.

Antibiotics are needed prior to dental surgery in patients with previous heart surgery or heart damage (but not if you have had a "broken heart" from an old boyfriend!)

VIRTUAL ELIMINATION OF DENTAL CARIES THROUGH PRENATAL FLUORIDE SUPPLEMENTATION

The beneficial effect of sodium fluoride supplementation to infants and small children for the prevention of dental caries is well known. Glenn, et al, have reviewed the literature and report a study of 492 children which demonstrates that *prenatal* supplementation with sodium fluoride results in a 99% reduction of caries formation in deciduous and permanent teeth.

The children studied were aged three to twelve. They were divided into five groups to allow for comparisons of the prenatal fluoride children with matched controls having fluoridated water only. The prenatal fluoride children consistently showed a 99% reduction in dental caries. Interestingly, fluoridated water during pregnancy does not confer similar protection since a greater blood level of maternal fluoride is required for placental transfer. Incidental findings in the study were that the prenatal fluoride children were slightly longer and heavier, possibly due to fluoride deposition in bone. The prenatal fluoride group also had fewer birth defects and lower rate of prematurity.

The recommended dosage is a 1 mg. fluoride tablet (2.2 mg. sodium fluoride) daily on an empty stomach beginning with the third month of pregnancy (12 weeks). This is the same size tablet given to children age three and older. A 1 mg. fluoride tablet results in 0.25 mg. fluoride transferred to the fetus.

The conclusion, therefore, is that prenatal supplementation with sodium fluoride beginning in the third month results in the virtual elimination of dental caries in the offspring. This treatment is safe and supported by the Food and Drug Administration, the American Medical Association and the American Dental Association. With widespread application, there is the potential for a generation virtually free of dental caries.

REFERENCE: 1) Glenn, et al, Am J Obstet and Gynecol 143:560-564, 1982. 2) Stollerman, et al, (Editorial) Hospital Practice 6:39-40, 1982.

Prenatal Dental Care

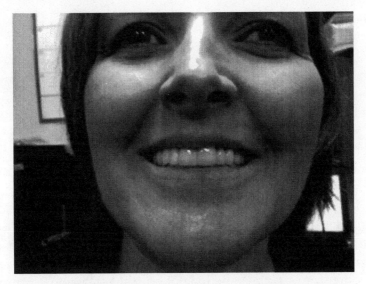

Figure 5-1 Dental care during pregnancy

During your pregnancy, every effort should be made to focus on good health practices. Proper prenatal care will help you enjoy optimum health during and after your pregnancy and the promise of a healthier baby. Such a program of prenatal care involves the combined efforts of your obstetrician, nurse, dentist, dental hygienist and YOU, the expectant parent. Most obstetricians recommend that needed dental care be completed early in pregnancy. Almost all dental procedures can be performed during the fourth to seventh months since the fewest problems of pregnancy occur during this period.

Your Baby's Teeth

Your baby's teeth begin to form about the fifth to sixth week of pregnancy. The baby needs calcium, phosphorous, minerals and vitamins as he/she grows and develops. Contrary to an old belief, however, the baby does NOT absorb calcium from the mother's teeth. Nutrients must be supplied from the foods you eat. Therefore, it is essential for you to follow your physician's and dentist's advice about diet.

Gum Problems and Pregnancy

Gingivitis

The condition of your gingiva (gums) is directly related to the presence of local irritants, namely plaque, calculus, and broken-down rough fillings. Plaque is a soft, sticky, colorless germ-filled layer which forms on your teeth each day. It makes your teeth feel "fuzzy" when you rub your tongue over them, yet it can be removed with a toothbrush. Calculus is a hard formation on the teeth that cannot be removed with a toothbrush, but needs to be removed in the dental office. These irritants can cause an infection in the gum tissue called gingivitis. The gums can get red, swollen, sometimes bleed, and be tender. Pregnancy, with its accompanying hormonal changes, tends to aggravate an existing gingival condition and can cause pregnancy gingivitis. A thorough prophylaxis or cleaning of your teeth early in your pregnancy coupled with daily brushing, flossing and proper diet are therefore most important to help you avoid such painful complications.

Summary

Working together with your physician, your dentist can and should provide for you close dental supervision to help you avoid undue discomfort caused by tooth decay, gum problems and improper diet. Seek their help early to assure proper prenatal care for you and your baby.

4. Eye Care and Changes

Vision may change during pregnancy. With the accumulation and retention of fluid during pregnancy, the eyeball may swell. Visual accuracy may become poorer. Do not, however, hurry down to your optometrist (or ophthalmologist) for new lenses or contacts.

After childbirth, the swelling of the eye dissipates and returns to normal. Vision usually returns to its previous level. If, after six to eight weeks postpartum, vision is still suboptimal, then an eye examination would be appropriate.

"I guess I need to cancel my eye appointment now because I didn't know it could take up to 6-8 weeks for the changes in my eyes to return to normal."

Lastly, extra secretions and chemical changes during pregnancy require that contact lenses be cleaned more frequently in order to prevent "clogging" to the porous surfaces.

5. Seat Belts

Before we go any further in this book, I want to be sure you are going to be around to read the rest of it! Answer me honestly! Did you wear seat belts when you rode in the car today? Yesterday? If you did, that's great. I hope you always do. Nothing has contributed more to the safety of people in automobiles than the seat belt. I know you are a good driver. I know you are usually only going a short distance, but you are being a negligent mother to your unborn child if you don't buckle-up. (When nothing else works, I've always found guilt works wonders!)

The seat belt is a safe and recommended precaution to take, even during early and late pregnancy. It may not be the most comfortable feeling, but you can place the seat belt underneath the uterus or across the upper thighs. The lap belt should be across your shoulder and there should be at least three inches of belt slack across your body. The lap and seat belt will not hurt your baby. Studies prove that the leading single cause of fetal death is the death of the mother.

In many states, it is now a law that children under four years of age must be placed in an approved car seat in a car. Even though the baby is quite small, it is not safe to hold the baby in your arms. At ten miles an hour, at impact, it has been shown that a baby has the force of up to 150 pounds. No person can hold on to that kind of weight in an automobile accident. The babies first ride home from the hospital should be in a baby safety seat.

You may have experienced troubles with your other children or may have trouble with this baby complaining about the car seat. They may cry and try to squirm out. Be firm and consistent: the car does not move without safety seats and belts. Use your lap and seat belt every time you put the key in the ignition. Children eventually realize that safety seats and belts are as much a part of riding in an automobile as putting gas in the tank. In the best interests of you, your family and your unborn child, please begin to use your car safety belts now! Besides, it is the state law!

6. What about Sex during Pregnancy?

Questions concerning sex during pregnancy are often difficult for an expectant mother to ask. Many women feel that if they desire sexual relations during pregnancy they must be nymphomaniacs or, if they lack interest, that they have become frigid.

Although sex is a very private part of one's life, it should be a positive and fulfilling one. Sex is not something which you need to be embarrassed talking about with your obstetrician. After all, without sex your friendly neighborhood obstetrician would be out of business!

Obstetricians are currently in agreement that sexual intercourse has no harmful effects on a *normal* pregnancy (exceptions are the conditions of placenta praevia, preterm labor, and preterm cervical dilatation or cervical incompetence). The uterus during pregnancy is situated far above and somewhat perpendicular to the vagina. There are no anatomic structures such as the cervix or pregnant uterus that can be "bumped" or "hit" during sexual intercourse. The uterus and the baby are out of the pelvis and in the abdominal cavity until the last week or so of pregnancy. Penetration cannot hurt the mother or baby. The frequency of love-making, orgasm, breast stimulation, vaginal lubricants, positions and even oral stimulation will not affect pregnancy. Semen may contain hormones, i.e. prostaglandins that may cause uterine contractions. These contractions will usually subside in less than an hour. Orgasm, too, may stimulate contractions, but these contractions, too, will subside quickly.

In certain high-risk pregnancies, sexual intercourse, stimulation and orgasm may cause the onset of premature labor and, consequently, early delivery. These high-risk cases include women who have a history of premature labor, women carrying twins and patients with anatomical abnormalities of the uterus (such as fibroids). So, if you have been told that your pregnancy is "high-risk," it is important to ask your obstetrician about the advisability of sexual intercourse.

Your partner (husband, etc.) is just as concerned about having sex during pregnancy.

Communicate your feelings, enjoyments and discomforts to each other, so that a more satisfactory sexual relationship may continue. Many couples must change their usual or preferred positions during love-making in order to feel more comfortable. Many books will illustrate some optional positions in great detail. These illustrations may flame some spicy excitement, but these illustrations and notes are nothing compared to your own creativity that, as a couple, you both are capable of!

7. Incompetent Cervix and Early Second Trimester Loss

Most (about 90%) pregnancy losses, or miscarriages, occur in the first trimester of pregnancy. Most of these losses occur due to a genetic or other anatomical abnormality in the baby, i.e. fetal causation.

Losses in the 2nd trimester are usually due to abnormalities in the mother, i.e. maternal causes such as:

1. Anatomical abnormalities of the uterus such as myomata (or "fibroids") or other congenital malformations of the uterus

2. Infection such as Listeria, Group B Streptococcus, Chlamydiae or other bacteria/viruses.

There are a small number of patients that will have a loss of pregnancy between 16 to 20 weeks of pregnancy due to "cervical weakness." In this clinical syndrome there is a "painless" dilatation of the cervix. Patients have no pain. The only clinical signs are as follows:

1. An increased amount of mucus passed vaginally or increased vaginal discharge
2. A small amount of spotting
3. Pelvic pressure as if "something is trying to come out."

The cervix is designed to hold the baby inside the uterus (much like a cork in a wine bottle) until the baby is fully developed: "all systems go" or mature humanoid capable of external life. However, the strength of the cervix can be compromised by the following situations:

1. Cervical Conization procedures (such as Cold Knife Cone Biopsy or occasionally LEEP conization)
2. Previous D&C's and miscarriages
3. Other congenital or inherited abnormalities of the cervix

Most patients will experience some increased mucus or spotting and will report such changes immediately to their OB. This "cervical weakness" can be treated surgically by placing and tying a suture around the cervix in order to keep it closed. The suture is similar to a "purse string" in securing the cervix: the procedure is medically known as a "cervical cerclage."

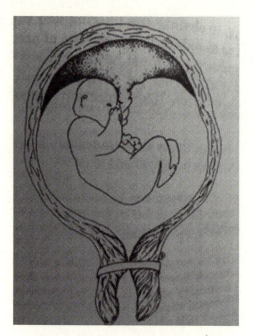

Figure 5-2 Suture around cervix

Bed rest is advised for a short period of time after the suture is placed. Physical work activities are curtailed depending on the individual situation of the patient.

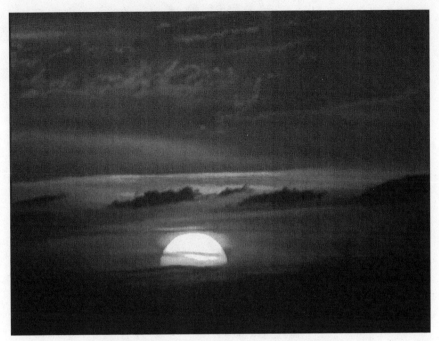

Figure 5-3 Sunset in Southwest Oklahoma

Well I never been to Heaven, but I have been to Oklahoma
Well they tell me I was born there

--"Never Been to Spain," by Elvis Presley and Three Dog Night

CHAPTER 6

Mostly Third Trimester Pregnancy Issues or "The Final Stretch"

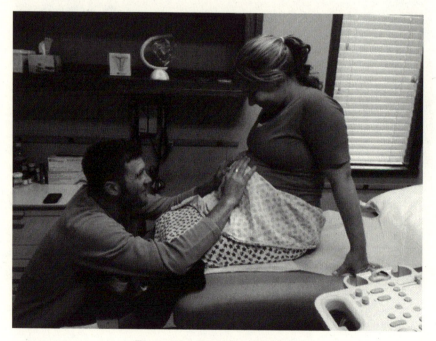

Figure 6-1 "Daddy's Hands".

I remember Daddy's hands, how they held my Mama tight,
But I've come to understand,
There was always love in Daddy's hands.

---Lyrics written and Song sung by Holly Dunn

1. "Baby-Moon"

Just as a newlywed couple takes a trip (or a cruise) for the period of time after the wedding (traditionally a month, i.e., lunar month or "honey-moon") many couples are taking time off in the last trimester to find "alone time" together to experience some leisure, fun and intimacy before (or occasionally after) the baby arrives.

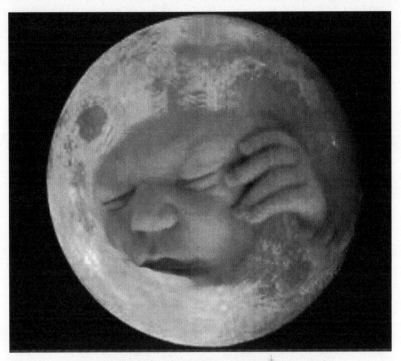

Figure 6-2 "Baby Moon"

The term was first used by Sheila Kitzinger in her 1996 book *The Year After Childbirth* with reference to the *husband* taking the month off after the baby was born in order to make his psychological transition from married man to fatherhood. In 2004, Lisa Lewis converted the meaning of "Baby Moon" to the following:, i.e. just like a honeymoon except while pregnant in your last trimester, in this instance the couple has one last "hurrah" the baby is born (from her article in the *Athens Banner Herald* per Wikpedia.org).

Many couples are taking their "Baby Moons" to locations such as Las Vegas, Hawaii, Mexico or the Caribbean. Because of the possibility of a preterm labor or labor itself, it is recommended that couples take long distance trips early in the 3rd trimester. Local trips to vacations spots 1-2 hours away from home can be taken closer to your due date. The "new-mom-to-be" below took her Baby Moon to nearby Oklahoma City, enjoyed the many restaurants in the Bricktown section as well enjoyed her daily strolls down the River Walk taking in many of the tourist attractions.

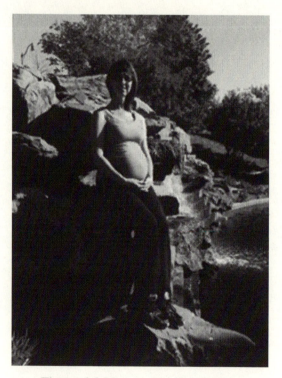

Figure 6-3 Mom on her Babymoon.
Expectant Mom enjoying her time away at the OKC River Walk

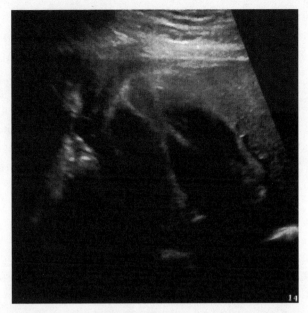

Figure 6-4 Baby "Mooning." Not your typical Baby Moon. The author took this picture during a routine ultrasound

2. Preparing in advance for your Hospital Stay

Pre-Registration.

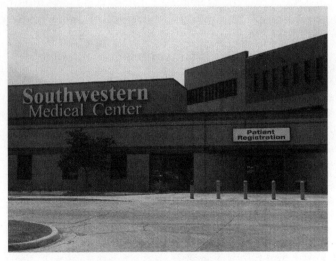

Figure 6-5 Registration Office at Hospital

Patients should pre-register at the hospital where they plan to deliver by the beginning of the 3rd Trimester. Many patients may already be registered into the hospital computer system because they have had their laboratory testing or ultrasound examinations there. If you have not already been pre-registered, you can call or go to the Admissions Department to fill out any necessary forms. Many hospitals may already be doing the Registration process via their website on the internet. Patients can also request that their OB's office print out their demographic and insurance information so that you do not have to go through filling out similar forms at the hospital.

Pregnancy Classes.

Patients can also call the OB or hospital Education Department regarding OB tours and Prenatal Classes. Most hospitals providing Obstetric care will offer classes in breastfeeding, Lamaze or Bradley Childbirth methods, anesthesia and pain control, etc. Again, you can check the hospital's website for any information that may be posted there.

Your Bags Need Packing.

Patients need to plan to pack in advance all items that they will need at the hospital. Going into the hospital for a few days is not too dissimilar from a weekend trip away from home. A "short list" of items is as follows:

Toiletries: Toothbrush, toothpaste, shampoo, conditioner, blow dryer, hair brush, combs, mouthwash, deodorant, perfume, etc.

According to the nurses, the most common items requested by new moms are pads, panties, soap, toothpaste, toothbrushes, and telephone charging cords.

Most hospitals will supply overnight maxi-pads (the "2 by 4's"), but if you are accustomed to thinner pads, you should make a mental note to include your pads of choice in your suitcase.

Medications: bring all medications that you are taking to the hospital so the nursing staff can make a medication record. Nurses routinely do a "Medication Reconciliation" document into the hospital computer system so that necessary medication can be provided to you during your stay. The Hospital Pharmacist performs a check of all your medications to be sure your medications are compatible with each other and that previous medications you have been taken are re-ordered in the hospital.

Clothing: night gowns, underpants, "Going Home" outfit, T-shirts, pants, socks, shoes, slippers etc.)

Camera, Recharging Cords and Batteries (unless you use your phone): Do not forget your phone and camera recharging cords. Bring extra batteries for your cameras. Also make sure your SD card in your camera has sufficient memory capacity

"Going Home" outfit for your baby

"Going Home" outfit for the New Mother

Baby Book for your Girl or Boy: to record the names and pics of the nurses, your OB, etc.

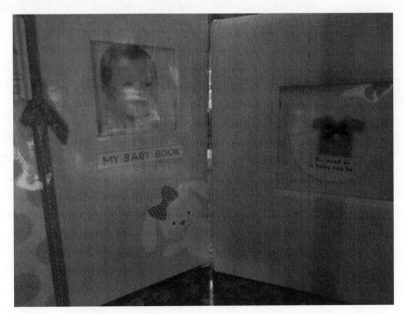

Figure 6-6 Baby Books for your Girl or Boy

Emory boards to file down the baby's fingernails so that they will not scratch themselves

Mittens for your baby's hands so that they do not scratch their face

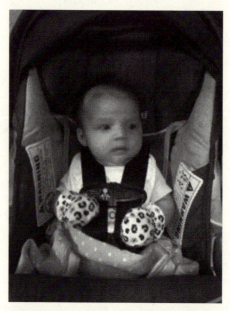

Figure 6-7 Newborn with her mittens on

Transportation: make sure you have a reliable way of getting to the hospital lined up: taxi cab, family or friends. Be sure your vehicle is regularly serviced and has sufficient gas.

Coupons: it is especially important to have your pizza, sandwich, and etc. coupons with you so that you can use them to buy food for the overworked and hungry OB nursing staff (not just your family and friends!).

Care for your other children. The last trimester is a good time to make arrangements for the care of your other children in the family when you go into the hospital. The hospital and its staff cannot take the responsibility of caring for your children while you are in labor. Most hospitals will not allow children to stay overnight in the hospital with you during labor and after you delivery.

3. Pre-eclampsia or Toxemia of Pregnancy

Historically and even today, pre-eclampsia is one of the *main* pregnancy-related conditions that dominate the practice of obstetrics. In a sense pre-eclampsia was probably the "Number One" disease that led to the creation of the specialty of Obstetrics itself. Pre-eclampsia is a disease that can cause severe complications to the pregnant mother as well as the baby: at its worse, potentially death of the mother and baby. Avoidance of these and any complications is focused on the *early* diagnosis of pre-eclampsia.

What is pre-eclampsia? By definition pre-eclampsia is a specific disease of pregnancy with the following medical criteria:

- High blood pressure (Hypertension with an increase of 30/15 mm Hg systolic/diastolic pressures over your baseline blood pressure in early pregnancy or a blood pressure exceeding 160/90
- Protein in your urine
- Edema (swelling of your face, hands and feet) with sudden weight gain (greater than 2 lbs. in a week)

Pre-eclampsia manifests itself mainly in the 3rd trimester or last 13 weeks of pregnancy. Physicians are still uncertain about the cause of the condition, but it is considered a *placental* disease. The only absolute treatment is removal of the placenta, i.e. the baby must be delivered. Of course, if the baby is too premature to deliver, there are still therapeutic interventions than can treat the disease until the baby can be born with the least amount of problems. It is predominately a disease of the 1st pregnancy. However, it can re-occur in subsequently pregnancies in a small percentage of patients with the following underlying associations:

a. Different father of the baby in the current pregnancy
b. Advanced Maternal Age (>35 years of age)
c. Long intervals of time between each pregnancies
d. Twin or other multiple pregnancy
e. Hypertension prior to pregnancy (kidney disease, other vascular disease)
f. Diabetes prior to pregnancy
g. Collagen Vascular diseases prior to pregnancy

    h. Kidney disease prior to pregnancy
    i. Fibrinolytic Syndromes such as Factor V Leiden, METHR genetic diseases, etc.
    j. IVF or ART (Advanced Reproductive Treatment) produced Pregnancy

Your OB office visits in the third trimester have been purposely set to be more frequent so that pre-eclampsia can be diagnosed as early as possible.

    27 to 36 weeks: 2 week intervals between appointments
    36 to 40 weeks: 1 week intervals

Of course, your OB may want to see you more frequently at any time during pregnancy depending on your health situation.

Prevention of Pre-eclampsia

There are no absolute preventative measures that can be taken to avoid the disease altogether. Medical studies have shown significant decreases in the incidence of pre-eclampsia when the daily diet of the pregnant mother contained 80 to 100 grams of protein. There have been conflicting reports regarding the use of "baby aspirin" daily prior to and during pregnancy with regard to prevention: a topic that you can discuss with your OB particularly if this pregnancy is your first.

Pre-pregnancy programs are also helpful:

    a. Attainment of ideal body weight
    b. Cessation of smoking
    c. Proper conditioning and muscle tone (improve physical fitness)
    d. Control of all of the above medical conditions prior to becoming pregnant

Pre-eclampsia hopefully will be diagnosed prior to you developing any symptoms of the disease. The following symptoms are the most common:

a. Swelling of the feet that progresses to the hands and face (cheeks and eyelids)
b. Headaches
c. Visual changes: blurring and perhaps "seeing spots"
d. Nausea progressing to vomiting
e. "Stomach" or Epigastric Pain ("Liver Pain" or Right upper quadrant pain)
f. Mental changes, i.e. slowness, inability to concentrate or focus, "fogginess"

The treatment of the disease depends on the week of pregnancy the disease starts as well as the speed of its progression. Hypertension or increasing elevation of your blood pressure during the third trimester is the usually the first *sign* of the disease. *Protein* in your urine is usually the second most common presentation of the disease but can be the only sign in some patients: you do NOT have to have all the signs of the disease to have severe pre-eclampsia.

Pre-eclampsia is taken very seriously by OBs because of many *uncertainties* posed by the disease:

- How quickly or suddenly the blood pressure increases and how well it responds to medical treatment
- How many organ systems are currently being affected: liver, coagulation or clotting ability, etc?

For the most part, treatment starts with bed rest and the cessation of employment. Elevated Blood pressure can be treated with anti-hypertensive medication as an outpatient. If the pregnancy is 39 weeks or longer, delivery should be considered. Your Ob will formulate a treatment plan if pre-eclampsia develops when your pregnancy is in the premature zone: between 27 to 34 weeks. There are so many different circumstances to take into account in any given pregnancy complicated by pre-eclampsia such that the author cannot realistically explain detailed treatment options prior to term pregnancy.

Eclampsia

Eclampsia is all of the above except the patients suffers a grand mal seizure or convulsion. Eclampsia is the most advanced part of the disease. Regardless of the number of weeks of pregnancy, eclampsia requires that the pregnancy be concluded and the baby delivered.

Eclampsia is a Greek word meaning "A Bolt of Lightning."

A patient with pre-eclampsia can deteriorate so quickly that, like a sudden "strike of lightning," she starts convulsing in front of you. One minute you can be having a conversation with her and the next *second*, her eyes roll up, she falls down on the bed and starts involuntary arm and leg jerking motions while drool and foam pour out of her mouth. Blood flow to the baby can be compromised during a seizure.

An increasingly more severe headache is the usual symptom experienced by the patient just prior to the seizure.

At this point medication (usually magnesium sulfate bolus and sometimes IV Valium) is given to stop further seizures from occurring. The patient is first stabilized and critical assessment of the mother and the baby is performed. Within a certain period of time, labor is usually induced. If labor and delivery is projected to be lengthy in time, a C-section may performed to expedite delivery and treat the disease.

Pre-eclampsia and Eclampsia usually develop during pregnancy *prior* to delivery (incidence 66%). However, 33% of the time the disease can manifest itself in the postpartum period (usually the first 72 hours after delivery).

Author's Notes: Pre-eclampsia and Eclampsia are very serious diseases of pregnancy: they can develop suddenly and progress rapidly. Further, the disease can be puzzling to diagnose early because it can masquerade itself by presenting with uncommon disconnected symptoms.

Case 1. Mary was a 28 year old female in her first pregnancy and was 26 weeks pregnant. She called her OB's office and said that she was having right upper abdominal pain. Her pregnancy was uncomplicated to this point. She was referred to a General Surgeon for probable gallbladder disease. Unfortunately, her blood pressure was not checked at this time. Gallbladder ultrasound study was negative for stones or inflammation. She continued to have the pain. She was then referred to internal medicine for evaluation of possible ulcer or pancreatitis. Her blood pressure was taken and was elevated. The internist made a diagnosis of hypertension but did not relay that information immediately to her OB. The internist, many years distant from his rotation on the Obstetrics service during his medical school training, did not make the connection of possible pre-eclampsia. It was not until the patient's next OB appointment 2 weeks later that her OB made the diagnosis and admitted her to the hospital for care.

Case 2. Ryan was an 18 year old having her second pregnancy with a different "baby daddy." She had delivered her first baby at 25 weeks gestation by C-section for eclampsia. The baby weighed 1 lb. 4 oz. and was in the NICU for 45 days. She was brought in by ambulance at 29 weeks gestation after having a seizure at her mother's home. She had no OB physician and had no OB care during this pregnancy. Two weeks earlier she had split up with the baby daddy and moved from Texas back home to Oklahoma. She had another seizure just after entering the OB suite. Neither RN on duty had ever witnessed a patient with eclampsia (eclampsia is rarely seen today because most patients are diagnosed early by their OB during prenatal care). The nurses called the author immediately. An IV had been started by the EMTs in the ambulance. The author told the nurses to give 10 mg of Valium IV in order to immediately stop the current seizures. Magnesium sulfate bolus was given followed by a continuous infusion. The baby was quickly monitored and was fine. Evaluation of the mother continued: physical exam of the mother combined with laboratory evaluation. The patient's blood pressure was 180/102 but came down quickly with the Magnesium infusion. Ultrasound and Biophysical profile was performed. Laboratory results showed she had 3+ proteinuria (Scale is 1 to 4). Her drug screen was positive for opiates. She was stabilized and transferred to the closest Medical

Center with a NICU that can care for very premature babies (OU Medical Center in OKC).

As stated previously, pre-eclampsia and eclampsia can be difficult to diagnose: not all parameters of elevated blood pressure, protein in the urine, sudden weight gain /swelling need be present altogether but just one of them by themselves. A severe headache, nausea and vomiting or visual blurriness may be the only initial symptoms: call your OB when these symptoms appear.

4. Pre-term Labor

> *Every OB patient should be aware that labor contractions can start many weeks prior to their due date. Labor is defined as contractions that cause cervical stretching and dilatation. Patients should notice hardening of the uterus: when there are more than 6-8 contractions per hour for more than 2 hours, the patient should notify her OB or go to the OB suite at their hospital. If there is passage of pink tinged mucus, the patient should go to the OB suite as soon as possible.*

Preterm Labor is defined as contractions prior to 37 completed weeks of pregnancy that lead to cervical effacement (thinning and shortening of the cervix) and dilatation (see Labor section).

More than 8 regular contractions per hour for more than an hour of time is a reliable sign of possible preterm labor.

Contractions associated with mucus or bloody discharges from the vagina are even more significant signs of premature labor. Notify your OB or proceed to the OB suite at your hospital.

There are many predisposing conditions that can lead to preterm labor such as:

1. Overly distended uterus (Twin or multiple pregnancy, polyhydramnios—excess of amniotic fluid)
2. Previous cervical surgery (Cone biopsy)

3. STD's such as chlamydiae
4. Systemic Infections: pyelonephritis, gastroenteritis, Listeria, dental abscess or other sepsis
5. Myomata (fibroids) or other congenital abnormalities of the uterus (i.e., uterine septum)
6. Trauma such as a Motor Vehicle Accident or a fall

Testing

At the office or more likely in the OB suite, First a urinalysis test will be performed to diagnose upper or lower tract urinary tract infection, i.e. pyelonephritis. Thereafter, a pelvic exam with speculum visualization of the cervix may be performed. Frequently, a swab will be taken for a "Fetal Fibronectin Test "(FFN). FFN testing provides objective testing whether "true labor" is occurring: the test provides insight and can help predict whether true labor will occur in the next two (2) weeks. Frequently other testing may be performed at the same time: Group B strep swab, DNA Sureswabs® for other infectious diseases.

Treatment

Depending on the presumptive cause of your contractions or preterm labor, your OB will advise you of appropriate treatment. Bed rest and fluid hydration (oral or intravenous) may be the first line of treatment. If these measures do not slow down the uterine contractility, your OB may attempt to stop the contractions with medication (terbutaline, nifedipine, indomethacin, magnesium, etc.). If the pregnancy is still under 34 completed weeks, Betamethasone will be given to help speed the development of the baby's lungs. Bed rest is a major component of initial treatment along with cessation of employment/work. If delivery is not likely to be delayed, the patient less than 34 weeks gestation may need to be transported to a tertiary center where a NICU (Neonatal Intensive Care unit) and neonatologists are available (unless your local hospital is so equipped along with a staffed NICU).

5. Premature Rupture of Membranes

The amniotic sac can rupture or leak prior to 37 completed weeks of pregnancy. There are some predisposing causes such as:

1. STD or other cervical infection (GBS)
2. Cervical Incompetence (weakness)
3. Over-distended uterus (twins or excess amniotic fluid, i.e. polyhydramnios) as noted in Preterm Labor
4. Preterm Labor in itself
5. Infection of the amniotic and chorionic membranes from systemic or local infection
6. Compression trauma of the uterus
7. Amniocentesis

The treatment of PSROM depends upon the point (which week) in pregnancy it occurs. When the membranes rupture, the barrier between the baby and the vagina is broken. The growth of bacteria from the cervical area spreading upward into the uterus and baby is the main focus of concern. Prior to 24 completed weeks of pregnancy, the prognosis for saving the baby is very poor: the baby is too immature to live. Between 24 to 34 weeks the management entails the following:

> Cultures of the cervix along with a GBS swab/testing
> Antibiotics
> Administration of steroids (Betamethasone)
> Bed rest
> Constant observation for infection of the uterus (i.e. "Chorio-amnionitis")

Every Medical Center has their protocols for proper timing of delivery depending on the clinical factors involved with individual cases. Most patients with premature membrane rupture will go into spontaneous labor and deliver within a 3-5 day window. Once the amniotic sac ruptures, medications to stop labor are not very effective. Delivery is just a matter of time and, as with preterm labor discussed in the last section, the patient that is less than 34 weeks gestation needs to be admitted to a hospital in which there are neonatologists and a NICU.

6. Twin and Multiple Pregnancy, Just a few important comments ("Double Trouble")

If you are carrying twins, there are a few more considerations with regard to pregnancy that you need to know.

Hyperemesis Gravidarum (extreme nausea and vomiting in Pregnancy) is more common with twin pregnancy. When the usual treatments for nausea are not being particularly effective, your OB may suspect that twin pregnancy is the probable cause and order an ultrasound as seen below.

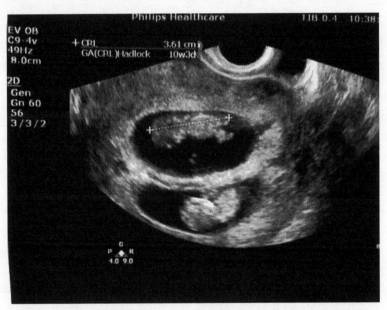

Figure 6-8 Ultrasound showing two babies in two different

Two placentas produce much higher levels of HCG and HPL (the pregnancy hormones) and nausea can be more severe.

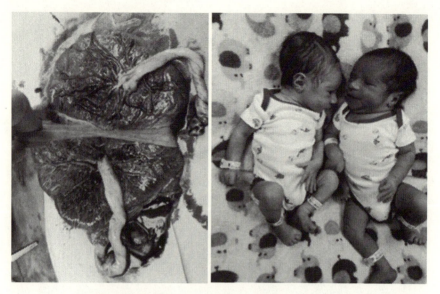

Figure 6-9 win Placenta with 2 umbilical cords from the birth of twin girls seen on the right

Your protein intake must be increased so that the babies fulfill their needs: 100 grams per day is a goal you should strive to attain (see a Registered Dietician for counseling).

- Your Iron intake must be increased: your iron is being siphoned off by two babies. Try to take Iron with Vitamin C three times per day. Of course, foods rich in iron include meat, liver, and cooking in an iron skillet. Anemia is quite common with twins and without adequate supplementation, the need for transfusion after delivery is even more a possibility.

- Gestational diabetes is increased with twins due to the increased demand for insulin on the maternal pancreas and the interference of insulin action from placental hormones. Overweight or obese patients further compound the incidence of gestational diabetes in twin pregnancy (and the likelihood for the need of insulin treatment).

- Approximately 50 percent of twins deliver prior to the last month (less than 36 weeks) of pregnancy. Premature labor is the most significant threat to the health of the babies. Most physicians recommend that patients with twins to drastically cut down on their physical activities and even quit their jobs in the last trimester. The most critical time for twin pregnancy is between 26 and 36 weeks of pregnancy: it is at this time that the babies become viable and are able to survive. The longer the pregnancy the lower the chance your child will be born with complications. The author tells his patients to stop working (unless they have a sedentary occupation) or work from home via Internet. Twins need to be incubated (just as if you were "a chicken sitting on her eggs!")

- If you have more than 6 to 8 contractions per hour, you need to get off your feet and drink fluids. If the contractions still persist, call your OB physician or go to the OB unit.

- Increased surveillance of twin pregnancy will be performed by your physician. Some of the parameters of evaluation will be performed regularly as follows:

a. Cervical lengths,
b. Individual growth of each twin along with any disparities of growth,
c. Amniotic fluid levels,
d. NST's and Biophysical Profiles,
e. Cord and MCA Doppler
f. The position, or lie, of each twin.

Pre-eclampsia (or toxemia) is particularly increased in incidence during twin pregnancy (especially if it is your first pregnancy or the twins were conceived with the assistance of IVF or other advanced reproductive technology (ART)

Many OB's will recommend preventative treatment of RDS (Respiratory Distress Syndrome) of the Newborn by administering Betamethasone in the 3rd trimester. Betamethasone is given as two injections of 12 mg usually 12 to 24 hours apart.

Triplets pregnancies, as one my patients told me who has triplets (my fertility treatment worked!), can cost a couple at least $400 per month in diaper expenses alone!

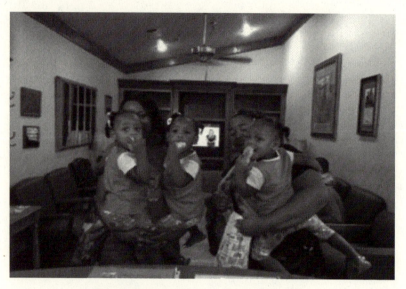

Figure 6-10 aruthers's Triplets at age 2
(Author used fertility medications in this couple).

7. Abruption of the Placenta

Abruptio Placenta means separation of the placenta from the uterine wall. The patient usually presents to the OB suite with "painful" 3rd trimester bleeding. Blood flow to and from the placenta and hence, the baby is directly affected. A major blood vessel bleeds between the placenta and uterine wall. A blood clot will form: it can stop bleeding or continue to bleed to the point where the entire placenta can be sheared off the uterine wall. If more than 50% of the placenta separates, the baby will usually not survive. Abruptions can occur at any time during pregnancy but mostly in the last 4 weeks of pregnancy. Some of the most common causes of abruption are as follows:

1. Cocaine drug abuse
2. Severe Pre-eclampsia
3. Severe blunt trauma to the patient's abdomen and uterus

4. Uncontrolled maternal hypertension
5. Fibrinolytic syndromes such as Factor V Leiden and METHR genetic variations
6. IVF/ART induced pregnancies

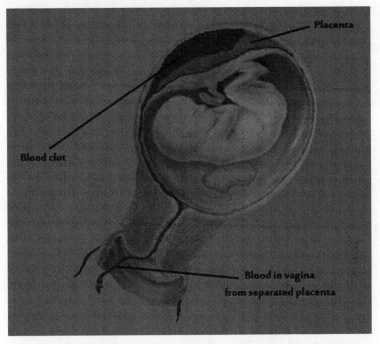

Figure 6-11-Placental Abruption with Illustration shows a large clot (Black area under placenta) with blood streaming down into vagina: Condition presents as painful 3rd trimester bleeding

Management depends on the extent of the abruption, the baby's toleration of decreased fetal-placental blood flow and the week of pregnancy the event occurs.

Case study: 22 year old female in her 5th pregnancy presents to the OB suite at 24 weeks gestation with vaginal bleeding and "labor pains." Fetal heart beat is absent on the monitor. Ultrasound confirms there is no fetal heart beat or circulation (*color-flow*) to the baby. She is 3 cm dilated and within a few hours she delivers a normal appearing stillborn baby girl. Her drug screen was positive for cocaine. It is learned that all of her previous children had been removed from the home because of chronic substance abuse.

8. Placenta Praevia

Placenta praevia is an obstetric condition in which the placenta is implanted just above the cervix: the patient presents with "painless" vaginal bleeding. Depending on the placement of the placenta with relationship to the cervical canal, placenta praevia is defined as follows:

Complete placenta praevia: the placenta completely covers the cervical canal

Partial Placenta praevia: the placenta covers part of the canal

Marginal Placenta praevia: the placental edge just touches the cervical canal

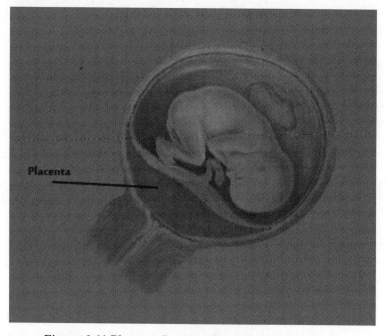

Figure 6-11 Placenta Previa. The placenta completely covers the bottom of uterus: the baby's pathway out of the uterus is blocked. If cervix dilates, the placental vessels can be sheared and cause excessive amount of painless bleeding

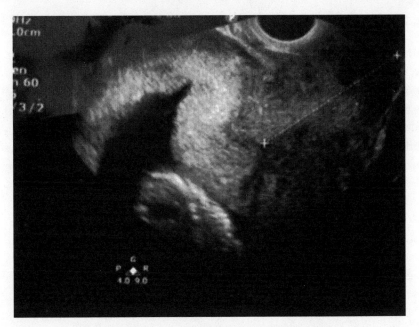

Figure 6-12 Placenta Previa on Ultrasound

Ultrasound picture showing the placenta covering the cervix: line shows axial measurement of cervix and the baby is above the placenta.

Further, there are "low-lying" placental locations that can also predispose to 3rd trimester bleeding. More often, the diagnosis may be made during the "anatomy" ultrasound between 18-20 weeks prior to any bleeding episodes.

However, bleeding can occur at any point in pregnancy after the first trimester. Sexual intercourse is obviously prohibited because penetration can disrupt the placental bed and bleeding can ensue.

The first bleeding episode usually stops with hospitalization and bed rest: it does not typically result in the need for delivery of the baby. Delivery is needed when the bleeding is relentless despite bed rest and transfusion therapy. C-section is the customary method of delivery (as the baby cannot deliver "through the placenta" without engendering extensive maternal hemorrhage).

9. Fetal Kick Counts and Fetal Movements

First time mothers will usually feel the baby's movement between 18 to 20 weeks of pregnancy. Second time mothers and others will feel the baby moving between 14 to 16 weeks of pregnancy. In the past prior to ultrasound exams coming into widespread use, OB's could "date" pregnancy by combining the day/week that the mother first felt fetal movements with fundal height (in centimeters) as well as the LMP (last menstrual period) and calculate the "due date" within a 2 week window of time.

Mothers will usually be conscious to the baby's activities: fetal kicks, fetal rolls, hiccups, etc. As is characteristic of children, a healthy baby moves around a lot. Sick children do not move but just lay around the house. Baby's that are "not well" are the same: their activities in the uterus decrease. Fetal kick counts are a way for the mother to check on the health of their unborn babies. Patients with high risk conditions, such as diabetes and hypertension, are asked by their OB's to do regular daily "kick counts." It is best to try and perform this "test," as follows:

<u>Fetal Kick Testing</u>. Start a journal with a pen close by: you need to be comfortable so that sitting in a chair might be best

Try to perform the test about the same time of day when the baby is most active: after meals or in the early morning

Record the date and time you start counting the baby's activities: rolls, movements, hiccups etc. all count as a "a kick"

Record the time you stop and count up the number of movements

Normal Test Results equal 10 movements in a 2 hour period of time

If the baby is not moving, he/she just might be experiencing a "sleep time." You might have a glass of orange juice or other source of energy and then restart the test. Most mothers will be "used to" feeling their babies in the background of their day to day activities and automatically sense that the baby is not moving as usual.

10. GBS Testing ("The Swab Test")

GBS (Group B streptococcus) is a bacterium that colonizes the rectal area in about 10-20% of pregnant women (depending on which population was studied).

At 36 weeks gestation cotton tipped applicator is swabbed from the vaginal opening down to the rectum. The test can be done earlier if a pre-term delivery is a risk factor.

Author Note: The timing of this test follows the study protocol as performed by the original NIH study. 36 weeks is not a "magical time" when Group B strep bacteria decide to manifest themselves. Further, in the original study, the swab was placed inside the rectum. Most OB's, including the author, just swab around the anal opening.

If a newborn baby comes into contact with the bacteria during the labor and delivery process, some babies can become contaminated and become infected. Newborn babies do not tolerate this infection and can become seriously ill. Because of the possibility of serious infection in the newborn, it is standard practice to take a swab from the rectal area of all pregnant women at 36 weeks of pregnancy. If the culture is positive, then the pregnant woman is treated with antibiotics when she is admitted in labor. Sterilizing the vaginal and vulvar areas prior to delivery virtually eliminates the infection in the newborn.

The bacteria are basically present in the rectal area permanently: it colonizes the area but does not infect the mother. The bacteria live in a *symbiotic relationship* with the mother due to her immunologic status. Treatment of the mother with antibiotics prior to delivery only eliminates the bacteria for a limited period of time. The bacteria re-colonize the same area within days: therefore, treatment is only administered at the onset of labor.

11. Vertex position in the 3rd trimester

Typically the baby's head will be positioned downward (upside down or the "vertex position") by the beginning of the 28th week. Once the baby's head assumes this downward position, it usually stays in this position. On the other hand, if the head is up or "breech," the baby's head will usually rotate into the vertex position by the 38th week of pregnancy. A discussion of breech babies late in pregnancy is discussed later in this book (External Cephalic Version section).

Beware of Author's Humor Spot below

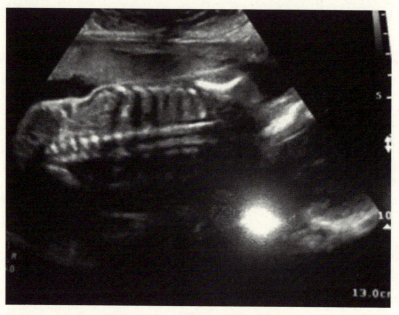

Above photo: Baby's Backbone

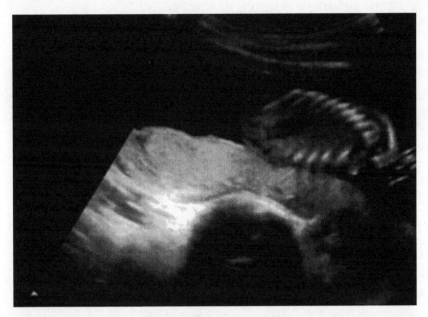

Middle photo: Baby's Ribs

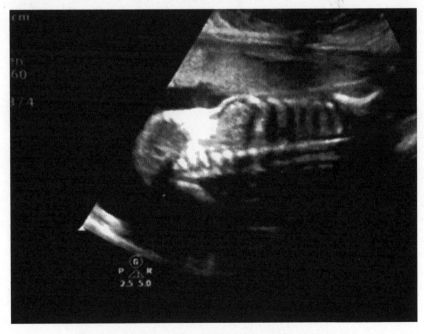

Figures 6-13, 6-14 and 6-15 Ribs and Backbone on ultrasound **Bottom photo**: "Baby Back Ribs"!

12. Fetal Surveillance testing (Baby "health checkups" while pregnant)

Besides checking on the health of the expectant mother, the OB office visits (OV's) is also directed to checking on the health of the baby at any given moment of time. Usually the OB will measure the length of the uterus (fundal height) and listen to the rate and rhythm of the fetal heart beat. In high risk pregnancy, further testing may be necessary as follows:

Fetal Heart Monitoring (the NST and the CST)

Fetal heart monitoring is a diagnostic examination of the baby's health status while pregnant. It is routinely utilized throughout labor (*Intrapartum*) but it can be also be utilized while still pregnant (*antepartum*) even when you are *not* in labor. I*ntrapartum* fetal Heart monitoring will be discussed in detail later in this book but the interpretation of the testing is the same. Fetal heart monitoring is performed for high risk pregnancies in which there is a possible risk that adequate circulation to the baby may be compromised. There are a number of medical and obstetrical conditions (diseases that affect blood circulation to the uterus, placenta and umbilical cord) in which antepartum fetal testing is helpful in the management of the pregnancy:

- Diabetes
- Pre-existing Hypertension and Pre-eclampsia
- Intrauterine Fetal Growth Restriction (placental or fetal causes)
- Oligohydramnios (low amniotic fluid levels)
- Twin or Multiple Pregnancies
- Collagen Vascular diseases (Rheumatoid Arthritis, SLE or Lupus, etc.)
- Placental diseases
- Umbilical cord problems (knot, cord wrapped tightly around neck, 2 vessel cord, straight cord or other cord anatomical abnormality)

The most important question is how the fetal-placental unit will provide circulation during a contraction. Remember: the circulation of maternal blood flow to and through the placenta and ultimately to the umbilical cord is impeded to a certain extent during a contraction. Blood supply to the baby is dependent on the mother's arteries to the uterus, blood flow through the uterine muscle to the placenta and through the placenta into the umbilical cord. Any compromise of blood can occur at any point in this pathway. Any disease or condition that affects the blood supply along this life support chain will prompt the need for fetal testing.

For the most part the Non-stress test (NST) is utilized during the last part of pregnancy when the pregnant is not typically in labor. The NST observes the baby's heart rate (FHT): its baseline rate and variability of heart rate and whether accelerations or decelerations of the fetal rate are present. Specifically the test looks for FHT "accelerations" in relation to the baby's spontaneous movements.

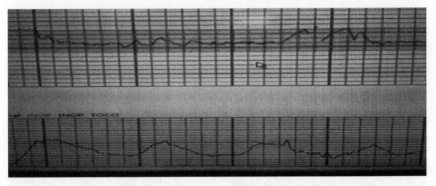

Bottom portions of graph showing "peaks" or contractions every minute. The upper tracing is the continuous plotted fetal heart rate. There are fetal heart accelerations above the baseline greater than 15 bpm for greater than 15 seconds. No decelerations are present.

The NST is considered normal if there are fetal heart accelerations (increase of 15 bpm over 15 seconds) with fetal movements

If there are any contractions, the test observes particularly for any fetal heart rate declarations. A contraction Stress Test (CST) looks at fetal heart rate variability as well as the presence of any decelerations/accelerations during a 10 minute window of time in which there are at least 3 contractions. CST's evaluate the baby's physiologic ability to tolerate labor contractions and ultimately labor itself. The CST was, in the past, the main test of fetal health but it was time consuming and expensive: it took at least 1-2 hours to perform. The NST supplanted the CST: it did not require an IV line and Pitocin infusion in order to produce uterine contractions. However, the CST did have the ability to *predict* that the fetal-placental unit would have sufficient reserve such that the baby would be safe to *survive in the intrauterine environment for at least one week*.

The Biophysical Profile (BPP). Real time Ultrasound is an important tool in evaluating the health of the baby. As described previously, anatomic abnormalities can be detected. Second, ultrasound can assess Fetal health by doing the "Biophysical Profile." There are 5 parameters of the test and each parameter is given a score of 2 points: amniotic fluid volume, fetal movements, muscle tone and reactivity, fetal breathing movements and the NST.

Criteria for BPP

Measurements done within 30 minute window	
☒ NST	Reactive
☒ Breathing	1 episode in 30 seconds
☒ Tone	1 flexion/extension
☒ Amniotic fluid	2 cm vertical pockets in L1 areas
☒ Gross movements	3 movements

Table 6-1 Criteria for Scoring a Biophysical Profile

Color Doppler Study of the baby's umbilical cord.

Even more helpful, when there is any ambiguity regarding the interpretation of the BPP or NST, a color Doppler can measure the systolic and diastolic blood pressure of the baby. The Systolic Diastolic ratio (SDR) is a reliable measure of the feto-placental circulatory capacity: especially if it can be measured during an actual contraction. The SDR ratio, of the fetal umbilical cord is most important in cases of oligohydramnios and intrauterine fetal growth restriction (these conditions can co-exist and be related). The S/D ratio of the MCA (middle cerebral artery) is most important in cases of fetal anemia (Rh or other ABO abnormalities, fetal hydrops and placental abruptions, etc.).

In clinical practice the NST is the "go-to" initial screening test for fetal surveillance for most high risk pregnancy conditions: diabetes, pre-eclampsia, chronic hypertension, advanced maternal age, post-dates pregnancy, etc. If the NST is "equivocal, "a Biophysical Profile (usually with an umbilical S/D ratio) may be helpful in determining if the baby is in imminent jeopardy.

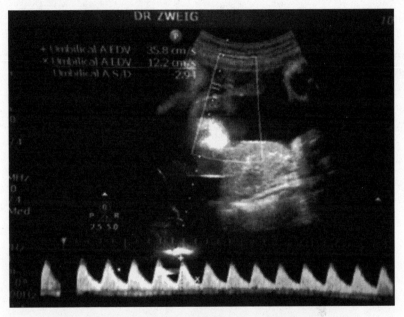

Figure 6-17 Color flow Doppler of cord The graph on the bottom shows peak and trough pressures and the S/D ratio is shown equal to 2.94 The Doppler window or equal sign in the color flow trapezoid is shown above.

13. 3D Ultrasound

3D ultrasound is another new development in the technology that allows physicians to see your baby better before it is born. 3D ultrasound may be the next advanced technological step your OB team will take in diagnosis a suspected abnormality or uncommon birth defect in your baby. It may be valuable in determining the *severity* of any given birth defect such as spina bifida or a heart abnormality. Real time 3D Ultrasound, i.e. "4D" is seeing the baby moving in 3 dimensions. In specific situations, such as imaging the constantly moving heart, physicians have further abilities to evaluate the anatomy of the baby's internal structures.

Today many physician offices and hospitals have ultrasound units that are capable of 3D renderings of your baby. It is good "PR" for physicians or hospitals to allow their patients see their baby as it would look after it is born. It allows parents to visualize the baby as being very much a real human and alive in appearance.

For these reasons, 3D ultrasound is used for commercial purposes or publicity. Many couples want "to see their baby" and their faces prior to birth. In some states, like Oklahoma, there are commercial stores (i.e. StorkVision) where you can obtain these ultrasound pictures and video without a physician's order.

3D ultrasound is best performed in the third trimester (30-32 weeks gestation) at which time the baby has accumulated enough weight, i.e. fat and other tissues, such that the baby can visualized more realistically.

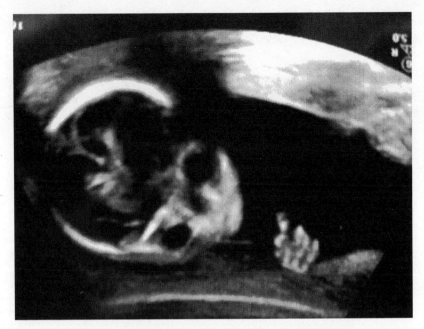

Figure 6-18 Ultrasound of baby's face and hand.

Ultrasound of baby in mid-pregnancy:

3D ultrasounds are best taken in late pregnancy so that your baby does not look like "Achmed, the Terrorist" (Credit, Jeff Dunham, Ventriloquist) as seen in the ultrasound picture above.

However, insurance companies will not pay or cover such ultrasound examinations. Depending on the "package" you purchase such photos of your baby will cost around $200. Many baby showers ("Grandparents to be") or Gender Reveal parties may gift the prospective parents such a 3D exam.

Bear in mind that in at least 30% of the examinations it is difficult to see the head clearly because the baby loves to keep its hands in front of their face. Some of these stores will allow you a second visit in order to capture better images of your baby and their "portrait."

These commercial Ultrasound stores have disclaimers that they are not liable for any defects or abnormalities that they may see. Most of the ultrasound techs are licensed and certified and most likely will refer you back to your physician if some abnormality is suspected.

The author's point of view is "just save your money and get a really great stroller. You are going to be seeing your baby almost every day for the coming years (except when they become teenagers!).

14. How long after my due date will my OB allow me to stay pregnant?

Most patients (>90%) will deliver within one week prior to or one week after their due date. Very few patients will go more than one week after their due date (assuming that their "due dates" are correct by early exam and 1st trimester ultrasound). If your cervix is not ripe for induction of labor at 41 weeks of gestation, your OB will perform "health surveillance" checks on your baby:

Non-stress testing

Biophysical profiles with or without Doppler (SDR) ultrasound of the umbilical cord

Labors that start naturally on their own are usually shorter and less invasive. Most OB's will recommend induction of labor if you go one week past your confirmed due date.

15. When can I stop working?

Most OB patients can work all the way up to their due date if they are so inclined. Most patients can take their "maternity leave" at 36 weeks or 4 weeks prior to their due date. Many patients can receive *disability* payments that typically start four weeks prior to their due date and end 6-8 weeks after delivery.

Patients may have to be taken off work sooner due to developing medical complications of their pregnancy. The most common causes for early maternity leave are as follows:

- Preterm Labor
- Pre-eclampsia
- Twins or other multiple
- Gestational Diabetes Class B through R
- Preterm Spontaneous Rupture of Membranes
- Intrauterine Fetal Growth Restriction
- Other significant co-existing Medical conditions:
    - Chronic Hypertension.
    - Lupus,
    - Rheumatoid Arthritis,
    - Heart disease,
    - Pulmonary or Lung conditions,
    - Liver disease

16. Cord Blood Banking

The expectant couple should be aware that it is possible to obtain some of your baby's cord blood for storage at a Cord Blood Bank. There are both "public" and "private" banking options. The baby's "stem cells" may be preserved for later use if certain childhood illnesses should occur in the future. Private Banking fees may average $2500 for initial set up costs and $130 for annual maintenance. There are a number of certified and licensed companies (such as CBR© and ViaCord©). Please note that couples should make preparations for such banking at least 8 weeks prior to their delivery date.

The reader is referred to the internet for more detailed information available regarding this option for parents. In the author's experience very few parents can afford or will necessarily need these stem cells for their child in the future.

17. 3rd Trimester Testing

It is in the 3rd trimester that certain laboratory testing needs to be performed:

a. "Pregnancy-related diabetes" screening will be performed by checking your plasma glucose level 1 hour after drinking a 50 gm bottle of glucose. This "screening test" should be performed between 24 and 28 weeks of pregnancy. It can be performed sooner if there are *increased risk factors* for diabetes as follows:

Obesity
Strong family history of diabetes
Glycosuria (glucose in urine),
History of large baby (greater than 4500 grams)
Previous adverse OB events such as stillbirths or congenital anomalies.

If your glucose level is higher than 135 mg then the standard 3 hour glucose tolerance test (OGTT) will be necessary for accurate diagnosis. The OGTT (100 gm glucose load) is performed after an 8 hour fast (usually overnight fast) so accordingly, most patients desire testing that is done in early morning. Hunger pains ("I'm starving!"), grouchiness and a lack of energy are not well tolerated by most people. Gestational Diabetes is diagnosed if two values are above the normal range:

- *Fasting level <95 mg/dl*

  1 hour<180 mg/dl

  2 hour < 155 mg/dl

  3 hours < 130 mg/dl

b. GBS (Group B Streptococcus) testing.

GBS testing is performed at 36 weeks of pregnancy. A cotton-tipped applicator is swabbed from the vaginal opening to and around the rectal opening. Should your test results show the presence of GBS, then antibiotics coverage will be initiated when you are admitted to the hospital in labor. Most OBs consider a patient GBS positive in a previous pregnancy always a "positive" GBS patient and not bother testing in future pregnancies. Testing may be done sooner for other indications: preterm labor or history of preterm labor, preterm rupture of the amniotic sac, etc.

Author Note: The above Guidelines are drawn directly from the NIH study on GBS testing in pregnancy. The test was performed at 36 weeks. Unlike common practice in the office, the swab is placed into the rectum during the study.

GBS positive patients live in a symbiotic relationship with GBS: it uncommonly infects the patient. GBS can initiate a urinary tract or vaginal infection. GBS is harbored inside the rectum. The 36 week timeframe is not a "magical time", i.e. GBS bacteria do not wait until this week in pregnancy to "hatch." GBS can spread from the rectum and colonize the vulvar and vaginal areas at any time during pregnancy.

18. "Nesting" Instincts

Sometime between 20 and 32 weeks of gestation the expectant mother will experience a natural urge to prepare her home for the baby. This maternal "nesting" instinct is produced by the varying levels of estrogen, progesterone and prolactin. Some of the behaviors that are exhibited are as follows:

> Cleaning and organizing the home
>
> Procurement of the "layette:" crib, changing table, blankets, diapers, clothing, etc.

19. Birthing Plans

A "Birth Plan" originated 4 decades ago in the 1970's. It was a time when obstetrics was practiced in a very controlled environment by the physicians and nurses. The 1970's were times when all previous routines and orthodoxy ways of childbirth were questioned. Questions quickly arose:

1. Why cannot the father of the baby be present in the delivery room?

2. Going one step further, why cannot the father of the baby be present in the C-section Operating Room as a support person for the mother?

3. Why do women need to be shaved or have enemas?

4. Why do I need to have an episiotomy?

5. Why do I need to have drugs or anesthesia such as an epidural?

6. Why do I need my labor induced?

There were many other questions. Consequently many expectant parents started doing their own research and education about childbirth. The practice of obstetrics changed dramatically:

1. ABC (Alternative Birthing Center) rooms were put into place in the late 1980's: now a woman could labor, deliver and recover in just one place without having to be moved from labor room to delivery room to recovery room and lastly, out to the postpartum floor. Hospitals and physicians saw the simplicity and the convenience of the birthing room.

2. Anesthesia was not always necessary: most moms in the 1970's and early 1980's were able to have an un-medicated birth.

Today obstetrics is a blend of the old and the new: most patients will labor and deliver in the same room and only later, be transferred to the postpartum floor: just a 2-step process. Most patients (>80%) today will desire the pain-free birth that an epidural provides. Most physicians are no longer shaving, doing enemas or cutting routine episiotomies.

There are the occasional patients that want a "Birthing Plan" so that the OB and the nurses can be aware of the patient's plans for her birth experience. Birthing Plan patients have researched information regarding their pregnancy (reading books like this one!) and well-educated in the process. Most patients want the birthing process to go as naturally as possible. Such patients request the following:

- Ability to be able to walk during labor
- Ability to take a shower
- Ability to suck on popsicles
- Ability to have supportive family and friends in the Labor Suite
- Ability to be free of IV's and fetal monitoring straps
- Ability to be able to interact with her OB and the nurses when "natural labor" is not proceeding "naturally" or as planned.

Most obstetrics today is practiced along *evidence-based* guidelines and protocols. Patients and OBs need to understand that these guidelines help achieve as much as a "natural "childbirth as can be possible. The *active management of labor*, as first promulgated at the Dublin Rotunda in Ireland, has been influential in lowering both the C-section and obstetrics complications rates in the United States and around the world.

The Ultimate Natural Birth Jinx

It is a well-known scourge among OB nurses and OB's that if a patient provides a written detailed birth plan, the plan in itself, is a curse to the patient. The birth plan seems to actually jinx a natural childbirth for the patient. It is "an old nurse's tale" that these patients increase their chances of ending up with a C-section.

It is okay to have a birth plan but it is more important that both the patient and her OB be very flexible: not everything works out just like you planned or what you thought nature intended.

Today's birth plans focus on the following issues:

1. When do you start Pitocin augmentation if my labor is not progressing?
2. When do you rupture membranes in the course of labor?
3. Will you use internal fetal monitoring: when and why?
4. How many people can I have present in the labor room? In the C-section room?
5. When will I be able to hold my baby and when can I begin breastfeeding and bonding
6. At what cervical dilatation can I have an epidural?

Please see the Appendix for a birth plan by one of our patients in 2014: we all planned her labor and delivery the way she did but, at the end, the baby was the person who was really in charge.

Though no one can go back and make a brand new start, anyone can start from now and make a brand new beginning

--paraphrased from Carl Bard

"Each of us has different talents, different dreams, different destinations, But we all have the same power to make a new tomorrow."

20. Other 3rd trimester Experiences and Feelings.

As the expectant mom gets closer to her due date, she will notice certain changes in her anatomy and physiology.

> Leaking Colostrum from the breasts (purchase those breasts pads sooner than later!)
>
> Walking is no longer possible but has changed to "waddling" from place to place (disregard people who make you feel self-conscious)

Pubic bone (Symphysis) pain. The weight of the pregnant uterus places pressure and pulls on all the ligaments of the bony pelvis. The pubic bone is separating to make more room: widening in response to hormone, relaxin. The discomfort can be severe and feels like your pelvis is being pulled apart. Further, the baby's head may be dropping into the pelvic inlet with pressure on your bladder. Consequently, there is less bladder storage capacity and more frequent trips to the bathroom.

Baby Hiccups. Yes, your baby can "get the hiccups" during the last month of pregnancy. The baby's diaphragm is trying "to work out" so this breathing muscle is ready when the baby pops out. The nerve supply to the muscle itself is maturing at this point in pregnancy.

Hemorrhoid Swelling: Hemorrhoids can swell and "pop out" particularly in the last trimester or last month of pregnancy. Drinking plenty of fluids (especially during the hot summer months), consuming enough fiber from fruits and vegetables, and avoiding prolonged standing can help prevent or decrease the severity of the swelling and pain during the last few uncomfortable weeks of pregnancy. Uncommonly, a thrombosis (or clot) forms in a hemorrhoid that may need surgical care prior to delivery.

Fetal Breathing Movements. Unlike the hiccups above, the baby's diaphragm is active and on ultrasound exams, you can see the diaphragm move up and down regularly. However, you cannot feel such movements. Fetal breathing movements (FBMs) are one of the 5 parameters of the Biophysical Profile: 10 breathing movements per minute indicate your baby is healthy.

3rd Trimester Check List

Pre-Registration at the hospital completed

Baby's Room is ready: crib or bassinette, diapers, receiving and baby blankets, clothes, etc.

Car Seat for Baby (baby can't leave hospital without it!)

Suitcase to be packed with normal over-night items (toothbrush, toothpaste, hair dryer, etc.)

Cell phone and camera chargers

Pads at home

Vehicle (or other arranged transportation) has gas and serviced to get you to the hospital

Child care, if any, for your other children has been arranged

If you have had a previous infection with herpes, start taking prophylactic medication

> **I finally understood what true love meant...love meant that you care for another person's happiness more than your own, no matter how painful the choices you face might be.**
>
> *— Nicholas Sparks*

21. Pregnancy Portraits

There is a special beauty of a woman when she is pregnant. There is a wondrous glow exuding from a woman who is expecting a child. Many women make an effort to capture that magnificence during their third trimester. As every trimester in your pregnancy is important to photograph, many women have chosen the last trimester as that special moment in her womanhood.

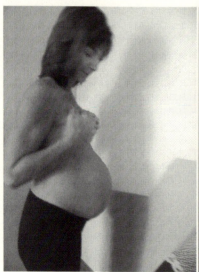 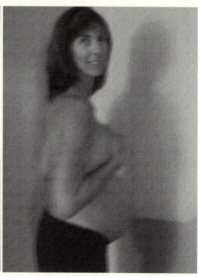

Figure 6-19 Pregnancy Portrait of Julie

Figure 6-20 Pregnancy Portraits of Julie

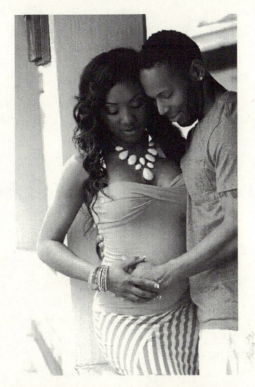

Figure 6-21 Pregnancy Portrait of Lataura

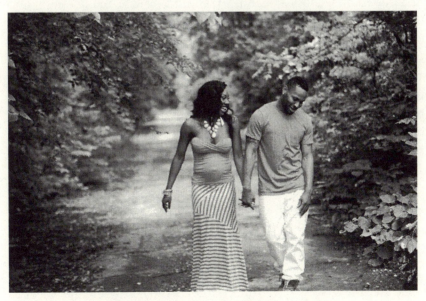

Figure 6-22 Pregnancy Portrait of Lataura

CHAPTER 7

Labor and delivery: How you can be "Birthing with the Stars"

The real climax to the long uncomfortable pregnancy is the process of labor with the "event"-ual delivery of your baby. "What is it all about?" is the question that is answered in this section. Labor and delivery conjures up images of women moaning and groaning in small hospital rooms. Their husbands or partners are seen at their side with little to offer except love, sympathy and emotional support. Realistically, labor and delivery in the US today can be as safe and as comfortable as you want it to be. Childbirth education, modern birthing rooms, labor-coaching techniques, safe medications and anesthesia as well as medical technology have made birthing a baby a positive experience. The following sections are intended to provide the information you need to understand the "miracle of birth." Each stage of the process is explained. After reading this material you may have had the wondrous vicarious experience of having just given birth yourself. The cloud of mystery will disappear. You and your partner can look forward to childbirth self-assured. You will be mentally and physically prepared.

1. Preliminary Remarks

Never a day goes by that a patient relates to this author some childbirth "horror story" that a friend or relative has experienced. The goal of childbirth is to transfer the baby out of your uterus and into your arms. Let me give you a "time frame" in which you can expect to deliver your baby:

- Primagravida (first childbirth): 12 hours
- Secundagravida (2nd childbirth): 8 hours
- Multipara (Third baby or more): even shorter!

I like to tell patients the following comparisons: having your *first* baby is like blazing a trail through the forest: it takes a long time to make a pathway. The *second* baby is like traveling down a country road. *Third* babies are like motoring down a highway. Having more than 4 babies is like speeding on the Interstate! You could get a speeding ticket (no, but your doctor might!).

Labor is managed by your Obstetrician and your OB nurses. OB nurses are the first to see if your contractions are adequate or not. The OB team is vigilant to be sure that your labor is "progressing." Your Obstetrician or OB nurse may insert an "IUPC," an intrauterine pressure catheter, to directly measure the strength of your contractions. If the proper the proper contraction strength ("Montevideo units") is not reached, your contractions may be augmented with oxytocin (Pitocin). Your OB team is on the alert to see if your baby is "too big" for your birth canal, i.e. your bony pelvic measurements. The OB team does not want you to be in labor any longer than necessary.

Painful labors and difficult deliveries are really "things of the past." Never has it been so safe, comfortable and satisfying to have a baby. But, the old adage is still true to some extent, "If there is no pain, there is no gain."

Through your research with friends and others, you have selected a most highly trained and compassionate obstetrician as well as a modern OB hospital birthing unit. You are now prepared to experience a wonderful birthing event.

2. When does Labor Occur?

For 80 per cent of patients, labor usually begins within two weeks of their due date. Ten (10) per cent of patients experience labor before the 38th week. Pregnancy usually spans forty (40) weeks from the last menstrual period (LMP). Ten (10) per cent of patients deliver after their due date.

First-time pregnancies (Primagravida) do not deliver "late" statistically—another old wives tale told too often told to many women.

In general, most OB's (and patients) desire to have their baby born no longer than two (2) weeks after the due date (unless there is a serious question about the accuracy of their due date). The placenta does not continue to grow or further develop after the fortieth (40th) week of pregnancy. However, the baby usually continues to grow at a rate of approximately a ½ to 1 ounce per day. After the 42nd week it is possible that the bay's growth and nutritionally requirements could outstrip its support supplier, i.e. the placenta. Obstetricians can evaluate and ascertain whether a decreased flow of oxygen and nutrients through the placenta is occurring after the 42nd week by biophysical and cord blood flow monitoring of the baby (see Sections on fetal monitoring). If the cervix is "ripe," perhaps you and your Ob may desire to induce labor by various methods (see section on induction of labor).

Remember that a "full moon, hot weather (your baby is not a chicken and not likely to "hatch"), castor oil, etc. will not make you go into labor any sooner!

3. But How Do I Know When I'm in Labor?

"Believe me; you'll know when you are in labor!" --Author

Author's Note:

I did not know the pain of a kidney stone or even knew what a kidney stone was until I had one. I was in incredible pain with nausea and vomiting. Even Demerol did not take the pain away. I have asked every one of my patients who have been pregnant and had kidney stones at one time or another, "What is worse: labor or the kidney stone?" Without a hesitation all my patients have said, "kidney stones!" So, as an OB, I can appreciate fully the pain you are experiencing. I know what it means when you say "that Demerol does nothing for the pain (but it just causes nausea)". Vomiting from Demerol along with the pain makes things even worse. The author has experienced labor vicariously with all five (5) of my own children (and some step children as well). He has almost passed out when he and his wife were holding their breaths and pushing together as she was pushing the baby's head out.

It is very unusual for patient *not* to know when they are in labor. Start timing your contractions.

Wait until your contractions are consistently down to 3-5 minutes apart for 45 minutes prior to going to the hospital.

<u>Author's Note</u>: I remember this 19 year old patient-teenager who presented to the ER with abdominal pain. She was pregnant and in labor. She delivered a healthy baby without problems. I remember making rounds on her the very first day after delivery. I looked at every non-verbal and body-language queue I could find after I asked her the real question, "So you really did not know you were pregnant?" She looked up at me and said, "No, I really did not know." To this day I believe her. There are a few women who will be in total *denial.*

Toward the end of pregnancy the uterus becomes more "irritable." It contracts and tightens up. The expectant mother feels "hardening of the uterus" or the abdomen. There periodic hardenings are known as "Braxton-Hicks Contractions. The uterus is toning up and gearing up for the "big events." With labor contraction the discomfort is "different." Instead of just hardening of the uterine muscle, the uterus tightens and constricts with a band-like 'squeeze" that involves both the front as well as the lower back. Theses contractions occur more frequently. There is a decided difference in their feeling and strength. At first contractions may be irregular, every 15 to 20 minutes. In other patients they may start out every 5 minutes and get closer together. Every woman and her labor is different and unique to her.

> *Just because your "mother had a "short" labor does not necessarily predict that your labor will be just as quick. It all depends to some extent on whether you inherited your body anatomy more similar to your mother than your father's family. Labor and delivery patterns and characteristics do not have any direct genetic or hereditary basis. However, if your mother had a C-section for "a small pelvis," there might be a slight increase in chances for a similar reason.*

There are a few situations in which the duration of labor can be shorter than normal:

1. Young mothers (18 to 26 years old) tend to have shorter labors due to their "younger" or "athletic" uterus
2. OB patients with pre-eclampsia or patients with a large gynecoid pelvis (author's observation)
3. OB patients with a history of endometriosis or prior D&C/Cervical surgeries (author's observation)
4. Small baby and mother with normal or large pelvis
5. Previous miscarriages, D&C's or LEEP/cervical surgery

I recommend that patients wait until the contractions are down to every 3-4 minute intervals for at least one hour before calling their physician or rushing to the hospital. First or second time mothers have 6-12 hours of regular contractions before they are most likely to deliver. Second or third babies are faster as your cervix has "stretched out" from previous labors. If you have had a quick first or second (or third, etc.) alert your OB so that you can report to the hospital "sooner than later!" Many OB's will do pelvic exams on their patients during the last 3-4 weeks of their pregnancy. These "cervical checks" ascertain how "thin" (or effaced, the medical term) as well as how "open" (dilated, the medical term), the cervix has become. If the cervix is already flattened and softened out, it can stretch easier and hence, quicker!

Table 6-1 the Four Stages of Labor

The Four Stages of Labor
First stage.
Latent Phase: the duration of time from the onset of contractions until 3-4 cm of cervical dilatation
Active Phase: the duration of time from 3-4 cm of cervical dilatation until 10 cm is achieved
Second Stage: The duration of time from complete cervical dilatation (10 cm) until the baby is born
Third Sage: The time from when the baby is born until the placenta is delivered
Fourth Stage: The most difficult and longest stage: it is the time from when the placenta is born until your child leaves home, graduates college and lands a great job!

Authors Note:

There is a somewhat of a humorous story about the question, "when exactly does a baby or human truly become *viable*, i.e. when it is truly "alive" and humanoid.

This moral question may be a legal or a religious argument. No matter. One day a Catholic, a Christian and a Jewish mother are discussing this particular issue. The Catholic mother states emphatically that a "human is life from the time of conception." The Christian mother hesitates and thinks about it. She finally remarks that she believes that "a human is life and viable when the mother first feels the baby move around inside of her." The Jewish mother is silent for a while. There is a prolonged and uncomfortable hesitation from the Jewish mother. Then, she exclaims to the other mothers, "I believe that a human is truly viable when she/he graduates medical school and opens her/his medical practice! (Yes, that was my Mom!)

4. Definition of Labor

Labor, to most people, means painful uterine contractions. However, a patient may have contractions and yet, not be in "true labor." Contractions, to be effective, must gradually thin and stretch open the cervix (the mouth of the uterus). Accordingly, labor is medically defined as contractions that cause progressive thinning, increasing dilation of the cervix and descent in the baby's head into and through the birth canal. Furthermore, labor contractions must cause the presenting part, usually the head, to descend deeper and further into the pelvis (i.e., the birth canal or "passageway"). "True" contraction must have "to do something." They must effect a true change in these three components:

1. Cervical effacement, or "cervical thickness of tissue thinning out"
2. Cervical dilatation, or enlargement of the cervical opening
3. Descent of the baby's head (or bottom!) further downward into the pelvis and through the vaginal canal

False Labor contractions may feel just as strong and as painful, but the main difference is that they do not cause any changes to occur in cervical effacement, dilation or descent of the head. In false labor, the contractions may start out at 15 minute interval, go to 8 minutes apart, and possibly even to 5 minutes. However, they do not become any more frequent. They can be very painful and therefore, the amount of pain the patient experience is not correlated with the act of being in true labor. In a short amount of time they begin to space out: they gradually become less frequent or slow down to 8 10 minutes apart. They eventually stop when one goes to sleep, lies down or rests for a while.

5. What is the Purpose of Labor? Your baby wants to Head Out!

The goal of labor is to get the baby out of the uterus (the womb). The nine month lease is "up" and the baby must vacate immediately!" Birth of the baby may be the first *rejection experience* that a human feels after being born! Basically, the uterus squeezes the baby out through the "mouth" of the uterus and pushes the baby out through the vaginal canal until the head bursts through the vaginal opening.

6. **What Does a Turtle-Neck Sweater Have To Do with Childbirth?**

It is sometimes easier to help patients understand the process of labor if one uses an example, i.e. an analogy. The neck of a turtle-neck sweater is a most appropriate "visual aid." I have always had a fascination with turtle-neck sweaters. When I have seen all those brightly colored sweaters on the counters in department stores, I have often wondered how anyone could put on one of those sweaters without first squeezing their brains out in the whole process! Even if one did manage to slip one of these sweaters on, I am sure they would strangle themselves to death by the time the turtle-neck reached down to the level of their necks! Some people with long necks look great in a 'turtle neck" but I was always worried that I would like my head was mounted on my shoulders!

A baby tries to squeeze his or her head through the cervix very similar to an adult stretching his head through the neck portion of a turtle-neck sweater. Just as you would put on the sweater and pull the narrow neck portion over your head, similarly the baby's head is performing the very same act: pushing through and expanding the cervical opening with the force of the uterine contractions behind it.

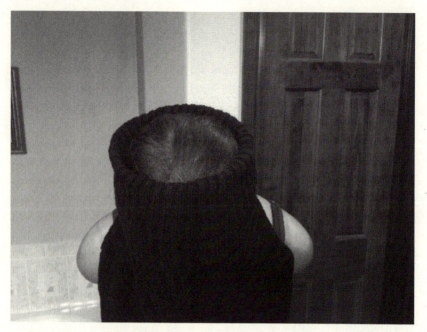

Figure 7-1 Cervical Dilatation Analogy. The neck of the sweater is dilating over "this babe's" head. Notice thinning of the neck portion.)

At first, the neck portion of the sweater is long and narrow. The cervix is also long and narrow until the last few weeks of pregnancy. As one pulls harder, the neck of the sweater becomes shorted. Similarly, the uterine contractions shorten and "thin" the cervix (the process of cervical "effacement"). When the neck portion of the turtle-neck sweater becomes completely flattened out on top of your head, it becomes much easier to pull your head through it. Similarly again, it is much easier for the uterus to **squeeze** the baby through a thinner barrier than a thick one. As one pushes your entire head through the stretched out neck of the sweater, the neck portion now can dilate or expand to fit over your head.

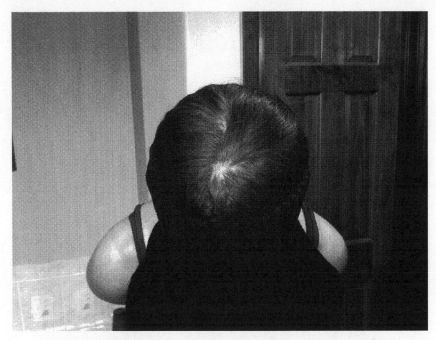

Figure 7-2. Notice that turtle neck like the cervix is now almost completely "dilated" and fitting over the neck.

The neck portion of the sweater expands and dilates until your entire head can fit through it. As in the case with labor, the cervix stretches over the top of the baby's head until it, too, can negotiate through the opening. Further contractions of the uterus push the baby through the vagina and out through the vaginal opening. The baby is thus born!

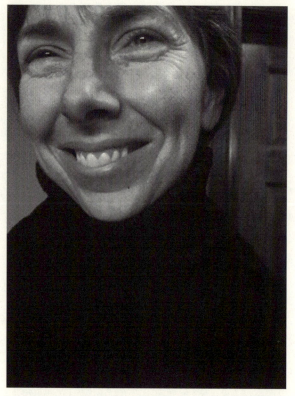

Figure 7-3 Cervical and Turtle Neck Dilatation The head is completely through the turtle neck sweater and "this babe" is ready to go!

Theoretically, one can surmise that the total length of labor depends on the following different factors (the four P's):

1. *The size or diameter of the baby's head (PASSENGER)*
2. *The rigidity or "stretch ability" of the mother's cervix (PERMISSIVENESS)*
3. *The strength of the labor contractions or "pulling/pushing strength"(POWER)*
4. *The diameter or size of the PELVIS (the birth canal or the PASSAGEWAY)*

7. "Engagement?" Doesn't that occur before marriage?

The medical term "engagement" means that baby's head has dropped into the true pelvis. For "primips," i.e. (primagravida or first time mothers) the baby usually drops downward into the pelvic cavity two weeks prior to labor. When the baby does drop or "engage," the expectant mother feels more comfortable and breathes easier now that the baby is no longer pushing up and compressing her ribs and constricting her breathing abilities. This "lightening" off the chest means that engagement has occurred. Engagement usually occurs in 80 percent of primagravida mothers within 2 weeks of their due date. It does not necessarily occur until the onset of labor in second or other subsequent pregnancies. It can be a red flag to the physician (and the patient!) if the baby's head does not drop or engage prior to labor in first time pregnancies, i.e. one can be suspicious that perhaps the head is too big or the pelvic entrance is too small for the head to drop in.

8. The "Mechanism of Labor"

The "mechanism of labor" is a medical term in OB textbooks describing how the baby "navigates" itself through the bony pelvis. As has been described earlier in this book, the baby must "jump through two hoops" that are in its pathway.

The baby's head is longer than it is wide. Further, the shoulders are wider than they are thick or deep. Fortunately our head and shoulders are perpendicular or 90 degree angles to each other. If you were a baby trying to get through the pelvis, you would have to figure out a way to "fit through."

First, you would flex your head onto your chin. Such flexion creates a smaller diameter of the head that has to fit.

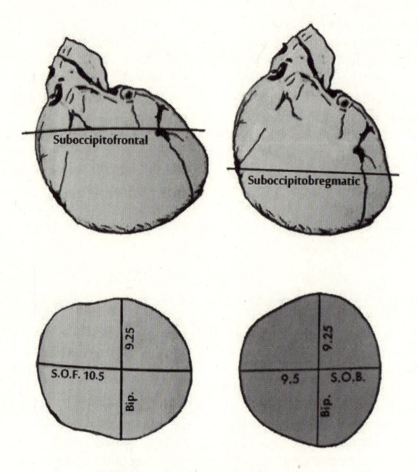

As flexion increases, anteroposterior diameter of head, which must pass through pelvis, becomes shorter. (From Beck AC: Obstetrical practice, Baltimore, 1955, The Williams & Wilkins Co.)

Figure 7-4 Labor, Head diameters.

The above illustrations shows that flexion causes the suboccipito-bregmantic diameter to be much smaller than the occipital-frontal diameter (Illustration reprinted with permission of Williams &Wilkins Co.)

Accordingly, the flexion allows the baby's head to fit through a smaller hole or accommodate to the small passageway. Because the top part or "inlet passageway" of the pelvis is wider than it is deep (in most women), the baby's head enters the pelvis looking to the right or the left side. The head further descends to the mid-pelvis. However, the mid-pelvis passageway is different: the ellipse rotates 90 degrees. Thus, the baby must turn his (her) head 90 degrees so that the long axis of the head (front to back) is now facing the mother's front or back. Just as the top of the head is turning to the front (or back) of the pelvis (internal rotation), the shoulders of the baby –which are perpendicular to the head, can now enter the inlet or upper passageway side to side. The breadth of the shoulders enters the top of the pelvis because the pelvis is wider than it is deep (as it was for the head).

When the baby's head is delivered through the vaginal opening (the baby's head extends or flexes upward) a very curious event occurs: the baby's head suddenly rotates so that the baby is looking sideways again (external rotation). There is a dramatic jerking around of the head, initially looking downward when it is born, and then suddenly turning looking to one side of the vaginal opening. The turning of the head sideways is caused by the shoulders turning in the mid-pelvis— where the ellipse is deeper than it is wide (the head had turned similarly when it encountered the mid-pelvic passageway's change in the elliptical direction). The shoulders must rotate 90 degrees just as the head did when it came to the mid-pelvic plane. The shoulder turn at the mid-pelvis causes the head to turn to the side as it is delivered through the vaginal opening. Thus, when the head is born, the shoulders are descending and hitting the mid-pelvis. The pelvic plane, the ellipse, rotates 90 degrees and the shoulders must face front and back in order to negotiate this change in the pelvic passageway. The baby's head and shoulders have thus jumped through 2 hoops: an ellipse wider at the top of the pelvis and another ellipse in the midpelvis that is longer front to back.

The mechanism of labor can be summarized by a definite 90 degree rotational movement by the baby's head and then the shoulders:

1. Descent
2. Flexion of the baby's head onto its chest
3. Internal rotation (looking to the front or back of the mother in the pelvis)
4. Extension of the head (un-flexing of the head or extension)
5. External rotation of the head (as the shoulders rotate front-back alignment in the mid-pelvic plane)
6. Delivery

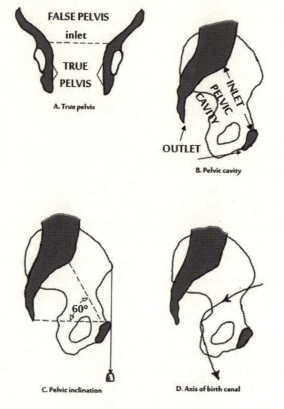

Figure 7-5 Birth Passageway.

Illustration above reprinted with permission (Oxorn-Foote, *Human Labor and Birth*) demonstrating the Inlet, the Mid-pelvis and Outlet planes of the pelvis.

The above illustration to really understand how the baby makes two major 90 degree rotations or turns as it travels its way through the bony pelvic tunnel.

9. Other Medical Definitions and Terminology

It is helpful to understand the medical language so that you, the patient, understand what is being discussed during your labor.

LIE. The baby normally lies up and down, i.e. longitudinally, with the baby's head in the pelvis and the bottom below the ribs. A transverse lie means that the baby is "side-ways" with the head on one side of your abdomen and the bottom on the other.

PRESENTATION. Most commonly, the head is pointed downward in the "launch" position. However, the baby's bottom can be the first part of the baby to deliver, i.e. breech presentations. The face, the brow and even an arm or shoulder can be the leading part of the baby in the birth passageway.

STATION. The station is the level at which the presenting part of the baby is located. "High station" means that the baby is still high above the half-way point of the passageway (the half-way point in the passageway is at the level of the pelvic spines, by definition). The midway point in the pelvis is called "Station 0." "Minus stations" (-3,-2,-1) indicates that the baby is 1 to 3 cm above the mid pelvic plane. "Plus stations" (+1, +2, +3) indicates that the baby's head is below the pelvic mid-plane by 1-3 centimeters).

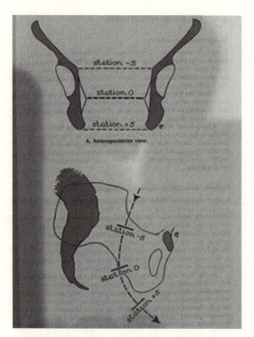

Figure 7-6 "Station" in the pelvis (reprinted with permission from Oxorn and Foote, *Human Labor and Birth*

Station is a very important parameter to understand: the baby's progress through the pelvic passageway is measured by each centimeter of distance it travels. It is also a measure of the effectiveness of the labor contractions.

POSITION. The position of the head, in which direction the head is pointed, can be quite variable. Obstetricians talk in terms of the "occiput, the back part of the baby head (because that is the hardest part of the baby's skull and is the most prominent part of the head – the head is flexed on the chest so the back of the head is easily felt). Consequently, the OB can feel the front or the back part of the baby's head during an examination. When the baby's head is facing downward, the top of the head, i.e. occiput is at the top (or the 12 o'clock position), i.e. occiput anterior or "OA." 90 percent of babies deliver with the baby's head facing downward in the OA position. The variation positions and their names are shown in the diagrams below.

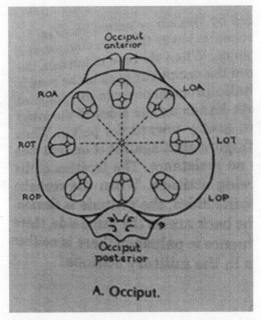

Figure 7-7 "Position" of the baby's head in labor (Reprinted with permission from Oxhorn and Foote, *Human Labor and Birth* Position of the baby's head in labor

When the back part of the baby's head is pointing downward (or is at the 6 o'clock position), the position of the baby is called "occiput posterior" or "OP." The author calls his babies that are looking "straight up" his "optimistic babies."

Author's Humor Moment:

Do you know the difference between an optimist and a pessimist?

A pessimist states the following, "All women are bad!"

The optimist says, in response, "I hope so!"

However, such OP babies have received a bad name. Most women have been told that "OP position" babies are responsible for harder and more difficult labors. Such OP, or posterior babies, has been implicated with the reputation in causing the infamous *"back labor."*

Back labor has the notoriety of being the most painful type of labor a woman can experience. Such an assessment is NOT *completely* true. First of all, almost all labor pain is radiated to the lower back, regardless of the baby's head position. Secondly, posterior babies eventually rotate to the anterior position in over 90 per cent of all labors. If rotation to the OA position does not occur, those babies can either delivered in the posterior position (sometimes requiring more stretching on the perineum or the need for an episiotomy). Further, if the baby does not turn to the OA position, the OB can attempt a manual rotation with his hands or even use an instrument to help guide the baby into the proper OA position—the position that results in a shorter 2nd Stage of labor and decreases the amount of stretching of the vaginal opening needed for the baby. Nonetheless, OP positions, in general, result in longer labors and lengthier times and efforts for 2nd Stage pushing.

10. True Labor: Sometimes may be difficult to diagnose!

As stated previously, labor is defined as contractions that cause progressive thinning and dilatation of the cervix. Unless one knows what the physical status of the cervix was before an examination, one pelvic examination may not determine whether the patient is truly in labor. Of course, if the cervix is fully effaced or over 4 centimeters (cm) dilated, these obviously advanced physical changes in the cervix can only occur in true labor.

Unless the patient has dilated passed 4 cm or has ruptured her membranes, the diagnosis of labor cannot always be made instantaneously: it is a diagnosis that can only be made over a given interval of time, i.e., two points in time.

The frequency and strength of the contractions must be evaluated. Still, uncertainty may exist, and the obstetrician may request that the patient return again to be checked in another hour or two. Two or more exams may be necessary to perform in order to fully determine whether a patient is indeed in "true labor." The contractions must be effective. They must first thin out or efface the cervix. They must open up or dilated the cervix. Contractions in true labor become closer together and stronger. They may start out at first being only 10 to 15 minutes apart but they get closer together and become 3 to 5 minutes apart within a few hours. Sometime they start out directly at 3 minutes apart and just keep getting stronger.

The frequency of contractions is timed from the start of one contraction to the very start of the next contractions. The duration of each contraction is timed from the first perception of the labor pain until the contraction is no longer felt.

Another sign of true labor is the substantial loss of mucus, sometimes mixed with blood that comes out of the vagina. The mucus plug that seals the cervix drops out when the cervix opens up or dilates. However, the loss of the mucus plug by itself does not consistently signify that you are in early labor. The cervix can be dilated by other causes than labor:

1. The weight of the baby's head on the cervix by its gravitational force
2. Relative weakness of the cervix with some dilatation as a result from genetic/constitutional factors, previous pregnancies or previous miscarriages, D&C's and/or deliveries

The loss of a large mucus plug with some bright red blood usually results from contractions. Labor is probably "just around the corner!" If the amniotic sac starts to leak watery fluid, you are considered to be *in labor*. When the cervix is in a state of advanced dilatation, i.e. over four (4) centimeters, then further stretching of the cervical tissue may cause the small blood vessels in the cervix to break and bleed a little. Bloody mucus fluid coming from the vagina and staining the inner thigh and pubic area, the so-called "bloody show," signifies that the cervix is in an active labor (greater than 3-4 centimeters).

11. The Amniotic Sac

In approximately ten (10) percent of all pregnant patients, the amniotic sac, i.e. "the bag of waters," starts leaking before the onset of contractions or labor. It is unclear what causes the membranes to rupture: labor contractions are not perceived by the patient- or there may be an underlying cervical infection. If a patient ruptures her membranes/amniotic sac prior to 36 weeks of gestation, "premature spontaneous rupture of the amniotic membranes (PSROM) is by definition to have occurred. The causes of PSROM include Infection, uterine anatomical abnormalities and footling breech presentations.

The closer the patient's pregnancy in weeks is to her duedate, the more likely she will go into spontaneous labor. At term i.e. near the "due date,") most patients will go into labor on their own within 12 hours of the membrane leakage. When the amniotic sac ruptures, the *sterile* compartment barrier between the vagina and the baby is broken. Bacteria in the vagina can easily spread upward through the cervix, through the hole in the amniotic sac and infect the baby and placenta. In 20 per cent of patients such bacterial colonization occurs within the first 24 hours of amniotic membrane rupture. Accordingly, most OB's prefer to have the baby delivered within that 24 hour window after membranes ruptures. On the hand, if pelvic exams are avoided and the GBS status is known and/or negative, watchful waiting ("expectant management") can also be an option. It is very difficult for an OB to "predict the future!" Some reasonable guidelines are as follows:

If the cervix is "ripe", i.e. thin and dilated: Pitocin (oxytocin) induction of labor may be a consideration

If the cervix is "un-ripe," i.e. thick and closed, *expectant management* (waiting patiently for contractions to start spontaneously --usually within 12 hours)is a consideration. Alternatively, oxytocin induction of labor may be started. The closer in time you are to your due date, the greater likelihood that your labor will start spontaneously.

A *favorable*" cervix is characterized as one that is:

Effaced (>80% thinned out or stretchy)
Dilated (open to a diameter of 1-2 cm)
Head is engaged ("dropped into the pelvis" at a minus 3 station or lower)

The author recalls a story by Jeff Foxworthy with regard to the childbirth of one his children: It was a story about SROM (spontaneous rupture of membranes) as it is summarized as follows

We had to go to childbirth classes. At the end of the last class we were given a "Labor Instruction Sheet." Under item number 3 it stated that "if your water breaks, you should refrain from any further sexual relations." He thought about this instruction and said, "I guess they would have never put this warning on the instruction sheet unless this scenario had become a *serious* problem. Hey, Honey, I know you're leaking fluid, but just before we go to the hospital I was thinking....."

12. The Bishop's Score

There is actually a Scoring System ("The Bishop's Score) that has been adopted by most OB's that assesses the likelihood of vaginal delivery success based on multiple factors as follows:

BISHOP SCORE N/A ☐

BISHOP SCORE	0	1	2	3
Dilation (cm)	Closed	1-2 cm	3-4 cm	≥ 5 cms
Effacement (%)	0%	40-50%	60-70%	≥ 80%
Station of vertex	-3	-2	-1/0	+1
Cervical Consistency	Firm	Medium	Soft	
Cervical Position	Posterior	Middle	Anterior	Total Score =

In general, the higher the Bishop scores, the greater likelihood of a normal duration of labor and the lowest chance of a C-section.

The Bishop Score is interpreted as follows:

<4 points: not favorable for induction of labor with increased risk of C-section

5 to 6 points: intermediate favorability for induction of labor

7 to 10 points: favorable for induction of labor with low potential of a C-section

13. Leaking Amniotic Fluid

Because of the risk of infection (from bacteria colonizing the placenta and baby from the vagina) as well as the risk of the umbilical cord falling into the vagina through the hole in the amniotic sac, it is prudent that the patient be checked at least once when such leakage occurs. Sometimes vaginal discharge, urine, semen or mucus may be confused with leaking amniotic fluid by the patient.

<u>Objective Testing for Amniotic Sac Rupture</u>

> The Amniosure™ Test
> The Nitrazene Paper test
> > Amniotic fluid is "basic" in acidity and turns the paper dark purple or dark blue
> Urine is "acidic" in acidity and the paper remains yellow
> Fern Test: amniotic fluid will crystalize on a dry microscope slide: crystals look like plant "ferns" when dried

Some OB offices may give their patients this "nitrazene paper" in order to avoid unnecessary trips to the Ob suite. The patient places this strip of yellow paper at the opening of the vagina where the fluid is leaking out. Normal vaginal secretion or mucus is usually acidic so the nitrazene paper usually retains its yellow color. Vaginal infections such as trichomoniasis can cause the paper to turn blue.

Author's Note:

It is not usually difficult to tell whether you have ruptured your membranes. If you continue to experience a constant leakage of fluid out the vagina and down your leg, you are most likely are leaking amniotic fluid. Rupture of the membranes does not usually stop: it is continuous whereas if the baby kicks your bladder, it is a one-time occurrence and stops. Much vaginal discharge or secretion that may accumulate overnight might "leak" upon arising: it may be confused with leaking amniotic fluid. Many vaginal infections such as yeast, BV and trichomoniasis can cause a profuse leakage of fluid.

Any suspicion by the patient that her amniotic sac is leaking should necessarily prompt an immediate call to her Ob's office or the Ob suite. During office hours (9-5 PM) call your physician's office for instructions. If there is some question about the membrane status many OB's prefer that their patients come to the office to be checked. After hours and on weekends, particularly if there is continuous drainage of fluid, even if you are not experiencing any contractions, the patient should proceed quickly to the hospital for an OB check. With the loss of amniotic fluid from the sac, very important "vital shifts" can occur:

1. Cord prolapse or compression: the "cord" can prolapse out the cervix or become compressed between the baby and the uterine wall

2. Fetal Blood vessels coursing through the amniotic membranes close to the site of rupture (vasa praevia) can be disrupted

In the OB suite the fetal monitor or ultrasound can be utilized to check whether any compromise has occurred to the baby due to the rupture.

<u>Danger signs of Amniotic Sac Rupture</u>

Significant bleeding

Color of the amniotic fluid is green

A loop of umbilical cord can be seen or palpated in the vagina

14. What do I do when Labor Starts?

If you think you are in labor or have ruptured your membranes, you should notify your OB's office during office hours or proceed to the hospital at all other times. Prior to going to the hospital it is customary to call the OB suite and "give them a head's up" that you are coming in. Frequently, if the OB nurses are tending to other patients, the OB suite will have to call in another RN to take care of you. Some OB's want you to call them at all times: the office during office hours or the answering service after-hours (usually the same phone number, i.e. the answering service picks up after hours).

Author's Note
It is important to keep your telephone line "open" after calling the OB's office. Your OB will usually call you back within 30 minutes. Remember that he/she may be taking care of other patients at all times during the day or night (doing a delivery or involved in emergency surgery). Wait until your OB calls you back before you start notifying the rest of your family that you are going to the hospital. OB's get upset when an "emergency call" comes in and the telephone line is continuously busy!

Options:

> Go to the Hospital. Regardless of day or hour, some OB's prefer that all patients proceed directly to the Ob suite.

> Go to your OB's office, if the problem occurs during office hours and the office is open. Such an option can avoid an unnecessary trip to the hospital (and charges!)

15. The Trip to the Hospital

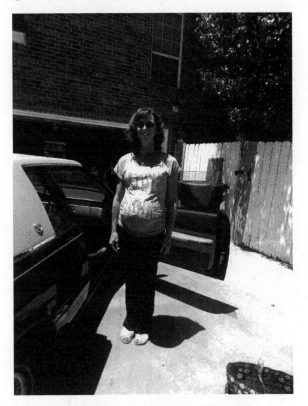

Figure 7-8 The Trip to the Hospital

Now that it is time to go to the hospital, please don't get over-anxious and over-excited.

Stay calm!

First-time mothers usually take an average of 12 to 14 hours to deliver their baby. Your husband (father of baby or SO, significant other) can grab your suite case, "labor bag" and camera and load everything into your vehicle. Buckle your seat belts and drive slowly and carefully.

During the last 4 to 6 weeks of pregnancy, you should be sure that your car is in good running order. Make certain that there is always enough gas in the tank. Better, yet, it is wise to have a back-up method of transportation (such as a relatives' or neighbor's car because "dad" may be at work or, if in the military, "out in the field"). As a very last resort, call the fire department, police or paramedics for help.

Make arrangements ahead of time for your other children. It is not appropriate to bring them to the hospital while your wife (baby's mother) is in active labor. The hospital staff cannot care for them. In an emergency you can proceed directly to the OB suite with your other children but you should be calling for their care providers at the same time.

When you reach the hospital, your husband (or relative, or whoever brings you!) should drive you to the emergency entrance to the hospital. Follow the signs posted "Emergency Room" or "Ambulance Entrance." During your pregnancy or your hospital OB tour, check out where the "ER" is located and the OB Departments directions on where to go when you are "in labor." If you are in "early labor and the contractions are not too painful, it is permissible to park in the main parking lot and walk into the ER or Admissions area. From that point both of you can take the elevator to the OB suite. Most of the time "labor patients" are brought to the ER and then wheel-chaired up to the OB suite while the driver parks the vehicle and goes to Admissions to check in—much like checking into a hotel! The OB nurses are going to take some time in admitting you to the OB suite (medical information gathering, undressing, fetal monitoring, consent process, etc.). Simultaneously, the driver can park the vehicle, go to the Admissions office to verify demographic data, bring up your suitcase and all other necessary belongings that have been left behind (phone and camera charger, blankets, pillows, and most importantly, cookies and brownies for the nurses!).

If labor contractions are too uncomfortable to permit walking, you should be driven directly to the ER. Whoever is driving should stop the car outside the ER entrance, go inside the ER and alert the ER clerk that you have a "mother in active labor" that needs immediate assistance.

Authors Note: An OB patient in labor gets the ER personnel's attention faster than any other emergency! No doctor or nurse in the ER wants to be involved in this "mysterious complicated process" of birth that just might happen immediately in front of them! Never will you see a patient get transported out of the ER faster than that of an

OB patient. Transit times from ER to OB suite are as reportedly as fast as the Indy 500 qualifying times!

At this point the ER personnel will come out to your car with a wheelchair or gurney. From the ER you will be transported to the OB suite. The husband or driver can now re-park the vehicle in the visitor's parking area. Depending on the circumstances, your suitcase and labor bag can go with "mommy" or brought to the labor suite later. If the neighbor has brought you to the hospital, then hopefully someone has been able to reach the father or left a message at his job to let him know that you are at the hospital.

When the *husband* has driven to the ER and after he has already dropped you off, he should re-park the vehicle and check in with the Admissions office (or ER Admissions after 5 PM). He will notify the Admissions clerk about his wife's admission to the OB Suite. Because most patients have pre-registered at the hospital during the last part of pregnancy, there should be a very minimal amount of paper work be left to be filled out and signed. The husband can then proceed to the OB suite to join his wife. If not pre-registered, the Admissions Clerk will obtain the necessary personal information, i.e. full names, address, phone numbers, age, employment, insurance plan information, etc. If the OB patient is in "hard labor," i.e. contractions every 2 minutes with some bloody show, delivery is probably "imminent." The expectant father should accompany his wife to the OB suite (and not worry about "the bags"). The OB staff does not want the new father to miss "the Grand Finale" to the pregnancy! Admission forms can always be filled out later.

Patients should plan the following:

1. Pre-Register with the hospital at the beginning of the 3rd trimester (about 30 weeks)
2. Sign up for the OB Tours or "Teas." Call the hospital and ask to be transferred to the Education or OB Department for the schedules and times. Check the Hospital Website for important information.
3. Do a "Dry-Run." Do drive to the hospital as if she were in labor. "Practice makes perfect." Be aware of traffic conditions

in your area at different times of the day. Drive to the ER entrance and the Visitor's Parking lot. Find out where the Admissions office is located. Visit the OB suite. If you have questions, ask them!

Getting back to our patient in labor, she will be checked in by one of the OB nurses. She will be weighed and then brought to the labor room to undress. She will have her vital signs taken and the fetal monitor belts will be applied. The OB suite usually gets a phone call from the emergency room that Mrs. "So and So," a patient of Dr. "What his name," is on her way up from the ER. While the expectant mother is being wheeled up to the OB suite, simultaneously the OB nurse will go to the Prenatal Files and pull out the OB chart (either on paper or on computer Electronic Medical Records) along with the doctor's standard admissions Orders.

The labor nurse will have you undress and put on a hospital gown. She will take your weight, blood pressure, pulse and temperature. She will strap the fetal monitor (2 external belts) to record the baby's heart rate and the frequency of your contractions. She will confirm (from the prenatal records and from your own verbal information) your age, gravidity (the number of pregnancies), and parity (number of deliveries), status of your amniotic sac (ruptured or not) and your due date. If there is any possibility that the amniotic sac has ruptured, she will test for membrane rupture with the Amniosure© test or other testing that is available. The degree of cervical effacement and cervical dilation, as well as the baby's station, will be assessed. The frequency and strength of the contractions, if any, will be observed. This "Labor Check" evaluation by the labor nurse will then be reported to your physician. Depending on the situation you may or may not be admitted to the hospital. If not admitted, you may be asked to return when your contractions are more frequent or stronger. If admitted, a more extensive medical interview will be taken by the labor nurse. Routine items include the time your contractions started, allergies to medications, etc., presence of other medical conditions, complications of your pregnancy to date, previous pregnancy problems if any, medications presently being taken and your last ingestion of fluid or food. She will review your birth plan and ask about your expectations during labor and delivery. She will inform you about the various medications that are available for pain relief as well as the types of anesthesia that are available during your labor.

Reason for not being admitted during this time: You are not "in labor:"

1. Irregular contractions
2. No or minimal cervical effacement or dilatation
3. Membranes (amniotic sac) have not ruptured
4. Normal Fetal Heart Tracing

At this point, your husband (or SO, Baby's daddy=BD) will usually arrive in the labor room. He will check with the nurse and then question you about the status of your labor. He may bring items such as the camera, cooler/thermos or a packed meal from the car.

The labor nurse will put on your hospital wrist band. The wrist ID band is very important. It identifies you as a patient so that hospital personnel are performing tests and other examinations on the right patient. All Laboratory, X-ray, nursing and operating room personnel must check your wrist ID bracelet before any procedure is performed on you. Of particular importance is blood drawing and testing. ID's bands must be checked prior to the following nursing actions:

a. Medications given
b. Baby brought into the room for feeding
c. Any IV solutions
d. Any blood or blood products are given to the OB patient.

On the postpartum floor no baby is given to a mother for a feeding until that mother's ID bracelet is check with the ID bracelet of the baby. If your bracelet or the baby's ID bracelet comes off at any time, please notify the nurse so that a new bracelet can be mad made and placed around your wrist.

16. Video camera or other recordings of the baby's birth

Please check with the nurses regarding the official Hospital policy of video-recording of the baby's birth. Most hospitals will not allow actual recordings of the baby's birth whether it is a normal vaginal birth or by C-section due to liability issues. It is equally important that the husband or other support persons to not allow such private picture-taking to interfere with the mother's privacy, concentration, excitement or her medical care. Check with your OB as well as the hospital in advance about the recording and photographing polices. Sign the necessary permits, if any, as early as possible. Organize and have all such equipment ready to go to the hospital when labor begins. In advance, designate who is going to be operating this recording equipment.

17. How many people can I have in my Labor and Delivery Room? Can we have Cameras and Videos?

Each hospital and physician has their own rules regarding the number of adults that can be present in the room. Please check with your hospital OB nurses and your physician for their policies.

Labor and delivery of a baby is the most stressful and uncomfortable event that a woman will feel in her lifetime. It is advised *not* to have minor children present as they cannot understand the pain you are experiencing. It can represent a very frightening experience for them.

When you are in labor, you cannot "be yourself." You cannot disguise your physical pain and your emotions. You cannot hold back and "entertain" your family and friends while you are laboring. Unless these folks present are "comforting" to you, I would restrict their presence. As Eldridge Cleaver once said (re-phrased), "If they are not there to be part of the "solution", then they will be there to be part of a "problem."

The picture below illustrates how many people show up for your *birthing event*. As Gretchen Wilson states in her country song, "I'm just here for the Party." Believe me, they will not be there for you at 2 am when your baby is crying and you cannot do anything to console her.

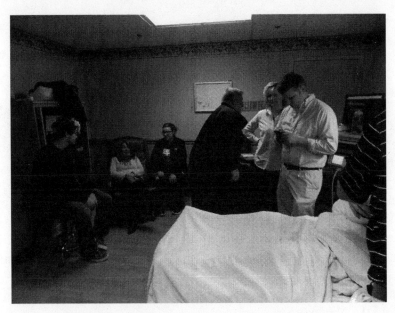

Figure 7-9 The typical Delivery Room Audience

Each hospital and physician has their policy regarding photography and video of the labor and birth. Each patient has to think seriously about the very personal nature of these "pictures" (especially if they get posted on Facebook and other sites!).

Author's Note:

I am somewhat surprised how many patients have their birth videoed. I had always advised patients to just point the camera on the baby and avoid not capturing the mother's "private parts." There are several "Kodak moment" shots that should be taken, such as the moment when the baby placed on the mom's abdomen, the father cutting the umbilical cord, the kiss the father gives to the new mom after she has delivered his baby and lastly, the baby being weighed on the scale.

I sometimes joke about folks who video record the baby's birth. I might say to the couple that, "Videoing the baby's birth is like reading the final chapter of a book without reading the first chapter. I mean, should you not have also videoed the conception as well as the birth?"

18. What if my doctor is not there?

It is true that your doctor may not be the doctor who delivers your baby. Pregnancy is a nine (9) month "construction project" and your doctor may be at a medical conference or on vacation when you go into labor. Illness, weekend trips or sudden family obligations may prevent your physician from being able to attend your delivery. Even if he/she is in town, he may have been up the previous entire night with another patient and is too exhausted to be with you. Occasionally, he may be doing surgery at the very moment you are ready to deliver. Because he cannot always be sure that he may be available 365 days a year and 24 hours per day, all physicians have "back up" coverage arranged so that any situation will be addressed. Usually this back-up physician is his/her associate or partner. If your doctor's back-up physician is not in the same office, he may have you meet him/her by arranging a courtesy appointment with him/her during your pregnancy.

When an obstetrician cannot be available to his/her patient because of vacations, meetings, etc., he usually "signs out" to the on-call physician. He informs them of which patients are likely to go into labor and which patients are having certain medical problems. He tells them about any important personality characteristics of his patients. Five (5) weeks before your due date your physician will have forwarded a copy of your prenatal records to the hospital or other birth center. Your complete medical history, physical examination, laboratory testing and any other studies are documented and sent to the OB suite so that they may be available at all times when you come into the hospital. Any significant medical conditions, social circumstances and individual features of a patient are usually recorded in the medical chart. Increasingly the OB's records and the Hospital electronic computer records are integrated or accessible by the OB nurses.

Most OB physicians associate with other physicians who have similar training and education. They usually share similar attitudes and views about childbirth. In smaller communities in which only one or two other physicians practice, there may be little choice for both the patient and her doctor about who will be covering in your doctor's absence. A "Birth Plan" or "Preference Sheet" is an ideal way of communicating your thoughts and plans for your childbirth for the substituting physician on-call. Examples of Birth Plans are reproduced in the Appendix of this book. The on-call OB usually cooperates and honors such birth plans as much as possible.

There is no question that your physician has mixed-feeling about not always being available to his patients. The emotional and personal relationship is felt equally by him/her. For the patient to feel that a vacation or conference is more important than the birth of your child is unfair to your OB. His/her personal time off is absolutely necessary for his mental and physical well-being. Otherwise, he cannot continue to give his patients the quality and personal care they desire and deserve.

19. Eating during Labor? I don't think so!

With the onset of your labor contractions solid food should not be consumed. In a very real sense, the entire body's attention and energies are directed toward the contracting uterus. Blood flow is redirected away from other organs, especially the stomach and intestine. Oxygen, nutrients and glucose is delivered to the contracting uterus. Accordingly, the stomach and intestines (the gastrointestinal tract) must "shut down" to give the uterus the "priority." Digestion almost ceases and food that was eaten just sits in the stomach. Furthermore, during the most intense phase of labor, the nervous system becomes highly irritable. The overwhelming number of nerve signals from the uterus stimulates the vagus nerve which, in turn, reflexes such stimuli back to the stomach. Nausea and vomiting ensue. It is because of the frequent nausea and vomiting during labor that physicians (and the nurses who have to clean up your mess!) caution their patients not eat at any point during labor. One of the stories in the section, "Old OB's Tales," entitled *Typhoon Yaling/Patsy* addresses this issue of eating during labor.

<u>Author's Anecdote</u>: It is really not thoughtful for family and friends to bring food into the labor room when a patient is in labor. In 2015 Oklahoma passed "The Consumption of Food in the presence

of a Woman in Labor Act." It is strictly prohibited by State Law. Under the provisions of this new law, a patient in labor can legally kill anyone who brings food, especially pizza, into the labor room (see the "insanity defense clause" of the law, OK Criminal code § Section253, p.931). On the other hand, the new law specifically describes the responsibilities of all birth attendants (family and friends) the appropriate types of food and deserts that they need to bring and furnish for the starving nurses!

20. The Umbilical Cord

During the late stages of pregnancy many patients ask the author frequently if "my baby's umbilical is around his/her neck?" Studies show and, in the author's experience, that there is a loop of umbilical cord around the baby's neck in 25% of all deliveries. 80% of the time the cord loop is "loose" around the neck. Even if the cord is "snug" around the neck, uncommonly are there any serious consequences. If there is significant compromise of blood flow to the baby by the "nuchal" (or other compression by the baby's body), such problems will manifest themselves on the fetal heart tracing. Category 3 FHT strips will be managed appropriately by the OB staff. C-Section intervention is available at any time when there is any potential harm for the baby's health.

A "true knot" in the cord is very uncommon. Again, 90% of the occurrences do not impact the labor and delivery. In the illustration below, the patient delivered a very healthy baby after pushing for over 90 minutes:

There is no intervention the OB can perform to effect unwrapping or otherwise manipulate the cord during pregnancy. During Labor and Delivery "cord compression" can be treated by repositioning of the mother, and or an amnioinfusion. Lastly, if severe cord compression is occurring, the patient may have to be delivered by an immediate C-section.

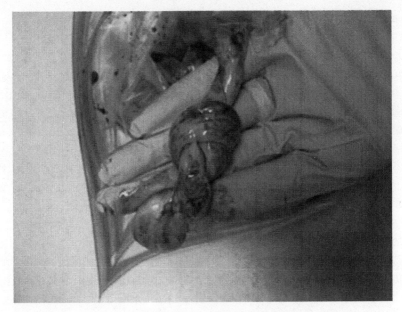

Figure 7-10. True Knot in cord.

21. The Emergency C-section and the prevention of Aspiration

(Aspiration is the vomiting up of stomach contents into the Lungs)

Further, because it is never known whether or not a patient may need an emergency C-section at any given moment (and may need to be "put to sleep," i.e. a general anesthesia), a full stomach of food can be aspirated into the lungs during the initial push of medication. The patient can vomit even before a tube can be put down the trachea to protect the airway. When the baby is "in distress," a baby can become asphyxiated and acidotic within 5-10 minutes depending on the individual clinical situation. The OB staff must use a "general anesthetic" as the fastest and most effective way to anesthetize the patient for a "stat" C-section delivery (as opposed to the longer set up times for a spinal and epidural). In many emergency situations the patient is already in advanced labor and an epidural has been placed: it just needs to be reinforced with more anesthetic.

All patients in labor should restrict themselves to a "clear" liquid diet: ice chips, broth, soup, juices, teas, etc. If a general anesthetic becomes necessary for an immediate C-section during labor, it is possible that all solid foods present in the stomach could be regurgitated into the lungs in the unconscious patient (*aspiration*). Food particles can be inhaled deep into the lungs and enter the small airway passageways. Of much more serious concern, acid liquids and enzymes (peptic and hydrochloric acids) can digest way lung tissues. Oxygen absorption and gas exchange can be drastically compromised. Pneumonia, lung damage and subsequent respiratory failure could ultimately lead to the patient's death. To prevent such a sequence of events, anesthesiologists and nurse anesthetists (specialists in this field) routinely place a small breathing tube into the trachea (windpipe). Such intubation effectively seals off the respiratory tract from the mouth and stomach so that vomited liquids and solids bypass the tracheal opening and continue up into the mouth. When such solids/liquids reach the mouth the anesthetist can then suction them out of the way. However, there are two (2) special times when aspiration, i.e. the regurgitation of acid liquids and solids, can occur despite the routine practice of intubation:

1. Just after sleep is induced when the body's muscles are temporarily paralyzed with drugs, reflex regurgitation can occur while trying to pass the tube into the trachea, i.e. during the initial attempt to intubate.
2. Just as the sleep and paralyzing drugs are wearing off and all reflexes are coming back, the labor patient may become nauseated and vomit just as the tub is being removed, i.e. during the immediate time just after extubation.

22. The Process of Labor

Many patients have asked me to describe how a "labor pain" feels. Phyllis Diller, a very popular comedian in the 1970's, humorously answered that question as follows,

> If you take your upper lip and then pull it up over the back of your head, you may get an idea how painful the stretching pain of labor feels like!"

Labor is truly felt and experienced differently by women of different ages and across ethnic groups and races. Dr. Ferdinand Lamaze, on the other hand, would "take exception" to my use of the term "pain." In his opinion labor pain is a "learned reaction." No pain would be experienced by a labor patient if she were not told over and over again that "labor is painful." With due respect to Dr. Lamaze, I disagree. Uterine contractions and the stretching of the cervix impact stimulate the very sensitive nerve ending in the cervix. Those nerves send real pain messages (stimuli) to the brain via the spinal cord. How these pain stimuli are interpreted is more of a "hard-wired" instinctive human sensation than a learned response. Yes, the sensation of one's pain can be modified by several variables: one's education, culture, race, upbringing, coping mechanisms, etc. and somewhat significantly, the "fear of the unknown."

Author's Note

The author himself has experienced several kidney stones. The first kidney stone he experienced when he was a 2nd year medical student. The pain, along with the reflexive nausea and persistent vomiting was not a "learned response." It was "real pain" emanating from the blockage of his ureter and the contractions of the muscles in my ureter trying to squeeze my stone into the bladder. I have asked all my patients who have had babies and kidney stones, "What is the worse pain?" Without hesitation they have all said kidney stone pain was "the worst" pain. I can reiterate the same statement that all of my labor patients have relayed back to me: "Demerol does not help the pain. It just takes off some of the sharp edge of the pain and makes me sleepy."

The length and course of labor is a crucial variable in the "pain experience." As President Franklin D. Roosevelt (FDR) said long ago, "the worst thing we need to fear is fear itself." It is the purpose of this section is to help you understand the process of labor and to know what to expect during childbirth (especially the usual length of labor). Armed with knowledge you will be in control of your labor, rather than labor controlling you. This childbirth education arms you with information and expectations, with no fear of the unknown. You are more mentally and physically ready for your impending childbirth experience.

23. The Typical Scenario of Childbirth

This brief scenario which is played out daily in delivery rooms across the country gives the reader an idea of the usual childbirth experience (please refer back to Pictorial Tour of Labor and Delivery in Chapter 4):

Mrs. Mary Smith experiences the onset of her labor contractions at home at 6 a.m. The contractions are approximately five minutes apart. At 8 a.m. she is checked by her physician. Her contractions are now three minutes apart and moderate in strength. The cervix is ninety percent effaced and three centimeters dilated. Her discomfort is moderate and she requests something to "take the edge" off her sharp labor pains. Stadol, a non-narcotic analgesic is injected into the small intravenous (IV) catheter placed in her hand (or can be given IM). She begins to feel relaxed and the contractions are less uncomfortable. At 10 a.m. her cervix becomes 5 centimeters dilated and one hundred percent effaced. At this point the Stadol has worn off and the pain is very intolerable. She requests an Epidural. An Epidural is placed and her labor pains are just "hardening of her abdomen" and barely perceived. The amniotic sac is bulging with fluid. A small hook is utilized by her physician to put a small hole in the sac and release the fluid pressure. Releasing some of the amniotic fluid in the uterus decreases the volume inside the uterus. The uterine muscles can now contract more efficiently (physics principle: squeezing down or pressure against a smaller volume, i.e. the baby, results in a greater force and effect). Also, at this time the color of the fluid is checked. Occasionally green-tinged or meconium-stained fluid may be present. It may be a sign that the baby may have been stressed. Pelvic examination at this point reveals that the cervix is currently seven centimeters dilated. The contractions become more effective — two minutes apart and moderately intense. At 2 PM the cervix is completely dilated and the head is at a plus one station. The occiput, or the back of the baby's head, is facing upward (OA). The pressure of the head against the rectal tissues gives the patient the sensation that she needs to go to the bathroom (as if she needed to have a bowel movement). Due to this rectal pressure she pushes just as if she were pushing out a large stool. In this case, however, mother is pushing out the baby's head. Within 45 minutes she feels the burning and stretching discomfort of the head ballooning open the vaginal orifice. Preparations for the delivery are made. Depending on the degree of numbness on the patient's bottom, a "local" skin block may be given to anesthetize the vulvar skin between the vaginal opening and the anus (less commonly used today, a pudental block may be given to numb the vaginal and vulvar tissues). This area bears the brunt of the vaginal opening stretch and can be torn. A cut into the skin directly at the bottom of the vaginal opening downward is made with a scissors. Such a deliberate cut is called an "episiotomy" and is only performed by physicians wishing to avoid irregular tearing of vulvar and vaginal tissues. With further pushing efforts on the part of the patient, the head is delivered over the episiotomy. The baby's nose and mouth are suctioned with a bulb syringe. Any loops of cord around the neck (present in about 25 percent of all births) are pulled back over the shoulders. The patient is asked to push again and the rest of the baby (the shoulders, abdomen and legs) are delivered in consecutive order. The baby cries automatically almost as soon as the shoulders deliver.

The need for an "episiotomy" is dependent on several important factors:

1. The size of the baby's head
2. The stretch ability of the vaginal outlet tissues (epidurals help relax the vaginal outlet and reduce the need
3. The length of the perineum (distance from bottom of vagina to rectum)
4. Position of the baby's head, particularly if it is "OP," posterior position (looking up rather than down)
5. The size and width of the shoulders, particularly in patient with diabetes
6. The size of the mother's pelvis or outlet (the size of the "donut hole")

Author's Anecdote:

After the author delivers a baby, he occasionally asks the family in attendance the following question, "Why does a baby cry after it is born?"

They all shake their heads "no" and gesturing that "they have no idea."

He then tells them, "The baby cries immediately after birth because I whispered into the baby's ear at birth that the US Treasury Debt is now at about $19 Trillion dollars! All babies cry when they hear this information!

If they still don't cry, I tell the baby, "Welcome to Lawton, Oklahoma: The Home of the Lawton Rangers' Rodeo!" They usually cry loudly after hearing this fact! The baby looks back at me puzzled and dumbfounded as if to say to me: I was hoping to be born in Hollywood, New York City or Las Vegas!

Frequently, a family member or friend in the Birth room may exclaim to the nurses, "The baby is blue!" The author then answers with this reassuring point, "Boys are blue and girls are pink!" Most baby's arms and feet are blue at birth. The baby tries to preserve their heat and spare losing calories by decreasing blood circulation to the hands and feet: it is a phenomenon medically called *Acrocyanosis*.

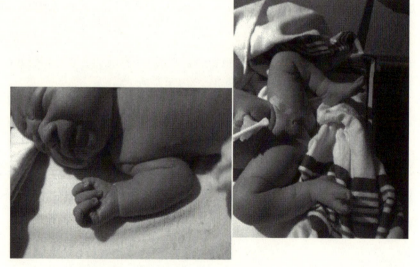

Figure 7-11 **Acrocyanosis: Blue hand and toes in this newborn baby**

One more story:

I was taking care of a patient in labor. It was long and arduous labor. It was very trying for the patient. She had an epidural in place. Her labor progressed very slowly but it did progress. After a long day the author checked the patient in the late afternoon. The patient was tired, sweaty and distressed. Her sister was standing next to her on the other side of the bed. She had a very serious and stern look on her face. I did the exam. A big smile then appeared on my face. I exclaimed to everyone in the room, "She is completely dilated!"

Her sister looked at me in a very critical manner and said, "Well, doctor. How far is that?"

I replied, "She is 10 centimeters!"

The sister then proceeded to tell me, "Well, doctor, I was 13 centimeters when I delivered!"

I asked quizzically, "You were 13 centimeters when you were completely dilated?"

She then stated, "Yes, the nurse said that I was 10 and plus 3!

Apparently the sister did not understand that she was 10 centimeters, i.e. the measurement at complete cervical dilatation but she also added "Plus 3" which indicated the plus *station* of the baby, i.e. number of centimeters of the baby's head below "0" station. Maybe not so funny: I guess you just had to be there!

The baby is placed at a lower level than the mother and is dried off with a warm towel (placing the baby lower than the mother allows for the baby's blood in the placenta to drain down by gravity to the baby: the "natural placental transfusion"). After about two minutes the cord is doubly clamped off and the obstetrician (or the husband, SO, BD or other support person) cuts the cord. The baby then is handed over to the mother so that she can hold her newborn.

Frequently the cord can be doubly clamped and the baby can be placed on a baby blanket on the mother's abdomen. At that time photos or videos of the cord cutting can be done. After the cord is cut, the OB will take a sample of blood from the cord for testing (baby blood type, hemoglobin and occasionally *nrbc's*, i.e. nucleated red blood cells).

Author's Anecdote: After a long and arduous labor with the mother being completely exhausted, I will tell the new mom as I gently place the baby on the mother's abdomen, "OK, that was just a "practice run." We are now going to put the baby back inside. We are going to try this all over again!" You would be surprised at the ugly look on her face at that point: I think I see daggers in her eyes at that point!

Variations to the above story are numerous, but basically the same sequence of events occurs. Instead of a second injection of Stadol™ (or Nubain™/Stadol™), the mother may have opted for an epidural anesthetic. Also, instead of progressing steadily to complete cervical dilation, the cervix may have stopped dilating due to fatiguing uterine muscle contractions. In such a situation, Pitocin (oxytocin) augmentation of labor would have been started to strengthen the intensity and increase the frequency of contractions. The arrested labor, having plateaued, would again be energized and the cervix would again begin to dilate all the way to completion, i.e. ten centimeters (10 cm). In most well-managed labors, delivery should be accomplished within twelve hours.

24. The First Stage of Labor

The **first** stage of labor is really comprised of two phases, the latent and the active phase. The beginning of labor, the **latent** phase, is defined as the time from when the uterine contractions begin until the time the cervix is three to four centimeters dilated (one centimeter equals one-half inch). The latent phase can be the most frustrating phase of labor to most parents. Little cervical dilation occurs. It is a time when the cervix thins out, or *effaces*. This phase can last nearly up to twenty hours for the first-time mother (primagravida) and up to twelve hours for previously-delivered patients (multipara).

The process of **effacement** involves making the cervical tissues thinner, softer and more stretchable. The latent phase of labor can have its own problems. It, too, can be complicated by a total lack of change in the status of the cervical tissues even in the face of continued uterine contractions. Lack of change, by definition, means that the patient is not in "true" labor. *False* labor is really a layman's term for the dysfunctional latent phase. This abnormal labor pattern is best treated by rest. It is significantly associated with large babies and high anxiety upon the part of the labor patient. Often the patient needs to be hospitalized and rested (occasionally with injections of pain relievers and sleep-inducing medications). Alternatively, **the uterine** muscles may be made to contract more effectively and in a more coordinated manner, by the administration of oxytocin (Pitocin). In the latent phase, the uterine contractions are anywhere from three to ten minutes apart and lasting thirty seconds. They are fairly well tolerated. Dysfunctional labor contractions can be very painful. The muscle contraction does not spread uniformly from the top of the uterus to the bottom. It pulls in many directions, even against itself. Try to picture two horses pulling a rope in opposite directions. One no longer has to visualize why false labor is so painful and why no labor progress occurs.

In the active phase of labor uterine contractions are usually two to three minutes apart, last forty-five to sixty seconds and are more intense. In general, the primagravid patient dilates at a rate of at least one centimeter (1 cm) per hour. The multiparous patient dilates faster, greater than one and a half centimeters (1.5 cm) per hour.

The author remembers his frustration in diagnosing true labor in a grand multiparous patient (more than five babies) when he was a resident at UCLA Medical Center. He cautiously admitted the patient to observe her for true labor (after five babies the patient herself smiled at me). I asked the nurse to give her an enema. Even though her contractions were very irregular, seven to eleven minutes apart, she knew from her own experience (my inexperience) that she was in true labor. Ten minutes later, among screams in the bathroom and the hustling of nurses and medical students, she delivered her baby while on the toilet seat! She went from three centimeters to complete cervical dilation and even to delivery **within ten** minutes.

Any labor progress slower than one centimeter per hour is considered abnormal. Such slowness calls for immediate evaluation and treatment. In the face of adequate contraction frequency and intensity, it must be assumed that some factor of disproportion exists; abnormal flexion or rotation of the head, external obstruction by a pelvic or fetal tumor, or the head is just too big for the maternal pelvic passageway.

If the contractions are not adequate, they can be strengthened (augmented) with the use of Oxytocin (Pitocin). More often than not, Pitocin administration results in the forward progress of the labor; further cervical effacement, dilation and descent of the head into the pelvis. It must be remembered that everyone's labor and delivery is individual and different. Many variations exist, depending on the baby's weight and head size, the size of one's pelvis, the uterine contractions, and many other factors.

Dr. Emanuel Friedman at Harvard Medical School is a noted expert and researcher in the various aspects of labor. After exhaustive study, he was one of the first physicians to study and to delineate the "average" labor process from the time contractions begin until the baby has delivered through all 3 stages of labor. He diagramed cervical dilatation as a function of time: thus graphing normal "labor curves." The labor pattern of a patient's progress can be mathematically graphed and characterized (see Friedman labor graph below). On average, a 1st time labor patient progresses at about 1 cm per hour after 4 cm of cervical dilatation is reached. The 2nd time pregnancy (secunda-gravida or multipara) progresses faster: at least 1.5 cm per hour. Departures from the normal labor graph have been defined and analyzed. Treatment and obstetrical management protocols that have been most effective in treating the various abnormalities of labor have been developed.

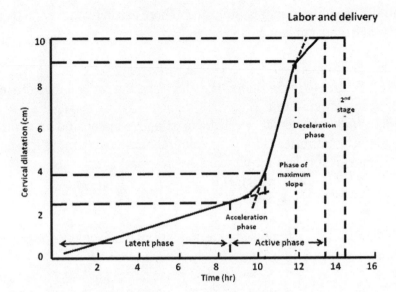

Phases of labor in primigravida. (From Friedman EA: Obstet Gynecol 6:567, 1955.)

More recent research has been done on the normal "progress" of labor: not all patients will travel along the same "labor curve" whether it is your first or subsequent pregnancy. Some experts are saying that the "active phase" of labor starts at 6 cm rather than at 4cm(see OBG Manag. 2013 December;25(12):12,15., based on Zhang J, Landy HJ, Branch DW, et al; Consortium on Safe Labor. *Contemporary patterns of spontaneous labor with normal neonatal outcomes.* Obstet Gynecol. 2010; 116(6):1281–1287).

The Active Management of Labor

In the everyday real world of obstetrics most labors that are not progressing by at least 1 cm per hour are augmented. Patients and their physicians desire to have their baby "sooner than later." It is true that labor can progress slowly and still wind up delivering a healthy baby. Most OB's have adopted the "active management of labor" principles." Progress," defined as cervical dilatation and descent of the head, should be followed very closely by the OB staff. If there is "no change" over 1 to 2 hours of labor, then augmentation of labor with the use of oxytocin is indicated. There are many advantages to the active management of labor:

1. Your labor and delivery time is shorter
2. With a shorter labor the development of a labor-related infection is less
3. With a shorter labor you are in pain for a lesser amount of time
4. With a shorter labor your epidural anesthesia time is less and the cost is less for you and the hospital
5. Your hospital stay may be shorter
6. Your hospital expenses may be less

Every pregnancy patient is unique and individual. Her labor variables are as follows:

1. Size and shape of her pelvis. Each patient's anatomy is a composite of their genetic inheritance. With such intermarriage and ethnic diversity in the United States and around the world, each patient's pelvic and abdominal anatomy is unique.

2. The size of the baby is also variable. As stated elsewhere, the baby's size is most related to the weight of the mother at the time of conception, how many pounds she gains during the pregnancy, and her own birth weight. The father of the baby's size and height must also be factored in the equation.

3. The muscle contractility of the uterus is special to each patient.

Every patient's progress in labor is special. Every OB gives his patients some latitude in the progress of their labor. The labor curves are just guidelines: deviations do and can occur. However, a "plateau" in the labor curve, i.e. lack of progress despite adequate contractions (as documented by an internal pressure catheter) does call for careful analysis and treatment.

How does one deal with painful uterine contractions?

Most new pregnant mothers believe that they will be able to withstand a normal labor and childbirth without any or little medications.

Other couples may want to attend childbirth preparation classes. Bradley, Dick-Reed and Lamaze methods have been the most popular in the past (particularly the 1970's and 1980's). If the couple is motivated, such classes are encouraged. Not only are they educational by furnishing you much factual information about your pregnancy, labor and delivery, but they provide you with the tools and techniques necessary for you to cope with your labor contractions and discomforts. Today these classes are not as available as in the past. Couples may have to purchase a DVD to do the classes at home.

There are three important principles that these methods employ:

1. Concentrating on a *Focal Point*.

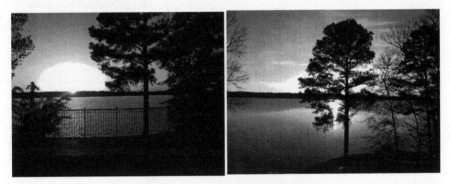

Figure 7-12 Labor Focus Points

Vacation Picture (Lake Oconee, GA) can be used as a focal point when contractions are hurting: mental substitution of happy memories in the place of labor pain.

It is important to focus on a peaceful scene rather than concentrating on the pain and contractions themselves.

One can also concentrate on certain special objects, like a Teddy bear, etc.

2. A definite breathing pattern. By breathing in a certain prescribed rhythm she can bear and harness the intensity of the contractions. Physically, she can "breathe through the

labor contractions." She can stay on top of the contractions. She is able to be in control of the contractions, rather than the contractions controlling her. It is only when control is lost that the fear, anxiety and more painful labor develop.

3. A coach is provided. A coach provides the emotional and physical support and encouragement needed to get her over the painful hump of her labor contractions. She is not alone. Someone else understands the breathing patterns and both can go through the labor together.

With such childbirth preparations, the discomforts of early labor are handled quite well by most couples. However, most couples, including husbands, tire after five to six hours. Both partners begin to fatigue, and lose their concentration as well as their determination. First-time labors generally last an average of twelve hours. Second-time labors may last only five to six hours—half as long! Consequently, most patients are able to get through their second labors with Lamaze alone or with only one or more injections of pain medication.

"Ring of Fire" during the delivery of the head

After complete cervical dilatation, the patient will push the baby's head through the vagina. When the head starts "to crown," the vaginal opening is the next anatomical area that needs to dilate.

When the OB patient has desired to have childbirth without anesthesia, the stretching of the vaginal opening and tissues, creates a burning sensation that many patients have described as a "Ring of Fire."

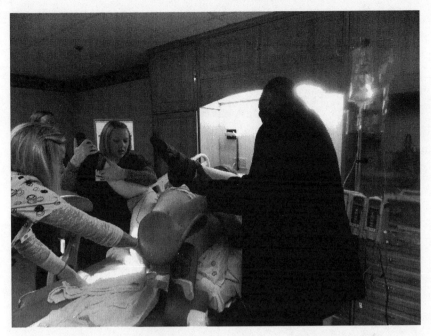

Figure 7-13 Southwestern OB Nurses "at your cervix!"

When the head dilates the opening to the vagina, such stretching of sensitive tissues gives the patient the feeling that the vaginal opening is "on fire." It is very temporary pain as the baby's head, shoulders and body deliver within a minute or two.

Authors Note: During the first labor the baby is literally "blazing" a trail through the mother's pelvis ("blazing a trail through the forest"). It takes a long time. The second baby has a trail or road to go down and therefore, the travel time is shorter. The third labor can indeed be very fast—like cruising down an interstate highway. Sometimes the doctor cannot keep up and be there to "catch" the baby!

Other factors also influence labor; the mother's age, the time interval between pregnancies and the number of pregnancies a mother has had.

It was always frustrating for the OB residents at UCLA Medical Center to have to perform a C-Section on a patient who had delivered five previous babies "at home," usually in Mexico. Many of the OB patients had deliberately immigrated to the United States from

Mexico in order to deliver their babies safely in an American hospital. However, the uterine muscles in these patients seem to be impaired and worn. Despite oxytocin the muscles are too tired, or "refuse" to open up the cervix. Also, babies tended more often to be in abnormal "lies," such as breech or transverse lies. Accordingly, after five babies, "Grand Multips" patients may have more difficult or complicated labors with the increased need for C-Section deliveries. With advancing maternal age and more pregnancies, babies tend to become bigger in size. A long interval of time between pregnancies, such as five to ten years, causes the cervix to become rigid. Accordingly, such labors often behave like "first-time" labors even though they really are the second one.

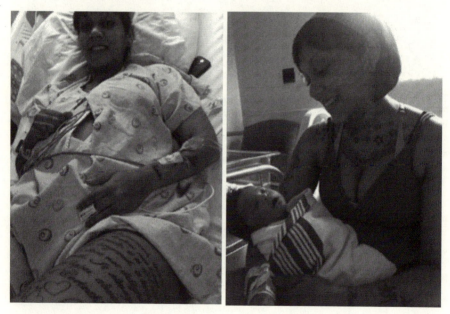

Figures 7-13 and 7-14 Our tattooed mom who said she hated needle sticks

Our tattooed OB patient, Valencia is pictured above. When the RN told her she needed to start an IV in left arm, she said "she was very afraid of needles." Seriously!,

25. Delivery

Prior to the birth of the baby, the baby's head is looking down at the floor. The back of the baby's head is the first part of the baby to deliver. As the head extends through the vaginal opening, one sees the forehead, the eyes, the nose, mouth and chin in that sequence. As soon as the head is completely delivered, it will rotate 90 degrees and the baby will look to the left or right side. As mentioned before, the shoulders hit the mid-pelvic floor just as the head is delivered. Since the mid-pelvis is deeper than its width, the shoulders rotate so that the baby will be positioned "sidewise" in the pelvis.

The rotation of the shoulder concurrently rotates the baby's head so that it too, looks at the side or inner surface of the mother's thigh. By gently pushing the baby's head down toward the floor, the baby's anterior "front" shoulder is delivered (or guiding upward the posterior shoulder to deliver first) from under the pubic bone. Then the baby's head is pulled gently toward the ceiling, thus delivering the baby's posterior or "back" shoulder. The mother is allowed to push with each of these steps. Further pushes or gently pulling by the obstetrician, help deliver the chest, abdomen and feet in that sequence. The baby's mouth and nose are suctioned with a bulb syringe as soon as the first shoulder is delivered. The baby is then dried off with a warm towel. The cooler air of the room with drying and touching of the baby all stimulate the baby to breathe its first breath and start crying. Obstetricians do not, if rarely these days, "spank" or hold the baby straight and upside down these modern days.

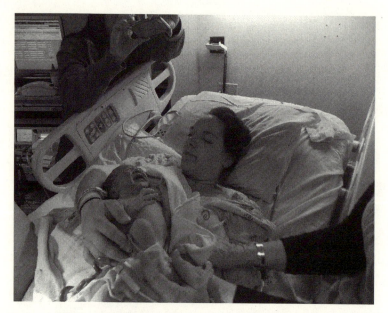

Figure 7-15 Baby is placed on mother's abdomen

If the baby is vigorous at birth, the baby is placed immediately onto a warm baby's blanket on the mother's abdomen. The baby is dried off and the mouth suctioned of fluids. The father, family and friends may be snapping pictures and videos of the first minutes of the baby's life. Patient's mother is snapping pictures from above.

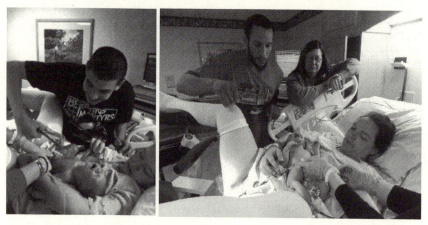

Figures 7-14 and Figure 7-15 Birthing Tradition being performed: the father of the baby is getting ready to cut the cord with the nurse

Both of the pictures above and below illustrate the RN showing the fathers how to cut between the two cord clamps.

The OB is usually exhorting to the father, "Don't cut anything else off—that is my job!"

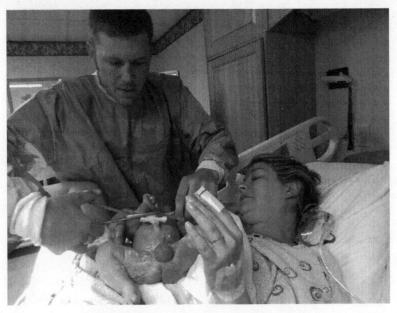

Figure 7-16 Cutting the umbilical cord.
Father, extremely focused, in cutting his son's umbilical cord

I knew when I met you that an Adventure was going to Happen!
Sometimes the smallest things take up
the most room in your Heart

--A.A. Milne, Winnie-the-Pooh

During the first minutes of life the baby is held below the mother's abdomen so that blood in the placenta can flow by gravity down into the baby's body (the "placental transfusion"). After two or more minutes, most of baby's blood in the placental vessels has been transferred back into the baby's circulation. After the placental transfusion the cord is doubly clamped and cut ("delayed cord clamping). The baby is cleansed further, wrapped in a warm blanket and handed to its mother in bed. Interestingly, the baby is quiet and rarely cries while it is cuddled in its parent's arms. The eyes are open or slightly closed because of the bright lights. The babies are curious and alert, yet very comfortable and reassured as they again hear the melodic and familiar voices of mom and dad that are no longer muffled by the abdominal wall barrier of the past nine months.

The baby will be immediately banded with a bracelet on one hand, and a second bracelet will be snugly applied to one leg just in case either bracelet falls off. A third identical identification bracelet will be applied to the mother's wrist. No baby will be given to a mother unless the ID bracelets match perfectly.

After the baby is banded, the mother may choose to breastfeed her newborn. Nipple sucking stimulates the pituitary gland to release oxytocin, which in turn causes the muscles both in the breast and in the uterus to contract, Muscles around the breast glands contract, pushing colostrum into the breast ducts. The baby sucks on the areola, squeezing the colostrum into his mouth. Similarly, oxytocin causes the uterus to contract and become smaller. The placenta, already buckled from the baby's delivery, is further squeezed out of the uterus into the vagina.

It is traditionally for the father of the baby to give the mother of his child "the classic kiss" that she deserves for the birth of his baby.

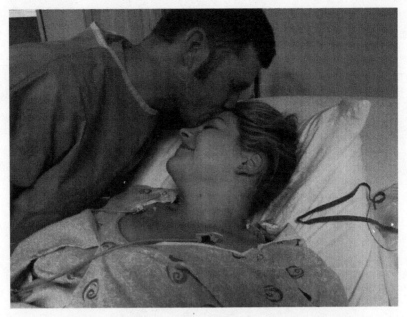

Figure 7-17 The "Birthing Kiss."

Author's Note: "Labor Losers" and "Labor Winners"

Your Labor Nurses and your OB are very conscientious about getting their "Moms" to deliver. If there are a number of patients in labor, the nurses can be quite competitive about getting their patients to deliver first. The author had a first time Mom in labor and, when he made rounds at 5:30 pm he found out that the other patients had already delivered. The RN looked at me with a very disappointed look in her face and said to me sadly, "I know, I am a *labor loser.* My patient has not delivered yet."

More frustrating, your OB physician and the nurses also feel like "labor losers" when their patients do not progress and, for whatever reasons, have to be delivered by C-section. The OB team at your hospital is always striving for only *normal* vaginal deliveries!

When everyone has a quick and normal vaginal delivery, then the OB team and the patient are all "Labor Winners!"

Author Anecdote: Not every support person in the labor suite can handle the emotional and physical stimuli and excitement that occurs with the birth of a baby. In the picture below is the father-in-law of the mother who had just given birth.

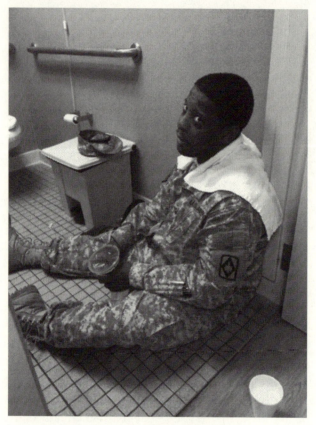

Figure 7-18 Emotional Delivery

In the above picture he said to me as the picture was snapped, "What happens in this room has to stay in this room."

> **Occasionally in life there are those moments of unutterable fulfillment which cannot be completely explained by those symbols called words. Their meanings can only be articulated by the inaudible language of the heart.**
>
> — *Martin Luther King, Jr.*

24. The Immediate Care of the Newborn in the Delivery Suite.

After the initial bonding of the baby with the mom, the baby is taken over to the Newborn warmer. The baby is further dried off and the wet or soiled blanket is discarded. To prevent any heat loss the baby is wrapped in a new warm blanket and the head is covered with a small cotton cap.

a. ID bracelets are immediately placed on the baby's arm and leg and the same ID's are given to the mother and other designated care giver. No other person can take the baby from the Nursery without the identical ID bracelet. There is a NEWBORN ALARM system in every OB unit such that any baby with a bracelet cannot leave the unit without the alarm system being tripped.

b. The baby's footprints and handprints are taken and a copy given to the parents on the Hospital Birth Certificate. The nurses may also put footprints on a "Father Scrub Shirt" so that the new father can show everyone that he is a New Dad. Later the scrub shirt can be sprayed and framed if so desired.

c. The baby is given an injection of Vitamin K in order to prevent bleeding in the newborn period. The baby's liver is still immature and has not had sufficient time to form all the clotting factors necessary to stop bleeding if any type of injury were to occur.

25. Third Stage of Labor

The third stage of labor principally involves the delivery of the placenta. However, despite what could occur at any time during your pregnancy and the first two stages of labor, the third stage is the most risky to the mother's health. The danger of obstetric bleeding and hemorrhage is most prevalent at this time.

The main time-frame during an entire pregnancy in which the most serious complications occur to a pregnant patient is the <u>time after</u> the baby is born, i.e. the 3rd stage of labor when the placenta is being delivered. Hemorrhage (loss of excess amounts of blood) is the main cause of maternal morbidity in the United States today.

After the baby is delivered, the uterus contracts to a much smaller size. The placenta "buckles" at the center. Blood wells up behind the placenta and, with further uterine contractions, the placenta gets pushed out of the uterus. There are 2 maneuvers that help with delivery of the placenta:

1) Gently massaging the uterus from the pubic bone upward and,
2) Gentle downward cord traction,

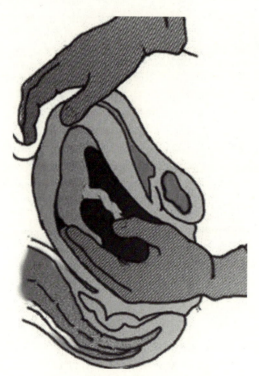

Figure 7-19 Retained Placenta

As the placenta separates, the uterus forms into a more globular, wider shape. The umbilical cord lengthens. Finally, as the uterus further contracts and pushes the placenta farther down in the uterus, that "well" of blood behind the placenta escapes - the so-called "gush of blood" that signals partial placental separation.

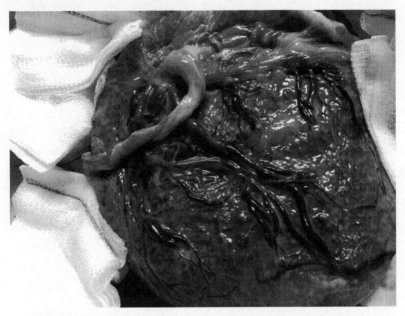

Figure 7-20 Placenta with acentric cord insertion. There is an off-center or acentric cord insertion in the above pictured placenta.

The fetal side of the placenta shown above illustrates the smooth membranes and cord (or "Shiny Schultz" side of placenta). Occasionally the placenta delivers showing the maternal side which looks similarly to liver ("Dirty Duncan).

Approximately ten percent of the time this normal sequence of placental delivery does not occur. Either no or partial detachment of the placenta from the uterine wall occurs. If no detachment ensues despite gentle uterine massage and cord traction, then the placenta is probably adherent to the uterine wall. Worse yet, if partial detachment occurs, brisk bleeding flows from that part of the uterine wall. Whether partially or completely adherent, the placenta must be manually sheared from the uterine wall by placing the obstetrician's hand into the uterus. Prior to manual removal, adequate anesthesia must first be given to the patient unless bleeding is severe and emergency life and death conditions prevail. Anesthesia can be given in one of three forms:

1. Intravenous analgesia: Ketamine, Demerol, Valium, combined with nitrous oxide and oxygen.
2. General anesthesia: (with or without intubation).
3. Regional anesthesia: epidural or spinal block.

After satisfactory anesthesia is established, the physician gently places one hand in the vagina and the other on the abdomen to steady the top of the uterus. The physician's sterile gloved hand reaches further into the uterus while his fingers are used to separate the placenta off the interior surface of the uterus. After complete shearing has occurred, the intact placenta can be brought out of the uterus and thus delivered. Occasionally the placenta must be removed in pieces. Rarely, should the placenta grow into or through the uterine muscle, no cleavage plane exists. Placenta accreta is the medical term for such a situation, and usually requires a hysterectomy in order to stop the hemorrhaging associated with it.

After delivery of the placenta oxytocin (Pitocin®) is usually given intravenously (IV) or intramuscularly (IM) if an IV has not been established). Pitocin® helps to contract the uterine muscle and, as the muscle contracts, blood vessels are bent and squeezed shut. Bleeding lessens. Breastfeeding and uterine massage alone may accomplish similar results, but since there are rarely any problems or side-effects from oxytocin, physicians routinely recommend it postpartum. If, after a long or arduous labor, or large baby, the uterus becomes atonic; i.e., remains flaccid despite massage, oxytocin can be lifesaving and save unnecessary blood loss, as well as avert the need for possible blood transfusion. Should uterine atony occur, an IV line is started and a dilute solution of IV fluids containing oxytocin is infused intravenously.

TMI Section (Too Much Information)

If you are further interested in the causes of uterine atony and postpartum hemorrhage, the reader can continue to read this section. If not, proceed to the next chapter!

27. Causes of Uterine Atony (TMI section)

The following are the most common causes of Postpartum Hemorrhage due to a "tired" or atonic uterus:"

Long, arduous labor
Large baby
Grand multiparity
Retained amniotic membranes
Retained placental cotyledon or fragments
Chorio-amnionitis (endo--myometritis)
General anesthetics (particularly Halothane)
Hematometra

Treatment of Uterine Atony

Intravenous Pitocin infusion	Balkri Balloon insertion into uterine cavity
Intravenous or intramuscular methergine	B-Lynch Suturing of the uterus
Intravenous of intramuscular prostaglandins	
Uterine packing with gauze (rare)	
Hysterectomy (rare)	

For the most part, placentas separate and deliver without much difficulty within five to ten minutes after birth. Thereafter the uterus contracts down vigorously and bleeding slows down. Surprisingly, about one-half to one pint of blood loss is associated with the average delivery.

To cut down on the loss of blood associated with delivery, it is of utmost importance that the uterus be gently massaged immediately after delivery as well as later during recovery. Optimally, it would be nice to have continuous massage, but a nurse or husband may not be available to do so. After the initial massaging, the physician is busy inspecting the vagina or sewing the episiotomy. The contracted uterus relaxes and blood vessels start bleeding into the uterine cavity. A *hematometra* may form, i.e. a uterine cavity full of blood and clots. As the uterus expands from the volume of clots, further relaxation of semi-contracted uterine muscle occurs. More blood vessels open up and bleed. Therefore, It is no wonder that when the uterus is massaged or *expressed* at the conclusion of the delivery, one can witness the amount of blood and clots that can be expelled from the uterus into the vagina.

Remember the 3 M's: Maintain Maternal Massage (or "How to Rub Mommy the Right Way")

It is helpful that husband, relative, friend or nurse gently massage the uterus with light stroking or rubbing from the pubic bone upward to the top of the uterus after the placenta is delivered. Maintain massage during the first hour after birth. Less blood loss and decreased risk of postpartum hemorrhage due to atony and hematometra will result.

28. The Delivery Room "Shivers and Shakes"

Within a few minutes after birth, the patient may experience intense shaking. These involuntary muscle movements last approximately ten to twenty minutes, and do not necessarily accompany all deliveries. They also tend to occur after C-section births. There are many theories to explain the postpartum "shakes," but no one knows for sure as the following explanations have been postulated:

1) Fetal blood to mother's blood transfusion reaction; i.e., baby's blood cells entering the maternal circulation during the third stage of labor

2) Amniotic fluid entering the maternal circulation

3) Local anesthetics entering the maternal circulation

4) Bacteremia, i.e. bacteria entering the mother's circulation from the new placental site (after the placenta is delivered)

5) Room temperature (colder)

6) Intravenous fluids running into the maternal circulation after delivery (if an IV is used)

No treatment is necessary for the "shakes" reaction, but if truly distressing, your physician can order an analgesic such as Demerol or morphine which usually alleviates the symptoms rapidly.

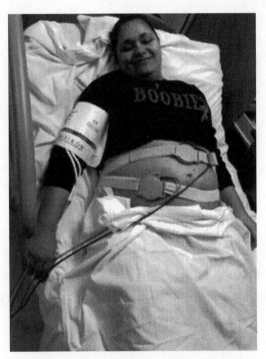

Figure 7-21 External Fetal Monitoring belts on patient in early labor

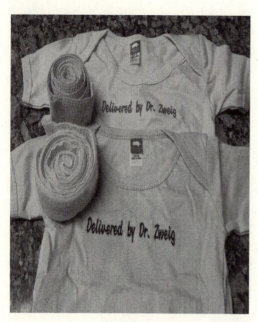

Figure 7-22. External Monitor Belts. Patients can keep their fetal monitoring straps and put them together with the hospital or OB's "gift T-shirt" in a shadow box for memory keepsakes

George Strait touched the emotional reality moment and the epiphany of the birth event in his popular country song "I Saw God Today" (author recommends internet search and reading all the song lyrics)

Got my face pressed up against the nursery glass,
she's sleepin' like a rock
My name on her wrist, wearin' tiny pink socks
She's got my nose, she's got her mama's eyes

Lyrics by Rodney Clawson, Monty Criswell and Wade Kirby and sung by George Strait

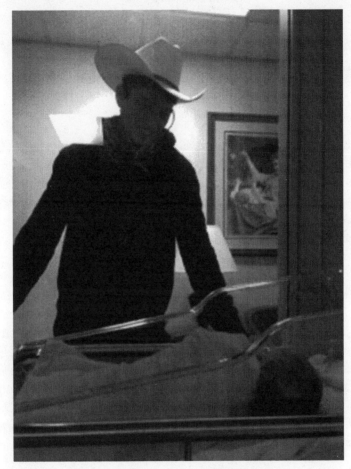

Figure 7-23. Cowboy saw God today

CHAPTER 8

Analgesics during Labor and Delivery: Medications available for Pain Relief

If you become tired of the discomfort of labor, perhaps a little medication may be all that you need to take the sharp edge off your contraction pain. Not only may you begin to feel better, but by feeling the relief, you may again gain back your concentration and determination. You may even dilate faster! When you become frightened and anxious, the body's adrenal glands (which sit on top of the kidneys) make a hormone called adrenalin. Adrenalin has many functions. It increases your heart rate and relaxes the muscles in the lungs airway passages so that asthmatics can breathe easier. It also relaxes the muscles of the uterus. Contractions are not as frequent or strong. With high adrenalin levels the uterus contracts less effectively. However, if your pain is relieved by medication, adrenalin levels fall and your contractions become more efficient. Therefore, you may dilate faster without the same intensity of pain. Doctors and nurses see this phenomenon regularly and call it the "pain relief effect." Any method, device, medication or anesthetic that results in pain relief produces the same effect, "true gain without pain!"

1. What Are the Most Commonly Used Medications?

Unfortunately, there are very few safe drugs to use for the pregnant woman in labor. Moreover, it is important for everyone to understand the following facts:

➢ There are no ideal or perfect drugs for the labor patient.

- All medications used in labor cross over into the baby's circulation through the placenta.
- Depending on the dose, route of administration (IV or oral), and timing of administration proximate to delivery, all medications can potentially produce respiratory depression (sleepiness in the baby at birth).
- All medications, if given too early in labor, during the latent phase, can potentially decrease the strength and intensity of the uterine contractions or slow down labor.

The obstetrical patient who is most motivated is the patient who goes to all the childbirth classes. She reads many of the books devoted to pregnancy information. Also, she will most likely require the least amount of medication during her labor and delivery. The patient who has the most desire to have and love a baby (particularly fertility patients) and those who have the solid support, both mentally and physically, from their husband and family, also tend to need the least amount of medication. The education, the understanding and the confidence that is obtained, along with her trust in her obstetrician, make labor and delivery a simple task for everyone involved. Most importantly, it makes labor and delivery less frightening for the patient herself.

Medications that are utilized most frequently can be categorized into three groups:

- Analgesics (pain-relieving) drugs
- Tranquilizers (relaxes and calms the nerves)
- Sedative-Hypnotics

The *analgesics*, or pain relievers, lessen the intensity of contraction pain. The most frequently used medications are Stadol and Nubain. In the past Demerol (Meperidine®) was one of the most commonly used medications in labor. It has a well-known track record in the sense that it has been used longer and studied more often than any other analgesic used for labor pain. A brief outline is given of all the analgesics currently available.

Stadol (Butorphanol®)

    Dose: IM 1 to 2 mg

              IV 1 to 2 mg

Duration of action: approximately one to two hours Side effects: sleepiness, sweaty/clamminess, dizziness, headache

Fetal effects: as opposed to Demerol, Stadol is one of the safest medications that can be used and yet not produce a "sleepy" baby (respiratory depression) at birth. If given just prior to birth, occasional respiratory effects are seen, but are most easily manageable. No short term effects seen on attentiveness or other newborn behavior, no long term consequences.

Timing of administration: 3 to 9 centimeters depending on labor progress.

Nubain® (Nalbuphine Hydrochloride) 5 to 10 mg IV or SQ

In general, this medication is very similar to Stadol but clinically tends to decrease the intensity and strength of the uterine contractions to a much greater degree than Stadol. Because of this slowing of the labor, Nubain may be used if Stadol is not producing the desired pain relief effect in labor.

It is the common practice in most OB units across the United States to use Stadol or Nubain during the latent and early active phase of labor. If the patient has dilated more than 3-4 centimeters and is requesting more relief of her pain in labor, the OB team will usually proceed with an Epidural at this juncture. If the patient is not dilated 3 centimeters, then more Stadol or Nubain is given. Frequently, the OB team will go forward with epidural despite the status of cervical dilatation. There are many studies that show that epidural anesthesia does not slow the progress of labor or lead to an increased C-section rate. If labor does not progress with an epidural, the contractions will usually be augmented with Pitocin. Labor may not progress due to inadequate contractions (frequency and strength). Contraction frequency and strength is obtained objectively with introduction of an IUPC (intrauterine pressure catheter).

Demerol® (generic: Meperidine)

Dose: IM (intramuscular): 50 to 75 mg every three to four hours

IV (intravenous): 25 mg every hour Duration of pain relief: two to four hours

Onset of effect: IM dose in twenty to forty-five minutes/ IV dose in ten minutes

Maternal side effects: nausea, occasional vomiting, and sleepiness

Fetal effects: sleepiness of the baby at birth only if given within two to three hours prior to birth

Occasional behavior disturbances such as attentiveness or suckling abilities

There are no long term effects or problems

Timing of administration: from two to eight centimeters depending on clinical course of labor

Demerol has a small role in today's obstetrics due to its prolonged duration of action. It is frequently used today to treat dysfunctional latent labor in order to give pain relief and rest to the patient. Demerol is utilized for pain relief when other medications cannot be utilized or have not been effective *and* delivery is remotely on the horizon, i.e. not expected to occur within 4 to 6 hours.

Morphine®

Time of administration: usually given in early or dysfunctional labor to rest a patient. Otherwise it is administered in the early part of "active phase" of labor so that its effect will be worn off at the time of delivery.

Route: IV 2 to 5 mg every hour.

   IM 10 to 15 mg every four hours.

Duration of action: one to four hours

Onset of action: approximately twenty to forty minutes

Side effects: nausea with occasional vomiting

Effects on fetus: newborn's breathing center is very sensitive to its depressant effects. Consequently, baby may be sleepy if morphine is given within four hours of birth. Similar to Demerol, the shorter acting drugs such as Stadol are given preferentially over morphine in OB suites in today. Morphine may have a prolonged neurobehavioral effect on the mother. Like Demerol, morphine is used in the few situations in which other short acting drugs would not alleviate the pain or achieve the desired result.

Fentanyl®

Because of its relative infrequent use, this narcotic has had limited use in obstetrics.

Doses: 25 to 50 micrograms IV causes peak analgesic effect within minutes and lasts thirty to sixty minutes

   50 to 100 micrograms IM causes peak analgesic effect within thirty minutes and lasts one to two hours

This drug does cross over to the placenta and to the baby but has minimal neurobehavioral effects on the baby.

Pentazocine (Talwin®)

This older and established narcotic has decreasing clinical use in obstetrics due to its unpredictable psychological effects on a patient while in labor. Also it has uncertain pain relieving properties depending on the patient's response. When it works, it works wonders. When it does not have any effect, it is disappointing to all.

Dose: 20 to 30 mg IM with an effect in ten to twenty minutes
10 to 20 mg IV with an effect in two to three minutes
Duration of effect: two to four hours

Sedatives and Tranquilizers

Vistaril® (Hydroxyzine)

Hydroxyzine is a tranquilizer in the sense it calms the nerves and makes the patient less anxious. This medication is usually used in early labor when narcotics could decrease the strength of labor contractions. It relaxes the patient who is very nervous in the early phases of labor. It also makes the patient a little sleepy. Some physicians may use the medication to produce rest in those patients who are in early labor at bedtime. Because of its anti-nausea properties, Hydroxyzine can also be used together with a narcotic to counteract the narcotic-associated nausea and vomiting. At the same time it can potentiate the effects of other pain relievers such as Demerol. The fetal heart rate variability is affected slightly but produces no real significant prolonged effect. Lastly, it has anti-itch properties such that any irritated, dry skin (even stretch marks) becomes less itchy during labor. The dose usually is 25 to 50 mg IM or 25 mg IV and its effects last approximately three to six hours.

Versed (Midazolam) is a new member of the Benzodiazepine drug family which possesses many superior advantages over Valium within the realm of obstetrics. First, Versed is water soluble (whereas Valium is oily: Valium may be more painful when given by injection). Versed starts to have an effect on the patient more rapidly than Valium but Versed also wears off quicker so that the baby is not affected by an earlier-than-expected birth time. Lastly, Versed does not readily diffuse into the fetal circulation via the placenta. Consequently, the mother can benefit from the medication without affecting the baby to the same degree.

Valium® (Benzodiazepines)

Valium is used in labor to relax anxious patients. It produces a soothing and calming effect on the patient. It also has a sedative effect and is used to "rest" patients in early and dysfunctional labor (erratic or false labor). It can be used simultaneously with a narcotic so that smaller doses of both medications can be utilized. It rapidly crosses through the placenta to the baby. Valium has a longer duration of action and consequently has decreasing utilization in modern day obstetrics. Valium, too, can decrease fetal heart rate variability, but this effect has no real physiological consequences. The main concern with valium is that it produces a sleepy baby if administered within four to six hours of birth. Also, in large doses, it is known to have definite effects on the newborn: decreased suckling abilities, alertness, and sleepiness.

Valium is given in doses:
- 2 to 5 mg IV
- 5 to 10 mg PO
- 5 to 10 mg IM

Its effect usually lasts four to eight hours.

Ambien®: Medication used to "sleep patients"

This medication is used principally to induce sleep. Patients in a "false labor," i.e. dysfunctional labor may be very exhausted from their contractions. In order to provide rest, Ambien is given in the Obstetrics Suite to "rest" patients. Frequently Ambien is given along with Morphine or other analgesics listed above to provide "pain relief." With relief of the contraction pains as well as the sleep induced by Ambien the patient in false labor will be "rested." Two subsequent events will occur:

- The patient will wake up and her "false labor" contractions will have stopped
- She will wake up rested and be in "true labor."

These two medications produce a very good sleep in the patient without any "hangover" effect. It is not uncommon for patients to remark the next morning, "That is the best night's sleep I've had in months!"

Barbiturates

The main barbiturates used in labor are Nembutal® and Seconal®. Some senior OBs may have occasional used Phenobarbital® for patients being hospitalized on the antepartum floor for pre-term pre-eclampsia. It is utilized for seizure prevention and to help patients sleep when they are confined to bed rest. These medications are used infrequently in today's Obstetrics because safer medications, i.e., Ambien, have been developed to take their place. If the patient is allergic to Ambien or has had other intolerable side effects from previous Ambien use, then barbiturate class medications may be called into play.

Nembutal® is used mainly to induce sleep in patients in early labor. However, it has a very short duration of effect: about two to three hours. Patients may be awakened in the middle of the night by their contractions. If labor ensues and is rapid, then Nembutal's effect would have already worn off. Accordingly, Nembutal should be used for patients who have quick labors but who also desire a little rest. For the patient in false, dysfunctional, or very early labor in which delivery is most likely many hours away, Seconal may be the drug of choice. It induces sleep that may last six to eight hours. The main disadvantage is that some patients may complain of its occasional hangover effect the next morning.

Pentothal® (Thiopental) is an ultra-short acting barbiturate that is used to put patients to sleep during the induction of general anesthesia.

Phenobarbital is an ultra-long acting barbiturate that is used mainly for its anti-convulsive properties. Patients with epilepsy or other seizure disorders may be kept on previously prescribed Phenobarbital until the onset of labor. Keppra® (Gaba-pentin) has now become one of the preferred drugs in the treatment of seizure disorders during pregnancy. Thereafter, Magnesium Sulfate or other safer medications may be used. Because of its long duration of effect, i.e., six to twelve hours, it is most likely that a baby would be born sleepy if it were to be given even in early labor. It must be remembered that barbiturates are sedative-type medications that induce sleep and relaxation. They do not relieve pain. Because they do relax patients, perhaps lesser doses of other narcotic medications can be administered. . Lastly, Phenobarbital may prescribed for seizure prophylaxis in pre-eclamptic patients in the postpartum period.

CHAPTER 9
Obstetrical Anesthesia

Many patients are able to get through labor with Lamaze, Bradley (or other childbirth methods), along with some medication. However, patients who are having their first baby or those having a difficult time with a subsequent birth, frequently desire better and deeper pain relief. Fortunately for these patients, regional anesthesia in the form of Epidural anesthesia is available. Regional anesthesia provides better pain relief than any other method. It is called the "Beverly Hills" method of childbirth because so many movie stars utilize it. It is also called the "Cadillac" of all pain relieving methods in childbirth. A regional anesthetic produces its effects by numbing the nerves coming from that part of the body experiencing the pain. Most painful stimuli are sensed by the peripheral nerves which transmit their pain messages to the spinal cord. From there the messages go to the brain to be received and perceived. Regional anesthesia numbs several nerve trunks that enter the lower backbone. Anesthetic drugs, related to the Novacaine family, are placed into a space within the patient's backbone. In this space the drug is sequestered and is not considered to be in the general circulation of the mother. Slowly the Novacaine-type of medication is absorbed by blood vessels in the backbone. However, the medication is eventually slowly absorbed into the circulation. In the circulation the medication is transported directly to the liver. In the liver it is taken out of circulation so that very little of the drug gets into the general circulation, and therefore, to the baby. In general, patients do not feel any effects, such as drowsiness or nausea, from a regional anesthesia. Better yet, the baby is exposed minimally to any drug that does get into the general circulation. The baby (and mother!) comes out of the delivery room screaming and alert. Regional anesthesia such as Epidural (or Caudal block) can be given at any time during labor. Most often, analgesic drugs are given in early labor to combat the pain. After four or five hours of labor, most patients have "had it" and want something better than just medications. At about four to five centimeters dilation an Epidural is requested and placed.

Epidural Anesthesia

Epidural anesthesia for obstetrical patients is available at most hospitals with an active delivery service (greater than 50 births per month). During their pregnancy it is recommended that patients check with their physicians regarding the availability of epidural anesthesia at the hospital at which they plan to deliver.

Currently, most OB services will provide epidurals "on demand," i.e. when the patients requests one when she is in labor. Most OB services will provide epidurals around the clock on all days of the week. The availability of epidurals was never as "so available "as it is today across the United States.

Authors Anecdote about past OB times: A few decades ago when epidural anesthesia was not so accepted as part of the delivery experience, patients had to ask the following questions during their pregnancy:

Does an epidural service exist at the hospital?

Is it available 24 hours per day (or just during the daylight hours)?

Does your physician allow his patients to have this form of anesthesia?

When does your physician allow his patients to obtain the anesthesia? Choices could be:

In the active stage of labor (greater the 4 centimeters),

At delivery time only,

At any time the patient requests it.

Is the epidural continuous (constant infusion by electronic pump) or intermittent ("top-up" doses given every two to three hours)?

Does your OB physician want the anesthesia to wear off so that the patient can feel and push in the second stage of labor?

In general, most obstetricians recommend that patients use the aforementioned Lamaze (or Bradley) shallow breathing techniques and try to cope with the labor contractions as long as possible. Sequential injections of pain-relieving medications (discussed in the chapter previously) can be used to complement coping techniques learned in childbirth classes. Only if the pain-relief is considered inadequate (by the patient), after the previous analgesic methods have been tried, should epidural anesthesia be offered and afforded to labor patients. The epidural provides pain relief by numbing pelvic nerves just as they traverse the epidural space to enter the spinal cord. The epidural space lies outside of the spinal cord and fluid sac: *Spinal headaches* should not occur with *epidural* anesthesia. If the *epidural* needle is advanced accidentally past the epidural space into the spinal space and into the spinal fluid, only then will an attempted epidural result in a postpartum *spinal headache*. Even then, an epidural "blood patch" could be given later to relieve the headache.

Once in place, an epidural results in incredible pain relief within three to four contractions. The characteristic "epidural smile" appears on every labor patient's face. She feels the hardening of the contractions but they are no longer uncomfortable. At the same time she does *not* feel sleepy, dazed, or otherwise "out of it." She is conscious, awake and mentally alert.

Technique of Epidural Anesthesia

Prior to placing an epidural, a CBC with platelet count is checked by the anesthetist (a CBC, or complete blood count, is ordered on all patients after they are admitted to the Labor suite. A CBC provides important blood information about the patient: anemia, or low red blood count as well as thrombocytopenia, or low platelet count. Rarely, does a patient have thrombocytopenia, i.e., a "clotting disorder" that would lead to a patient's tendency to bleed: particularly after the placenta is delivered or from lacerations in the vaginal tissues. Bleeding may also occur during placement of an epidural needle into the patient's back. Though there are not any major blood vessels where the epidural is typically placed, a blood vessel could be present in the path the epidural needle takes. Blood vessels could inadvertently be injured during an epidural placement. Without adequate clotting abilities, a patient could not stop bleeding sufficiently such that a blood clot, or hematoma, could form in back.

An epidural anesthetic can be performed within five to ten minutes depending on the skill of the anesthesiologist and the cooperation of the patient. Epidurals are classified by the anatomical area of the back in which the needle is inserted. If the epidural space is approached just above the tailbone, it is call a "caudal" epidural. If the needle is placed in the "small of the back," it is called a "lumbar" epidural. The technique is simple:

1. The patient is positioned correctly. For a lumbar epidural, the patient lies in the fetal position on her side or sits bending over on the side of the bed. For a caudal epidural, the patient can also be placed in the knee-chest position.
2. The skin is cleansed with an antiseptic such a alcohol and/or Betadine.
3. The skin and deeper tissues are number by injecting these areas with a Novocain-like anesthetic. A very fine needle is used so the patient does not feel this injection. During the injection a slight burning or "bee -sting" may be felt as a result of the anesthetic medicine itself.

The epidural needle punctures the numbed skin area. It is pushed through the deeper soft fatty tissues between the spines. The needle is then stopped by the tough ligament running between the backbones. When the anesthetist further advances the needle slowly through the ligament, he can feel a "loss of resistance" when the epidural space is entered. At this point the anesthetic solution easily flows into the correct area. A small amount of anesthetic medication (a "test dose") is allowed to go in. After a few minutes, the epidural catheter is threaded through the Touhy needle and further "test dose" is given through the catheter ("catheter test dose"). The catheter is then taped in place. After a period of time the epidural dose medication can be injected safely.

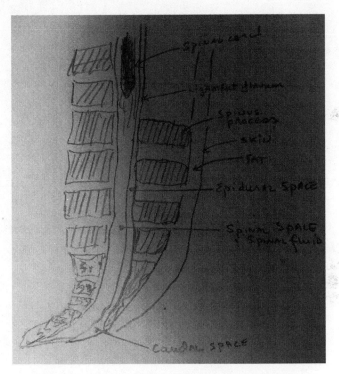

Figure 9-1 Epidural and spinal spaces backbone.

A small tube ("catheter") is then threaded through the needle into the epidural space. The needle is then removed. The catheter is taped to your back. More medication can be injected through this catheter. No more needles are necessary after this point.

Warning: The illustrations that follow may be too graphic for the reader to see.

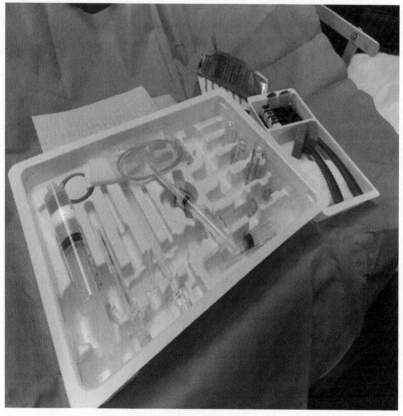

Figure 9-2 Epidural area prepped with Betadine and barrier

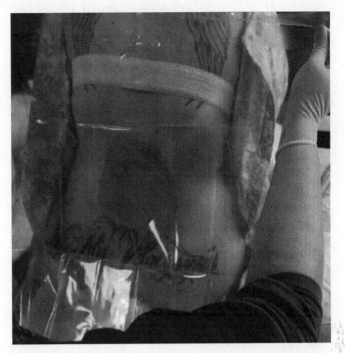

Figure 9-3 Epidural area prepped and draped

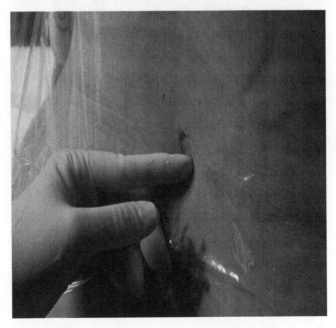

Figure 9-4 Epidural space between spines

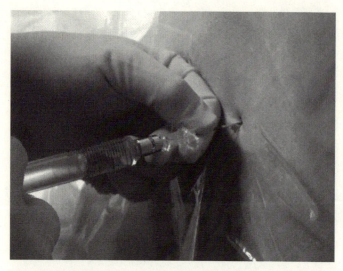

Figure 9-5 Epidural needle being placed between the spine.

Picture shows area of skin that was numbed and the "loss of pressure" technique being performed with a syringe attached to the needle about to enter the epidural space.

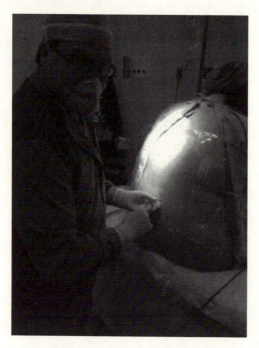

Figure 9-6 Epidural placement

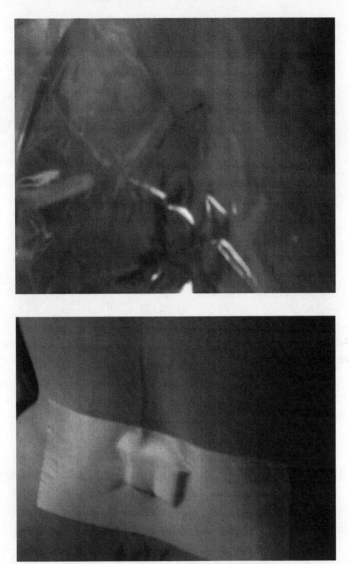

**Figures 9-7 and 9-8 Epidural procedure.
Left side: Catheter has been inserted into epidural space and
needle withdrawn. Right picture shows catheter taped into place.**

Epidurals can be continuous or intermittent. In continuous epidural anesthesia, the outside end of the catheter is attached to an electronic infusion pump containing a very dilute solution of anesthetic medication. Accordingly, the nerves are constantly bathed with the anesthesia medication so that the anesthesia does not wear off.

The amount of drug infused is equal to the amount of drug that is lost and inactivated by the body. On the other hand, the epidural can be intermittent. A "labor dose" can be given at the time the epidural is initially placed. This labor dose may last two to four hours. Consequently by the time the labor dose wears off, the patient may be already finished with the first stage of labor and be completely dilated. Accordingly, further "top-up" doses or continuous anesthesia may not even be necessary. The choice of epidurals, whether lumbar or caudal, continuous or intermittent, should be left up to a discussion by both the patient and the anesthesiologist.

It is crucial that the anesthesiologist get to know you as well as your established contraction pattern and labor curve. He/she must prescribe the correct type, concentration and amount of anesthetic medication to alleviate the labor pain, as well as produce the least physiological effect on your labor. A common criticism of epidural anesthesia is that the patients cannot feel adequately in order to push effectively in the second stage of labor. Without any anesthesia the patient can feel when the baby's head pushes against the vaginal and rectal tissues. By anesthetizing the vaginal and pelvic area too deeply, the epidural could interfere with this natural urge to push. If the patient cannot push the baby through the vagina after a certain length of time, many obstetricians accomplish the delivery with the aid of forceps or a vacuum extractor; accordingly, the common comment by many people that "epidurals may result in operative vaginal deliveries." By careful observation of the epidural's effect on labor after placement, the epidural can be adjusted to correct for too shallow or too deep an effect. Also, by turning off the continuous infusion pump, the epidural can be allowed to wear off. Accordingly, epidural anesthesia need not result in operative vaginal deliveries if appropriate modifications are made.

Epidural anesthesia has become very "exact" science: combination medications in the epidural give pain relief but do not completely paralyze the muscles. The vaginal pressure to push is felt by the patient but does not hurt.

More often than not, if vacuum (or forceps) are required to accomplish delivery in the presence of epidural anesthesia, they are required because of *existing* obstetrical conditions (big head, small pelvis, and maternal exhaustion). In these situations the epidural is "just the innocent bystander," yet becomes associated with perhaps more operative vaginal deliveries (sometimes a middle ground needs to happen: less pain relief and more ability to push).

Epidural anesthesia has a double bonus. Not only can it be used for labor, but also it relieves the pain of vaginal (and even cesarean) delivery. Vaginal delivery is accompanied by tremendous pressure against the vaginal and vulvar tissues. Without anesthesia, the stretching of these tissues is experienced by the patients as a burning, tearing and/or even a ripping pain. A delivery dose of epidural anesthetic medication given just prior to crowning of the baby's head completely alleviates the pain of childbirth. The patient can sit up and observe comfortably the entire birth of her child whether it be vaginal or even Cesarean. Should an episiotomy be necessary, the initial cutting and the suturing after birth will not be felt by the patient.

Epidurals can be given at almost any time during labor.

Lastly, it should be remembered that an epidural can and should be given at any time it is needed during labor and delivery: it can be given in early labor, and if desired, can be given minutes prior to delivery (depending on the skills of the anesthesiologist).

Indications for Epidural Anesthesia

1. Painful labor contractions not alleviated with analgesics and other childbirth coping techniques.
2. Painful labor contractions caused by induction or augmentation of labor with Oxytocin.
3. Most operative deliveries: vaginal and Cesarean.
4. Most intrauterine manipulations: removal of trapped adherent placenta, external podalic version (turning of a breech or second twin)
5. Some extensive repairs, i.e. suturing of vulvar, vaginal and cervical lacerations.
6. Treatment of all pelvic hematomas (Large blood collections from bleeding).

7. Mostly, whenever the patient requests it.

Risks and Side Effects of Epidural Anesthesia

The <u>most common</u> side effects of Epidural are pain in the back where the needle was placed and occasionally some redness of the skin in that area. The needle placement may be sore for a few weeks but the skin heals quickly.

<u>Uncommonly</u>, the epidural needle inadvertently enters the spinal fluid area and a "spinal headache" develops the next day. Spinal headaches can be treated with analgesics, bed rest and caffeine. Most patients will be treated with an epidural blood patch: the patient's blood is drawn and placed into the epidural space. The blood forms a clot over the hole in the spinal sac. The spinal fluid stops leaking and the headache is alleviated within 30 minutes.

<u>Very rarely</u> are there any serious complications with epidural anesthesia. There are potential risks as would be expected from any anesthesia:

<u>Too high a level of anesthesia</u>, i.e., the level of the anesthesia could rise to the chest nerves. The ability to breath could be hampered. Rarely does a patient need a ventilator machine to help them breath until the anesthesia wears off.

<u>Accidental entry of medication into the blood stream</u>. With proper test doses and appropriate monitoring, it is very uncommon for an anesthesiologist not to diagnose bloodstream entry of anesthetic medication before larger labor and delivery doses are given. Bloodstream entry of the anesthetic in large amounts is a potentially lethal complication that could lead to convulsions, brain damage, cardiac arrest and death.

The above complications are indeed rare and are tracked to supervisory medical committees and quality assurance personnel. More commonly, the only side effect from epidural anesthesia is a little soreness in the area of the back where the needle was placed. Epidural anesthesia does not cause any short or long term back problems or pain. Epidural anesthesia does not aggravate any pre-existing back conditions. Previous back injuries and surgery (with attendant scar tissue and adhesions) may prevent an epidural anesthetic from working satisfactorily. The spread of the medication may be hampered by the distorted anatomy in and around the epidural space.

In summary, childbirth under epidural anesthesia is one of the safest and most comfortable ways to have a baby today. It is also the most humane service a physician can provide for a woman in labor. An epidural should never be withheld from someone who needs and requests it.

SWMC Anesthesia Department Labor Epidural Information Sheet
--From Albert Arrendondo, CRNA, Southwestern Medical Center

What is an epidural?

An epidural is an anesthetic technique using a small tube placed in the lower area of your back/ lower than where the spinal cord ends, to deliver local anesthetic or other pain medicines near the nerves that cause pain in labor. You will not get sleepy from this type of anesthesia.

Will it hurt my baby?

If you have an epidural anesthetic, your baby will be safe. The epidural will not depress your breathing or put your baby to sleep.

How long does it take to do?

Placing the epidural takes about 10-20minutes, with good pain relief starting in another 10-15 minutes. In patients who are obese or have scoliosis, more time or attempts might be required to place the epidural. Once the epidural is in place, medicine will go through the tubing continually to maintain pain relief through the rest of your labor and the delivery of your baby.

Will it hurt?

Compared with the pain of contractions, placement of an epidural results in minimal discomfort. As the epidural is placed, you will feel a brief bee-sting on the skin where local anesthesia is placed under the skin. After this, you should feel only pressure in your back during the procedure. The needle is then removed entirely. Once placement of the epidural is completed, you will feel only the tape on your back that keeps the tubing in place for the duration of the labor.

How is it done?

The anesthesia provider will ask you to sit up or lie on your side, keeping the lower part of your back curved towards him/her. You will be asked not to move at all during some parts of the procedure. Your nurse will help you get in the correct position. After the anesthesia provider numbs your skin with a local anesthetic, he or she will insert a needle between the bones of your spine into the epidural space and then leave a tiny tube (catheter) in place while the needle is removed. A test dose of medication is given to ensure the catheter is in the correct space. The tube is secured in place with an adhesive and bandage, and the tube stays in place for the duration of labor and delivery. You should be comfortable in a short period of time. It is safe to move around in bed, but it is recommended that you do not drag or slide on your lower back as these motions may cause the catheter to accidentally slide out.

Does all the pain go away?

Epidurals make the contractions feel less strong and easier to manage. Some pressure might be felt in the rectum and in the vagina later in labor. Being totally numb during labor is undesirable because you need to know when to push at the end of your labor. At SWMC, we adjust the medication type and amount to meet each patient's needs. Most of our epidurals allow the patient to give herself a couple of extra doses of medication each hour. Such self-administration is called patient-controlled epidural analgesia or PCEA. The anesthesia team sets specific limits so that safe doses are administered. For the majority of patients, these safe extra doses will provide satisfactory pain control. If you start to develop more pain after the epidural is in place and your labor progresses we will add more medicine to your catheter. If you are too numb, we will decrease the amount of medication you are receiving. Ask your nurse to call the anesthesia provider with any questions you have about your pain relief. An anesthesia provider is available for labor and delivery 24 hours a day, usually immediately, but sometimes there is a small wait. Within the limits of safety for you and your baby, we will work with you to obtain the comfort level that you desire.

Does epidural anesthesia always work?

The majority of patients experience significant pain relief from an epidural. Occasionally (5% of the time), pain relief is one-sided or patchy. The anesthesia provider can usually address this problem without the need to redo the procedure. Very rarely, there are technical/anatomical problems that prevent the anesthesia provider from getting the needle into the epidural space. These patients may not get adequate pain relief; other arrangements for analgesia can be explored.

Are there any side effects?

Common side effects:

    a. Your legs might tingle or feel numb and heavy. This is normal and will disappear soon after delivery.

    b. Your blood pressure might fall slightly but this is easily and rapidly treated.

    c. Some back tenderness might occur at the site of the insertion, and it might last for a few days. However, no evidence exists that epidurals cause chronic back pain. Mothers with preexisting back issues have a higher incidence of post epidural back pain.

    d. Headache can occur after delivery in 2-3% of patients, due to unplanned puncture of the lining containing spinal fluid. This headache can be moderate to severe, but is not permanent or life-threatening. Specific treatment (conservative or invasive) is available for severe headaches. Mothers with preexisting treatment of headaches/migraines have a higher incidence of post epidural headaches.

e. Itching, very mild sedation, and difficulty urinating are also occasionally noted.

f. You might have temporary temperature elevations that are not significant. No evidence exists that the increased temperature is due to an infectious source.

Rare side effects:

a. After delivery of the baby, some women might develop minor neurologic problems (e.g., a small patch of numbness on one leg). Such problems are rare, and most patients have complete resolution of their symptoms. The exact cause might be impossible to determine and these problems might occur both with and without epidural anesthesia. The delivery of the baby can itself cause pressure on nerves, as can some of the pushing positions used, that can cause these rare side effects.

b. Permanent neurologic problems, such as paralysis, can occur with ANY type of anesthetic procedure, but they are exceedingly rare. The drugs and equipment used for these procedures are thoroughly checked, and our placement technique is very cautious.

Can I walk with my epidural?

The anesthetic solution used for control of labor pain can sometimes make it difficult to walk without assistance. For this reason, most women do not ambulate following epidural placement. Please be sure to check with your labor nurse before attempting to get out of bed.

What is a CSE?

CSE, which stands for combined spinal-epidural, is similar to an epidural. Sometimes we use this technique when a faster onset of pain control is needed. CSE uses the same types of drugs and has similar side-effects to those of epidural pain control. This technique has higher incidence headaches afterwards.

Does an epidural affect the progress of labor?

   a. The first stage of labor (until the cervix is fully dilated): The effect of an epidural on this stage is impossible to predict in an individual. Labor might not be affected at all; or labor might slow down and a drug (oxytocin) will be needed to speed it up, especially in some patients who develop poor labor patterns and are progressing slowly; or labor might go faster.

   b. The second stage (the pushing stage, after full dilatation and until delivery): This stage may be slightly longer with an epidural, but there is no evidence that this harms mother or baby. If the patient experiences loss of complete feeling in her pelvis, she might not push effectively. For this reason, the anesthesia team attempt to balance pain relief so that the patient is comfortable but still feels some pressure in the rectum and vagina during contractions.

Does using an epidural for pain relief in labor increase my chances for a cesarean section?

There is no evidence that epidurals increase the risk of cesarean section. This is also supported by the American College of Obstetrics and Gynecology (ACOG), who state that "fear of unnecessary cesarean delivery should not influence the method of pain relief women choose during labor". At SWMC the anesthesia team uses dilute solutions of local anesthetic; studies show that these dilute solutions do not affect labor. You should speak with your obstetrician about his or her beliefs and feelings about pain relief during childbirth.

Are there any patients who cannot have an epidural catheter?

Yes. For example, patients with the following conditions may not safely undergo epidural anesthesia:

a. blood clotting problems or if the patient has recent use of blood thinning medications
b. heavy bleeding
c. neurologic disorders
d. patients who have had certain types of lower back surgery
e. patients with skin infection at the insertion site
f. Allergies to the local anesthesia medications

Do I have to have an epidural?

Certainly not! If you are coping well with labor pain you might choose not to use any kind of pharmacologic pain relief. If you find the pain too unpleasant, the anesthesia provider is available every day and night to help you. Many women try having no pain medications at all in the beginning; they might then request a shot in their intravenous (IV) line; some will be quite happy with this, while others might desire the stronger pain relief that comes from an epidural. Remember, the choice is yours.

What if I have more questions or need more information about epidural anesthesia?

If you have specific questions or concerns that are not covered here, we would be glad to speak with you.

For more information, visit this website: www.soap.org (select Patient Education). We also encourage women who have unusual and/or complex medical problems to come talk with us during the latter part of their pregnancy. Above all, our strongest desire is that you have a safe and rewarding experience during childbirth.

Spinal Anesthesia

Today spinal anesthesia is primarily used for C-section delivery. It is placed prior to scheduled repeat C-sections or it may be placed for a

1st time C-section if the patient's epidural is not providing sufficient anesthesia at the time of C-section.

Occasionally a spinal or caudal anesthesia will be used for an operative vaginal delivery (forceps or vacuum) when the epidural is not providing sufficient pain relief or the patient has had no epidural during labor.

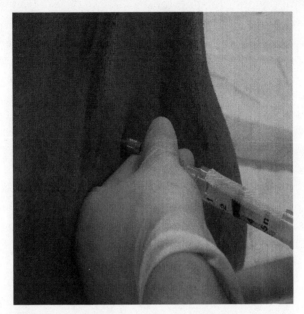

Figure 9-9 Illustration of Spinal Anesthesia being placed

General Anesthesia

In order to provide pain relief when other methods are not available or effective, general anesthesia is used in modem obstetrics in the following situations:

Cesarean Section

Removal of a trapped and adherent placenta after vaginal delivery, and

To suture lacerations of the cervix, vagina and vulva that have occurred with vaginal childbirth.

In brief, the patient is given a sedative medication (Pentothal), followed by a muscle relaxant, followed by placement of an endotracheal tube. A "balanced" anesthesia is provided: a little of each medication to provide sleep, hypnosis (forgetfulness), analgesia (pain relief) and muscle relaxation. Other medications include anti-nausea prevention and relief, drying out of mucus production, etc. Nitrous gas is a frequent component of the anesthesia.

The patient is completely prepped and draped prior to the induction of general anesthesia. The OB will be able to cut through all the layers of the abdominal wall and uterus within 5 to 10 minutes and deliver the baby. The longer the" incision to delivery time" the more likely the baby will be affected by the medications given.

General anesthesia is not used commonly but mostly in the following circumstances:

1. Spinal anesthesia cannot be performed due to technical reasons (obesity), spinal conditions or previous spinal surgery, infection of the skin in the lower back, etc.

2. An OB Emergency in which the baby is in extreme distress, i.e. hypoxia and/or acidosis, such as placental abruption, prolapse of the cord, breech presentation with imminent delivery

3. Failed Epidural in which the medication is not completely effective in anesthesia of the skin or deeper layers.

4. The OB patient is unable to cooperate with placement of spinal or epidural anesthesia: psychiatric conditions or other mental conditions.

5. Maternal medical conditions in which the OB patient could not physiologically withstand a sudden drop in blood pressure that commonly occurs with epidural and spinal anesthesia.

CHAPTER 10

Operative or Assisted Vaginal Delivery

There are occasional times when the patient cannot push sufficiently over a period of time to accomplish delivery of her baby. Circumstances are quite *variable* from patient to patient. Usually there are some guidelines to length of the 2nd Stage of Labor:

- Primagravida (1st pregnancies) 2 hours (up to 4 hours if an epidural is in place)
- Secundagravida or Multipara (2nd or more pregnancies): 1 hour

Again, guidelines are variables and situations are specific to each patient and how their baby is "tolerating labor."

Each OB is trained differently and their experience is also variable. The author was trained to perform forceps and vacuum deliveries: in the author's opinion and other experienced OB's, there is a *place* for these operations in the practice of Obstetrics today. Most forceps or vacuum deliveries in the United States today are done as outlet or low procedures: the baby's head is near crowning or can be seen but the mother just cannot push past this point. Most of the time she will be both completely physically and mentally exhausted. With the vacuum or forceps a "mother push" and an "OB tug" will help faciliatate the baby "to slide" the baby out safely.

1. Vacuum Extractor

Most OBs will select the vacuum cup over the forceps to affect delivery. The vacuum extractor is an obstetrical instrument designed to place a suction cup on the head of the baby. Perfected in Sweden, it gained slow acceptance by American obstetricians. Basically, it is a "toilet bowl plunger" that sticks to the baby's scalp. A vacuum pump keeps the plastic attached to the baby's head. By pulling on the vacuum cup, in conjunction with pushing efforts on the part of the patient, the push-pull combination gives the added force and leverage to produce forward movement in an otherwise immobilized situation in the second stage of labor. The advantages of the vacuum extractor are numerous:

Built-in safety (if excessive pulling force is utilized, the vacuum cup is pulled off at a low pulling pressure).

No compression force on the baby's head (the vacuum is attached to the baby's scalp and no pressure or compression can be transmitted to the baby's brain).

Maternal vaginal injuries are minimized. Because the vacuum cup goes on directly on top rather than around the sides of the baby's head when forceps are applied, there is little risk of lacerating or damaging the sidewalls of the vagina or cervix).

Minimal discomfort to the mother during application of cup compared to forceps.

The vacuum is valuable in the following clinical scenarios:

1. Category 3 Fetal Heart changes (Fetal Distress: delivery reduces the time the baby's oxygenation could be compromised

2. Cessation or Failure of Progress, i.e. further movement when the head is "stuck" in the vaginal canal over a period of time

3. Maternal Compromise Potential: if delivery is delayed: Heart conditions in the mother, Pre-eclampsia,

4. Fetal Compromise Potential: chorioamnionitic

5. Maternal Exhaustion and the inability to push effectively any longer

6. Second Twin delivery: expediting the delivery of the 2nd twin down when there is potential compromise

There are certain drawbacks as well:

1. A red mark, as well as swelling of the baby's scalp, usually occurs. However, the swelling or "caput" goes away in days and the redness within a week or two. Occasional bruising or blistering can also occur.

2. Sometimes not enough pressure can be generated without pulling off the cup to affect delivery. Consequently, technical problems with the vacuum (leakage, inability to flex head) may lead to use of "trial forceps" or may lead to C-Section: depending on your OB's experience and judgment.

The vacuum cup extractor is a simple and effective obstetrical instrument to end an arrested second stage in an exhausted mother who is unable to push any further to produce delivery. The added pull-push combination slides the baby out in 3 or more contractions. Furthermore, in a relatively tight situation, the vacuum cup can be introduced into the vagina under local or pudental anesthesia. Forceps usually require epidural and/or spinal saddle-block. Such major blocks numb the patient so completely that she cannot feel the pressure of the baby's head in order to push effectively and adequately. The vacuum cup can be applied with minimal maternal discomfort without such major nerve blocks. Her pushing abilities are not affected and can be enlisted to produce the push-pull (or "slide-out") desired to effect delivery.

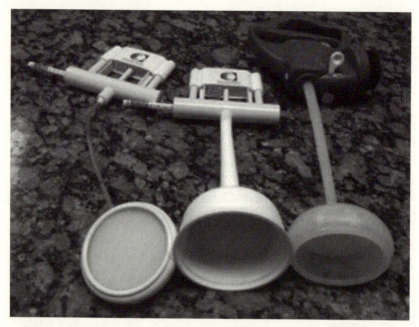

Figure 10-1 Illustration of Vacuums cup instruments. Illustration of Mystic II Mityvac with permission from Cooper Surgical.

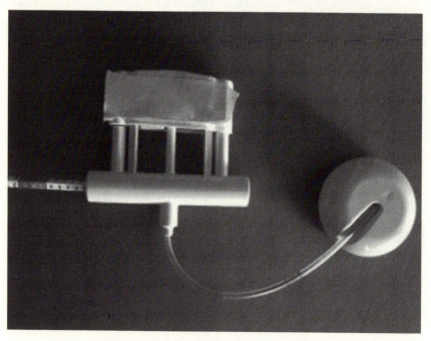

Figure 10-2 Kiwi® type of vacuum cup

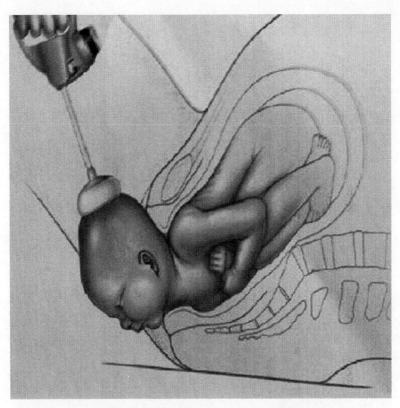

Figure 10-3 Illustration of vacuum application (Reproduced with permission from Cooper Surgical)

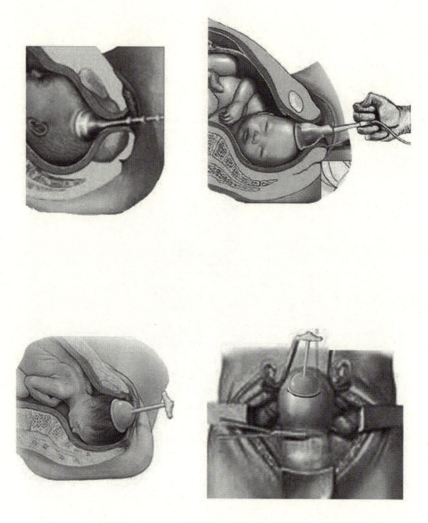

Figure 10-4 Vacuum Delivery. Illustration demonstrating use of vacuum to help guide the head out of the vaginal canal

2. Obstetrical Forceps

There are clinical scenarios when forceps, rather than the vacuum, is a better choice as an instrument for delivery.

The first scenario is when the baby's head is no longer" budging" or moving any further toward delivery. Despite the best pushing efforts on the part of the exhausted patient and the greatest coaching by the nurses, the head is basically stuck. The OB concludes that the use of the vacuum in this situation would not provide enough flexion of the head and the pulling forces on the babies scalp would put too push pressure on the babies scalp. In this case the forceps can provide better flexion and traction with less pressure on the baby's head and skin.

Forceps are utilized to help deliver the baby and conclude the duration of the second stage of labor. Contrary to popular belief, the forceps *protect* rather than compress the baby's head. The forceps go around the baby's head much like a football helmet goes around and protects the football player's head. Like a football helmet, the forceps touch the baby on the cheeks exactly the same way the helmet is strapped to the football player's face. In this way the OB pulls on the "face guard" and can flex, pull and thus move the entire head without putting too much pressure just on one part. Gentle use of the forceps flexes the baby's head further: thus resulting in a decreased diameter and dimension of the baby's head-sphere. With a smaller "sphere" to negotiate the birth canal, the head can be moved further down. Such gentle flexion and pulling, in conjunction with the mother's pushing efforts, provides the added mechanical advantage to finally move the baby's head from its arrested position in the pelvis.

There are only two choices of management in these difficult situations that come up daily across the country:

1. Operative Vaginal delivery with the vacuum or forceps

2. C-section

A C-section is a major operation and it involves more risks, in general, than an operative vaginal delivery. The OB is treating two patients at the same time: the mother and the baby. The OB must way the risks to both patients and decides how to optimize the outcome for the two of them.

Forceps deliveries are categorized according to the station or level of the head in the mother's pelvis.

<u>Low forceps delivery</u>: one in which the head is facing straight up or down and "25 cents worth" of the baby's scalp can be seen poking through the vaginal opening.

<u>Mid-forceps delivery</u>: when the baby's head is higher in the pelvis, but below the pelvic spines.

<u>High forceps deliveries</u>: when the leading edge of the head is above the pelvic spines. The use of high forceps in delivery is almost rarely done because of the high risk of birth injury to the mother or the baby. In an emergency situation (baby's life in immediate danger) without the immediate availability of the OR and staff, an experienced OB may attempt to deliver the baby.

It must be remembered that all obstetricians care greatly about your baby. OB's deliver each baby with the same consideration as though they were delivering their own daughter or son. They would never jeopardize the health or safety of your baby by pulling too vigorously with the forceps or vacuum extractor. The author always tells his patient that if he feels that too much pressure or force would need to be applied to affect a vaginal delivery, he will abandon such efforts and perform a C-Section.

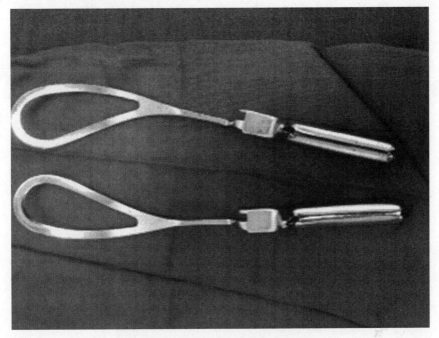

Figure 10-5 The Simpson Forceps

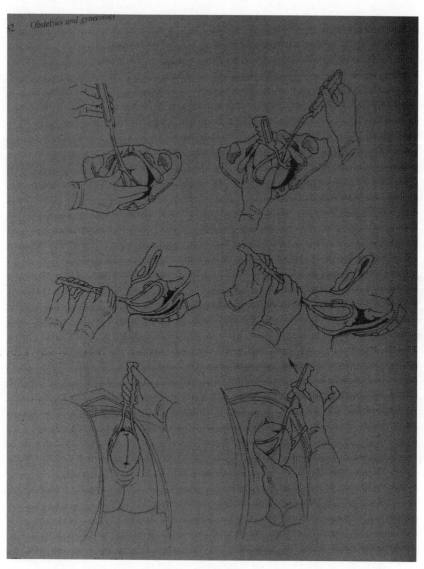

Figure 10-6 Low Forceps Application to effect delivery of the Head, reprinted with permission from *Obstetrics and Gynecology*, Willison and Carrington, Mosby Year Book, 9th edition, 1991

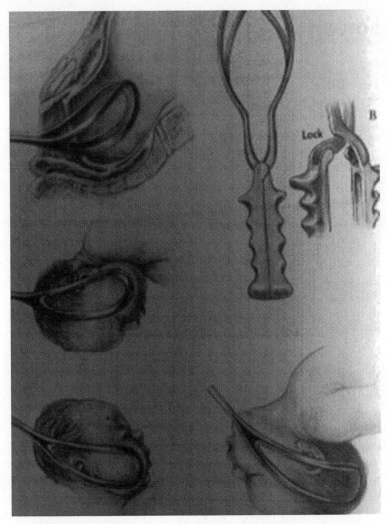

Figure 10-7 Illustration of forceps application for delivery

CHAPTER 11

Fetal Monitoring

The fetal monitor machine continuously records the fetal heart rate of the baby. It simultaneously records the frequency and intensity of the mother's uterine contractions. Measuring the fetal heart rate alone truly provides only a rough index of the baby's health and well-being during labor and delivery. Fortunately, over the past twenty years, it has been shown to reliably predict any dangerous situation developing to the baby during childbirth.

Parameters of fetal health evaluation are:

1. Fetal heart rate and heart rate changes.
2. Measurement of fetal blood gases (CO_2, HCO_3, pH).
3. Respiratory rate (fetal breathing movements by ultrasound).
4. Fetal echocardiographic changes.
5. Fetal movements (by ultrasound).

Today, and in the future, medical scientists are studying new ways and parameters by which we can judge and predict the future well-being of the unborn child. The fetal monitor has the capacity to indirectly or directly measure the fetal heart rate and uterine contractions of the mother. Indirect measurements such as external monitoring, involves the placement of two belts around the pregnant mother's uterus. One belt ultrasonically detects the fetal heart rate and the other belt "feels" the frequency and relative intensity of the uterine contractions. Direct measurements, or internal fetal monitoring, involve the placement of a wire electrode into the superficial skin of the baby's scalp. In addition, a small fluid-filled catheter or "show" is placed through the vagina into the uterine cavity alongside the baby's head.

On admission to the labor room, most patients are initially placed on the external fetal monitor. The fetal heart rate, heart rate changes, as well as the frequency and relative strength of the contractions, are recorded. If no apparent abnormalities are seen, the fetal monitor may be removed from the patient at that time. Most obstetricians prefer that the external fetal monitor remain on their patients as long as it is comfortable and acceptable to them. If their patients desire to walk around the labor area or go to the bathroom, the monitor's belts can easily be removed from the patient.

During a uterine contraction the blood circulation through the uterine muscle is slowed. In essence the baby "holds its breath" during a contraction. If there is decreased flow of blood from the uterine artery or decreased placental surface to receive the blood that does come through the uterine muscles, the baby consequently receives less blood. Less blood flow to the baby usually results in decreased transport of oxygen, glucose, etc. to the baby, and carbon dioxide and other wastes away from the baby. Labor, specifically uterine contractions, represent the most stressful and critical time of a baby's intrauterine existence. If there is any threat to the baby's health during the nine-month long pregnancy, that threat usually comes at the time of labor. Therefore, it seems most appropriate to carefully monitor the baby with the most accurate means that is available today, i.e., the fetal monitor. A baby's prayer might be "I hope and pray that my mother forgoes the minor discomfort and inconvenience of the fetal monitor to be sure that I receive all the oxygen and nourishment I need during my twelve-hour trip through the birth canal."

Factors Affecting Blood Supply To Baby

Caliber/size of uterine arteries

Maternal blood pressure

Maternal blood volume (i.e. anemia)

Placental surface area

Oxygen/carbon dioxide composition of maternal blood

Fetal circulation

Frequency of uterine contractions

Intensity/strength of uterine contractions

Permeability of tissue surfaces

Fetal Heart Monitoring Crash Course

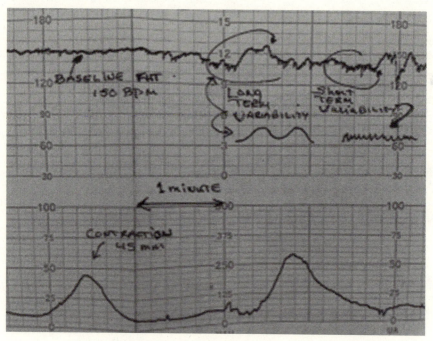

Figure 11-1 Illustration of a fetal heart strip with descriptions

The thick green or red <u>vertical</u> lines (if your book is color version) on the fetal heart strip represent one minute intervals of time. The top part tracks the fetal heart tones (FHT's) or beats per minute (BPM). The bottom part tracks the contractions.

The fetal heart rate varies from 120 to 160 beats per minute. The fetal heart rate is NOT constant, but is "variable." Technically, the "variability" has to do with the modulation of the heart by the human nervous system (sympathetic and parasympathetic systems).

"Variability" itself is split into two types:

"Short-term" variability, i.e. the normal scratchy beat-to-beat up and down second by second recording of the heart rate

"Long term variability" as seen in the wavelength patterns (oscillations or cycles) over a few seconds of time.

"Variability" of the heart rate is normal and is the chief parameter of fetal health and oxygenation. In the tracing below there are peaks of increased heart rate, i.e. accelerations that are at least 15 beats higher in rate for over 15 seconds. "Accelerations" are a parameter of fetal health and well-being.

In the strip below the bottom parts shows the contractions coming about every 2.5 minutes. The top graph shows thicker horizontal red lines graduated to represent 30 beats per minute intervals.

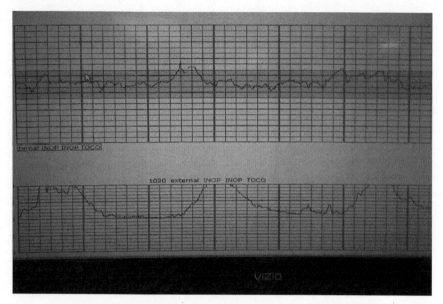

Figure 11-2 Typical "Normal" Fetal monitor tracing with "peaks" of the fetal heart rate depicting "accelerations"

Each vertical red line (color book version) represents one minute. Contractions are represented by the "peaks" on the bottom and are 3 minutes apart (from the beginning of one contraction till the start of the next one). Fetal heart rate is illustrated on top tracing. The fetal heart rate is NOT a straight line but is *variable*. The fetal heart rate oscillates from 120 to 160 beats per minute. The peaks on the top tracing represent "accelerations" and are a sign of a normal varying heart rate.

In order to evaluate the fetal heart tracing there are a number of parameters that must be checked for accurate interpretation:

FHT Baseline rate (and if FHT is a "stable" baseline and not "wandering" or undeterminable)

Determination of short and long term variability

Presence of FHT decelerations

> if present, the type of FHT decelerations: Type I, II or III

> Depth of decelerations, Recovery time and slope, presence of "shoulders" either before or after contractions or both

Frequency of Contractions

> "Resting Tone" of the contraction, i.e. baseline contraction strength or pressure in mm Hg (determined only with internal pressure catheter)

> Peak Strength of Contractions in mm Hg or "Montevideo Unit Score"

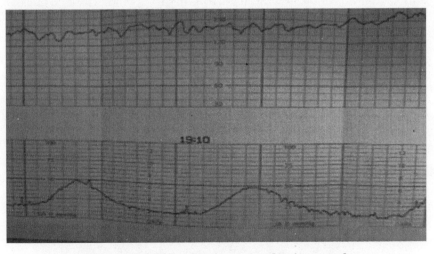

Figure 11-3 Strip showing normal to increased "Long term variability as more oscillations or waves per minute"

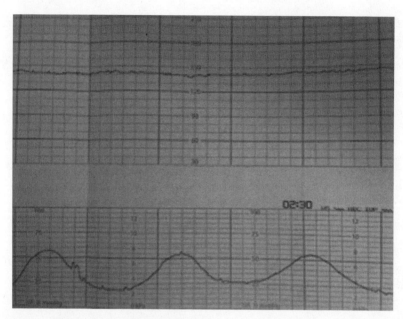

Figure 11-4 Fetal Strip showing no "long term variabilityi.e. wave-forms in the heart rate and diminished "short term variability," hardly any up and down movements of the heart beat at any given 1-2 seconds. If the strip had been normal previously, this baby could simply "be asleep at this time!"

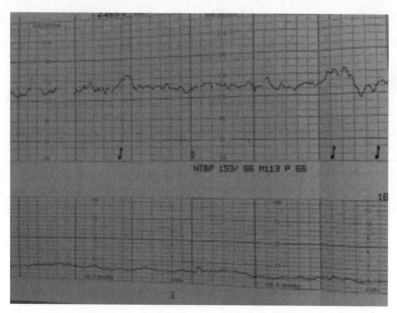

Figure 11-5 Fetal strip showing normal short and long term variability

In Figure 11-5 above no significant contractions are seen on the bottom part of the strip. There are musical notes to mark when the baby has moved: accelerations of 15 BPM for 15 seconds is "the standard" for meeting the requirements of a "normal" NST (Non-stress test)

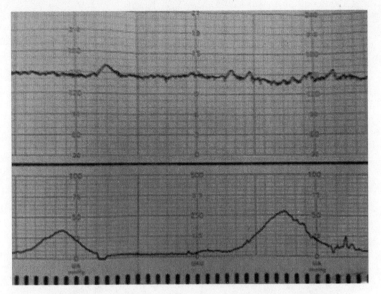

Figure 11-6 Normal short and long term variability.

This fetal heart strip in Figure 11-6 shows a baseline heart rate of 150 beats per min with normal short (small oscillations "chicken scratch" movements of the cursor) as well as normal long term variability with "acceleration curves" above the baseline of 15 bpm lasting 15 seconds. There are no fetal heart decelerations. The above pattern is classified as a normal or Category I strip. Baby acid-base status and oxygenation are normal.

There are 3 types of fetal heart rate "Decelerations Patterns.

Type 1 "Head Compression" Decelerations

The fetal heart rate dips down from the beginning of a contraction and ends with the end of the contraction. It is usually a *smooth symmetrical* concave shape and the fetal rate does not usually drop lower than 100 beats per minute (bpm). This type of pattern usually occurs with the baby's head being applied to the cervix with the contractions. Variability is not affected and this pattern does not cause any loss of oxygen to the baby.

Type II "Late" Decelerations

These decelerations (heart beat drops or slows down) have their onset half way through a contraction but the heart rate does not return to the baseline until the contraction is over. It is a very *smooth symmetrical* curve that forms under the baseline heart rate. The drop in heart rate can be very minimal, i.e. 10 to 15 bpm. This pattern is associated with blood supply to the baby. The baby can tolerated these decelerations for a long time as long as the variability is normal. In today's standard definitions, such "late decelerations" are considered Category II patterns. They are considered Category III when the variability is decreasing slowly over time.

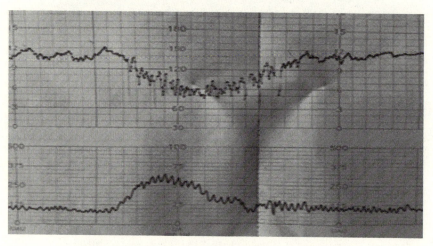

Figure 11-7 Late Deceleration Pattern, Type II.

The deceleration occurs after the onset of the contraction and ends after the contraction is over. The decrease of the FHT (fetal heart tones) is more than typical: in the strip above is it down to about 80 BPM. Further, note the loss of the "short term" variability and decreased "long term" after the deceleration. This baby needs to be delivered soon!

Type III "Cord Compression" Variable Decelerations

The types of dips in the fetal heart rate are truly variable: variable in onset with regard to the contraction, variable in shape and variable in the amount of drop in heart rate from the baseline. These types of decelerations are rather dramatic, angular in shape and can return to the normal baseline in a short few seconds of time.

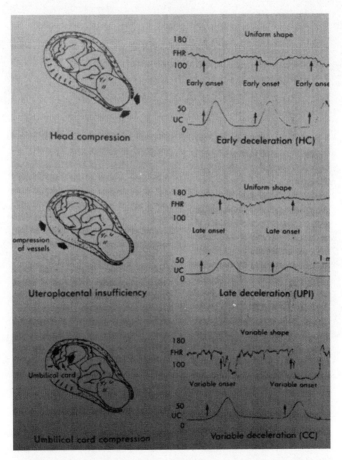

Figure 11-8 FHT pattern Summary, reprinted with permission from Obstetrics and Gynecology, Willson and Carrington, Mosby Yearbook, 9th edition, 1991

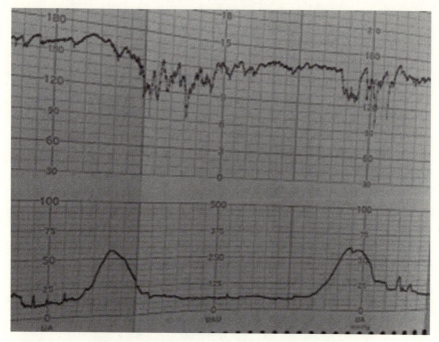

Figure 11-9 Variable or Type III decelerations.

They are very angular (or "spikes") with abrupt returns to the baseline. The short and long term variability is normal. This pattern should be watched. It would be classified today as a Category II pattern.

However, these type of angular or "spike-looking" decelerations are of significant importance (Category III) when they

   a. drop down significantly below 100 bpm,

   b. return to the baseline 15 to 20 seconds after the contraction is over

   c. have small 10 to 15 bpm accelerations above the baseline <u>after</u> they do return to the baseline("shoulders")

   d. the short and long variability is affected and is "being lost" altogether

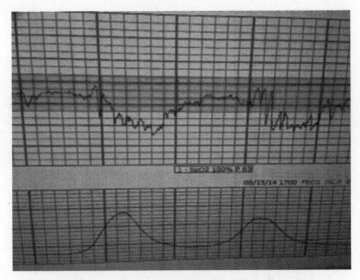

**Figure11-10 Variable Cord Compression Decelerations
(see photograph below of double loop around neck**

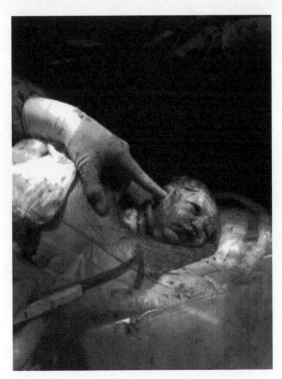

**Figure 11-11 Cord around neck twice at C-section (see preceding
FHT strip: baby could not further time in labor)**

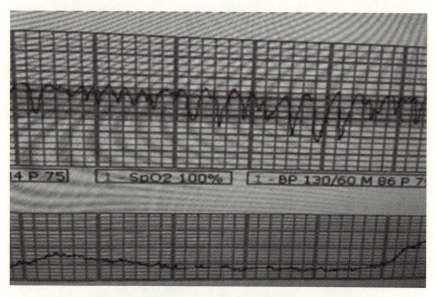

Figure 11-12. Extreme long term variability Tracing shows extreme (90 to 155 bpm) "long term" variable decelerations

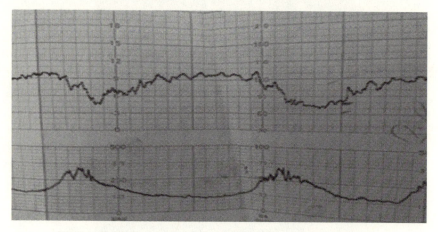

Figure 11-13. Type II and Type III decelerations with slow return of the FHT to baseline. This is a Category III type of strip. This baby delivered vaginally about 10 minutes later. Notice that the FHT's still retain "long term" variability but short term variability is decreasing toward the end of the strip.

As long as there is "variability" in Category III fetal heart strips, the baby's oxygenation (receiving adequate intake of oxygen) may be becoming slightly impaired. The important point or parameter is that the baby is NOT becoming *acidotic*. Oxygenation is being affected in Category III strips. Over a period in time, compromised oxygenation can lead to *acidosis*. When there is decreasing variability or loss of variability, then the baby can develop *acidosis*. If left untreated and not addressed *immediately, acidosis* is not tolerated by a baby and may lead to permanent problems with the baby.

When there is a question about the oxygenation and possible acidosis in the baby, the baby's blood can be tested directly: fetal scalp sampling (FSS). Much of the original work on fetal monitoring and FSS was done at USC-LA County Medical Center. One of the senior residents realized that when the fetal scalp sample was performed there was an acceleration of the fetal heart rate from the noxious stimulation. He made the clinical correlation that, whenever there was fetal heart acceleration with the FSS, the baby's oxygenation test came back normal. Now, instead of doing a FSS, nurses and physicians will "rub" the baby's scalp and look for accelerations. Such accelerations provide reassuring information that the baby is tolerating the labor adequately.

Additional Modern Monitoring Techniques of the Baby during Labor

Furthermore, just like the thumb pulse oximeter (similar to ET's finger in the Disney movie)used routinely on surgical patients and in the ICU's, Nellcor Corporation developed a continuous *fetal* pulse oximetry in the 1980's to provide similar information. It is *not* used routinely in labor because there are very uncommon instances in which it may be needed.

During a pelvic exam the OB can insert the pad through the vagina and the cervix. He subsequently maneuvers that the electrode pad such that the pad can be placed against the baby's cheek while the mother is in labor. A fairly exact approximation onto the cheek skin is essential in order to record the baby's oxygenation through the skin sensors.

When Category II or III fetal heart pattern manifests itself during labor, several forms of treatment are immediately instituted (Intrauterine Fetal Resuscitation Maneuvers):

a. Place oxygen via facemask on the patient

b. Reposition the patient: she is placed completely on her left side (the baby is not resting on the vena cava or the main blood vessel bringing blood back to the heart). If the heart beat does not return to the normal rate then the patient can be switched over to her right side or even in the "knee-chest" position.

c. IV fluids are infused rapidly or "bolused" in order to increase fluid volume and blood pressure: particularly if the blood pressure is running low

d. A pelvic exam is performed to check for a prolapsed cord and assess cervical dilation and station. At the same time the "fetal scalp stimulation" test can be performed to assess fetal response and oxygenation

If vaginal delivery in not imminently expected, within 30 minutes, then your OBs may recommend that an emergency C-section be performed as soon as possible.

CHAPTER 12
Induction of Labor

Induction of labor is utilized frequently by physicians in these modern times. However, national standards of care have recently dictated that "elective," i.e. non-medical and "convenience factor," inductions of labor should not be performed prior to 39 completed weeks of pregnancy. Labor can be started prior to its natural time of onset if necessary by the physician for medical reasons. Induction of labor prior to your EDC may be necessary to protect the health and well-being of the fetus or the pregnant patient herself.

Labor can be started by various methods. Usually if the cervix is ripe, rupturing the membranes with a small hook will initiate labor contractions. It is felt that the loss of amniotic fluid through the cervix decreases the intrauterine volume. Uterine muscle fibers shorten and this triggers off more uterine muscle contractions, i.e. labor starts. Furthermore, cervical manipulation releases a prostaglandin-type hormone which further stimulates uterine contractions. Should labor contractions be infrequent or poor in intensity, intravenous infusion of gradually increasing Pitocin concentration further augments the frequency and intensity of contractions. These two methods, rupture of membranes and Pitocin infusion, are the traditional medical approaches to induction of labor.

Cervical ripening of the cervix is different than *induction* of labor. Cervical *ripening*, i.e. to make it softer, thinner and more dilated, prostaglandin hormone suppositories and gels are placed in the vagina or cervix. By placing prostaglandin gel against the cervix, a long, closed, hard cervix may painlessly become almost completely effaced, soft and two centimeters dilated overnight while the patient sleeps.

It is a common misconception that induced labor is harder or more painful than "natural" labor. The goal of any induced labor is to simulate the natural process itself. If labor starts and progresses with AROM (artificial rupture of membranes), then that labor pattern is natural and represents the uterus' own contracting abilities. If oxytocin is utilized to augment the labor contractions, its concentration should only be increased to the point of producing a natural labor pattern, contractions every two to three minutes of moderate intensity (40-50 mm of mercury or Hg.). Intensifying labor contractions, (i.e., *frequency* of contractions every two minutes with a strength over 60 mg. Hg.), by increasing the infusion rates of Pitocin results in a harder, more painful labor. This labor may not be easily handled by patients without use of analgesics. Lamaze or Bradley techniques of coping would be significantly compromised.

Techniques of Labor Induction

Surgical amniotomy (AROM): 80% effective alone with ripe cervix

Oxytocin infusion

Prostaglandins (intra-vaginal Cytotec® i.e. Misoprostol or Cervidil®)

Foley Bulb dilatation

The induction of labor also carries certain inherent risks. Prematurity with respiratory problems and jaundice may occur if due dates are not certain **or** have been miscalculated. Sometimes prematurity cannot be avoided if the mother's health dictates early delivery. Furthermore, if one is over-vigorous in the use of oxytocin, hyper stimulation or even titanic contractions may result in fetal distress and decreased oxygen transport to the fetus. Lastly, induction of labor may fail to produce enough cervical dilation and vaginal delivery. A failed induction results in a C-Section delivery. It goes without saying that medical reasons for labor induction must be sufficient to justify a possible C-Section delivery if so needed.

Proper Conditions for Induction of Labor

Ripe cervix: soft, effaced, dilated, adequate station and descent of head

Correct due date

Appropriate medical indications

Experienced nursing personnel

Fetal monitor with both internal and external monitoring capacities

Electronically controlled infusion pump

Ancillary medications tray to treat hyper-stimulation

Scheduling within a week or two of due date

Mature fetal pulmonary test: mature L/S (Lecithin/sphingomyelin) ratio and phosphatidylglycerol (PG) tests from amniocentesis

On the other hand, there should theoretically be few problems with induction of labor under the proper conditions. Many physicians and patients desire to induce labor at or near term for the convenience of all involved. For the sake of the patient, a date can be selected so that babysitting arrangements, husband's leave from work, as well as a good night's rest can be accomplished. For the sake of the physician and hospital, proper numbers of nursing personnel can be arranged to cover the patient's care. In England, induction of labor is done in the majority of pregnancies. Admitting the patient to the OB suite in the early morning for induction of labor helps to effect a *daytime* delivery. A daytime delivery translates into an hospital that is fully staffed: all the hospital's personnel such as laboratory, imaging services (ultrasound), respiratory therapy, anesthesia and OR nurses are present. This daytime staff is rested. Accordingly, an alert, awake, and complete medical and nursing staff are available to handle any problems with the patient and her newborn baby. Having such a hospital team available during the daytime insures your baby a safe entrance into the world.

The sequence of events surrounding labor induction goes as follows: Patient enters labor & delivery suite. The patient is admitted to the unit: the patient changes into a hospital gown and an ID bracelet is placed. The patient's medical and OB history is taken. An IV route is established. Laboratory tests are performed: blood is drawn and urine specimen is obtained. The patient's OB chart is reviewed and a medical/nursing history is taken. The external fetal monitor is placed on the mother and held in place with the elastic straps. The baby's heart rate strip and the mother's baseline uterine activity is completed. If the mother's Group B strep test is positive (done at 36 weeks in the OB's office) penicillin prophylaxis is given intravenously. The nurses further evaluate that the proper conditions for induction; i.e., correct due date, ripe cervix, adequate fetal weight.

A blue chux and a towel are placed under the patient so that any amniotic fluid that runs out of the vagina is caught and soaked up so that the bed sheets do not get wet. The OB ruptures the amniotic sac: a small hook on his glove or on a stick snags the membranes that lie just above a slightly dilated cervical opening. Rupturing the amniotic sac is not a painful procedure: it is just slightly more uncomfortable than a regular cervical/vaginal examination. The amniotic fluid runs out of the vagina: it feels like you are "peeing" on yourself.

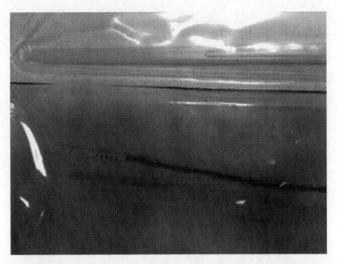

Figure 12-0-1 Fetal Scalp electrode and amniohook stick

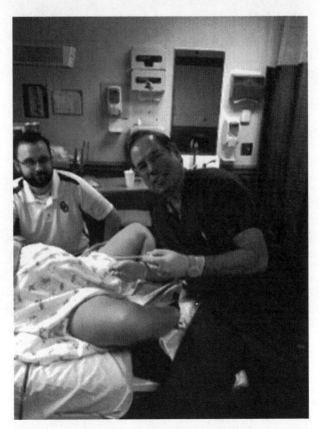

Figure 12-0-2 Rupturing the membranes and placing monitors

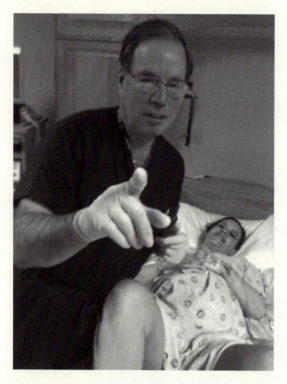

Figures 12-3.

Figure 12-1 in the above picture illustrates a fetal electrode to monitor the baby's heart rate. The amniohook is beside it. The bottom left picture shows the "crochet hook" about to be inserted into the vagina through the cervix to break the amniotic sac. The bottom photo shows a hook-finger cot placed on a sterile gloved hand. The cot on the finger has a flexible small hook with which to puncture the amniotic sac.

Author note: The conception of pregnancy at the beginning as well as the delivery of the baby at the end of pregnancy are both generally messy affairs!

Usually contractions start within one to two hours. Labor, i.e. cervical thinning and dilatation begins. Should labor not start or contractions or be infrequent, a Pitocin augmentation is started. An ampoule of 20 units of Pitocin is placed in an IV bag. The IV tubing is placed through an electronically controlled mechanical pump to allow the Pitocin solution to flow into the patient's circulation at a given rate. The rate of flow is increased just to the point to produce an adequate labor pattern, moderately intense contractions every two to three minutes.

"I've learned that people will forget what you said, people will forget what you did, but people will never forget how you made them feel."
--Maya Angelou

Being deeply loved by someone gives you strength, while loving someone deeply gives you courage."
---Lao Tzu

CHAPTER 13

CESAREAN DELIVERY:
Babies born that are "A Cut Above!"

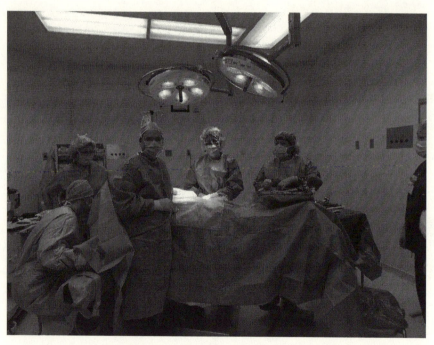

Figure 13-1 Typical OR Scene during C-section (Author is facing reader and the husband is sitting down next to his wife)

Childbirth by means of Caesarian section is increasingly being more utilized by today's obstetricians. There are a number of reasons for this increased C-section rate:

1. Previous C-section in the patient and the decreased availability at hospitals to do VBAC deliveries
2. Continuous fetal monitoring with the ability to make an earlier diagnosis of fetal intolerance to labor
3. Increased prevalence of obesity (>33%) with the attendant gestational diabetes, pre-eclampsia and larger babies
4. Decreased utilization and training of OBs in the use of forceps and vacuum deliveries as well as patient's increasing un-wiliness to undergo operative vaginal delivery
5. Malpractice risks: OBs are un-willing to take *any* risks that might lead to a lawsuit

OBs must avoid any possible risk to the baby that might occur during a difficult labor or delivery. At this time 20 - 25% of all babies first time born in the United States are being born by C-Section. In this chapter we will discuss the history, the medical indications and the operative details of C-Section.

Author's Note regarding the History of the C-section: Contrary to popular beliefs, Julius Caesar was not born by C-Section. The term arose from the Roman law (the "Caesarian Law") that, should a woman die in childbirth which was quite common in ancient times, no pregnant woman should be buried with her unborn child left inside her. Accordingly, after the mother's death, an incision would be made and the dead baby would be delivered from the womb. The mother and unborn fetus would be buried in separate graves. It was not until the 15th and 16th century when anesthesia and other pain control methods became available that the operation was tried on live women during childbirth. In the early reported cases, the women usually died from the operation, but most of the babies were saved. Not until advances in surgical techniques, sterility and anesthesia were developed, along with fine suture thread, could the operation be performed without loss of the mother. In the early part of the 20th century, the operative technique was further perfected and the operation was utilized for very strict reasons: to save the woman's life in cases of obstructed labor or severe bleeding.

Not until later in early 20th century, when blood banks and other advances occurred, was the operation performed to decrease birth injury to the baby or to save the baby's life.

The operation itself involves making an incision in the abdomen above the pelvis in order to affect delivery when the baby cannot or should not be delivered through the pelvis. More than 95% of all C-Sections are performed by "bikini," i.e., horizontal incisions on the abdomen as well as the uterus. Only in cases of extreme emergency in which time is extremely critical for the baby (fetal distress or oxygenation issues) or the mother (i.e., hemorrhage) does the obstetrician need to do a "vertical" or up and down, incision on the abdomen and the uterus. The vertical, or "up and down," incision is the fastest way to open up the abdomen and expose the uterus. At this point, the obstetrician needs to decide which way to make the incision on the uterus. Most commonly, the incision is horizontal and low in the lower uterine segment. However, if the placenta covers the opening to the uterus and occupies the lower part of the uterus, the physician may need to do a vertical incision higher up on the uterus in order to avoid cutting through the placenta itself.

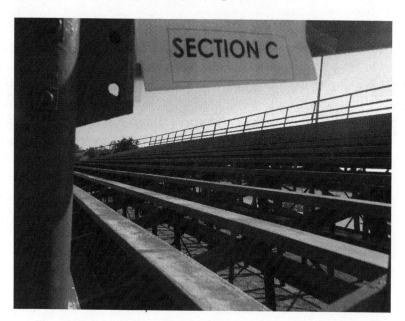

Figure 13-2 We are *not* talking about this kind of C-section!

Abdominal Incisions:

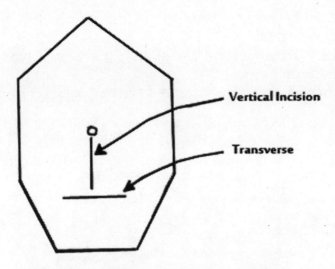

Figure 13-3 Types of Abdominal incisions

<u>Author Note</u>: The reader should realize that the incision on your lower abdomen may not necessarily be the same horizontal cut on the uterus and vice versa. Most OBs usually do a transverse incision on the lower abdomen and a horizontal cut in the lower part of the uterus.

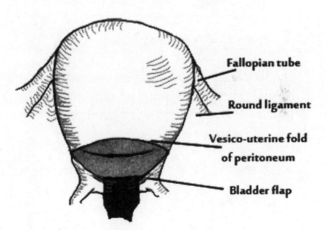

A. Lower segment transverse incision

Figure 13-5 Typical low "bikini cut" uterine incision transverse seen below

Other types of Uterine Incisions

1. Classic (used for placenta praevia, transverse lie, fetal distress)
2. Low Vertical
3. Low Transverse or" Bikini cut"(Pfannenstiel type--most common incision)
4. Combinations of horizontal and vertical or higher transverse or vertical

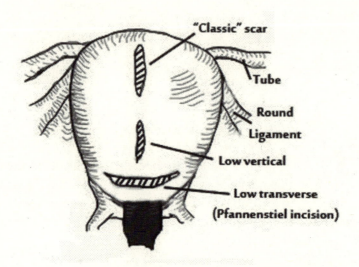

Figure 13-6 Types of *Uterine* Incisions

Occasionally an OB has to "T" the incision when there is not enough exposure or there is not enough room to deliver the baby from the crisscross or horizontal incision in the lower narrower portion of the uterus.

From a surgical perspective, there are approximately eight layers of tissues through which the obstetrician must traverse in order to reach the baby. Likewise these tissues must be placed back together so that the mother heals properly. The following chart shows the layers that must be sutured in order to complete the operation: there are seven (7) layers in total.

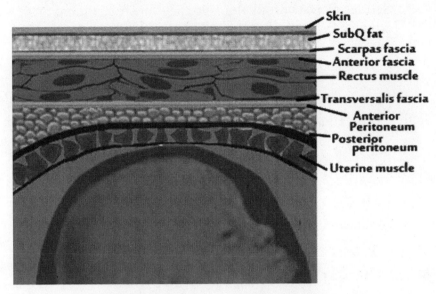

Figure 13-7 C-section surgical planes:
The 7 layers that must be traversed in order to deliver baby by C-section as can be seen from above sketch:

Skin
Subcutaneous fat
Scarpas fascia
Anterior fascia
Rectus muscle
Transversalis fascia
Anterior peritoneum
Posterior peritoneum
Uterine muscle
Chorioamnionitic membranes

Closure of the Incision: the Skin Layer

Sutures in all of these layers (except possibly the skin) are usually of the "self-dissolving" type. The skin can be closed in a variety of ways:

1. Staples or clamps of stainless steel that are removed early in the post-operative period (rarely used today).

2. Sutures of nylon or silk (removed anytime from the 3rd to the 5th post-operative day depending on the rate of the healing process.
3. Sutures under the skin (self-dissolving or re-absorbing suture).

Medical Indications for a C-Section

1. Maternal, i.e., when the mothers health is jeopardized by continued trial of labor.

2. Fetal, i.e., when the baby's health would be jeopardized by continued labor or the delivery process

Obstetrical Legal Indications.

Today's obstetricians are charged with a very difficult or impossible responsibility: a perfectly healthy mother and baby without any complications.

<u>Author Anecdote</u>: *The author had long ago read a Letter to the Editor of the OB-GYN NEWS from a recently trained and talented OB from a reputable University Ob-Gyn Program: She wrote in her Letter that she was quitting the practice of Obstetrics because she could not practice in a field in which the "Standard of Care" was perfection. If you want a perfect pregnancy and a perfect baby, then you need to make an appointment with God in order to get such results.*

More so than ever, either the baby comes out smoothly (via the pelvic-vaginal route) or it does not come out that way at all (thus a C-Section). It is important for every patient to know that the clinical practice of obstetrics is not a precise science. Obstetricians cannot know the exact size and weight of the baby. Nor can they measure the dimensions of the female pelvis. Furthermore, both the baby and pelvis can change during the process of labor: the baby's head can "mold" and take on a new shape. Likewise, the pelvic bones and tissues can spread a few millimeters more so that the baby can eventually "fit" through the pelvis. Therefore, the obstetrician never knows for sure whether a baby can be delivered vaginally. There are too many variables and thus, unanswered questions:

Should the patient "push" for a longer period of time?

Should the strength of the uterus contraction be augmented with the use of oxytocin?

Would vacuum or forceps be needed now to effect the proper angle of traction in order to accomplish delivery without resorting to C-section?

If the baby's head is not in the right position and subsequently causing the delivery to be delayed, should the head of the baby be rotated?

Can the baby withstand a longer labor or do a vacuum/forceps delivery?

Will the mother incur any injury to her vaginal and supporting tissues from a vaginal delivery?

Will the mother suffer any complications from performing a C-Section?

These are a few of the many questions an obstetrician must ask himself/herself during an abnormal childbirth. The problems are further compounded when the mother has such health problems as diabetes, hypertension or other serious medical diseases.

Obstetricians have two patients to think about during childbirth: the mother and the baby. Usually both tolerate the childbirth process well. However, when the baby starts to show signs that may place his/her life in jeopardy, the mother may be subjected to a major surgical operation with its own inherent risks and complications for the sake of the baby. In clinical practice, the majority of C-/Sections are done because there is a lack of progress in labor. Essentially, the cervix stops dilating or there is failure of the baby to progress downward through the pelvis. Failure to progress is usually due to the **four P's:**

Pelvis: too small

Passenger: too large or baby's head is rotated in a posterior or transverse position

Power: inadequate uterine muscle contractility

Permissiveness of the tissues of the pelvic sidewalls and cervix to expand

In reality, all the four P's usually operate together: too large a baby cannot fit through the small pelvis and the uterine muscle tires out.

The second most common indication for a C-Section is "fetal Intolerance" to labor, i.e. Category III FHT strip that does not improve with conservative maneuvers and treatment. The other common indications include the following:

Previous C-section (s)

Abnormal presentations, i.e., breech or transverse lie

Placenta Praevia or Abruption

Failed Induction of labor

Maternal medical conditions such that there is "maternal intolerance" to labor

Patient choice or option (patient wants to avoid damage to her pelvic support)

Author Observation of Patients with Polycystic Ovarian Syndrome (PCOS) –His Special Concern

Many patients with Polycystic Ovarian Syndrome have an "android" (we are not talking about electronics and phones here!) type of pelvis. The Android pelvic shape closely resembles that of a "male" pelvis: convergent sidewalls to the pelvis (or funnel shaped) with a short front to back dimensions and a coccyx/tailbone that is less concave.

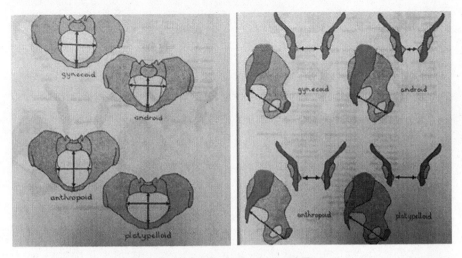

Figure 13-8 Pelvic Shapes and Types

PCOS patients are heavier than most patients or may be obese. They have a higher frequency of having pre-existing diabetes or may develop gestational diabetes during pregnancy. Depending on diabetic blood sugar control, these patients may consequently grow a larger baby. Furthermore, these patients are likely to have increased incidence of pre-existing hypertension and, if not, have a higher rate of developing pre-eclampsia during pregnancy.

It is the author's opinion that these patients must have an inherited "genetic sequence" that is activated during fetal development that produces the anatomic male shaped pelvis rather than the female-shaped *gynecoid* pelvis. As the predisposed PCOS goes through puberty and develops during the teen years the increased levels of free testosterone levels produced by her ovaries lead to increased appetite and weight gain(obesity), oily skin, and hirsutism (hair on chin, pubic area, etc.).

The android pelvic shape lends to the formation of a smaller pelvic passageway and an increased C-section rate." Because of the relative increased *weight* of the baby (due to pre-pregnancy weight and their increased rate of gestational diabetes) PCOS patients have further increased incidence of C-section. An increased rate of pre-eclampsia can also increase the incidence of C-section.

In the later adult years, PCOS patients have an 33 to 50% incidence of developing diabetes and hypertension. PCOS patient make up a disproportionate share of the mix of patients undergoing gastric bypass surgery. PCOS patients are more likely to develop uterine leiomyomata in their future and, with their small pelvic dimensions, more likely will require abdominal approaches for their surgeries.

The Uterine Incision

The Uterus is a muscular organ that varies in its muscle and tendon composition from top to bottom. The lower part of the uterus mainly consists of elastic tendons so that it can stretch and expand open. It is a "passive portion" and does not contain many muscle fibers to contract. The upper part of the uterus is mainly muscle. It actively contracts in its attempt to pull open the stretchable mouth of the uterus. Like the mouth and cheek muscles, the lips are pulled open by the jaw muscles. When the OB sews the tendons (i.e. the fascia) together with sutures, a strong scar usually forms. Muscles, on the other hand, do not heal together and weak scar tissue is formed between muscle edges. Accordingly, a healed incision made through the top part of the uterus cannot withstand much pressure against it: it splits apart easily. A healed incision in the lower part of the uterus, which is designed to expand and stretch, can hold and tolerate the pulling forces of the upper part of the uterus. The lower uterine segment is also thinner and stretches easily.

The Risks of a C-Section

Like any other major surgical operation, a C-Section has the same anesthetic and post-operative complications that any abdominal surgery can incur. Fortunately, C-Sections enjoy a very low risk profile, and are one of the safest abdominal operations performed in the U. S. today.

The most common problem associated with a C-Section is bleeding. As with any surgery, an incision through the abdominal wall involves some bleeding. Blood loss from the skin edges and subcutaneous layers is usually very minimal. The transverse, or "bikini," incision is made in an area where no major arteries and veins exist. Small vessels are usually "bovied or cauterized," that is coagulated with the electrical scalpel before they are cut. The most dangerous area to cut through, however, is the uterus. The uterine muscle wall is very similar to a soft sponge soaked with blood. Accordingly, any incision into the uterus is accompanied by rapid bleeding. When the obstetrician gets ready to make the incision in the uterus, he makes a small opening initially so that bleeding is minimized. When he is sure he is through the uterine wall (because he can see the amniotic membranes bulging through much like an inner tube through a crack in a rubber tire), he extends the incision quickly cutting laterally to the right and then to the left side. Note that the surgeon places his index finger inside the uterus and cuts the uterine wall above his finger so that no part of the baby is cut in the process.

The second most common problem with a C-Section is infection. After labor starts and the amniotic sac is ruptured, bacteria can spread up into the uterus, placenta and baby. The rhythmic contractions of the uterus act much like a blender sucking up bacteria from the vagina. After many hours of labor and multiple pelvic examinations that push vaginal bacteria up through the cervix, there is clearly a natural contamination of the uterus and amniotic membranes. Accordingly, if a C-Section should be done, one is necessarily opening up a partially contaminated uterus. During surgery this bacteria can spread upward through all layers of the abdominal wall and the surgical incision. To counteract this problem, obstetricians usually administer antibiotics through the intravenous line prior to surgery (or in the past, just after the baby is delivered). Any bacteria in the uterus and incisional layers are usually sterilized by the antibiotics. The antibiotics are continued for two or three more doses just to be sure all bacteria are killed. Should the bacteria persist, the blood and sutured tissues of the uterus provide an ideal environment for the bacteria to grow and spread. Endometritis, or infection of the uterus, will develop. Such an infection is signaled by fever and a very tender uterus. A pelvic exam is performed and a culture of the uterus through the cervix is taken. Antibiotics are usually continued until the infection is gone.

Other problems can occur with a C-Section. Some of these are:

  a. Infection (uterus, incision, bladder, kidney)
  b. Bleeding (uterus, incision)
  c. Organ damage (bladder, ureter, intestine)
  d. Anesthesia (convulsion, nerve damage)
  e. Thrombophlebitis or DVT (clots in legs and pelvis that can travel to lungs)
  f. Drug reactions (rash, psychological effects)
  g. Pneumonia (aspiration during anesthesia)

Approximately 15 to 20 percent of women experience complications from a C-Section. The most common complication is a bladder or urinary tract infection. These infections are easily treated with antibiotics. They may result from urinary catheterization during labor and after placement of an epidural. Whenever a catheter is placed in the bladder, there is a twenty percent risk of infection despite the very sterile technique during insertion. Pre-operatively, a Foley catheter is placed in the bladder for two reasons:

First, the bladder sits above the uterus and over the area where the uterine incision is made. Keeping the bladder empty provides better exposure and helps prevents the bladder from being injured.

Second, the catheter drains the bladder in the immediate postoperative period so that the patient does not have to get out of bed to go to the bathroom when her incision hurts the most.

Endometritis, or infection on the tissues lining the cavity of the uterus, is also quite common. Infection of the incision is another common occurrence after a C-Section. It may involve just the skin edges or it may lie deeper in the subcutaneous tissue layer. Deep infections usually need to be opened up so that the infection can be drained. Even without infection, the C-Section incision can ooze fluid or small amounts of blood while it heals.

Thrombophlebitis or DVT of the leg veins is also a possible complication after a C-Section. One of the more important changes that occur with pregnancy is what is called the "hyper-coagulable state." Coagulation factors are produced in abnormally large amounts to protect the pregnant patient from any bleeding during bleeding. After delivery, there are still increased clotting factors present in the blood: the blood is *thicker* and blood clotting in the veins can form. DVT's, or clots in the leg or pelvic veins, are four times more likely to form than they were during the pregnancy. Thrombophlebitis is signaled by calf or thigh pain when walking, swelling of one leg, or a painful and reddened area over a vein. Occasionally, a part of the clot can break off and travel to the lungs (pulmonary clot or *embolism*, i.e. PE). Pulmonary embolism is characterized by the sudden development of chest pain, labored breathing and coughing up of blood.

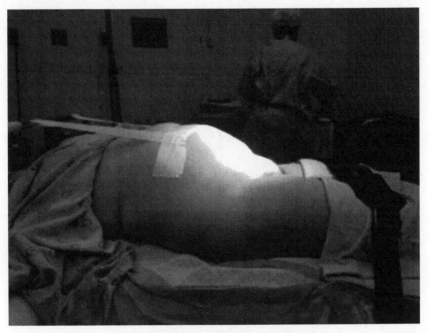

Figure 13-9 C-section Preparation.

Because of the significantly increased prevalence of obesity in pregnancy (>33%), the abdomen might need to be taped up (see illustration above)in order for the OB surgeon to make incisions in the lower abdomen.

C-Section Complications

Common complications:

1. Bleeding
2. Endometritis
3. Cystitis (bladder infection)
4. IV site phlebitis
5. Drug reaction (usually an itchy rash)

Infrequent complications:

1. Thrombophlebitis and/or DVT
2. Wound infection
3. Spinal headache
4. Need for a blood transfusion
5. Intestinal obstruction requiring a nasogastric tube
6. Keloid scar formation on incision
7. Injury to bladder or intestine during surgery

Rare complications:

1. Pelvic thrombophlebitis
2. Hepatitis or AIDS from blood transfusion
3. Need for hysterectomy

The Cascade of Events for a C-Section

Once the decision is made to deliver the baby by C-Section, many pre-operative preparations must be performed. First and foremost, operative permits for the C-Section must be signed. By this time, the patients and her husband are informed of the reasons for the C-Section as well as the usual surgical risks. Consent forms must also be signed for anesthesia. Most C-sections in the United States are done under epidural nerve block, occasional spinal block, and rarely under general anesthesia. General anesthesia is usually employed for immediate emergencies such as fetal distress or when a patient requests it.

Depending on individual hospital policies, the father (or designated support person) may be able to go into the operating room to provide moral support to the patient. Whichever support person (or persons) that will be in the Operating room with the patient may be required to read an informational sheet (protocol) that details their role in the operating room. Each hospital spells out the rules for support- person behavior in the OR. Further, a required consent form might be signed by the father/support person stating that they have read, understand and agree with the hospital's policies.

Melanie's Story

Melanie was a 36 year old Lab Tech that worked for the local Laboratory. On a rare vacation she and her husband went back to her home country of the Philippines to be with family. They were not trying but she became pregnant while they had some "alone time."

She had had 2 normal vaginal deliveries: a girl that was 15 and a boy that was 8. Her pregnancy was uncomplicated and all of her testing was normal. Two days before she was supposed to be induced, she came to the office to discuss the procedure. By happenstance, I did an ultrasound on the baby. The amniotic fluid levels were extremely low: actually little fluid could be seen. I told Melanie that I wanted to do further testing on the baby: a NST (non-stress test). I instructed her to go immediately to the OB suite at the hospital. She sensed the concern and instantly became worried. She was so nervous she knew she could not even drive. She asked her husband to come to the office and drive her to the hospital as she was just too anxious. Within 5 minutes after she was placed on the fetal monitor, the fetal heart tracing of the baby was showing several significant variable decelerations.

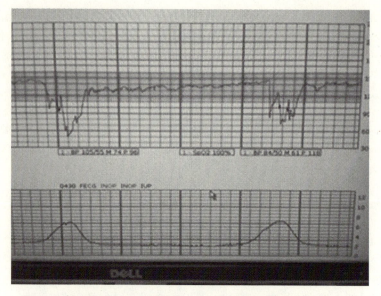

Figure 13-10 Melanie's FHT strip showing the angular cord compression decelerations (Variable Decelerations)

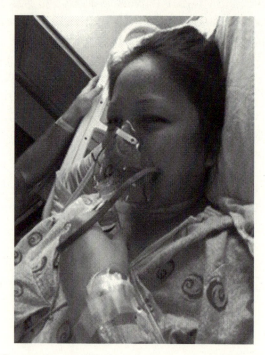

Figure 13-11 Oxygen by mask being given to patient for better oxygenation

I was called and saw the strips on my phone. I told the nurses to call a "Code C" and I instantly left the office and headed to the hospital. Melanie called her husband back who was already on his way back to work. Within 30 minutes, she was wheeled into the OR, a spinal anesthetic was placed, and she had the C-Section delivery. The baby came out fine. Melanie stated to me at her 6 week checkup, "These types of events don't happen to me, Dr. Zweig, they happen to someone else. It was like watching me on a TV show. It all occurred so fast!"

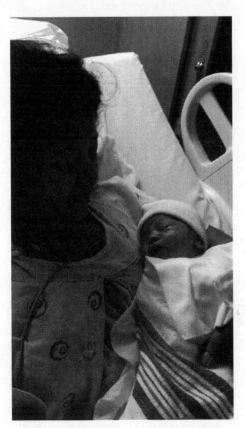

Figure 13-12 Melanie and her new baby after C-section

When the OB nurses see a baby in a life-threatening situation, the entire hospital staff becomes mobilized. Phone calls go out to the OR, to anesthesia, lab, etc. (a Code C for stat or immediate C-section is blurted out on all the speakers in the hospital). The patient is placed on her left side and oxygen is administered with a face mask. An IV is started and information regarding the baby and what needs to be done is given to the patient and her family.

Non-emergent (or "elective") C-sections

If a C-section is being done on a scheduled or even semi-emergent basis, the author will inform the patient and the family exactly what to expect, see and feel when the surgery is being performed. He will also discuss briefly the common complications that most frequently are associated with the surgery.

<u>Author anecodote.</u> The author always counsels the support person who is planning to go into the OR on what they might see: "You may see blood, amniotic fluids and even internal organs when you are there. If you feel dizzy, faint-like or nausea, please close your eyes. That's what I do!

Next an intravenous line is started. The fluid used in most intravenous bottles contains salt and water. Since the fluid is at room temperature, the patient may experience some shivering as the body tries to warm up the fluid to body temperature. The pubic area is shaved and a catheter is placed in the bladder,

The anesthesiologist will interview the patient, reviewing her medical history, any allergies, and the pros and cons of the various anesthetic techniques. Laboratory personnel will draw blood for a complete blood count.

The operating room nurse performs your final "check-in." She makes sure all consent forms are signed, lab results are back, and the patient understands what will shortly transpire.

Prior to all of the above, the obstetrician has makings sure everything is prepared properly for surgery. He/she must arrange for the following in order to do a C-section:

The anesthesiologist/anesthetist to administer anesthesia
The pediatrician or Nursery RN to examine the baby

The assistant surgeon and OR Technician to assist with the surgery
The operating room supervisor to call and assemble the necessary personnel.

Once the patient is in the operating room, she will be transferred to the operating room table. EKG leads that monitor the heart will be attached to the chest. An oxygen pulse oximeter that measures capillary oxygen content will be attached to a finger. The regional anesthetic block, epidural or spinal, will be administered with the patient either lying on her side or sitting up (depending on the anesthesiologist's preference). The skin will be prepped with a germicidal solution (which is cold!). The skin and subcutaneous tissue will be injected with a local anesthetic solution. The epidural (or spinal) needle will be placed through the numbed area into the appropriate location. The patient will usually only feel pressure as the needle and anesthetic is given.

After the anesthetic is administered, the patient is placed on her back but tilted to the left side (to avoid vena cava compression). A plastic oxygen mask is placed over her nose and mouth. The abdomen is prepped with alcohol or betadine.

Prior to any surgery being performed in the hospital, a "Surgical Pause" must take place: the name of the patient and the exact kind of surgery to be done is stated to all the medical personnel in the room: nurses, technicians, physicians, and nursery staff.

Before surgery commences, the surgeon tests the skin with an instrument to make certain that everything is properly numbed. At this point, the husband/support person is allowed to enter the operating room and sit down next to the patient at the head of the table. (Should the husband/support person feel light headed or sick, he should notify the anesthesiologist or scrub nurse immediately)

While the abdominal wall is being opened surgically, patient should be prepared to listen to the obstetrician's latest jokes or his most recent golf scores (this verbal information could be more painful than the surgery!). Hopefully, the next voice you will hear is your baby's crying his/her entrance into the world. The cord is clamped and cut, and the baby is shown to you, the proud parents. The baby is then handed over to the nursery team to be dried off, weighed and placed in a blanket. Over the next thirty minutes, the incision is sewn up and you are transferred back to the OB suite (or to the recovery room in some hospitals) for close observation. The baby is taken to the nursery by the new "father." The nursery team usually allows the father to carry the baby from the OR to the nursery (and show off the baby to all the family and friends nearby).

Visual Tour of a C-section

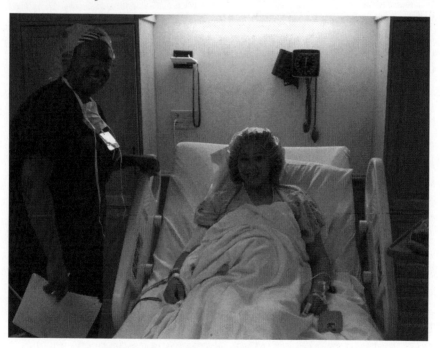

Figure 13-13 Patient Ready for C-section

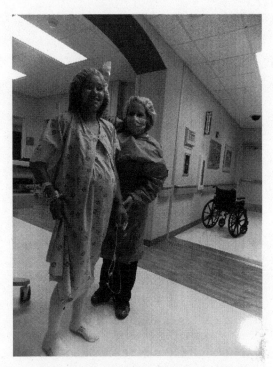

Figure 13-14 Patient Going to OR

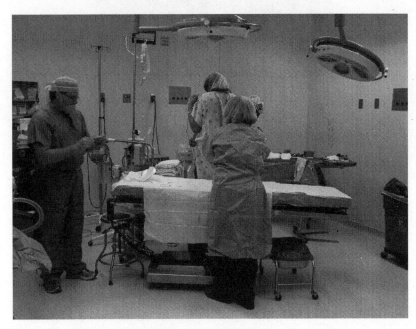

Figure 13-15 Patient being positioned for Spinal

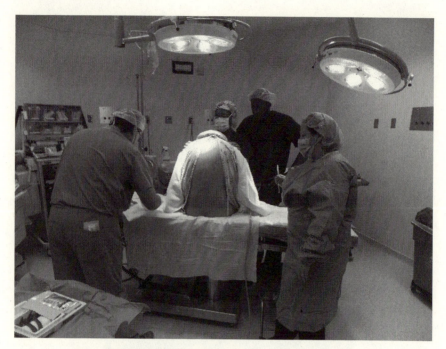

Figure 13-16 Patient in Bent- Over Position for Spinal

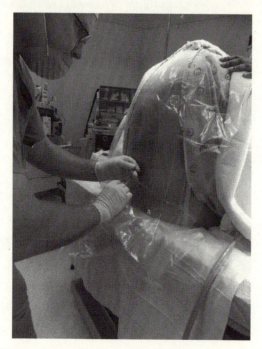

Figure 13-17 Local anesthesia injected into skin

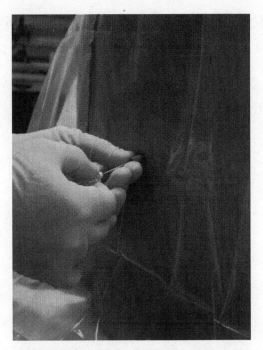

Figure 13-18 Spinal needle going through needle guide

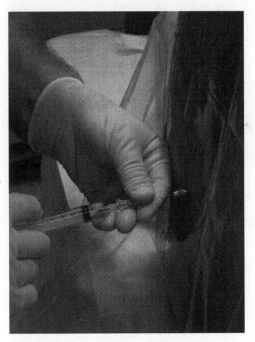

Figure 13-19 Injection of Spinal Anesthetic

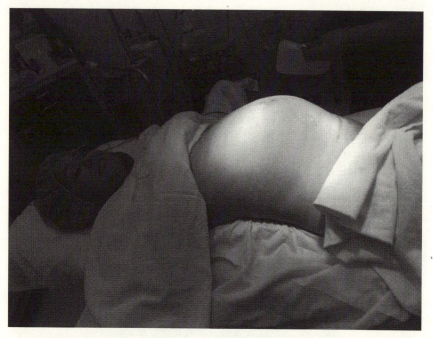

Figure 13-20 Abdomen Prepped for Draping

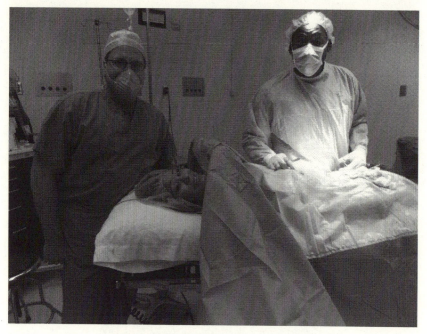

Figure 13-21 Draped for C-section

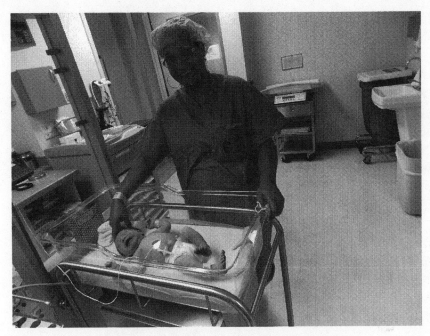

Figure 13-22 Baby in cradle after C-section

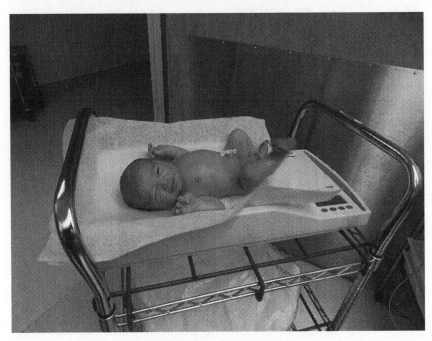

Figure 13-23 Baby being weighed after C-section."

Priceless "Kodak Moment when your baby is being" weighed in" for the first time

In the nursery (or in the OR), the baby is weighed, examined and cleansed. A heel-stick blood test is done to check the baby for anemia and low blood sugar. The baby may be given water to be sure that the stomach anatomy is normal prior to the commencement of breast or bottle-feeding. Later, after the baby has had a period of "bonding" with the parents, the baby's eyes are treated with erythromycin ointment and vitamin K is given to prevent "hemorrhagic disease of the newborn."

As the anesthesia wears off, you will start to experience some pain. Most spinal and epidural blocks have combinations of local anesthetics and Dura morph. Consequently, the patient has satisfactory pain relief without any other medications. The first day after surgery, the patient can be started on oral analgesic pain pills.

Without use of spinal narcotics or if a general anesthetic was given, patient can be given Demerol™ and Morphine™-- the most common pain medications used post-operatively. Injections can be given every two to four hours depending on their need. More recently, patient-controlled administration (PCA) machines have become available so that the patient herself can "push a button" and receive a dose of pain medicine directly into her intravenous line. These machines are set-up so that the patient cannot over-dose herself. Be sure to check with your insurance company to see if the additional charge for the machine is covered.

On the first post-operative day, the patient is recommended to walk around as much as possible. The urinary catheter is removed and normal urination is usually possible (the first time may be accompanied by some "stinging"). A liquid diet is served because the intestinal tract is not usually ready for solid food. Frequently, nausea and occasional vomiting is experienced as a result of the surgery and the pain medications. Because of the volumes of intravenous fluids given and the natural postpartum diuresis of retained salt and water accumulated during the last months of pregnancy, frequent trips to the bathroom to empty the bladder are common.

By the second post-operative day, the intravenous line is removed (and the patient is finally free of all lines and tubes!). Gas has started to build up in the intestinal tract, resulting in burping and intestinal cramps. Early feedings of solid food and lack of walking (ambulation) may make the "gas pains" worse. Accordingly, it is recommended that a liquid diet be continued until the gas is finally expelled through the rectum. At this point, the intestines are ready for solid food. The need for intravenous (PCA) or other injectable pain medication tapers off and much of the incisional discomfort can be blunted by pain pills. Many physicians use combinations of Tylenol (or aspirin) with codeine or codeine-derivatives. Though most of the pain medications filter in small amounts into the breast milk, the baby is not significantly affected. All the medications noted in the following table are safe to take in the post-operative period, Ibuprofens (brand names: Advil™, Motrin™, etc.) are not recommended for use at this time.

Commonly Used Medication for Post-Operative Pain

Percocet™ or Norco 5™ mg to 10 mg (contains Tylenol)

Percodan™ or Norco™ 5 mg to 10 mg (same as above but contains aspirin)

Hydrocodone or Oxycodone 5 mg to 10 mg (Lortab™, Norco™)

Demerol™

Tylenol #3™ (Tylenol with codeine)

Aspirin with codeine

Aspirin or Tylenol

Most C-Section patients are discharged from the hospital on the third or fourth day after delivery. By this time the pain is tolerable with infrequent doses of pain pills, and the intestines are functioning satisfactorily. If staples or sutures were used to close the incision, they may be ready to be removed at this time. Obstetricians usually make rounds in the morning and, at this time, any special instructions or advice may be given. Most patients need several medications during their recovery at home. First, pain pills may be required to dull the incisional pain. Hemorrhoid suppositories and external ointment may be necessary to reduce hemorrhoid swelling and pain. (Stool softeners may also be recommended.) If more than the normal amount of blood was lost at the time of surgery, an iron supplement may be prescribed.

Lastly, if a patient is not nursing, the patient is advised to wear a tight bra and not to express milk. The breasts will swell and become very hard. Ice packs may provide some relief for the swelling. The engorgement of the breasts will abate in 3-4 days. Medication is no longer given to prevent the initiation and production of breast milk.

OB History Tidbit or TMI: Medications used in the past for OB Lactation Suppression

In the past estrogens (Deladumone, ™ Delestrogen, ™ Tace, ™) and bromocryptine class (Parlodel©) medications were prescribed. The most popular medicine prescribed for lactation suppression was Parolodel™ (generic, bromocryptine). The prescription of these medications was halted when possible increased complications were reported: at the worse, possible stroke. Such milk production ceases shortly if a tight bra is worn and no attempts are made to express the milk.

If a well-balanced diet cannot be followed or attained, a prenatal vitamin or other multivitamin may be prescribed for the patient.

Diet instructions after a C-Section are fairly simple: whatever is desired and tolerable. You should ask your physician whether any special dietary advice applies in your case. Until the intestinal tract recovers to its normal status, it may be best to avoid fruit and vegetables that produce a lot of intestinal gas. Coffee, tea and even an occasional alcoholic beverage are permissible. Eggs, cheese, yogurt, milk, meat and fish are highly recommended.

Physical activities are naturally limited by the pain of the incision. It takes at least eight weeks for 90% of the C-Section wound to completely heal. Accordingly, activities or exercise that put tension on the incisional edges might weaken the incision. Rarely, however, can the incision "open-up." If the patient is doing excess weight lifting or puts increased tensions on the abdominal wall, the supporting tissues might be weakened. Increased abdominal tensions and increase abdominal pressures can predisposed toward hernia formation.

The kind of closure of the skin in C-sections varies among OBs. Most OBs use a "subcuticular" stitch that is essential under the skin and cannot be seen. Depending on the suture material used, these stitches dissolve in 3-5 weeks. If the incision cuts into hair glands, there may be some red "spots" above or below the incision. Not all patients can dissolve delayed absorbable sutures and the suture may "spit" or be pushed out of the skin. Weeping, moisture and some redness will be seen. Use a panty liner in your underwear to absorb the moisture. Staples are usually removed in 3-5 days depending on the stage of healing. After staples are removed, steri-strips are placed to keep the skin edges together.

Questions Most Frequently Asked After C-Section Surgery

1) Will the post-operative pain medications affect my baby if I am nursing?

All medications given to the mother can filter into the breast milk to a certain extent. The breast milk does not usually come in for at least three days post-operatively. By that time, most patients only need oral pain medications or antibiotics. Because these medications do not affect the baby to any significant degree, breastfeeding is entirely permitted.

2) Can I break any of my stitches?

Rarely can anyone break their stitches open. Occasionally, wound edges may separate, only to grow back together in a few days. Only high risk patients, such as diabetics or very overweight patients, are more predisposed to poor wound healing and rupture.

3) When can I take a shower (or bath) and wash my hair?

Most patients are permitted to take a shower and wash their hair once the IV line and urinary catheter are removed. Patients with significant anemia, fever or other post-operative problems may have to wait a little longer.

4) When can I go home?

Most patients can go home as soon as their physician determines that going home could be safely tolerated by the patient. Barring any fever, infection, wound or intestinal problems, most patients go home on the third or fourth post-operative day.

5) When can I drive a car?

Patients can be allowed to drive whenever they feel they can safely operate their car. It must be remembered that stepping on the clutch or brake pedals, even turning to look for cars over your shoulder, puts tension (and pain!) on the incision.

6) When can I exercise?

Because 90% of all wound healing takes at least eight full weeks, it is best to avoid any exercises that put tension on the incision for that period of time. Walking and upper body toning exercises are permissible.

7) When do I need to see my doctor again?

Visits to the office (or clinic) after C-sections vary from doctor to doctor, and with the needs of the mother. Some physicians prefer to see patients for an "incision check" in two weeks while others prefer four to six week postpartum check-ups. It is best to ask your doctor.

8) When can my husband and I resume sexual relations?

Most patients will still have a brownish discharge for about three to four weeks after a C-section. Furthermore, the vulvar and the vagina tissues become extra *sensitive* in the immediate weeks after delivery. Accordingly, the couple should use an extra amount of lubricant and "go slow" if intercourse is going to be attempted. From a medical stand point, it is probably safe to resume sexual activity four to six weeks after surgery. Because of incisional pain, fatigue and the constant attention to the baby, most couples refrain from intercourse for about four to eight weeks after delivery. It goes without saying that sexual activity depends on the needs and feelings for each other.

9) What kind of birth control can I use?

For bottle-feeding patients, birth control pills can be started on the second Sunday after delivery. The regular combination Birth control pills are not recommended to nursing mothers because they can interfere with milk production. Breastfeeding patients can take the progesterone only pills for birth control as they contain no estrogen to interfere with milk supply.

For patients who cannot or do not desire the pill, contraceptive foams and suppositories are entirely safe to use. Diaphragm users can still utilize their old diaphragms until the obstetrician can re-check you at the post-operative visit. An IUD (Intrauterine Device) or Nexplanon can also be inserted at the postpartum visit. The patient must check with their insurance carrier for their benefit information, obtaining the proper pre-certifications and any primary care referral that may be necessary.

10) What other kinds of medications do I need to take?

It is best for all women to take an iron supplement daily regardless of pregnancy. A vitamin supplement during lactation may also be encouraged by your doctor. The patient may simply continue using her prenatal vitamins. Stool softeners may also be recommended because they prevent unnecessary painful straining as well as decreased hemorrhoid irritation.

11) When will I stop bleeding?

The uterine bleeding that ensues after birth tapers gradually over a three to four week period of time. By the second post-operative day, the bright red color of the flow turns to a dark purple. Clots and flow diminish rapidly so that by the fifth post-op day, pads may only need to be changed five or six times in a day. Pads, rather than tampons, are recommended for at least the first two post-operative weeks. By the end of the third week, only a brownish to blackish discharge remains. Any return to a bright red and heavier flow, especially with clots, should be reported immediately to your doctor.

VBAC: Vaginal Birth after C-Section

When Cesarean surgical deliveries became a safer operation in the 1920's, it became apparent early that such incisions in the uterine muscle would tend to pull apart if the patient was allowed to go through labor in a subsequent pregnancy. Even the lower transverse uterine incision had a 1 to 3% disruption rate. In today's medico legal environment, the obstetrician knows that he can take no risks in the care of the mother or the baby. Consequently, the dictum "once a C-Section, always a C-Section" held up until the early 1980's.

What Were The Risks of VBAC?

The main risks of VBAC were that the uterus would rupture and the baby would be expelled into the mother's abdominal cavity. The old uterine scar would not only open up but extend itself further laterally to the right and left sides of the uterus where the large blood vessels entered. The blood vessels could be lacerated during uterine rupture causing life-threatening blood loss to both the mother and the unborn child. Should rupture occur, prompt emergency surgery would become necessary to stop the bleeding. A ruptured uterus with its disrupted blood vessels usually could only be treated by a hysterectomy. The mother would therefore lose her capacity to become pregnant in the future.

In the early 1980's, several medical centers started looking at ways to decrease the climbing C-Section rates. Almost exclusive use of transverse incisions in the lower (non-muscular) portion of the uterus, the presence of advanced antibiotics, newer suture materials and safe blood banks made obstetricians take a hard look at the real versus the theoretical risks of a VBAC. Other countries, unable to financially afford repeating all C-Sections, were finding VBAC a safe alternative in most situations. The results of such studies were revolutionary. Prior to these studies, it was felt that only patients with a non-repeatable cause for C-Section could be candidates for VBAC. If the first C-Section was done for fetal distress or a breech presentation, patients with an adequate sized pelvis should be able to deliver vaginally the second time around. These conditions usually do not reoccur in subsequent pregnancies. On the other hand, patients with a repeatable cause for C-Section, such as a small pelvis, could not be expected to deliver their second baby vaginally if the first baby could not make it through. The pelvic capacity does not increase in size from one pregnancy to the next.

Medical studies have revealed the following facts:

Patients who underwent a primary (1st time) C-Section because of FTP (Failure to Progress) or CPD (Cephalopelvic Disproportion) had a 50-60% chance of a subsequent vaginal birth.

Patients whose main indication for C-Section was an abnormal "dysfunctional" labor pattern tended to have only a 30-40% chance of vaginal birth. Those same patients with dysfunctional labor contractions during their first pregnancy tended to have the same recurrent labor problems in a subsequent pregnancy (with arrest of progress and repeat C-section). Those that did not have a recurrent dysfunctional labor were able to deliver vaginally.

Those patients with a *non-repeatable* cause for the first C-Section had the best chances for vaginal births: 70 - 80% special circumstances, patients with two or more previous C-Sections could also become candidates for a trial VBAC attempt.

The risk of uterine rupture was less than 1 per cent. The risk of needing a hysterectomy for uterine rupture was 0.05%, i.e. one in 6000. Accordingly, not all uterine ruptures were serious: less than one in four. The uterus could be surgically repaired so that the uterus could be saved for subsequent pregnancies.

The risk of losing the baby was 0.05%, i.e., one in 5000. No mothers were lost during any of the studies.

When compared to the control group of patients, i.e., those patients who were designated to undergo repeat C-Section, it was found that there was a *relative* eleven times greater chance of maternal complications from a repeat C-Section than from having either a successful or failed VBAC.

Furthermore the studies showed that epidural anesthesia could be safely utilized in patients undergoing a VBAC attempt. The anesthesia did not mask the pain of uterine rupture or lead to any other complications. Lastly, any hospital with an obstetrics service should be able to also perform VBAC's. Except for large University Medical Center or other large OB units, most other medium to small OB hospitals cannot afford the cost of keeping an OR and anesthesia staff waiting for hours while the patient labors for hour to see whether or not the patient will deliver vaginally. Less than 5% of C-sections are performed for emergency or stat reasons: usually the baby is not tolerating labor contraction from an oxygenation standard. It is true that an immediate C-section may be needed for a patient with a previous C-section than one who is having her first or other number) baby. Most OB units can start a C-section in 30 minutes (sometimes more quickly depending on the urgency). However, with the current 30% C-section rate in the United States, it is more likely that the patient will need an immediate C-Section for other unexpected obstetrical events.

Hospitals and medical institutions follow ACOG Guidelines with regard to VBAC protocols. Each Hospital has a written protocol under which all patients and medical personnel must follow. A sample protocol is listed in the Appendix of this book. The reader is also recommended to google other VBAC protocols at other medical institutions (e.g. University of Michigan VBAC protocol).

VBAC Protocol

Patients must be given information regarding the risks and benefits of VBAC as well as a repeat C-Section. No guarantee can be made with regard to the success of surgery of either procedure.

Risks of: Repeat C-Section and VBAC

1. Bleeding
2. UTI anesthesia
3. Uterine rupture with Hysterectomy
4. Post-op pain
5. Post-op uterine infection
6. Post-op phlebitis

Benefits: VBAC

1. No incisional pain but possible episiotomy pain
2. Decreased post-op problems
3. Anesthesia may not be necessary but still can have epidural
4. Earlier return to home and family
5. Easier recovery
6. less hospital expense

VBAC candidates must do the following:

- Sign consent form for repeat C-Section and anesthesia during early labor just in case a repeat C-Section becomes immediately necessary.
- Lab work such as a CBC type and screen blood type and Rh factor
- IV route must be established
- Continuous fetal monitoring when in active labor: internal fetal and uterine monitoring if oxytocin stimulation is utilized

VBAC patients who require an *emergency* C-Section for VBAC complications must realize that the following may be necessary:

General anesthesia may be necessary.

The husband or support person may not be able to go into the operating room with the patient.

Photographing or video-taping may not be permitted.

Should the VBAC attempt should fail for any reason a repeat C-Section can be performed on *a non-emergent* basis, i.e., there is no immediate rush to the Operating Room and the need for general anesthesia.

How can someone deliver a baby vaginally the second time around when the mother was "too small" to deliver her first baby?

There are probably several explanations to the above question. Although it may seem trite to say, "No two pregnancies are alike." In a sense, no two babies and no two labors are the same. Babies vary in size and dimensions. Muscle contractions (labor) vary in their strength, rhythm and synchrony. Each baby's head, which is the first and usually largest part of the baby to push through the pelvis, differs in shape, flexion and ability to mold to the mother's pelvic shape. Consequently, even a bigger baby could deliver vaginally during a second pregnancy because its configuration was conducive to delivering through that size and shape pelvis.

There are also two other theories on how babies can deliver vaginally the second time around. First, there is the "maze theory" The mechanism of labor, the physiology of how the baby maneuvers through the various levels and shapes of the pelvis may be quite different from one pregnancy to the next. Like going through a maze, a baby must make appropriate turns and movements in the right direction so that he does not "get stuck" in a corner. Some babies can "make the right motions" just as they are required. Other babies are unable to twist or bend at the right point in order to negotiate a "tight spot."

The second theory is the "balloon theory." The first time someone tries to blow up a new balloon, it can be very difficult. Each attempt thereafter becomes easier and easier. It is the same situation with the uterus. Once the cervix, or opening to the uterus, is stretched the less force is necessary to stretch it open the second time around. The "balloon theory" is based on physics: the force necessary to dilate an opening is conversely related to its diameter. The ability to rupture or bend a pipe depends on the size and thickness of the pipe itself. Obstetricians are well aware that each labor is usually easier and quicker with each pregnancy.

A copy of a typical VBAC protocol is available for review in Appendix C.

Breech Babies

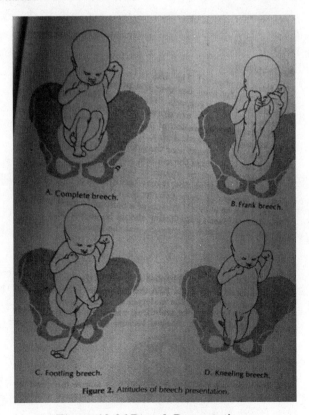

Figure 13-26 Breech Presentations:
Illustrations of the different types of Breech presentations

Most babies settle into the head-down (or vertex) position by the last month of pregnancy. Gravity, uterine shape and tone, as well as the larger space of the pelvis favor such accommodation by the fetal head. The head is the largest and heaviest part of the baby.

In approximately five (5%) percent of all pregnancies, the baby remains in the breech position, i.e., head in the top part of the uterus with the "breech," i.e. "the butt," sitting downward in the pelvis. Except in special circumstances, breech babies have fewer complications statistically if they are delivered by C-Section. Accordingly, if the baby remains in the breech position in the last two to three weeks of pregnancy or if the patient is in early labor, a caesarean delivery is the standard route of delivery.

Many institutions and OB's will not deliver breech babies vaginally due to liability issues: malpractice insurance carriers provide explicit guidelines to their hospitals and physicians. If your baby remains in a breech position near term, you can discuss with your OB the complex issues involved with vaginal breech births.

External Cephalic Version (ECV)

In the early 1980's, new medical studies showed that external cephalic version, that is, turning the baby around by external application of pressure, was a practical method of avoiding a C-Section. Approximately 50% or more of all breech babies can be successfully turned and be maintained in the normal head-down position.

External cephalic version is performed in the last two to three weeks of pregnancy in the labor suite. The patient is undressed and placed in bed. Consent forms are signed. An intravenous route is established and the operating room is placed on "stand by" in case an emergency C-Section becomes necessary. Because it is more difficult to turn the baby through a tense and contracted uterus, most physicians "relax" the uterine muscle by the administration of a uterine "tocolytic" medication (medications such Terbutaline® that are similarly used to stop preterm labor contractions). Some OBs prefer that epidural anesthesia be placed prior to version: epidurals provide more comfort to the patient, The relaxation of the abdominal wall may be more conducive to version and a higher success rates may be effected. Further, with an Epidural already in place, anesthesia is available for a possible C-section if an emergency occurs during the version or if the version is not successful.

Prior to attempted version, an ultrasound examination of the uterine is performed to confirm the baby's position, the location of the placenta and to detect any other abnormalities (such as a septum or myoma). By simultaneously lifting and pushing the baby's buttocks up and to one side, while the other hand directs downward pressure on the head, the baby can be maneuvered and turned. Most often the procedure "goes easily." Sometimes persistent effort is required.

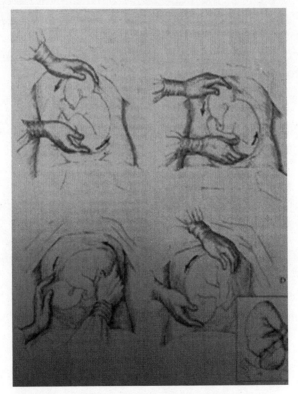

Figure 13-27 Illustration of External Version

If there is very "little give" after several attempts in different somersault directions, the version attempt should probably be abandoned. Serious consideration should be given to caesarean delivery because there may be some internal obstruction (i.e. uterine septum, placental band or fibroid) preventing rotation in the first place.

The risks of the procedure can be potentially serious. Because the baby may not tolerate the manipulation, the procedure is performed mostly within the hospital setting. The most feared complication of the procedure is "fetal distress," and may necessitate an immediate C-Section delivery. Fetal distress occurs when the baby's heart rate drops to an abnormally low rate. Fetal distress can result when pressure on the uterus during the procedure causes the placenta to detach or separate from the uterine wall. Also fetal distress may occur when, as the baby is turned, the head or other body part, compresses or tightens the umbilical cord. During the procedure, the baby's heart rate is monitored so that the procedure may be stopped or pressure from one hand stopped in case a low heart rate is detected. In actuality, an emergency c-section or serious harm to the baby or mother uncommonly transpires.

After a successful version, the patient may be observed and monitored for a short time prior to being allowed to go home. If ideal circumstances exist, labor may be induced before the baby has the opportunity to revert back to the breech position. Most of the time, however, the baby will remain in his/her new "vertex" position. Both the expectant couple and the obstetrician can now wait until labor starts on its own accord.

Author Note: Molly Alonso Method of External Cephalic Version

After being informed that her baby was still in the breech presentation, Mary Alonso decided to try another way of "turning her breech baby." She thought about the physical dynamics of the situation and came up with the following solution: she did a "handstand in her swimming pool." And, it worked!

The author is not advocating this method of version nor has it been shown in any medical study that it has a higher than random success rate. However, if the handstand is performed for a long enough period of time, it is indeed certain that you will *drown*!

CHAPTER 14

Exercise and Physical Fitness in Pregnancy

Pregnancy is not the time to "get into shape." On the other hand, it is not a time to lounge around on the couch for nine months. In general, there are common sense guidelines to physical activities during pregnancy.

Exercise Don'ts:

Do not do any bouncing maneuvers that can jerk the womb up and down such as jumping on a trampoline, water-skiing, jumping jacks, four wheeling in a jeep, motor-biking and horseback riding.

Stop or slow down physical activities when you start to become "winded" (short of breath).

Stop any activity that makes you "hurt" or sore, particularly if in the abdomen or pelvic area.

Stop any activity that causes dizziness or faintness.

Stop or decrease any activity that prevents you from "talking" or "singing" while exercising.

Unfortunately, there is a lack of documented information regarding exercise and pregnancy. Contrary to popular belief, one cannot exercise the uterine muscle so that the length or pain intensity of labor is shortened. However, certain exercises that increase the muscle tone of your front abdominal wall, back, pelvis and chest may significantly lessen back and hip discomfort during pregnancy, labor and delivery. Such exercises may also improve your strength and ability to push your baby through the birth canal in the second stage of labor.

There are certain *inescapable facts* that must be taken into consideration during pregnancy.

First, there is a fifty percent increase in the amount of "work" that the heart has to perform during pregnancy just by itself. The added pregnancy weight, increased volume of blood, the expanded circulatory vessels in the placenta, kidneys and intestines all make your heart perform twice as much "work" as it did when you were not pregnant. Just by being pregnant, a woman is necessarily performing a weight-bearing aerobic exercise.

Second, the enlarging uterus and baby get in the way of certain activities such as jogging, racquetball, sit-ups and knee bends.

Third, as a result of the added weight, protruding uterus and increased curvature of your spine, your center of gravity changes, creating balancing problems. The pregnant athlete is in danger of falling, stumbling, tripping and injuring herself.

Exercise Do's:

There are many exercises that can be safely performed during pregnancy.

Swimming is one of the best exercises during pregnancy and can be continued until the time labor ensues.

Walking (at a fast pace or "race-walking"), bicycling (stationary or on a path), rowing or other aerobic exercise increase the tone of your muscles. These activities also burn excess calories from previous indiscretions and give you an improved sense of well-being and self-image.

Cardinal Principles of Exercise during Pregnancy:

(1) Avoid twisting, turning; or bouncing motion (non-impact)

(2) Do not start an exercise program or activity for the first time during pregnancy. Consult your obstetrician first.

(3) Maintain adequate fluid intake (bring your water bottle with you.)

(4) Exercise for 30 minutes at least three times a week to maintain "training".

(5) Pregnancy, because of increased heart work and extra weight bearing, is an "exercise" in of itself. By being pregnant, you are in fact, "in training".

(6) Exercise or training programs do not make "an easier labor" or "help you avoid a C-Section". They chiefly maintain muscle tone and more important make you feel healthier and happier (mental lift).

Exercise Cautions:

When exercising, follow a few simple rules:

1. Do not exceed a pulse of 140 beats per minute. A lower pulse may be necessary if you are anemic, overweight, out of shape or dehydrated.

2. Do not perform strenuous activities continuously for more than 15 minutes at a time. Your baby may be subjected to decreased oxygen and waste products from your blood. Furthermore, your core body temperature may rise to a high level (102 F or 39 C). High-core temperature levels may, theoretically, affect your baby's cell metabolism and development. Humid and/or hot weather may dictate shorter exercise intervals.

If you have been inactive prior to pregnancy, then begin an exercise program slowly, gradually and preferably, under a physician's or other health professional's guidance. Many hospitals, athletic clubs, adult schools and community colleges offer prenatal and postpartum fitness classes.

When initiating an exercise program for the first time during pregnancy, there are three types of activity that are recommended most:

1. Swimming
2. "Wogging" (i.e. walking at a brisk pace)
   a. 2 1/2 mile Wog equals a one mile jog or
   b. 1/4 mile swim.
3. Bicycling (indoor or outdoor)

You should not perform any exercise while lying flat on your back after the fourth month of pregnancy. The vena cava (the largest vein in your body that carries all the blood from your legs and intestines back to your heart) can be compressed and obstructed by the heavy overlying uterus and baby ("Caval Syndrome"). Such an enormous blockage of blood back to your heart is analogous to losing half your blood volume. Decreased blood volume makes your body go into circulatory "shock." Subsequently, your heart rate speeds up to compensate. There is less blood coming out of the heart to go to your head and, consequently, you may become dizzy and faint. Further aggravation of this situation by lying flat on your back can lead to possible more profound medical situations.

Exercise during pregnancy is most beneficial when done on a regular basis. Most physiologists agree that muscle tone is maintained when exercise is performed for 20 minutes at least three times per week. Tone is increased when exercise is performed more than three times per week and decreased when performed less than three times per week. There are many excellent books available in your bookstore or library (or on-line) regarding specific toning regimens. This book does not intend to duplicate their efforts. The reader should refer to the bibliography at the end of this book for assistance.

Water or Snow Skiing

Water Skiing should be avoided during pregnancy because of the potential dangers of falling with a direct hit on the uterus.

Rarely, there has been reported a "douche effect", i.e. water can theoretically enter the vagina (and *rarely* further upward through the cervix into the pregnant uterus by excessive water pressure).. This dangerous occurrence could occur if a water skier "hit the water" at the right angle at 40 MPH.

Snow skiing involves other problems. First, at higher altitudes there is less oxygen in the air, 70% at 5000 feet (normally 100% saturation at sea level). Second, skiing puts one at risk for falling directly on the abdomen that is protecting your "baby bump." Abdominal wall trauma on hard snow or ice is possible. Lastly, the twisting and turning motions as well as bouncing over moguls can cause such forces to be relayed directly to the uterus. Fracture of blood vessels with bleeding and disruption of the placenta have been known to occur. Bottom-line, it is important to maintain conditioning and tone during pregnancy but these goals can be achieved in non-impact exercise activities.

Scuba Diving

Scuba Diving below 35 feet has been associated with a threefold increase in birth defects (10% in some studies; first trimester of pregnancy). As with other sports, use proper equipment. Use the buddy system. Be properly covered and dressed. Watch for dangerous "fish attacks" and sharp rock formations. Stay above 35 feet.

Weight Lifting Programs

In general toning muscles of the arms, legs, and trunk can be continued but at a reduced level during pregnancy. The same end point of any exercise, i.e., a pulse greater than 140 or fatigue, must be constantly born in mind. If beginning a weight program for the first time go slowly and gradually under expert supervision.

CHAPTER 15

Other Questions most asked about during Pregnancy

Saunas And Hot Tubs . . . Can I Use Them?

Currently, it is not recommended that expectant women use saunas or hot tubs *with any fre*quency. The developing fetus has no way to rid itself of excess heat except through its mother's body and bloodstream. If you sit in a sauna or hot tub that raises your core body temperature significantly (over 100 F), over-heating of the baby may occur. Chemical reactions and cell-to-cell relationships theoretically could be altered. Birth defects might theoretically ensue (no conclusive studies to date). Furthermore, dehydration and pooling of blood to the vast skin surface can result in shock and fainting. Loss of consciousness might result in falling down with subsequent injury to you or your baby. Without anyone else around in the sauna, such fainting might result in further prolonged exposure and other complications. Rarely, drowning similarly might result in the hot tub should a fall result in a head injury and there is no other person present to help you. Avoid hot tub temperatures over 104 degrees: you might get burned!

However, it is safe to dangle your legs in a hot tub or sit in a sauna as long as your core body temperature is not raised above 100 F. Be careful never to go into the sauna or hot tub alone!

Electric Blankets

Electric blankets do not raise the core body temperature and therefore are safe to use (as long as the wiring is intact!).

Can I Sunbathe or Tan? No, unless you use Sunscreens!

For those of you who are avid sun worshippers or those of you who may spend much time in the rays of the sun because of your occupation, care and protection of your skin should be a greater concern during pregnancy. Melanin producing cells (melanocytes: the cells that lay down the dark pigment into your skin) are under heightened stimulation during pregnancy by MSH (Melanocyte Stimulatory Hormone) produced by the placenta. Exposure to the sun causes generalized tanning of the body; but, certain specific areas of the body such as the face (*Chloasma*), midline (i.e. *linea nigra*), moles and nipples are more affected. Such darkening, particularly on the facial areas of the forehead, cheeks and jaw may be cosmetically displeasing and may remain permanently darkened.

Pregnant women are just as susceptible to sunburn and skin damage as anyone else, particularly those of you who are fair-skinned (Northern European and Scandinavian descent). Accordingly, the principles of skin protection apply. Wear sunscreens before such exposure. Sunscreens are commercially available and graded 1 through 50 so that the proper sunscreen is used. Use sunscreen of about 25-50 on the "white" (or rarely exposed) portions of your body; i.e., breasts, bottom, tops of your feet, etc. Also, use this grade of sunscreen if sun exposure is intense and/or prolonged. Sunscreen of a lower grade can be utilized if sun exposure is limited or if only the tanned areas of your body (arms and legs) are involved. SBF (Sun Block Factor) scores are directly correlated with protection: 50 SBF is not twice as protective as 25. The SBF system is a curve such that SBF 30 to 50 provides minimal extra protection. See the Appendix for more information regarding Sunscreen formulations and new product labels.

After coming in out of the sun, it is important to moisturize your skin with emollients. Creams that are of aloe base, etc., prevent your skin from drying out. Vaseline Intensive Care, Nivea and other commercial products are perfectly satisfactory.

Skin tinting, rather than actual tanning, is permissible than sun tanning. The reader is also referred to the Appendix for more information regarding skin protectants.

Can I Smoke?

It goes without saying that if smoking is not good for you, it cannot be good for your baby. Pregnancy is a good time to finally stop smoking. Indeed, many thousands of women have quit smoking because they became pregnant and did not want to endanger the growth and future health of their babies.

For those of you that cannot completely quit smoking, it is important to understand that the nicotine in smoke causes a generalized constriction of the arterial blood supply and stops, or decreases, the flow of blood to all parts of your body. It therefore, decreases the flow of blood which contains oxygen and nutrients to the placenta and to your growing baby. Chronic and continued smoking slows and affects the development of your baby. Hence, babies of smokers weigh less than average full-term infants.

Smoking has not been proven to produce any specific birth defects to date. It does not cause mental retardation or any other specific abnormalities of the brain, heart, kidney or genitourinary tract.

Needless to say, however, smoking has pronounced effects on the pregnant woman's lungs, cardiovascular and genitourinary systems. It is a promoter of cancer in all organ systems, and over fifty percent of women with genital tract cancer (i.e., cervix, vagina, and ovary) do smoke. It accelerates the atherosclerotic process (plugging up of the blood vessels), as well as the aging process itself.

If you would like to quit smoking and need help, do not hesitate to ask your physician or contact your local American Heart Association or the American Cancer Society. Your hospital may contain a

"Smoke-Enders program". You, your family and your physician will be glad you did!

> Author Note: I have informed my teenage son that smoking is associated with increased risks of ED (Erectile Dysfunction) in the hope that he will not take up the addiction. Nicotine has been implicated as a co-factor in causing atherosclerosis of small arteries and hence, decreased blood flow to organs. In the later middle age men are more likely to have decreased flow through the penile artery resulting in the most common cause of ED. Similarly, women are more likely to develop decreased clitoral blood flow and lack of arousal and possible decreased orgasmic response.

Can I Travel During Pregnancy?

It is my personal recommendation that patients do not travel during the first three and the last two months of pregnancy. Why? In the first three months, the chances for miscarriage of the pregnancy are greatest. The first four weeks are a particularly important developmental period of time for your pregnancy: I recommend that travel be restricted to local distances from your home.

There is less risk and more freedom to travel during the first three months if an ultrasound has been performed in early trimester and the embryo has been seen. If the heartbeat (or two!!) has been seen (it can be seen as early as six weeks), then it is probably safer to travel from that point on in your pregnancy. Travel is likewise unrestricted if the doctor has heard the baby's heartbeat. Once the heartbeat has been seen or heard, then the pregnancy is a viable one and it is unlikely that you will have any major problems with your pregnancy (less than 2% miscarriage rate).

When traveling long distances, you should take frequent "pit stops." Sitting in a car for a long period of time necessarily slows blood circulation in the body. Your blood gravitates downward in your legs and "pools" there. Fighting gravity and hydrostatic pressure, circulation of blood back up to the heart becomes sluggish. Clots may start to form in your legs and be the set-up for potential problems later. Fortunately, most patients cannot tolerate long car rides because of their decreased bladder capacity. Nature, in this way, steps in and forces you to stop so you can get out of the car and walk to the restroom.

It is also quite safe to travel by plane (unless a terrorist is on-board!). Airplanes are now pressurized so that there is plenty of oxygen for the baby. Should a sudden loss in cabin pressure occur, the plane has emergency oxygen masks that will drop down and provide oxygen to you. Again, it is important to get up and move about frequently about the cabin after the seat belt sign has been turned off. Once again, I stress the importance of using seat belts and lap restraints in any vehicle of travel (make sure the lap strap goes under your bump).

Fortunately for the pleasure seekers, cruises and boat trips are also permissible. Because of an increased tendency toward nausea in pregnancy, I would recommend having medication on hand in case the nausea becomes severe or prolonged. Consult your doctor for anti-nausea medication. Needless to say, travel by water necessitates use of life vests and all other water safety precautions. Boating and jet skis activities can could result in severe bouncing motions and hard falls: it has a potential of disrupting the placental attachment.

Today, train rides are back in fashion and railway travel is safe during pregnancy. All the preceding advice applies. Move about frequently. Be careful and protect yourself against all the sudden jerks and stoppage of the train.

The moving motion of any kind of vehicle does seem to increase the tendency of nausea. A simple, but very effective remedy is to carry some plain soda crackers with you in your purse. The crackers absorb the acids and enzymes in the stomach and help relieve the nausea.

Whether traveling by car, plane, boat or train, exercise common sense and safety. And don't forget to have a good trip!

Any Wardrobe Changes?

In general, clothing should be chosen to match weather conditions as well as your comfort. Warm clothing such as gloves, hat, coat and sweater should be worn in colder temperatures; whereas cotton "air-breathing" underwear, blouse, shorts and hat are appropriate for warmer summer weather.

Specific articles of clothing need particular emphasis. Underwear or panties (as well as bras) should almost always be made entirely of cotton or possess a cotton crotch. Cotton "breathes" and circulates air, preventing wetness. Moisture and wetness set up conditions ideal for producing yeast infections, vaginal, in your groin creases and under your breasts.

Use cotton or other high tech "breathable" undergarments, tops and shorts.

Breasts enlarge tremendously during pregnancy, particularly during breastfeeding. Purchase a bra that is comfortable and loose. Be mindful that it must have extra capacity to accommodate your expanding chest size. It is not uncommon to have to buy several larger-size bras during pregnancy and lactation. Remember to purchase a cotton bra. Be careful of bras colored with dyes, fashioned with lace, or, made with rubber elastic supports that may be irritating (or worse, cause allergic reactions) to your skin.

Pants and dresses should be loose-fitting. Too often, physicians see their patients trying to wear their hip-hugging designer jeans. Undue pressure may be exerted on their abdomen and internal organs such as the stomach, liver and kidneys. The same constrictive force can be caused by belts that can impede circulation of blood from the legs back to your heart.

CHAPTER 16

Foods And Nutrition

Nutrition during Pregnancy

During your pregnancy you need to remember that the food you eat will eventually provide the nutritional building blocks from which your baby is made. Both your body and your baby's body need about fifty nutrients. No one food or pill can supply all these at one time (your prenatal vitamins usually contain just fifteen vitamins or minerals your baby needs). By following a few simple rules, you should be able to meet all the requirements for both you and baby.

One of my patients had read this book and said she could not find out any nutritional information about "smoked salmon." Fish, like all food sold in the US, is carefully inspected by the appropriate Federal Agencies (FDA, EPA, etc.). Such inspections also cover "raw fish," such sashimi, etc. Vendors and supermarkets are especially careful but it is best to consume "cooked" seafood such as shrimp, crab, scallops and lobster. Fish is a very lean source of protein and Omega-3 fats.

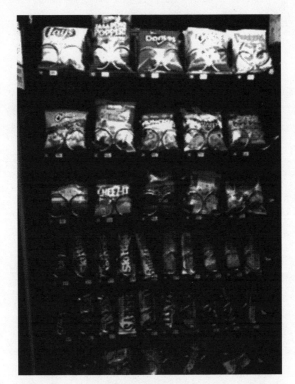

Figure 16-1 The Snack Machine. This is NOT the place to obtain nourishment for your baby.

It has always been taught that fish is a very good source of protein and Omega -3 fats. A 2 ounce serving of canned chunk light tuna contains 11 grams of protein and .5 grams of fat. In early 2014 the FDA and ACOG believed that the incorporation of more fish protein in the US diet and particularly pregnant patients would improve the quality of protein in their diet. They recommended that *a pregnant patient could consume up to 12 ounces of fish per week without significantly increasing her consumption or exposure to mercury.*

Source: *ACOGPracticeAdvisory,* http://www.acog.org/About_ACOG/News_Room/College_Statements_and_Advisories/2014/Seafood_Consumption_During_Pregnancy

However, *Consumer Reports* (October 2014 issue) reviewed the FDA data and disagreed.

Consumer Reports recommends that pregnant women avoid eating tuna altogether.

Tuna is the second most consumed kind of fish in the US: right behind shrimp. However, there are other fish that contain very low levels of mercury that pregnant women can eat without worry as follows:

Lowest-mercury Fish	Low-mercury Fish
Wild and Alaska Salmon (canned or fresh)	Haddock
Shrimp (most wild and U.S. farmed)	Pollock
Sardines	Flounder and sole (flatfish)
Tilapia	Catfish and Trout
Scallops	Atlantic mackerel and croaker
Oysters	Crab
Squid (domestic)	Crawfish (domestic) and Mullet

Caloric Requirements

Now that you are pregnant, you have probably heard, "you are eating for two." This statement is an old adage that does not really tell the whole truth. It takes about 80,000 calories to "build a baby." Sound like a lot? In actuality, 80,000 calories can be translated into an additional 300 calories per day. Not a large amount, considering that your nutritional needs are so much higher during pregnancy. Thus, the proper diet for a pregnant woman stresses quality versus quantity. Here are some simple examples of some food *additions* that would increase the quality of your diet, yet keep you near your goal of 300 calories:

Example A

Two soft boiled eggs		160 Cals
One cup low fat (2%) milk		140 Cals
	Total	300 Cals

Example B

Two cups low fat (2%) milk		280 Cals
One fresh fruit		40 Cals
	Total	320 Cals

Example C

One slice whole wheat toast		70 Cals
One slice cheese		100 Cals
One cup low fat (2%) milk		140 Cals
	Total	320 Cals

Weight Gain

More important than the total amount of weight gain is the rate at which you gain weight. You can anticipate about a one-half pound weight gain per week during your first two trimesters of pregnancy, and one pound per week during your last trimester. Remember, pregnancy is not the time to attempt to lose weight as weight loss can adversely affect the baby. You should expect to gain between twenty to thirty-five pounds during your pregnancy (overweight woman should gain much less weight).

Staying within this weight gain range promotes an uncomplicated pregnancy and delivery of a healthy baby. The patient can approach full term at a good weight.

In general, a newborn that is at or near the average birth weight (seven and one-half pounds) thrives better. As a result, proper weight gain decreases the risk of having an underweight or a "low birth weight" baby. Studies have shown that a mother's weight gain during pregnancy does influence the infant's birth weight. Women who are underweight prior to conceiving and gain less that the recommended weight, (ninety percent of ideal), more often give birth to babies under five and one-half pounds (2500 grams and are termed "small for gestational age, i.e." S.G.A). In comparison, women who are overweight prior to conceiving and gain more than the recommended amount (one hundred twenty percent of ideal), frequently have babies weighing greater than eight pounds, thirteen ounces (4000 grams). These babies are called large for gestation age (L.G.A).

A woman who is underweight should gain more weight during her pregnancy than the woman of average weight. Such underweight women should have gained approximately thirty-five pounds by the time labor ensues. Appropriate weight gain should help reduce the many risk factors of pregnancy: anemia, premature rupture of membranes, endometritis, postpartum hemorrhage, pre-term labor and an infant with low Apgar score. Contrary, for a woman who was overweight (one hundred thirty percent of ideal weight) before becoming pregnant, keeping the weight gain between twenty and twenty-four pounds may help reduce her risk of developing diabetes, hypertension, pre-eclampsia, postpartum hemorrhage, Cesarean section delivery and assisted labor.

It may help you to understand your weight gain if you see the *sources for weight increase*:

Infant	7.5
Placenta	1.5
Amniotic Fluid	1.8
Uterus	2.0
Increased Breast Tissue	1.0
Increased Blood Volume	4.0
Increased Extracellular Fluids	2.7
"Other Tissue" (fat stores)	3.5
	TOTAL: 24.0 pounds

Nutrients

Protein

Protein supplies material for building, maintaining and repairing body tissues. You need protein every day. You need it in greater amounts while you are pregnant and breastfeeding. It is of utmost importance that you plan to get all the protein you need in your diet. Protein is a food component that is not included in your prenatal vitamins. From the protein you eat, your body will make the additional blood needed for pregnancy. Also, protein makes the baby's muscles, nerves, body tissues and brain cells. Protein is used to make enzymes and hormones used to regulate body processes during pregnancy. Antibodies that fight infections are formed from proteins. This natural immunity is important as any "medicine" that may be prescribed.

Proteins are made up of amino acids. Although there are many different types of amino acids, nine of them are "essential amino acids." These must be supplied by the foods you consume because the human body cannot produce them.

Proteins that contain the essential amino acids are classified as "complete proteins." These are the highest quality proteins and come from animal sources such as fish, poultry, meat, eggs or dairy products. Other sources of quality protein foods may lack one or more of these essential amino acids: hence their designation as "incomplete proteins." This group includes proteins from plants such as legumes (beans and lentils) and nuts. To add variety, these proteins can be substituted for some of the animal proteins in your diet. For example, peanut butter on toast can be substituted for eggs in the morning. If you intend to follow a vegetarian diet during your pregnancy, you need to know how to combine various plant (incomplete) protein foods to get all nine of the essential amino acids. Consult a registered dietitian or obtain further information by reading *Diet for a Small Planet* by Frances Moore Lapai.

In order to obtain enough protein in your daily diet, drink four (eight ounce) glasses of milk and eat three ounces of a protein-rich food at lunch and dinner. It is important to discuss these protein foods in more detail at this time.

Eggs: Eggs are an "Egg-cellent" source of protein.

Eggs are the highest quality of protein and the cheapest source available. They are a good source of vitamins A and E and iron. Eggs can be an easy, practical and economical way to get the protein you need. You can eat them as an entree, such as an omelet. Boil up a dozen eggs and use a hard-boiled egg throughout the day: as a snack by itself, over your salads, in your soups or as egg salad sandwiches.

Poultry, Veal and Fish

Poultry (turkey and chicken), veal and fish provide the protein you need in your diet without adding a lot of fat or calories. Poultry and veal are called "light meats" and, in comparison to red meats they contain less calories, cholesterol and saturated fat (lard).Fish also contains less cholesterol than red meats and provides our bodies with a very healthy fat called EPA (Eicosapentainoic Acid). Researchers believe this type of fat helps our body make the right type of prostaglandin, a substance that helps regulate body processes. EPA decreases the risk of heart disease, cancer and many other long term illnesses. In addition to being a low-fat, protein rich food, both light meats and meats may alleviate the heartburn and indigestion that are so common during pregnancy.

"Good food depends almost entirely on good ingredients."—Alice Waters

"It's bizarre that the *produce manager* (at my supermarket – author added) is *more important* to my children's health than my Pediatrician."
    --Meryl Streep

"My doctor told me to stop having intimate dinners for four—unless there are three other people."
    --Orson Welles

  --Above quotes from *The Family Chef,* by Jewels and Jill Elmore

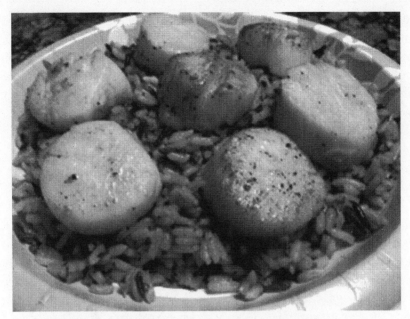

Figure 16-2 Lightly sautéed on a bed of wild rice:
Seafood as an excellent source of protein in your diet scallops

Red Meats

Red meats (beef, pork and lamb) supply high quality protein and can add variety to your diet. Red meats are an excellent source of iron. Iron is important to have during pregnancy as it is a very important component of the red blood cell. The demand for iron by red cells is great during pregnancy because blood volume nearly doubles.

One should remember that the majority of red meats are higher in fat and calories than the light meats and fish mentioned above. Most red meats, even the leanest "cuts", contain between 60 to 70% of their calories as fat. Therefore, when purchasing meat, try to buy the lean cuts (see Table 1), trim away any visible fat before cooking, and limit yourself to less than 4 ounces at a serving.

Lean cuts of meat tend to be tougher and you may use different cooking methods to make them moist and tender. For example, slow cooking (as with a crock pot), marinating meats before cooking, or braising meat by cooking with some liquid in the bottom of the pan, are cooking styles that should be used with lean cuts of meat. One can also slice lean meat across the grain and stir-fry, thereby reducing your consumption of cooking oil. In preparing other cuts of meat you might try to bake, broil, boil or barbecue so that you allow the grease within the meat to "burn" off. It is the fat within the meat that adds most of the calories.

Calorie Concerns and Sources

Protein and carbohydrates (starches and sugars) provide four (4) calories per gram. Fats provide more than twice this amount; nine (9) calories per gram (see Table 2). If you are concerned about weight gain during pregnancy, cut down on all fats in your diet. Decrease (or avoid) fried or oily foods such as pizza, chips, French fries, bacon, sausage, fatty cold cuts. Avoid excessive amounts of butter, margarine or mayonnaise. Do not worry! You are still able to obtain all the fat necessary for the baby from other foods in your diet, (such as cheese, milk and salad dressings.

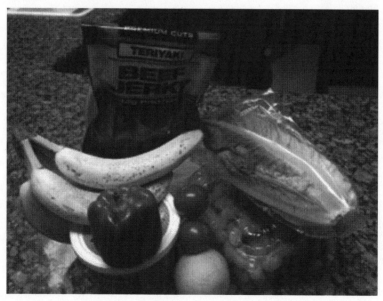

Figure 16-3 Vegetables, fruit and protein sources

Author's Anecdote with regard to eating;

I am always careful about eating very tidily. I always keep my napkin very handy. But, I have always been amazed that after a meal, the person on the other side of the table from me still has a crease in his napkin. It is still clean and neatly folded. In fact, he has no food stains on it at all. But if you gaze down at the author's napkin while he is eating, it looks like he must have passed all his food he has eaten right through it!

TABLE 1

Fat Content of Protein

Lean Meats	Medium Fat Meats	High Fat Meats
55 calories	75 calories	100 cal.
3 gms. fat	5 gms. fat	8 gms. fat

Poultry

Chicken, turkey	poultry with skin	duck, capon
Cornish hen,	skin goose, franks	
Pheasant without skin		

Lean Meats Veal	Medium Fat Meats	High Fat Meats
All cuts are	cutlets	breast
Lean except		
Cutlets		

Beef

Flank steak	cubed steak	sausage,
Tenderloin,	porterhouse,	bologna,
Ribs,	T-bone extra	franks,
Eye, bottom	lean ground(15% fat)	cold cuts,
Or top round,	rib eye	brisket,
Rump, tripe, tip	corned beef, lean ground.	

Roast, sirloin, Top loin, rib Roast blade pot roast	roast (rib,(20% fat), chuck, rump) most USDA prime cuts of beef Meatloaf	
Lamb	loin, breast, roast, shoulder mutton rib, chop	
Pork Smoked center Chops, loin Canadian bacon	Ham, tenderloin, roast, cutlets, Ground pork, shoulder arm, Boston butt sausage	spareribs, country shoulder blade ham Deviled ham

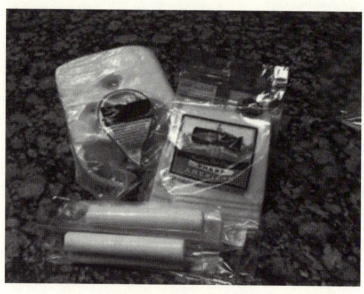

Figure 16-4 Cheese Choices

Low Fat	Medium Fat	High Fat
Cheese		
Cottage cheese (2 or 4 %)	mozzarella, ricotta,	cheddar Monterey,
Farmer's cheese Neufchatel,	Blue,	
Edam, Swiss, Parmesan	Brick	
Fish		
Fresh, frozen	tuna in oil	any fried
Canned sole, tuna in water	salmon,	
Scallops, crab	Lobster, sardines,	Oyster
Miscellaneous		
Dried beans	eggs (whole)	peanut butter
Peas, tofu	95% fat-free	
luncheon meat		
Egg whites		
Organ Meats	liver, kidney, Meats	heart & sweetbreads

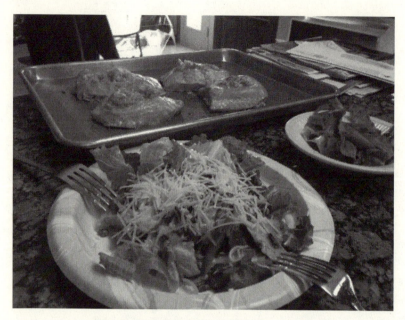

Figure 16-5 Example of Balanced Meal

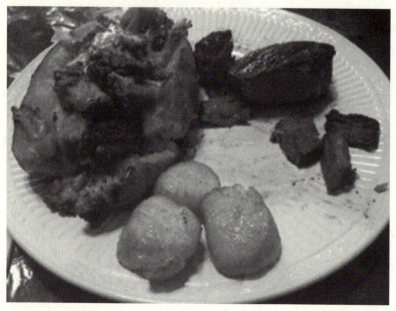

Figure 16-6 Balanced Meal Example of a balanced Meal with fiber (broccoli), carbohydrate (baked potato) and protein (steak and scallop).

Milk and Dairy Products

Milk is an extremely important food during pregnancy because it contains all three of the basic food groups: protein, carbohydrates and fats. Many vitamins and minerals, such as calcium, zinc and Vitamin D are also present in milk. In addition to these vitamins and minerals, there are other nutrients found in "trace" amounts within milk that are needed for chemical reactions to occur in your body that are not included in your multivitamins. Chemical reactions bring protein, carbohydrate and fats together to build baby's body cells. Body cells build the baby's tissues and, as these tissues group together, they form the baby's organs such as the brain, stomach, kidneys and liver.

Calcium obtained from milk or dairy products is easily utilized in the body. Calcium gives structure and strength to bones and teeth. Calcium also helps your blood to clot, keeps nerves, muscle and heart tissue healthy, aids in wound healing and helps fight infections - all of which are necessary for your healthy labor and delivery. The recommended amount of calcium a pregnant woman should consume is 1200 milligrams (mg.) each day. One glass of milk has about 300 mg. of calcium. Four glasses of milk (or four servings of a high calcium alternative) satisfies your daily requirements for calcium.

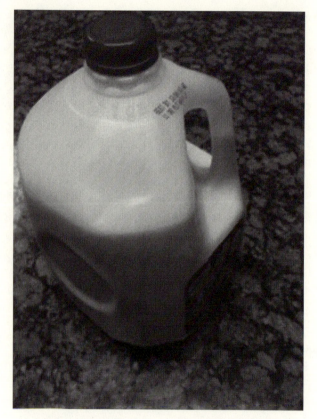

Figure 15-7 Milk is a very important source of protein and calcium

If you are unable to drink milk or tolerate dairy products, you should consider taking a calcium supplement in addition to your prenatal vitamins. You can purchase calcium supplements in many forms. Select a supplement made from calcium phosphate, calcium lactate, calcium gluconate or calcium

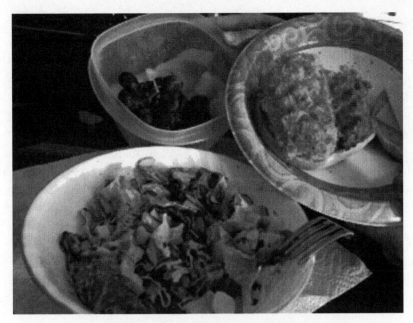

Figure 15-8. Balanced meal plans. Balanced meal with salad, fruit and protein (tilapia fish) and bread

carbonate (Tums, Rolaids, etc.). Check the dosage so you take 1200 mg per day. The pharmacist at your local pharmacy should be able to assist you if you have further questions regarding Calcium supplements available at your pharmacy.

Note: Avoid taking calcium supplements made of bone meal or dolomite as a few samples of these were found to contain lead. Some sources of "Oyster" or other shell calcium has had reports of contamination with bacteria.

Iron

Iron is a mineral that is used by the red blood cells to carry oxygen to all the tissues in the body. As mentioned previously, your blood supply will double in volume during pregnancy. Consequently, your requirements for iron needs be doubled as well. The average woman needs 18 mg of iron per day. The body only absorbs a small amount from the food you eat. You must eat three times as much iron as your body needs: 90% of all the iron ingested as food or from a pill supplement is never absorbed and "goes out the other end." Dark or black stools (caused by iron itself) result from adequate iron supplementation but also illustrates out how much of the iron you ingest is poorly absorbed by the intestinal tract. During pregnancy, you therefore need approximately 60 mg of iron per day to prevent anemia. It is impossible to obtain this much iron from food alone. Therefore, a supplement should be taken by all pregnant women. If taking an iron supplement upsets your stomach, try taking it a different time of the day (for example at night before you go to bed). If you feel more constipated after taking the iron supplement, increase the amount of fiber in your diet (stool softeners and laxatives can be taken to counteract any constipating effects of Iron.

You may be interested to know that iron found in meat products is called "heme" iron. It is absorbed and utilized more efficiently than the form given in a iron pill supplement.

Therefore, an iron-rich diet is important. We can obtain iron not only from supplements but also from the food we eat.

Therefore, iron obtained from your food is an important source of iron along with the iron pill you take as a supplement. You should become familiar with foods naturally high in iron and include them frequently in your diet. Such examples of iron rich foods are meat and liver. Cooking in an iron cast skillet is also a possible source of elemental iron.

Fiber

Dietary fiber is also known as "bulk" or "roughage." Foods with fiber in them are not completely digested and absorbed. They are eliminated in the stool, resulting in softer and looser stools. Eating high-fiber foods can help pregnant women avoid constipation and hemorrhoids. During pregnancy, changes in hormone levels (i.e. elevated levels of

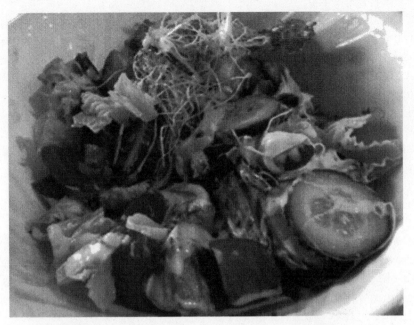

Figure 15-9 Salad with sprouts, lettuce, etc. to help fiber intake

progesterone which relaxes smooth muscle function) causes the stomach and intestines to relax and slow down. This is the main reason why women have a natural tendency toward constipation during pregnancy. The growing uterus will also take up much of the working space of the digestive system, further aggravating elimination problems. In addition, iron supplementation affects some women by causing harder stools. There is also greater pressure in the rectal area from an expansion in the number of congested blood vessels. When extensive pushing occurs during constipation, hemorrhoids (congested and swollen "varicose veins" in and outside the rectum) can develop.

To prevent constipation and hemorrhoids, eat foods that are high in fiber such as whole grains, fresh fruits and vegetables. Eat at least four servings of either a fruit or vegetable each day. *Fresh* or *raw* fruits and vegetables are higher in fiber than if they were canned. If you are unable to tolerate them because of nausea or heartburn, canned or frozen fruits and vegetables will give you less roughage, but will still have significant amounts of fiber.

Whole grains include foods such as whole or cracked-wheat bread, bran cereals, brown rice and oatmeal. Eat at least four servings from this group each day. You can accomplish these "fiber needs" by eating a bran cereal for breakfast; have two slices of whole wheat bread for your sandwich at lunch and perhaps some brown rice with dinner.

Old fashion Toasted Oats can contain 4 grams of dietary fiber. Nutrition bars at 190 calories each can supply up to 12 grams of protein and 2 grams of fiber.

Breads and Cereals

Breads and cereals have several nutrients important for you and your baby: B vitamins and iron. These foods may be either whole grain or enriched. It is best to eat whole grains: they contain more vitamins and minerals. Whole grains also provide fiber which helps prevent constipation as discussed above.

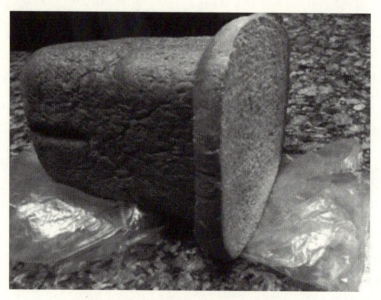

Figure 15-10 100% Whole wheat bread
(made by the author –Recipe is in Appendix)

<u>Author's Anecdote</u>. For the past 20 years the author has stopped purchasing bread at the supermarket and has made his own. He

cheats a little: he uses an electric bread maker. It takes only 5 minutes to throw all the ingredients into the loaf pan and 4 hours later, *voila!*, you have homemade wholesome bread! And, there is nothing like the aroma of freshly baked bread in the home.

Choose four servings of bread and cereal each day. A serving is any of the following:

Whole Grain Items	One Serving Size
Bread, cracked, whole wheat Or rye	1 slice
Cereal, hot: oatmeal, rolled or cracked wheat, wheat and malted barley	1/2 cup cooked
Cereal, ready-to-eat: puffed Oats, shredded wheat, wheat Flakes, granola	3/4 cup
Rice (brown)	1/2 cup cooked
Wheat germ	1 tablespoon
Enriched Items Bagel	1 small
Bread (all except those listed above)	1 slice
Cereal, hot: cream of wheat, Rice, farina, corn meal, grist	1/2 cup cooked

Cereal, ready-to-eat: (all Except those listed above)	3/4 cup
Crackers	4 pieces
Macaroni, noodles, spaghetti	1/2 cup cooked
Pancake, waffle	1 medium (5 inch diameter)
Rice (white)	1/2 cup cooked
Roll, biscuit, muffin, Dumpling	1
Tortilla	1 (6 inch diameter)

Doughnuts, cakes, pies and cookies are not included in the Bread & Cereal groups. These foods contain mostly calories and very few nutrients.

After delivering a 10 lb. 12 ounce baby boy vaginally, my patient, Megan Ellsworth stated to me, "Do you think that my having bowls of cereal each night during my pregnancy had anything to do with my baby's excessive weight?"

Fluids

Drinking enough fluid during pregnancy is important to meet the physical needs created by your increased blood supply and increased functioning of your body processes. You should drink at least eight to ten glasses of fluid each day. Fluids can be in the form of milk, juice, water, herb teas, decaffeinated coffee, soda water or seltzer-type drinks. Try to avoid sugar flavored drinks like soda pop, fruit punch or sugared lemonade that contain little nutritional value. Laboratory evidence surrounding artificial sweeteners, such as those used in diet sodas are considered safe with moderate use. It is recommended to limit the excess use of artificial sweeteners (Splenda, NutraSweet, Aspartame, and Saccharin). A moderate amount (perhaps limiting these "diet" products to 1 or 2 servings a day) would probably be prudent.

Limit your intake of caffeine and avoid alcohol. The potential harm of these products is listed in a later chapter titled Disease and Dangers.

Salt/Sodium

Sodium is a mineral with many functions. It is important in maintaining bodily fluid balance. Having too much salt can make you retain more fluid, causing swelling in your feet, legs, face or hands. Salt contains a large amount of sodium (forty percent). Sodium is found in all foods, even water. The problem with sodium today is that American diets contain too much of it. The majority of food manufacturers add salt to their products when they process them (as occurs in frozen dinners or bottled spaghetti sauce). Restaurants and fast food places also commonly "spice up" their plates by adding salt to their food. As we eat less home-cooked meals (where we can control the salt we add to our food) and as we rely more on pre-prepared and restaurant meals, we are consuming sodium in greater amounts than recommended. These simple rules may help you keep your sodium intake to a desirable level.

1. Cut back on using the salt shaker, especially at the table. Instead, use a lot of other herbs and spices such as oregano, dill and nutmeg. Consider sprinkling "Light Salt" on your foods instead of regular salt. Light salt (e.g., Lite Salt®) tastes like regular salt but contains 50% less salt itself. Other options for spicing up your food are using No Salt (potassium chloride) or Mrs. Dash.

2. Limit cured and pickled foods in your diet such as ham, corned beef, frankfurters, sausage, linguisa or foods like pickles (sweet, sour or dill), pickled herring and sauerkraut. Huge amounts of salt are used in curing and pickling which is then absorbed into the food.

3. Use more fresh foods and avoid processed foods.

For example, avoid frozen dinners and pizzas.

Nutritional Notes

Pregnancy and lactation create special nutritional demands which can usually be met by consuming a nutritionally-adequate diet. The National Research Council recommends on the average an additional 300 calories per day for a pregnant woman. If the mother-to-be is physically active or underweight, more may be needed. Protein needs increase during pregnancy. An additional 30 grams of protein per day is recommended. For most other nutrients, the small extra amounts which are required can be met by the aforementioned nutritionally-sound adequate diet.

There are exceptions with the following minerals:

Iron

Since a typical diet fails to provide the iron needs of the pregnant woman, Iron is recommended in supplemental amounts during the nine months of pregnancy. Many women who become pregnant already have low iron stores and may already be "anemic" because of previous iron losses during their previous heavy menstrual cycles. Most experts recommend about 30 mg of elemental iron per day during pregnancy and lactation. This amount is believed to prevent iron deficiency anemia. It also allows adequate iron stores in the newborn baby!

Folacin (Folic Acid)

The U. S. Public Health Service and CDC recommend that **all women of childbearing age consume 0.4 mg (400 micrograms) of folic acid daily** to prevent two common birth defects: spina bifida and anencephaly.

All women between 15 and 45 years of age should consume folic acid daily. Half of U.S. pregnancies are unplanned. Common birth defects occur *very early* in pregnancy, i.e. 2-4 weeks after conception: it is a time before most women miss their period and know they are pregnant.

If these folic acid supplement recommendations were followed before and during early pregnancy, the CDC estimates that most of these birth defects could be entirely prevented. The Recommended Daily Allowance (RDA) for folic acid during pregnancy is doubled. Folic acid deficiency during pregnancy has been linked with neural tube birth defects, noted above, in a small percentage of children born.

Another medical study showed that as the amount of daily folic acid went from 0 to 4 mg, the rate of birth defects declined in a linear manner.

Zinc

Zinc concentrations in the blood have been shown to decrease by 30-40 percent during pregnancy. Low serum zinc levels have been associated with a higher incidence of complications during pregnancy.

Your body needs zinc for the production, repair, and functioning of DNA (the body's genetic blueprint and a basic building block of cells). Consuming enough zinc is particularly important for the rapid cell growth that occurs during pregnancy. This essential mineral also helps support your immune system, maintain your sense of taste and smell, and heal wounds.

Zinc Deficiencies in the United States are rare, but studies link a zinc deficiency to miscarriage, toxemia, low birth weight, and other problems during pregnancy, labor, and delivery. How much zinc you do you need?

Pregnant women, 19 and older:	11 milligrams (mg) per day
Pregnant, 18 and younger:	13 mg
Breastfeeding women, 19 and older:	12 mg
Breastfeeding, 18 and younger:	14 mg
Non-pregnant women:	8 mg

You do not have to get the recommended amount of zinc every day. Instead, aim for that amount as an average over the course of a few days or a week. Fortified cereals and red meat are good sources of this nutrient.

Pregnant women should therefore consume adequate amounts of zinc-containing foods (seafood, liver, whole grain cereals).

Calcium

Several studies have associated low calcium intake with preeclampsia, i.e. pregnancy-induced hypertension. To counter any potential problems and also to allow for the needs of the growing fetus, 1200 mg of calcium allowance per day is recommended. (This provides a total of 30 grams of calcium during the pregnancy, most of which results in the calcification of the fetal skeleton.)

Conclusion

Pregnancy and lactation create special nutritional demands which can usually be met by consuming a nutritionally-adequate diet. The National Research Council recommends on the average an additional 300 calories per day for a pregnant woman. If the mother-to-be is physically active or underweight, more may be needed. Protein needs increase during pregnancy. An additional 30 grams of protein per day is recommended. For most other nutrients, the small extra amounts which are required can be met by the aforementioned nutritionally-sound diet. Remember, you will be eating to nourish your baby and not just to gain weight. You will need to eat at least 1,800 calories a day to obtain all the nutrition you need. Set a goal to include four glasses of milk each day (or an alternative from the dairy group), three servings of protein-rich foods, two servings of fruits, two of vegetables and at least four servings of starch. It is preferable to eat whole grains and fresh foods instead of processed foods. Processed foods contain more salt, food additives and preservatives. As the consequences of ingesting large amounts of these additives are unknown, you may want to limit them in your diet while you are pregnant. Some experts state that food additives and other chemicals cannot be handled by the human digestive system: they are stored in your fat (adipose) cells indefinitely making weight loss in the future difficult. Keep in mind that you should cut back on fatty foods and sweets as they are high in calories and low in nutrition.

Eating nutritiously does not have to be boring. Be creative and experiment with some of the foods we discussed. Remember that "variety is the spice of life". So if one food does not appeal to you, try it in a different form or find a substitute. Eating well should make you feel better throughout your pregnancy and, therefore, it is basic to creating a healthy, happy baby and mom. Enjoy!

Daily Food Guide

Food Group   Daily Servings

	Not pregnant	Pregnant	Breastfeeding
Protein Foods (3 ounces each)	2	2	2
Milk/Milk Products	2	4	5
Breads and Cereals	4	4	4
Vitamin C Rich Fruits and Vegetables	1	1	1
Dark Green Vegetables	1	1	1
Other Fruits and Vegetable	1	1	1

SAMPLE MENUS AND FOOD GROUPS

Sample Menu #1

Breakfast
Scrambled eggs
Cracked wheat bread
Margarine, 1 tsp.
Banana
Low fat milk, 1 cup

Midmorning Snack
Cheese, 2 oz.
crackers, 10
Herbal tea

Lunch
Tuna salad sandwich
(2 slices bread)
With celery, lettuce
& tomato
Low fat milk, 1 cup
Orange

Midafternoon Snack
Low fat yogurt
Mineral water

Dinner
Barbecued chicken, 3 oz.
Baked potato
Margarine, 2 tsps.
Broccoli
Low fat milk, 1 cup

Snack
Raisin toast
Margarine
Orange juice, 1 cup

Sample Menu #2

Breakfast
Peanut butter, 2 Tbsp.
Whole wheat English muffin
Orange juice, 1 cup
Low fat milk, 1 cup

Lunch
Cottage cheese (3/4 cup)
Pineapple
Whole wheat roll
Margarine, 1 tsp

Dinner
Spaghetti with tomato
Sauce, 1 cup
Meatballs (3)
Buttered French bread
Mixed vegetables
Low fat milk, 1 cup

Midmorning Snack
Blueberry muffin
Low fat milk, 1 cup

Midafternoon Snack
Low fat milk, 1 cup
Cookies, 2

Snack
lightly buttered
popcorn, 3 cups
iced tea

Sample Menu #3

Breakfast
Oatmeal, 1 cup
Low fat milk, 1 cup
Grape juice, 1/2 cup
Decaffeinated coffee or tea

Midmorning Snack
Peanut butter, 1 Tbsp.
Graham crackers, 4

Lunch
Roast beef, 3 oz. sandwich
Low fat milk, 1 cup
Margarine, 1 tsp.
Small salad & Italian dressing, 2 Tbsps.
Apple

Midafternoon Snack
Bran muffin
Low fat milk, 1 cup

Dinner
Baked salmon
With dill, 3 oz.
Rice pilaf, 1 cup
Green beans, 1/2 cup
Low fat milk, 1 cup

Snack
Pudding

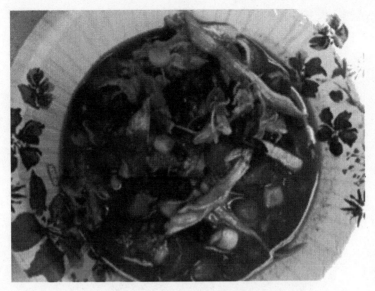

Figure 15-12 Chicken Taco Soup

The above photo illustrates another sample meal that contains chicken and beans (protein), corn (carbohydrate and fiber) as well as tomatoes (fiber vegetables).

What Is In A Food Label?

Why Is Food Labeling Important?

Before 1938 there was no mandatory labeling of food products. Without consumers' knowledge, manufacturers would add less expensive ingredients to extend or dilute a product such as adding chicory to coffee. Consumers would purchase products unaware of the contents. As the number of processed foods increased, the public welcomed regulations established by the Federal Government. The FDA (Federal Drug Administration) has monitored food wholesomeness and labeling and has established ingredient standards.

Food labeling was set up to help the consumer make better food choices; yet, food labels can be more confusing than helpful. Through explaining the different parts on a package, we hope to unravel the mystery behind food labeling.

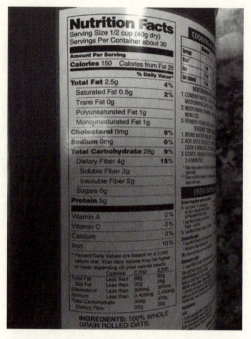

Figure 15-13 Example of Cereal food label

The law requires that a label contain:

- Name of the product (pears, beans, corn).
- Net weight of the product.
- Name and address of the packer or distributor.
- Style (crushed, sliced) and packing medium (heavy syrup, water juice).
- List of ingredients.
- Special dietary factors (no added salt, reduced calorie) with substantiating nutrition labels.
- Presence of any artificial color, flavor or preservative.

Nutritional information on the packaging is still voluntary. Foods which are enriched or fortified with vitamins or minerals and any foods making nutritional claims (like "reduced calorie") must provide nutrition information on the label. Because foods come in such a variety of sizes and shapes, the consumer must hunt to find some of this information.

Ingredient List

Ingredients must be listed in descending order, based on the quantity found in the product. The ingredient that weighs the most is listed first; the one that weighs the second most is listed second, and so on. The last ingredient listed is the item with the lowest concentration. You can use this information to help you assess the quantities of various food items within a product. For example, if sugar is listed as the second ingredient on one product, it will probably be in greater amounts than if it is listed as the fifth ingredient in another similar product.

There are a few recipes used in the food industry that are set by the government. If companies follow these recipes exactly, the ingredients do not have to be listed. Some examples of these foods are fruit jelly and ice cream. Standard recipes for certain foods explain why some products have no ingredients listed on the packaging.

Nutrition Information

Nutrition information is divided into two parts, nutrition information per serving and the percentage of U.S.

Recommended Daily Allowances (USRDA). Nutritional information includes:

- Serving size
- Servings per container
- Calories per serving
- Protein, carbohydrate and fat in grams per serving
- Sodium and cholesterol (optional in milligrams per serving)

USRDA must include information on five vitamins and two minerals: Vitamins A, D, thiamine, riboflavin, niacin, calcium and iron.

Nutrition Information per Serving

Serving Size is defined as the portion or the amount of food for which the nutrition information is listed. This may be one-half cup, one slice or three ounces. The serving size listed might not be the same amount that the consumer most frequently utilizes. Serving sizes vary from product to product as there is no standard serving size set for most foods. Therefore, the consumer needs to double check the serving size listed to figure out the nutritional value of the food. To do this, one should compare the actual amount one has eaten to the serving size listed.

Calories: a calorie is a way to express how much energy one obtains from a food. Calories come from the protein, carbohydrate and fat within a food. One gram of protein, or carbohydrate, gives four calories and one gram of fat gives nine calories. You can figure out the calories in a food by multiplying the grams in a serving by the calories provided by each nutrient (listed above). For example, two percent milk has:

Grams per Serving		Calories per Gram
Protein	10 x 4	= 40
Carbo	13 x 4	= 52
Fat	5 x 9	= 45
	Total	138

The 138 calories is then rounded to 140 calories per an eight ounce glass.

Protein: Protein is listed twice, once in grams and then under percent of the USRDA. As explained earlier, pregnant women and nursing mothers require more protein in their diets than the average person. The average woman needs 46 grams of protein, a pregnant female 76 grams, and nursing mother 66 grams. You can count up the amount of protein eaten at a meal if you know the grams. Thus, the amount of protein listed in grams may be more useful than the USRDA which gives the amount of protein listed in percent of your daily needs.

Carbohydrates: Carbohydrates are made up of two major groups: starches and sugars. Starch is obtained from grain products (cereal, flour, bread, and pastas), potatoes, and dry beans and peas. Sugar comes from beet or cane sugar, honey, molasses, syrup and corn sweeteners/solids. Carbohydrates are listed in grams. Remember one gram of carbohydrate yields four (4) calories.

Fat: Fat is the most concentrated source of energy and offers nine (9) calories per gram. Fats are listed only in grams on a label. Fats digest slowly and help to keep you from feeling hungry. You need to have some fat in the diet to help carry fat soluble vitamins (A, D, E and K). Yet Americans tend to eat too much fat. Recommendations for most people are to use foods high in fat sparingly. Examples of food high in fat are butter, margarine, oil, mayonnaise, shortening and salad dressings.

USRDA: Nutritional needs vary according to a person's age, sex, weight, height and health status. The nutrition a man needs varies from that of a woman or a child. In order for nutritional labeling to display what portion of daily needs are met when you eat a certain food, the government has established one set of standards: the U.S. Recommended Daily Allowances (USRDA). These USRDA's were set high enough so they could meet the nutritional requirements for all healthy persons. In most cases, the government simply selected the highest amount of protein, vitamins and minerals listed for all the groups. Generally, the USRDA for most nutrients prove to be the amounts recommended for men (men typically have the highest requirements for nutrients). However, in the case of iron, adult women need far more than men do. Accordingly, the amount of iron recommended for women was chosen as the USRDA (see Appendix 1). The USRDA is the symbolic abbreviation which the public sees the most: it appears on the packaging and wrapping of many food products.

But there are three additional USDRA lists for very specific populations. These are as follows:

1. Infants under thirteen months
2. Children under four years
3. Pregnant or lactating (nursing) women

These specific USRDA lists may be found on foods targeted for those special populations such as baby foods.

<u>Vitamins and Minerals</u>: FDA regulations specify that only a few vitamins and minerals must be listed as a part of all nutrition labeling. These vitamins and minerals are considered "lead" nutrients. If a "lead" vitamin or mineral is in a food, it is assumed that the food contains other important nutrients as well. For example, orange juice is high in vitamin C. Orange juice is also high in potassium, another important "lead" mineral that is not included in nutrition labeling. It is believed that if you eat a variety of foods high in vitamin C, you will obtain foods high in potassium and other vitamins and minerals.

What Else Might Be Listed On A Label?

<u>Sodium/Salt</u>

Salt is made up of sodium and chloride, but it is the sodium that we are concerned about. Sodium is a mineral found in all foods. It is important to have sodium in your diet. Yet, in recent years, Americans are eating excessive amounts of salt and foods high in sodium. It is recommended that people limit the amount of sodium to between 3,000 and 5,000 milligrams (three to five grams) of sodium per day. The following terms used in labeling define that amount of sodium found in foods:

Sodium free:	contains less the five mg sodium per serving
Very low sodium:	contains less the thirty-five mg sodium per serving
Low sodium:	contains forty mg of sodium or less per serving
Reduced sodium:	a food must contain seventy-five percent less sodium than the same product would if processed normally
Unsalted, salt-free	all these terms mean that no extra salt was added during processing

No salt: There is no added salt or products could be high in sodium (either without salt: naturally or from substances added for preservation, leavening or other purposes). Check the nutrition information panel for the specific sodium content per serving.

Cholesterol

Cholesterol is a sticky, waxy fat like substance that the body uses to make certain hormones, vitamins and digestive juices. You obtain cholesterol by producing it in your body (in the liver) or by eating foods with cholesterol in them. Some people have problems with elevated blood levels of cholesterol which can lead to arteriosclerosis (hardening of the arteries). For these people, the cholesterol content of foods is listed on food labels. It is recommended that these people limit their cholesterol intake to 300 milligrams per day. During pregnancy a woman's cholesterol level does increase as a result of all the hormonal changes occurring in her body. Eggs are one of the best (and cheapest compared to Filet Mignon) sources of protein for your growing baby. Despite the warning about the amount of cholesterol in the yolk portion of eggs, women need not be concerned about cholesterol consumption during pregnancy. Cholesterol is the basic building block necessary for the baby to make "steroid" and other complex hormones.

Beware!

Advertising agencies spend millions of dollars persuading consumers to purchase a specific product. As a result, some advertising may be misleading. An example is when a peanut butter manufacturer claims "their" peanut butter is low in cholesterol. This may be the truth, but not the whole truth. Cholesterol only comes from animal products and peanut butter is a plant product. Therefore, peanuts (or peanut butter) would never have cholesterol in it. What is not revealed is that the oil found in peanuts can be hardened (hydrogenated) turning the healthy peanut oil into a saturated fat which is unhealthy oil. Saturated fats, in turn, can elevate blood cholesterol levels.

Food products also use names to make the consumer believe that they are nutritionally beneficial. As an example, using the word "froot" and pronouncing it "fruit" can mislead the consumer. You would assume that there is fruit in it, when actually there is none.

The moral to this story is "Buyer Beware!" A wise shopper pays careful attention to food labels. Read ingredient lists and compare products based on the same serving size. If you have further questions, consult a Registered Dietitian (R.D.) by contacting a local hospital or using the yellow pages.

Food Preparation

What You Have Always Wanted to Know About Keeping Food Fresh but Were Afraid to Ask.

Through the ages, mankind has been concerned about trying to store uneaten food so that it may be eaten later and, therefore, not wasted. Because of weather and other natural events, man needed to gather enough food during times of plenty and learn how to store it through hard times. Early records have documented that the Romans stored food in ice that was brought down from the Alps. During the middle Ages, new techniques of smoking, drying and salting were used to preserve foods.

Today, keeping food "fresh" and safe becomes much easier because of the more recent developments of food processing and refrigeration. The federal government keeps a close watch on the cooking, processing and packaging of food during all stages of its preparation. Furthermore, the FDA (Food and Drug Administration) scrutinizes manufacturers and wholesale distributors to ensure that food is stored, dated and handled properly before it reaches the store. There is much more information the consumer needs to know in order to keep the food that he has just purchased fresh and wholesome. Insufficient cooking, improper storage and poor sanitation can allow bacteria in food to grow to a very high and dangerous level. The result is food poisoning. Approximately two million cases of food poisoning develop each year from improper handling of food in the home.

How is food preserved? Creating an environment that keeps bacterial counts in food down is the key point in preserving all foods.

There are five major food preservation techniques:

1. Canning
2. Drying
3. Pickling
4. Salting
5. Refrigeration and Freezing

Of course, the chief means of preserving food utilized today is refrigeration and freezing. Refrigeration does not kill bacteria in food, but works by retarding their growth and proliferation by the cold environment. Freezing is the most effective way of "stopping bacteria cold!" Bacteria do not reproduce and grow in adequately frozen conditions.

Many bacteria cause food to rot and become unpalatable to eat. However, there are specific bacteria and viruses that everyone should know about that lead directly to food poisoning. Most food poisoning-type bacteria like room temperature (60 to 90 degrees Fahrenheit). Their growth is retarded at low temperatures with refrigeration. They flourish at warmer room temperatures. The bacteria that cause food poisoning are very difficult to detect, most have little odor or taste and cannot be seen. There are four major bacterial food poisonings that will be discussed.

When Food is "Not Good"

Bacterial Food Poisonings

Staphylococcus Aureus ("Staph Infection")

Poor food handling that is, leaving food out too long under warm conditions or improper refrigeration (or worse yet, re-refrigeration!), allows the staphylococcus to grow in huge numbers. When ingested, the stomach acids can kill and neutralize only so many bacteria. Staphylococcus contains a powerful toxin: endotoxin. Endotoxin enters the bloodstream producing nausea, vomiting, diarrhea, chills and fever. Symptoms usually occur within two to six hours, and last one to two days. Healthy people usually can tolerate this brief illness without antibiotic therapy. Creamed pastries (such as éclairs) are notorious for producing this type of poisoning. Your bakery worker should never re-refrigerate these pastries after they have been in the display case all day. Most display cases are refrigerated to preserve these pastries longer (always ask when a particular piece of cake or dessert was made - hopefully that very day! Also, be careful of other rich foods, such as salads that have mayonnaise in them (potatoes and macaroni salads), salads with meat and cheese, and other creamed foods.

Salmonella

This type of poisoning comes from eating food in which large numbers of these bacteria are present. Raw and uncooked foods, such as poultry products, raw eggs, seafood and meat, are the special breeding ground for these bacteria. Re-refrigerated taco meat or fish that has been out in the summer heat all day are well known offenders in this infection. Severe flu-like symptoms of nausea, vomiting, diarrhea, fever and weakness ensue within 12 to 36 hours after ingestion. The illness may last two to seven days.

Clostridium Perfringens

("Gas Gangrene" Bacteria)

As the third leading cause of food poisoning, this bacterium differs from staph or salmonella in that it does not need oxygen in order to grow. These bacteria multiply quickly at warm temperatures. Gravy, dressings, stews and casseroles are mostly implicated as the prime sources for this infection. Again, gastrointestinal complaints of diarrhea and "gas pains" occur eight to twenty-four hours after ingestion and may last a day.

Clostridium Botulinum ("Botulism")

Though rare, the toxin produced by these bacteria is deadly. The toxin can enter your body without even swallowing the contaminated food in the first place: the toxin can enter your bloodstream through your cheek cells. It is crucial that you never even taste a food that may be contaminated with the botulism bacteria. The botulism toxin specifically attacks the nerve cells in your body. Paralysis ensues. Worse yet, the nerves controlling your breathing are knocked out and breathing may become difficult. Without proper medical care, death quickly results.

Botulism bacteria grow in foods that contain little or no air; such as packaged or canned foods. Improper canning, particularly home canning, receives the most notoriety in the press as the cause of botulism outbreaks. Low acid vegetables, such as corn, beets, green beans and peas, can house the botulism spores (bacterial seeds). It takes extreme high heat to kill these spores. Symptoms appear twelve to forty-eight hours after ingestion. The first signs of disease are manifested by double vision, dizziness, droopy eyelids, difficulties in swallowing, dry mouth and labored breathing. Medical help must be sought immediately so that an antitoxin can be administered. CPR and, possibly, a breathing machine may become necessary.

Accordingly, people should learn to inspect all of their food, particularly home-canned foods. Do not eat from any can or jar in which the top of the can is bulging. Toss away any food from cracked jars or damaged cans. Do not even taste the contents of a container in which a milky film or liquid floats or gives off a foul odor. Notify your local health department of the particular food, manufacturer and the store in which you purchased the food.

The bottom line is keep "hot foods hot, cold foods cold, and keep your kitchen clean."

Buy Quality Food

When you shop, be careful in your selection of perishable foods. Make sure frozen foods are solid and that refrigerated foods feel cold. The "sell by" and "use by" dates now printed on many products can also be helpful in deciding whether food is still safe to buy, provided you know how to use them. What do they mean? The "sell by" date tells the grocer, and you, how long the product should be kept for sale on the shelf. The "use by" date is intended to tell you how long the product will retain top eating quality after you buy it. While these dates are helpful, you can't rely on them absolutely.

Meat and Poultry Products

Make sure that meat is bright red or dullish brown. Return any package that has an off-odor when opened. The USDA (United States Department of Agriculture) stamp found on some meat and/or poultry products means that these items come from healthy animals and are processed under strict sanitary conditions.

Note: Many meat departments artificially color meat bright red so that it is more attractive to the buyer. Most meat is dark brown and checking the dating label is the most reliable indicator of freshness.

Canned Foods

Only buy canned food that is free of leaks, bulges, bad dents; jars that are free of cracks; and containers that do not spurt liquid when opened (a sign of botulism and, therefore, food should not be tasted).

Chilled Foods

Pick up chilled foods last when grocery shopping and put these items away first at home. Read dates printed on cartons of milk, orange juice, etc. Purchase before the date (most items are safe to use for one week after date). Do not buy cracked eggs. Cracked eggs can contain harmful bacteria.

Frozen Foods

Pick up frozen foods last when grocery shopping and put these items away first at home. Buy only those that are frozen solid. Never buy partially thawed frozen foods, or those which have been frozen, thawed and re-frozen.

Fresh Fruits and Vegetables

Buy when supplies are plentiful. Buy only what you need, since these fresh foods are perishable. Avoid damaged goods with sign of decay, skin punctures or other indications of spoilage.

Fresh-Baked Foods

Be alert for signs of spoilage, especially in the hot summer months when germs multiply fast. Only purchase custard and desserts with cream fillings if kept under refrigeration.

STORE FOOD PROPERLY

<u>Dry and Bulk Food</u>: store in a cool and dry area. You should store food away from contaminated areas that may have been visited by rodents and insects. Lastly, be careful to store foods away from cleaning materials and other possible sources of poison.

<u>Canned Foods</u>: most may be kept safely for a year if stored properly... BUT, if storage area is too warm, quality and taste may deteriorate. If it is damp, cans may corrode, allowing dangerous germs to enter.

<u>Chilled Foods</u>: refrigerate meats, dairy products and prepared foods immediately and continuously in a refrigerator set at 40 degrees F (or below). Egg-rich dishes, such as custards and cream-filled pastries, should be kept cold and served this way. Keep your refrigerator clean. Place foods in refrigerator in a way that maximizes proper circulation of cool air. Check the temperature by placing a thermometer in the warmest part of the refrigerator. It must be below 40 degrees F to inhibit the growth of food-poisoning organisms.

<u>Frozen Foods</u>: keep in freezer set a zero degrees F (or below) to prevent the growth of spoilage organisms. Frozen foods should not be thawed, then refrozen. However, if food is partially thawed and ice crystals remain, it is safe to refreeze the food.

Prepare and Serve Food Safely

Canned foods that spurt liquid when opened should not be used nor tasted: it is the foremost sign of botulism. Thaw meats, fish or poultry in the refrigerator or cook them frozen. If you must thaw poultry in a hurry, submerge it in cold running water. Use a meat thermometer when cooking meat or poultry. Insert it into the thickest part (but not in fat but make sure that it doesn't touch the bone either). On poultry, use it in the thick part of the thigh. Internal minimum temperatures of beef, veal and lamb should be a least 140 degrees F; fresh pork 150 to 160 degrees F (to kill trichinosis, a parasite found in some pork products); and poultry 165 degrees F. Wash poultry before cooking because salmonella organisms are often present in poultry, even when frozen.

Use separate cutting boards for vegetables/fruit, meats/poultry, and bread/pastries to avoid cross-contamination. Sanitize cutting boards after each use. Scrub vegetables and wash fruits thoroughly. Handle glasses by the base, dishes by the edges and silverware by the handles. Keep fingers out of food. Food prepared ahead of time should be covered until eaten in order to keep out airborne germs and insects. Never keep food more than two hours at temperatures between 40 and 140 degrees F. Cracked dishes and glasses can collect food particles in cracks which support germs, so discard them. Use a separate spoon for tasting food. Do not use the same spoon more than once.

Clean Kitchen and Equipment

Wash off cutting knives between uses, particularly if the knife is used on raw poultry or meat. This will help prevent cross-contamination. Wash utensils, pots and pans in hot, soapy water; rinse in hot, clear water and either air-dry or wipe dry with a clean cloth. Be sure to clean can openers along with other utensils. Scrub cutting boards with hot, soapy water, and rinse well. Be careful of steel wool and metal scouring pads; they may leave metal slivers behind. Rub a lemon rind on wood surfaces to prevent sour smell. Wooden cutting boards with many deep grooves should not be used. Plastic and/or rubber boards are safer to use. Scrub work surfaces with hot, soapy water, and rinse well. Give special attention to cracks, joints and edges where food particles may collect.

Use Leftovers Wisely

Cover, label and date all leftovers and place immediately into the refrigerator. Don't cool leftovers on the kitchen counter. Leftover hot foods should be placed immediately into the refrigerator (refrigerators are designed to withstand the excess heat from cooked foods). Divide large meat, macaroni, or potato salads as well as large bowls of mashed potatoes or dressing into smaller portions. Food in small portions cools more quickly to temperatures where bacteria quit growing. Reheat leftovers all the way through (to at least 165 degrees) and bring gravies to a rolling boil. Meat and poultry leftovers should be covered, stored in the coldest part of the refrigerator, and used in two days. If they are to be frozen, put them in a covered container or wrap them tightly. "If in doubt, please throw it out!" P.S. Don't feed it to your husband (but giving them to your ex-husband is okay!)

CHAPTER 17

Potential Hazards During Pregnancy

Environmental and Household Exposures

The pregnant patient should be careful to check the contents and ingredients of the following types of products. Most are safe and not harmful to you or the baby.

Household "Goods"

___ Cleansers

___ Disinfectants: Lysol, Pine-Sol

___ Waxes

___ Polishes

___ Strippers

___ Cleaners

Workshop Hazards

___ Paints, Shellacs, Varnishes, Thinners

___ Blow Torch and Soldering Fumes

___ Wallpaper and Pastes

"Personal" Products

___ Perfumes and Deodorants

___ Hair Sprays, Mousses

___ Shampoos

___ Coloring Agents and Permanent Chemicals

___ Soaps

___ Toothpastes and Mouthwashes

___ Eye Drops and Lens Cleaner Solutions

___ Facial and Body Creams and Lotions

Garden Products

___ Insecticides

___ Fertilizers

___ Gasoline and Oils

___ Barbeque Starters and Smoke

<u>Author Case Study in Point</u>: When I was a Resident at UCLA a pregnant patient presented to labor and delivery at 7 months gestation with significant amount of bleeding. The patient had unusual bruises on her legs and arms. Coagulation studies showed that the patient's bleeding time was significantly prolonged: she had a *coagulopathy*. The baby's heart beat was absent. After the baby was delivered stillborn the placenta basically fell out. The placenta had completely separated from the uterine wall, i.e., *abrupted* with complete loss of circulation to the baby. Further extensive questioning of the patient revealed that she was using "rat poison" to kill tree rats on

her property. Rat poison contains warfarin, the powerful anti-clot medication that causes hemorrhage in rats (it is used in minimal doses to prevent clots in your lungs or legs (DVT's(Deep Venous Thrombosis) in humans. Apparently, she had ingested or inhaled so much of the rat poison when she was handling it: the warfarin resulted in her blood not being able to clot when it circulated to the baby's placenta. Bleeding occurred between the placenta and uterine wall: the placenta separated from its attachment to the uterine wall and a large clot formed. The circulation to the baby was interrupted with the unfortunate loss of her baby.

Imaging studies during Pregnancy: X-Rays

X-rays should be diligently avoided during pregnancy. All women trying to conceive, or not using any reliable birth control method, should have their pelvis shielded prior to the taking of any x-rays. Better yet, such women should postpone all x-ray examinations until the time of their menstrual period - a time when pregnancy cannot occur. There are times however, during pregnancy, when x-rays must be performed for the sake of the mother's health; i.e., fractures of bones, kidney stones, gallbladder disease, to name a few.

If there is any possibility of pregnancy, please tell your chiropractor prior to taking full spinal films. Back x-rays produce the largest amounts of x-ray radiation and exposure.

If the part of the body needing to be x-rayed is outside the pelvis, then the pregnancy can be shielded by the use of the lead apron - the baby is protected. X-rays of the arms, legs, head, sinuses, ears, teeth, chest, breasts, fall into this category. X-rays of the abdomen and pelvis necessarily "radiates" the baby.

More importantly it must be pointed out that medical research has shown no linkage of x-ray exposure to any specific birth defect. Any radiation damage can be "patched up" quickly by the developing fetus. The Hiroshima nuclear bomb studies showed that radiation exposure had an "all or none" effect. Overwhelming radiation exposure to the fetus beyond tolerance resulted in miscarriage or stillbirth. Otherwise, the babies were born without any known damage. They repaired all affected tissues and healed normally. So far, medical research has been able to show a possible slight increase in the incidence of childhood leukemia in those children exposed in utero to the radiation of the magnitude of the Hiroshima nuclear bomb.

When x-rays of the abdomen do become absolutely necessary, both the radiologist (x-ray specialist) and the obstetrician try to minimize the dosage of radiation as well as the number of films. A kidney stone during pregnancy may necessitate a "one-shot" IVP to make the diagnosis. Although ultrasound has replaced x-ray in the diagnosis of gallstones, Gallbladder x-rays may be needed to diagnose the location and size of stones in the gallbladder or biliary tract. X-ray pelvimetry, i.e., x-rays to measure the pelvic capacity from bone to bone, is being utilized less frequently in today's obstetrics. Such x-rays were used regularly for assessing the anatomy and measurements of the pelvis as well as head flexion prior to vaginal breech delivery. CT scan pelvimetry now replaces x-ray pelvimetry when available at the hospital.

Other Diagnostic Imaging Technology

Ultrasound

As discussed in many parts of this book, ultrasound examination of the uterus is being performed in more than fifty percent of all pregnancies. To date, after forty years of clinical use, no adverse effects have been observed in the human fetus. No long-term effects or consequences have ensued. In fact, ultrasound as a diagnostic tool has only helped to diagnose serious birth defects while the baby still is inside the uterus. Ultrasound has made the field of "fetal surgery" possible. Only in early pregnancy (<12 weeks) can high dose ultrasound, i.e. power Doppler, for a prolonged duration could result in possible damage to the fetus: there are few times when power Doppler would even be considered.

The many benefits of ultrasound examination of the pregnant uterus are enumerated throughout this book.

CT Scans and MRIs

These imaging techniques may be performed during pregnancy in cases where the diagnostic benefit of a necessary diagnosis outweighs the risks to the baby. Avoidance of contrast in these studies makes them safer.

Occupational Safety and Environmental Exposures

More and more of today's women have become the "breadwinners" of American families. They work in a variety of industries and manufacturing plants. While pregnant, they come into contact with potentially toxic chemicals, solvents, gasses and radiation. In this section, pregnant patients are advised of the dangers of certain agents, as well as some principles of occupational safety.

Known Toxic Agents

Ethylene oxide (EtO) is a colorless gas used in sterilization of instruments in hospitals and other facilities.

Direct contact causes severe irritation of skin, mouth and respiratory system. Increased rates of miscarriages and cancer, as well as chromosomal abnormalities, have been reported; but the evidence is not substantial. OSHA (Occupational Safety and Health Administration) officials consider one-part-per-million (ppm) exposure of an eight-hour shift safe for women working with sterilization equipment.

Lead: is used in the gasoline and oil industries. Lead and its various byproducts are used in paints and printing. Lead has been implicated in increased rates of infertility and miscarriages, toxic anemias and neurological abnormalities in the children of exposed women.

Halothane and Nitrous Oxide are anesthetic gases. Anesthesiologists, anesthetists, physicians and nurses in the operating rooms across the country can be potentially exposed to these chemicals. Re-design of anesthetic machines has largely prevented the increased miscarriage rate associated with these gases in the medical and dental fields.

Asbestos was used in prior decades for insulation in ceilings, in wiring and around heating pipes. Primarily, asbestos is inhaled into the lungs causing chronic respiratory disorders in workers exposed over long periods of time. No fetal effects have been reported.

Coal and Forest Products. Inhalation of coal and other mining products can result in respiratory diseases similar to asbestosis. Pine tree dusts and ashes in the lumber industries may also cause skin and eye irritations, as well as breathing difficulties.

Farming and Dairy Industries Exposure. Bacteria such as tuberculosis and brucellosis are carried by animals. Listeriosis around hay can cause severe infection in the mother with the potential to infect the placenta and the unborn fetus.

Author Note: At the time the author was a resident at UCLA, the OB unit received a 7 month patient with a fever of 104, chills, sweating, and prostration. She was in sepsis: infection was present and circulating in her blood. When examined, the baby was found to be dead or stillborn. Her white blood count (WBC's) was 72,000 with normal being up to 16,000. The OB staff thought she had some fulminant type of leukemia. Blood cultures later revealed she had been infected with Listeria monocytogenes. She was exposed while she was working in the damp hay around the family barn.

Listeria most often contaminates various cheeses during their manufacture in the US and in other countries (more recently a ice cream manufacturer with product recall).

For very specific inquiries regarding any chemicals or other toxins, there are two main centers in the United States that are available for consultation:

1. Reproductive Toxicological Center in Washington
2. Dr. Victor McKusick's Laboratory at Johns Hopkins University, Baltimore, Maryland
3. Your local University Hospital Medical Genetics Unit.

All of these Centers, including the National Poison Control Center, may be reached by accessing their Internet websites. Google searches can provide even more in depth information.

Principles of Occupational Safety

There are hundreds of chemicals, gases and dusts in the working environment of women employees. Unfortunately, more often than not, physicians may have little knowledge of the effects of such agents because of the following compounding factors:

1. The particular substance is not listed in the usual references on reproductive hazards.

2. What information is available is not complete or statistically relevant. Much of the data is often conflicting either positive or negative about its potential dangers.

3. Data in animal studies may not be easily extrapolated to humans when excessive doses are utilized.

When reliable or no information is available, it is best that women request reassignment or comparable work in an unexposed area of the building while pregnant. If reassignment or other work is not possible, disability may be available to such pregnant women.

One cannot over-emphasize that workers take advantage of the protective gear given to them on the job. Ergonomic chairs and work stations in computer terminal operation, gloves when handling hot or toxic chemicals, protective eye wear in welding, helmets in construction, protective lead aprons in x-ray facilities and steel-covered shoes in material handling, provide the needed armor in hazardous jobs. Workers must pay attention to "warning" signs and "restricted" areas. Above all, follow directions and protocols without taking short cuts.

Wear plastic gloves when pumping gas from self-service gas stations. Be careful not to spill gas over one's clothing when maneuvering the nozzle to and from your car. Observe and make sure others obey "no smoking" in such designated areas. Check and test smoke alarms at the office and at home. Locate where fire extinguishers are placed at the job and be sure to have one in the kitchen at home. Be sure car exhaust pollution control devices and muffler systems are functioning properly.

Special Concern for Medical and Dental Fields

Day Care Centers and Other Institutions

Besides exposure to toxic chemicals, radiation, lasers and anesthetic gases, medical, nursing and dental personnel are at risk to contract a large number of infectious diseases. The following diseases also are quite prevalent in daycare centers, mental institutions, convalescent homes and correctional facilities.

1. CMV (Cytomegalic Inclusion Virus): This virus is prevalent in the laboratory, dialysis, oncology and nursery units of the hospital. Daycare centers, mental institutions and correctional facilities are also high-risk areas. Potentially serious fetal disease is remote: two to five per ten thousand maternal primary infections. It is recommended that workers in all risk areas undergo immunity testing for this virus.

<u>Author Note</u>: An 18 year old was in her second pregnancy. Her first baby was stillborn. When she was first seen in the second trimester, the ultrasound showed the baby had hydrops: fluid in the abdomen and chest. The "Torch Panel" was ordered: she was positive for CMV. She was currently working in a Day care center. The baby was born with deficits: he had a feeding tube in stomach and he had failed his hearing test. The author also notes a similar scenario with Parvovirus B19 (Slap Cheek Syndrome) detailed below. Pregnant mothers should avoid handling sick children in Day care centers.

2. Hepatitis B and C and HIV: Workers in direct contact with body fluids, such as physicians, nurses, medical and dental assistants or blood-handlers in blood banks, are constantly exposed to this virulent infection. Approximately ten to

fifteen percent of all persons who experience this disease never quite recover and suffer chronic active hepatitis. Another one to three percent of those so infected experience a fulminant disease, leading to liver failure and death. All workers should have hepatitis immunity testing and, if determined susceptible, be given hepatitis B vaccination. (Hepatitis B vaccine is now made by recombinant genetic engineering and not from pooled human serum. Accordingly, there is no risk of AIDS.)

3. Parvovirus B19 (Slap Cheek Syndrome) is also called 5th disease (after the 4 most common childhood diseases: measles i.e., roseola, rubella, mumps and chickenpox). This viral disease is commonly spread to non-immune adults in childcare centers or wherever children may be playing. It presents as a "flu-like syndrome," I.e. minor sore throat, congestion, low grade fever, but does NOT manifests itself in the classic red cheeks that are seen in children.

<u>Authors Note</u>: Eliza Chavez was 29 weeks pregnant with known ulcerative colitis when she presented to the office with a 7 day history of the "flu" but was experiencing high fevers and chills. She was admitted to the hospital for the possibility of a kidney infection, pneumonia, influenza, Cytomegalic Inclusion Virus (CMV) or mononucleosis. An intestinal wall crypt abscess was also a possibility with her ulcerative colitis. She was spiking fevers to 103 and all her tests results were negative for the preceding conditions. She was transferred to OU Medical Center for further consultation because of the possibility of premature labor due to sepsis. The Infectious Disease specialist considered Parvovirus as another possible infectious viral disease to which she could have been exposed while working at the day-care facility. The diagnosis was confirmed. She was carefully watched during her 3rd trimester and delivered a healthy baby girl!

Parvovirus B19 is a serious viral disease that can cause significant anemia in the unborn baby: especially in the 1st or 2nd trimesters. Pregnant women should be tested for their immune status if so exposed during pregnancy.

4. Rubella (German measles): Although most people have been vaccinated in childhood (or became immunized by having the "three-day measles"), it is uncertain how long the newer vaccines may confer immune protection for a given individual. Because of severe fetal damage to the eyes, ears and brain, all workers should also have rubella testing. If non-immune, such workers should be vaccinated. Although the attenuated rubella vaccine has not caused the rubella syndrome, it is recommended that reliable contraception be used for three months after vaccination before trying for pregnancy.

The vaccine is usually administered to postpartum patients if they were non-immune during pregnancy.

5. Tuberculosis (TB): Recent immigration of families from Mexico, Southeast Asia and the Middle East has brought back the specter of TB. This special bacterium lies dormant in the lungs, and infection may reactivate at times of decreased body resistance. Highly contagious, the bacteria can be inhaled if coughed up from the respiratory tract of a patient with tuberculosis. Newborns can be exposed by grandparents from the "old country" or hospital staff that has recently emigrated from other countries. TB skin testing and chest x-rays are mandatory in all hospital personnel on a periodic basis.

6. AIDS (Autoimmune Deficiency Syndrome): This viral disease is of special concern for those in the medical and dental fields. Also, workers in the pharmaceutical industries involved in the processing of human blood products (such as gamma globulin, RhoGAM and vaccines) should follow established health and safety guidelines. For further information, the reader should refer to the section on "AIDS.

Other Special Occupational Exposures

Computer or TV screens (VDT or Video Display Terminals): Research at the present time has shown that computer terminal workers are not dangerously exposed to electromagnetic radiation. Since 1974, such computer screens are constructed to standards that prevent leakage of such electromagnetic waves from the computer consoles. Furthermore, such electromagnetic waves are non-ionizing in contrast to x-ray radiation. Therefore, any leakage represents (theoretically) only a wave of energy. To date, studies have no evidence that VDT's are associated with fetal abnormalities or increased rates of miscarriage. More often, however, they are important causes of eye strain and headaches. Also, because of the keyboard operation, Carpal Tunnel Syndrome, i.e. numbness of the fingers caused by compression of the median nerve in the palm, is increasingly distressful to pregnant computer operators.

Smoking: Inhalation of "secondary" smoke may produce problems in exposed non-smokers. Large facilities may possess smoking and non-smoking work areas. Problems may arise in small businesses. Hopefully, fellow workers who smoke may be polite and smoke outside the facility (or better yet, stop smoking altogether!). Secondary smoke in the air contains nicotine, carbon monoxide, and other products. If so inhaled by expectant women, such substances may be transmitted to the developing fetus. Furthermore, some women may be highly allergic to such secondary smoke. Nasal congestion, eye irritation, coughing and wheezing may be experienced by such individuals. Pregnant workers should discuss any of these related problems with their supervisors or administrators.

Where to Go For Help

Lastly, it is important for the pregnant employee to know where to go for help when questions arise about the safety of the work environment. OSHA requires employers to furnish to their employees detailed information about the type and amount of substances used at work. First go to the plant medical or nursing station. If there is none, go to the plant's administrative offices. If satisfaction is not obtained, the following resources are available:

NIOSH (National Institute for Occupation Safety & Health) Occupational Health Services, Inc. (Oakland 415- 655-0535)

Occupational Safety & Health Administration (OSHA)

Poison Control Center (Oakland (415) 428-3248)

County Health Dept. (Alameda (415) 652-5566)

State Dept. of Health

Sanitation - Environmental Health (415) 881-6390 Guidelines on Pregnancy & Work (Published under NIOSH funding for the American College of Obstetricians and Gynecologists). Available from ACOG, 600 Maryland Avenue, S.W., Washington, DC 20024

AMA's Dept. of Public Health Policy in Chicago

(312) 645-4534 or (312) 645-4541

Barlow SM, Sullivan FM: *Reproductive Hazards of Industrial Chemicals* - London Academic Press, 1982

Council on Scientific Affairs, Advisory panel on Reproductive Hazards in the Work Place, AMA:

Effects of Toxic Chemicals on the Reproductive System, AMA, 1985 Council on Scientific Affairs, AMA: Effects of Physical Forces on the Reproductive Cycle JAMA 1984; 251:247

Council on Scientific Affairs, AMA: Effects of Pregnancy on Work Performance. JAMA 1984 and 251:1995

CHAPTER 18

Medications During Pregnancy And Breastfeeding

Quite often, an expectant mother wonders whether or not a certain drug or food can affect her unborn child. This section addresses these questions by outlining general principles, as well as detailing some information about frequently-utilized medications.

General Principles

During pregnancy and nursing, the following guidelines should be understood:

1. No medications, drugs or other chemicals should be taken unless prescribed by your physician.
2. No medicine or drug has been proven absolutely safe during pregnancy. Medicines should only be taken when the benefits, if any, substantially outweigh the risks.
3. There is little information about the risk of birth defects from any medicine, toxin, food additive or other chemicals. Information that is available has been obtained from experiments in rats (usually "mega-dose" exposure) or from inadvertent use during pregnancy. Results from these animal experiments may not be directly applicable to pregnant human subjects.
4. The most vulnerable time during pregnancy for drugs to exert their effects on the developing fetus is the first five-to-six weeks of pregnancy—the period of time before a

woman suspects she is pregnant and prior to even missing her period. Accordingly, couples trying to conceive should be very careful about taking any medicines or abusing any drugs (including alcohol) or other harmful substances during "unprotected" times of the menstrual cycle. Furthermore, couples attempting pregnancy should stay away from "sick" children or adults that have communicable diseases; i.e., viral, bacterial and parasitic diseases. Any chemical or biological agent can potentially produce an ill effect on the rapidly growing fetus and placenta

5. Most over-the-counter (OTC) medications are "safe" during pregnancy. Most have not been associated with any adverse effects--even when taken in the first weeks of pregnancy. The amount of active drug in these remedies is so little as to present a minimal risk to the fetus. Again, do not take any of these preparations unless you are very miserable from congestion, headache, constipation, heartburn, etc.

In 2014 an Israeli study reported that there was no increase in the risk of miscarriage with the ingestion of NSAIDS (aspirin, ibuprofen, and acetaminophen and naproxen sodium) during pregnancy.

To date there have been no reported statistical association with the use of NSAIDs in pregnancy and any adverse effects on the developing fetus: the exception being that NSAIDs may prevent the closure of the patent ductus arteriosus after delivery and therefore should not be taken in the last month of pregnancy.

Below is a table of select online resources that you may check out to research and know more about any medications you may be concerned with.

Table 2 Selected Online Resources for Safe Use of Medication during Pregnancy

Type of Information	Website Overview
Clinical:	
CDC: Pregnancy Information for Healthcare Providers and Researchers	Lists comprehensive resources on pregnancy issues, such as prenatal, maternal, and pediatric medical and preventive care.
National Center on Birth Defects and Developmental Disabilities	Provides resources on prenatal care, infant and child development, disabilities, and blood disorders.
CDC: Spotlight scientific articles on medications in pregnancy	Lists "spotlight articles" on medication use in pregnancy, disease management during pregnancy, and clinical guidelines.
Maternal risk	Healthcare professional-oriented site that provides such resources as information on safe medication use during pregnancy and breastfeeding and a link to clinical trials evaluating specific medications or disease states during pregnancy.
National Birth Defects Prevention Study	A study that seeks to determine causes of birth defects.
Mother To Baby	A service of OTIS that provides evidence-based information on medications and exposures during pregnancy and lactation.
US National Library of Medicine, Toxicology Data Network (TOXNET): Developmental and Reproductive Toxicology Database (DART)	Allows searching of drugs or outcomes (eg, neural tube defect) in the reproductive and developmental toxicology literature.

General:	
CDC: Digital Press Kit -- Safe Medication Lists on the Internet	Promotional materials about questionable validity of safe medication use lists found on the Internet.
CDC: Medication Use During Pregnancy	Discusses how common medication use during pregnancy has become.
CDC: Information on vaccines in pregnant women	Provides general information for the patient regarding vaccine use during pregnancy.
CDC: Medication and Pregnancy	Offers general information for the patient regarding medication use and safety in pregnancy.
CDC: Birth Defects	Discusses topics on birth defects.
Maternal risks	Patient-oriented site that provides general pregnancy and medication safety information.
FDA: Pregnancy	Gives medication, food, and product safety information to the patient during pregnancy.
Womenshealth.gov: Pregnancy	A project of the US Department of Health and Human Services Office on Women's Health that offers comprehensive guidance regarding optimal health for mother and baby before, during, and after pregnancy.
MedlinePlus: Pregnancy	A service of the US National Library of Medicine and National Institute of Health that provides comprehensive resource regarding health and other topics related to pregnancy.

CDC = Centers for Disease Control and Prevention; FDA = US Food and Drug Administration; OTIS = Organization of Teratology Information Specialists

Food Additives

Most foods and the additives in them (preservatives, colors, dyes, emulsifiers, etc.) are also safe to consume during pregnancy. Nevertheless, it may be wise to eat only those foods which come directly out of the ground, off the tree or from the bird, the fish and the animal. Be sure to wash all your fruits and vegetables thoroughly with water: they have usually been sprayed or otherwise chemically treated to retard the growth of microbiological organisms as well as other pests. Perhaps it may be best to avoid significant amounts of "prepared foods or fast food," such as luncheon meats, sandwich spreads, milk and butter imitators and other "chemistry set" concoctions that have been called "food" by my teenagers. Such convenience foods contain a whole host of chemicals, preservatives, coloring agents, stabilizers, and so on. Though probably safe because of their present use by the public, very little is still known regarding the consumption of these agents during early pregnancy. Read the labels for any warnings regarding their use during pregnancy.

Author's Note: My toxicology professor at UCSF gave a very important illustration of the amount of food additives to ordinary "wholesome" food. He presented a "healthy" breakfast of eggs, bacon, toast and orange juice. There were over 12 additives to orange juice alone! Pick up a loaf of bread and bacon and look at the food labels. It will surprise you.

Never take any medication that has caused you to have an allergic reaction in the past (i.e. rash, difficulty in breathing, edema or swelling of the eyes, throat or legs). If ever uncertain about a specific drug, its dose and how often it should be taken, do not hesitate to phone your physician's office.

Specific Harmful Drugs

The following drugs are known to cause birth defects in pregnancy:

Medication	Use	Effect
Thalidomide	sedative	limb shortening defects
Tetracycline	antibiotic	bone & teeth defects
Chloramphenicol	antibiotic	"Gray's syndrome" in newborn
Streptomycin	antibiotic	hearing, kidney damage
Coumadin	anticoagulant	bleeding in babies
Dilantin	anticonvulsant	cleft lip & palate
Accutane	acne drug	brain, nerve & heart
Ace Inhibiters	hypertension	increased risk of malformations

Commonly Prescribed Safe Medications

***Antibiotic Class*:**

> Penicillins: Ampicillin, Pen VK, Amoxicillin
> Cephalosporins: Keflex, Cefotetan, Ceclor, Mefoxin
> Macrolides: Erythromycin: Zithromycin(Z-pack)
> Sulfa: Septra DS, Bactrim DS, Gantrisin, Azo-Gantrisin
> Nitrofurantoin: Macrodantin

Analgesics (pain relievers) and Non-Steroidal Anti-inflammatory Drugs (NSAIDS):

> Acetaminophen (Tylenol, Datril, etc.)
> Hydrocodone, Oxycodone, Codeine (in Lortab and Percocet, Tylenol # 3, & Fiornal #3)
> Others: Pentazocine (Talwin)
> IV, SQ or IM analgesics : Stadol, Nubain, Demerol, Morphine, Dilaudid

> Under the direction of your physician during the 2nd trimester:
>> Aspirin (Bayer, Anacin, etc.),
>> Ibuprofen (Advil, Nuprin, Motrin, Tramadol or Ultram, etc.)
>> Indomethacin (used for Preterm Labor treatment)

Decongestants: Sudafed, Dimetapp, Triaminic

Anti-emetics:

> Diglegis (Doxyalamine and Vitamin B6)
> Doxyalamine 25 mg
> Phenergan (promethazine)
> Compazine
> Zofran (not FDA-approved in pregnancy but used by most OBs for treatment)

Antihistamines (allergy medications): Claritan, Zyrtec, Chlorphiramine (Chlor-tri-metron), Allegra, Actifed, etc.

Antacids: Maalox, Gaviscon, Riopan, Mylanta, etc.

Asthma Medications: Aminophyllin, Medi-Inhalers (Albuterol, Advair, etc)

GERD (Gastro-Esophageal Reflux Disease) or Peptic Ulcer Drugs: Zantac, Tagamet, Pepcid AC, Prevacid

Diabetic Medications: NPH, Lente, Ultralente, Regular Insulins U-100, Levamir, Lantus

Hypertension Drugs: Labetolol, Aldomet, Hydralazine, Diuretics, Potassium supplements

Anticonvulsants: Gabapentin, Zarontoin, occasionally Phenobarbital and Dilantin

Anti-Anxiety Drugs: Xanax conditionally and for limited duration of use

Sedative Medications: Ambien

Anti-Depressants: These medications should be discontinued when attempting pregnancy and used only cautiously if necessary after the first trimester: SSRI's (Selective Serotonin Receptor Inhibitors drugs such Paxil, Zoloft, Cymbalta, Celexa, etc.) and the Tricyclics such as Elavil, Tofranil, Desyrel

Local Anaesthetics: Novacaine, Lidocaine (Xylocaine), Marcaine, Nesacaine

Steroid/Cortisone Drugs:

Topical (Cortisone, Topicort, Kenalog, Lidex)
Injectectable (Betamethasone, SoluMedrol)
Oral such as Prednisone or Methylprednisolone

Tocolytics (Labor stopping) Drugs): Terbutaline, Nifedipine, indomethacin etc.

Stool Softeners: DSS, Surfak, Metamucil, Correctal, Colace

Laxatives: Dulcolax, Senakot, Milk of Magnesia, Doxidan, Pericolace, Fleets Enema

Thyroid Drugs: Synthroid, Anti –thyroid meds such as PTU (Phenylpropylthiouracil or methimazole)

Heart Medications: Digoxin, Labetolol

Vitamins: Prenatal vitamins with folic acid
Multivitamins: 1-A-Day, Centrum, Stress Tabs, etc.
Vitamin B-6 (no more than 500 mg/day)
Folic Acid (no more than 4 mg/day)
Vitamin C (no more than 500 mg/day)

Minerals:

Calcium (no more than 1500 mg/day), Tums, Calcium Gluconate,

Iron (no more than 1000 mg/day) Ferrous Sulfate, Ferrous Gluconate, Feosol, Fergon, Slow FE

Potassium

Ear and Eye Medications: most antibiotic and steroid drops/ointments are safe when used topically

Vaginal Medications: Miconazole creams (such as Terazol, Gynazole, monistat), Vagisil but, as follows:

Douches are a NO, NO during Pregnancy!

Hemorrhoid Preparations: Anusol, Preparation H, Nupercainal, Tucks, Witch Hazel

Sunburn Preparations: All SBF and anti-wrinkling preparations as well as "spray on" tans

"Cold Remedies": Cepacol, Listerine, Sucrets, Vicks, Hall's, Smith's, Scope, Ben-Gay

Deodorants: all topical preparations are acceptable.

Vaccinations during Pregnancy

The safety of specific vaccinations during pregnancy depends entirely on the type of vaccine to be given. In general, live and attenuated virus vaccines should not be administered during pregnancy. Inactive or "dead" vaccines can be given without concern (these vaccines are "not alive" and non-infective).

In general, an inactivated vaccine can be made from any part of a killed virus. When injected into a person, the viral fragment causes the body to react to it. The body's immune system forms particles, or antibodies, against the viral fragment. When the real "live" virus enters the body, these antibodies attack the virus and destroy it.

<u>The Process of Antibody Formation</u>. Vaccination with antibody formation is very similar to an enemy Navy vessel intruding into protected seaway. When a foreign ship enters the seaway (your body), your immune system attacks it with antibody "ammunition." The foreign intruding vessel explodes." Similarly, a 'foreign or infectious" virus is taken out of commission permanently (It is too bad our criminal justice system does not work the same way specific viruses kill foreign antigens, i.e., they are never allowed in the body again!) Therefore, killed or inactivated vaccines cannot infect the body and, when injected, pose no risk to the patient or fetus.

When the risk of catching a viral infection is very high and the health consequences of the viral disease are serious, vaccination with a "live" vaccine may become necessary. Examples of such vaccination include polio and yellow fever. Such high-risk exposure situations develop when the pregnant woman is traveling to a foreign country in which the disease is prevalent. Note that smallpox vaccine is no longer given in this country because of the rarity of this disease. Because patients are more likely to suffer more from the side effects of the vaccine itself than the risk of contracting smallpox, the United States stopped the routine smallpox vaccination of all children in the late 1970's.

Postpartum Rubella Vaccination/Immunization

Rubella vaccination is currently recommended to all postpartum mothers if their rubella blood test during the pregnancy shows a lack of immunity. Because rubella infection can cause severe damage to a fetus in the first trimester of the next (or subsequent) pregnancy, the safest time to give the rubella vaccine is postpartum (while the just-delivered mother is still in the hospital). Even though the rubella vaccine is a live virus, it is an attenuated strain. Though live virus is shed from the mother's body in the days following vaccination, such viral shedding does not represent a potential risk of infection to the newborn baby.

Breastfeeding is completely safe after rubella vaccination. When the breastfeeding mom goes home, she likewise cannot infect other members of the household. After rubella vaccination, she should is advised not become pregnant for at least three months. A reliable form of birth control should be utilized. However, accidental vaccination of an already-pregnant woman with the rubella vaccine has yet to result in a damaged fetus. Furthermore, rubella virus shed from recently immunized children in the same household (or neighborhood children) cannot infect the unborn fetus. Lastly, most other types of vaccinations are usually not communicable to the newborn baby. However, it is wise to limit exposure of the newborn to siblings and other neighborhood children who may be carrying other viral infections; i.e., colds, flu and other diseases.

I can remember a recently delivered mother whose newborn had a fever convulsion within the first few weeks of life. The baby had viral meningitis that probably resulted from contact from a contagious individual. It is especially important that other members of the household, relatives and friends, not "kiss" the newborn. The human mouth has the largest reservoir (variety and numbers) of potentially communicable bacteria and viruses. The newborn could care less if it is kissed or not. He, or she, only cares to be held and fed. The baby has no comprehension of the emotional or loving value of a kiss at this early age. Do not allow your baby to be kissed-particularly from strangers on the street who you do not know and who may be carrying around a disease.

<u>Author's Note</u>: When my wife and I had our first baby, Jennifer (who was four weeks premature), all visitors had to take their shoes off outside the door before entering the house. They were questioned about their recent and past medical health and then they were led to the bathroom where they scrubbed and gowned. They were allowed to hold the baby for a limited time. Although this may seem like "overkill," I am glad to report that Jennifer did not suffer from any colds or diarrhea during the first six months of life (but, her mom also breastfed her such that passive immunity, i.e. antibodies were transferred to her through her mother's milk).

SUBSTANCE ABUSE

Alcohol

It is recommended to avoid drinking alcoholic beverages during pregnancy. A few recent studies have downplayed the risks associated with occasional alcohol during pregnancy. The original studies were done on alcoholic women on skid row: these studies did not control for protein intake or smoking. A FA (Fetal Alcohol Syndrome) could be produced as a result of chronic (almost daily) drinking. Babies are damaged with facial and bony defects, mental retardation and stunted physical growth.

The patient should be assured that an occasional glass of alcohol (limited to one ounce of hard liquor or three ounces of wine) may be consumed. It is not really known when or how much alcohol is dangerous to the unborn baby. It is important to limit your use of alcohol, especially during the early and mid-part of pregnancy-the time in which the baby's brain cells, arms and legs are being formed.

Analgesics

Pain medication is a very troublesome addiction that can carry over if you are already addicted prior to pregnancy. Lortab and Percocet are the most commonly abused. Babies undergo *withdrawal* with marked physical and psychological symptoms after they are born. Many pediatricians will not accept and decline medical responsibility for such babies and they must be transferred to special units at major Medical Centers.

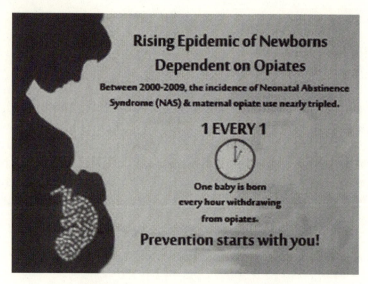

Figure 17-1 Newborn Drug Addiction

Marijuana: controversial with regard to pregnancy. In general, not recommended

Cocaine: habit-forming and not recommended whatsoever during pregnancy. Babies routinely withdraw in the nursery.

Methamphetamines: habit-forming and associated with placental abruption. It may cause preterm labor and fetal damage. Babies will go through withdrawal in the Nursery.

Tobacco: not recommended. It is associated with constricted blood flow to baby and thus, causing low birth weight babies

Xanax and other benzodiazopines: not recommended but can be used for a limited time as needed to treat severe anxiety

Caffeine Use

Caffeine is a stimulant and considered to be a drug. Caffeine increases heart rate and kidney blood flow and output, thus putting additional stress on these vital organs. Research shows that problems with pregnancy occur at a high level of caffeine intake (12 to 14 cups of coffee per day).

It is, therefore, recommended to use caffeinated products in moderation during your pregnancy. Consumption should be limited to three or less servings spread out through the day. The following Table is a list of some commonly consumed foods and beverages and their caffeine levels:

Product	Caffeine Levels (in milligrams)
Coffee - 5 oz. cup	
Drip	146
Percolated coffee	110
Instant, regular	53
Decaffeinated	2
Energy Drinks	
5 hour Energy	200 mg (equal to cup of coffee (Extra Strength = 12 oz of premium
Monster Beverage	86 mg
Tea - 5 oz. cup	
One minute brew	9 to 33
Three minute brew	20 to 46
Five minute brew	20 to 50
Canned ice tea	22 to 36
Cocoa and Chocolate	
Cocoa beverages (water mix, 6 oz.)	10
Milk chocolate (1 oz.)	6
Baking chocolate (1 oz.)	35
Carbonated Beverages/ Soda Pop (17 oz.)	
TAB	44
Sunkist	42
Dr. Pepper	38
Pepsi	37

Diet Pepsi	34
Coca Cola	34
7-Up	0
Sprite	0
Diet Sunkist	0
Fanta Orange	0

For further information the reader should consult the following resources:

Drugs during Pregnancy and Lactation by Briggs, Freeman and Yaffe

Drugs during Pregnancy and Lactation: Handbook by Schaefer, Peters and Miller

www.SafeFetus.com, www.cdc.gov/pregnancy/meds/ or www.drugs.com/pregnancy/

CHAPTER 19

Pre-existing Medical Conditions and Infectious Diseases during Pregnancy

1. Pregnancy and Diabetes

Although most people think that diabetes affects older people, there is a special kind of diabetes that occurs in pregnancy: gestational diabetes, or pregnancy-related diabetes. Diabetes is a medical condition in which the pancreas does not produce enough insulin hormones. This insulin hormone is responsible for keeping the blood "sugar" or glucose in the normal range. During pregnancy, other hormones of pregnancy (cortisone, growth hormones) interfere with insulin's ability to work. More insulin is required because you are carrying another "person," as well as increased weight on your own person. Increased insulin requirements, combined with interference in its action by other hormones, produce a relative insulin deficiency. Pregnancy diabetes results in elevated glucose levels in the maternal bloodstream. Higher glucose levels in the mother's blood diffuse readily into the baby's circulation via the placenta. The increased levels of glucose in the baby's blood (*hyperglycemia*) then stimulate the baby's pancreas to respond to by increased release of insulin. When the baby is delivered it is severed from the high level of glucose coming over from the mother's circulation via the placenta. However, the baby's pancreas continue to release large amounts of insulin after it is born (the pancreas is unaware that the baby is born and separated from the high circulating levels of glucose from the mother). Consequently, high insulin levels from the baby's pancreas produce "hypoglycemia" in the newborn. Babies must be placed on IV glucose in order to prevent the consequences of hypoglycemia in their baby. Increased amounts of glucose to the baby thus cause several adverse effects on the baby:

1. Increased birth weight of the baby.
2. Increased insulin levels produced from the baby's pancreas in the baby to "hammer down" the high level of glucose coming in from the mother's blood.

Large babies necessarily make for more difficult labors and deliveries: larger babies overwork the uterine muscles as well as require more "room" and "help" in order to be delivered.

Problems associated with "Large Babies:"

Pitocin (oxytocin) augmentation of labor
Internal uterine and electronic fetal monitoring
Larger episiotomies
Increased risk of "tears"

Difficulty in delivery of the baby's shoulders with injury to the baby's brachial plexus nerves or collar bone fracture

Increased use of forceps and Cesarean Section deliveries

Problems with control of baby's blood glucose and calcium in the nursery after birth

Stillbirths

Postpartum hemorrhage

Because of these problems associated with large babies (as a result of pregnancy diabetes), it becomes important to diagnose diabetes in pregnancy as soon as possible. Diagnosis is made by testing all women during pregnancy and testing earlier in pregnancy in those women who are at higher risk for pregnancy (or gestational) diabetes. Gestational diabetes does not mean that the patient will have diabetes forever. Over 98% of women with Class A Gestational Diabetes during pregnancy become *euglycemic* after childbirth and the glucose intolerance is alleviated: theyhave no more diabetes after the baby is delivered. However, gestational diabetes may recur in subsequent pregnancies and there is a 25% risk that the patient may go on and develop adult-onset diabetes later in life.

High-Risk Conditions Predisposing to Gestational Diabetes:

Overweight

Previous stillbirths, repeated abortions, or children with severe birth defects

Age 30 years or more

Previous delivery of a baby weighing more than 9 lbs. (4000 grams)

If any risk factors are present, you should be tested for gestational diabetes in the first trimester of pregnancy; and, if negative, re-tested in each subsequent trimester of pregnancy. Most obstetricians "screen" for gestational diabetes by a one hour glucose tolerance test in the second trimester of pregnancy (approximately 20-to-28 weeks). The test does not require any change in your eating pattern. You will be given a special 50 gm glucose bottle at the laboratory and asked to drink the bottle of glucose in the morning after an overnight fast. You will report to the laboratory within 45 minutes, so that blood may be drawn exactly one hour after drinking the glucose load. If your blood glucose is over 130-140 mg, then you'll be further tested by a standard three hour glucose tolerance test. The one hour test roughly *screens* for pregnancy diabetes, but it is the three hour test that makes the diagnosis of gestational diabetes conclusive. A high carbohydrate diet is prescribed for three days prior to the three hour test, followed by overnight fasting. The patient should report to the laboratory in the morning where a "fasting" blood glucose level will be drawn. A 100 gm glucose load (bottle of sweetened orange juice or cola) is then consumed and plasma glucose levels are tested at one-half hour, one hour, two hours and three hours afterwards.

Normal Values for Three Hour Glucose Tolerance Test (3 hour GTT)

Fasting	105-110
1/2	
1 hour	195
2 hour	165
3 hour	130-145

If any two values are abnormal, then gestational diabetes exists. If fasting glucose levels are very high, the testing is stopped immediately to prevent placing the patient into acute diabetes.

Treatment of Gestational Diabetes.

Gestational diabetes may be treated through diet, medication and/or insulin injections or possibly both. Mild "intolerances" usually can be managed by changes in diet and calories consumed. Large deviations occurring initially, or after diet therapy, require treatment. Patients with gestational diabetes require special "high risk" monitoring.

Author's Note: The increasing "obesity epidemic" in the US is the main cause of pregnancy-related diabetes. If you are "obese," i.e. greater than 25% over your ideal body weight by age and height, you will be screened for diabetes early in your pregnancy. On a given day the author saw 6 Diabetic pregnant patients in one day. Despite the advice of their doctors and nurses many Gestational Diabetic patients do not take their condition seriously. Heart malformations, newborn hypoglycemia, macrosomia, higher C-section rates with wound infections, stillbirth, etc. are just some of the complications diabetic pregnancies can experience.

2. The Rh Negative Factor

Approximately 87% of the world's population is Rh positive. That is, their red blood cells possess a factor (or antigen) that 13% of people do not carry. People whose red blood cells do not carry any Rh factor are called Rh-negative. Should an Rh-positive red blood cell enter the bloodstream of an Rh negative person, the Rh negative person's immune system will readily react to this "foreign intruder." The immune system acts much like a police department going after "intruders" (such as bacteria, viruses and Rh factors) that are different and do not belong in the patient's pregnant body. The immune mechanism goes after these "impurities in the system," hauls them in for questioning, analyzes their differences and, finally, takes them "out of circulation." Furthermore, after analysis is completed, the immune system develops specific weapons (or antibodies) to fight any similar aliens in the future (in this case future pregnancies and the baby).

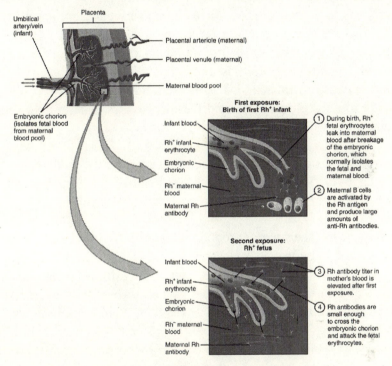

Figure 19-1 RH factor Illustration

	This is a file from the Wikimedia Commons..
Description	Illustration from Anatomy & Physiology, Connexions Web site. http://cnx.org/content/col11496/1.6/, Jun 19, 2013.
Source	Anatomy & Physiology, Connexions Web site. http://cnx.org/content/col11496/1.6/, Jun 19, 2013.
Author	OpenStax College

An Analogy as an Explanation for the RH Problem.

Assume you are a "RH Negative" Policeman. Your job is to hunt down "RH positive "criminals. You constantly search the entire circulation of the mother for them. When you see one, you can shoot and kill it with a RH Positive" antibody." If an RH Positive criminal gets by you, it will break and enter into the "Immune System Bank (the liver, spleen and bone marrow areas). When the Rh Positive criminal gets into these areas, the Immune Bank starts producing "antibodies" or weapons to defend itself: it forms RH positive antibodies. When the Immune Bank produces a large amount of these RH positive antibodies, they can slip or diffuse into the baby's circulatory system. These RH positive antibodies can "slip in" to the baby's system mainly because of their small size. Mother's and baby's red blood cells are too big to infiltrate or diffuse across the barriers between the circulatory systems.

"Sensitization" or "iso-immunization" occurs after the mother's body (RH negative) first encounter with the Positive Rh factor: usually after the first pregnancy at the time of placental separation.

It is only during the *second* pregnancy that the "Rh Problem" arises. If the second baby is also RH Positive, then RH positive antibodies developed from the first pregnancy will be again be generated, be released into the mother's bloodstream and cross over the mother-baby barrier. When these antibodies enter the baby's circulation they will start "attacking" and killing the baby's Rh positive red blood cells. The baby's red blood cells "die" and the baby becomes progressively "anemic" (anemia is defined as a low red blood cell count—red blood cells transport oxygen to the baby's growing tissues).

There are specific occurrences when the two circulations can be intermixed: the barriers broken between the two:

1. Blunt trauma (auto accidents, falls, etc.)
2. Separation of the placentas after birth of the baby or during pregnancy
3. Medical or Surgical procedures: amniocentesis, cordocentesis, fetal surgery, etc.

The RH Neg Police is always looking out for Rh-Pos "Intruders" in the maternal blood circulation.

Rh negative police will pursue and capture Rh-Pos "intruders" and bring them to "jail," i.e. into the hepato-splenic system where they will be destroyed (eliminated).

"The pregnant patient's circulatory system is completely separate and apart from that of the baby's (sees illustration). No intermixing occurs. Mother's blood flow to the uterus circulates to the placenta: maternal blood and fetal blood are in two different circulations that run past each other with a small membrane in between. Maternal blood circulates on one side of this maternal-fetal membrane and the baby's blood flows past the other side of the placenta. Accordingly, oxygen, proteins and glucose must diffuse or be actively transported across the membrane barrier that separate the two circulations.

Author's Note: Small molecules, not cells, can be transported back and forth between the mother's and the baby's circulatory systems. Because fetal hemoglobin is a small molecule, it can pass into the mother's blood. The fact that "fetal" hemoglobin enters the mother's circulation has become the basis upon which laboratories can extract these small molecules and analyze the chromosomes for genetic testing (NIPS, or non-invasive prenatal screening).

The Rh problem would not exist unless a "break" in the separating "barrier" membrane occurs. Frequently, such a major break occurs after delivery when the placenta detaches itself from the mother's uterine wall. It is at this time that fetal Rh positive enters the circulation of an Rh-negative woman. The Rh-negative woman's immune system reacts to the Rh-positive cells and develops antibodies against them. These antibodies, being very small, can easily cross intact circulatory barrier membranes. Consequently, in future pregnancy, should an Rh-negative woman again carry another Rh-positive baby, these antibodies will cross over to the baby's circulation and destroys the baby's red blood cells. The baby becomes progressively more anemic, as more and more of the red blood cells are eliminated. As anemia becomes more severe, the baby's heart has to pump faster in order to keep the limited number of red blood cells moving to deliver oxygen to the baby's organs. Eventually, the heart fails and the baby can die (stillborn). In the past, many stillbirths occurred prior to the 3rd trimester at a time when the baby is not sufficiently developed to survive outside the uterus. With early antibody screening tests and the almost universal use of RhoGAM, these babies can be saved. Intrauterine transfusions of blood can be life-saving and is available to those mothers previously sensitized.

Other circumstances present during pregnancy that can result in "breaks" between the two circulations. However, 98.5% of the time, the major break occurs during a diagnostic procedure, trauma or labor. However, it can occur during the following situations:

amniocentesis (a diagnostic procedure when a needle is passed through the uterine wall into the amniotic sac

external cephalic version (when a breech baby is turned to a head-down position by manipulation of the baby through the mother's abdominal wall) or

severe blunt trauma to the pregnant uterus (motor vehicle accident, falling down stairs, etc.)

In the late 1960's a major advance in the Rh problem was developed. By giving Rh-negative mothers an injection of antibodies that would destroy any entering Rh-positive cells before her immune system could react to them. The positive Rh red blood cells would be, basically, removed from her circulation as if they never had entered it in the first place. The antibodies against Rh-positive cell (Rho D "gamma globulin" or RhoGam©) are the same or similar antibodies that the mother herself would have produced if the immune mechanism had been called into action. Originally, these antibodies were obtained from the blood of Rh-negative mothers who had become "sensitized" (or self-immunized) to the Rh-positive red blood cells of their baby at the time of childbirth. Now, with advances in genetic engineering, these Rho D antibodies can be synthetically produced in the laboratory.

Until December of 1984, Rho D gamma globulin (RhoGam©) was given to un-sensitized Rh-negative women in the postpartum period. Studies showed that the injection could be given up until 72 hours after delivery (or miscarriage) and still be effective in eliminating any Rh-positive cells in the mother's body. 98.5% of the Rh problem was thus solved. But 1.5% of patients were experiencing "breaks" prior to delivery. In December of 1984, the American College of Obstetricians and Gynecologists (ACOG) began recommending the injection of Rho D gamma globulin before delivery (at the beginning of the third trimester). Therefore, if any breaks occur during late pregnancy, the mother, and future pregnancies, shall be finally protected from the Rh disease.

As far as the injection of Rho D gamma globulin itself, there have been few ill effects in the mother or in the baby. It is true that these Rho D antibodies may cross in small amounts into the baby's circulation and destroy a few of the baby's Rh-positive cells. It cannot destroy any Rh-negative cells, (should the baby be also Rh negative like the mother). Hepatitis and AIDS transmission were potential problems in the past; but with new manufacturing techniques (genetic engineering), the risk of these problems has been eliminated. To date, except for some minor muscle problems, no serious short or long-term effects have been reported with the use of Rho D gamma globulin in pregnancy (antenatal use or postpartum).

Obstetricians are offering antenatal and postnatal Rho D gamma globulin to their *Rh-negative* patients in order to eliminate, once and for all, the Rh problem. Accordingly, Rh-negative women may receive the injection if:

1. their husbands are Rh positive and, therefore, they are at risk of delivering an Rh-positive infant;
2. future pregnancies are anticipated;
3. Any procedures performed during pregnancy may result in the cross circulation of baby's blood into the mother's bloodstream; and

No previous exposure or sensitization to the Rh-positive factor has occurred in the pregnant mother.

Blood is routinely drawn from all Rh-negative women during the first, second and third trimesters of pregnancy to screen for the presence of Rho D antibodies that may have developed. If no such antibodies are found, then Rho D gamma globulin can be given. If the baby, too, is found to be Rh negative after delivery, then Rho D gamma globulin is not given post-delivery.

"The Sex of the baby has nothing to do with the Rh problem"

Rho D gamma globulin injections during pregnancy (28 weeks) and postpartum have virtually eliminated the disease.

No serious ill-effects from injection have ever been reported in mothers or their babies.

Rh disease only affects the second, and subsequent pregnancies (if not given Rho D gamma globulin); not the present pregnancy.

Lastly, in a similar situation to the Rh problem, the pregnant patient can develop antibodies to any foreign blood factor that is not present in her system. Again, a break in the circulation must occur and, if the baby's red blood cells carry a foreign antigen not present in the mother's system, she will develop antibodies against it. The sensitization affects the next, not the present, pregnancy and child. There are a multitude of other antigens (Kell, Kidd, etc.) carried on red blood cells that can result in anemia of the unborn baby. Unfortunately, gamma globulins to prevent their occurrence have not yet been developed. Accordingly, these babies may need to be transfused while still in the uterus (intrauterine transfusions) or delivered prematurely to prevent their untimely death.

Use of RhoGam while Pregnant

RhoGam, also known as Rho (D) immune globulin, has been used in this country since the early 1970s to prevent development of Rh antibodies in Rh-negative women. An antibody is a substance in the blood. Rhogam is effective only if given before the mother develops these antibodies. In most Rh-negative mothers, they do not develop until more than 72 hours after delivery. Rhogam is given routinely after abortions (or miscarriages) in Rh-negative women and, also, after an Rh-negative woman delivers an Rh-positive infant.

Rarely, an Rh-negative mother will develop antibodies to the Rh factor before delivery of the baby. If these antibodies form, they usually form during the third trimester of the pregnancy. It has been estimated that as many as 2% of Rh-negative mothers, carrying an Rh-positive baby, may become sensitized during their pregnancy. It would be too late to help these mothers by using RhoGam after the delivery.

There are also other procedures and medical events that could result in a transmission of the infant's blood into the mother's bloodstream, thereby sensitizing the mother. Such predisposing events are amniocentesis and antepartum hemorrhage (whether from placenta previa or placental abruption); or any manipulation of the uterus (such as an external version of a breech) Recent results of clinical trials in Canada, Australia and other countries have shown that prophylactic administration of Rhogam, during the antepartum period at 28 weeks of pregnancy, can further reduce the incidence of Rh sensitization in Rh-negative women. Now, many experts, including the American College of Obstetricians and Gynecologists (ACOG), encourage the use of Rhogam for all Rh-negative women at 28 weeks of pregnancy. However, this is only necessary in Rh-negative women who are at risk for delivering an Rh-positive infant. No ill effects have been noted among infants delivered of mothers receiving Rhogam antenatally. Many experts say that, since no risks to the fetus have been demonstrated and there may be benefit for up to 2% of future pregnancies, RhoGam should be given.

3. Herpes and Pregnancy

Synopsis:

Herpes Virus Family

HSV-1	Herpes Virus Simplex 1	Oral Herpes (mouth, lips, fingers—"whitlow")

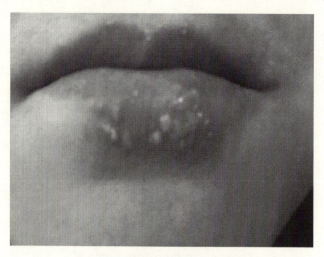

Figure 19-2 Herpes Type 1 Oral

HSV-2	Herpes Virus Simplex 2	Genital herpes or Herpes Progenitalis (Vulva, vagina, cervix, peri-rectal area)

Herpes Varicella: Chickenpox

Herpes Zoster: Shingles, i.e., Chickenpox varicella virus manifesting later in life along peripheral nerve routes and blisters and pain

Primary HSV Infection 1st infection and attack with HSV, can enter bloodstream, can become "systemic" and infect placenta, may require amniocentesis during pregnancy

Secondary HSV infection 2nd or other recurrent attacks of HSV, requires direct local contact of "open sore" to be contagious, minimal potential to become blood born or systemic

Management of HSV Infections

Secondary HSV infection: Pregnant mother with prior medical history of HSV is prescribed Acyclovir during last 4 weeks of pregnancy along with surveillance for active HSV infection with culture at 36 weeks gestation

Primary or HSV First Attack during pregnancy: Acyclovir treatment with determination if baby has been affected

Genital herpes (Herpes Simplex Virus-HSV-2) is a viral infection that has gained significant public notoriety since the 1970's. The incidence of genital HSV infection has significantly increased since the "Sexual Revolution" of the 1960's. With sexual barriers and stigmas of pre-marital sex left behind, along with the advent of "the pill," women were now liberated and free to experiment with relationships as much as men had in the past. Much media attention (television, magazine and newspaper articles) brought this uncommon infection to the "spotlight" and branded it more of a social stigma than any other infectious diseases. Because the infection can relapse at any time, it was difficult for anyone to hide the fact that they had contracted this infection. People were quick to condemn a person's "morals" based on their past sex life regardless of how they may have contracted the disease. Fears of spreading the infection to a loved one, perhaps their future husband)together with recurrent episodes of genital pain and sores (precluding sexual activity) only heightened the emotional upheaval associated with this recurrent infectious disease.

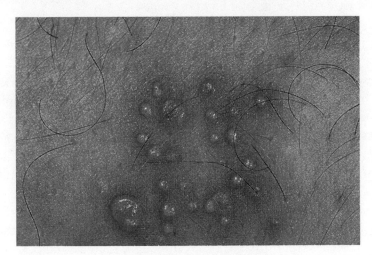

Figure 19-3 Herpes Blisters

"Herpes" usually refers to *herpes progenitalis* or HSV-2), a type of herpes virus that attacks the genital areas of the body (the vagina, vulva, cervix, penis and anus). As shown above HSV-2 is just one of the viruses of the herpes family that also includes chickenpox and herpes zoster (shingles). *Herpes simplex* or "cold sores" (HSV-1) attacks the lips, eyes and mouth. However, HSV-1 and HSV-2 can, on occasion, cross over and attack the opposite anatomic areas, i.e. HSV-2 can be transmitted to the mouth. When HSV-1 sores are present about the lips and mouth, the vulva and penis can be infected during oral- genital sexual activity. Primary herpes infection refers to the fact that one is experiencing the disease for the first time. Secondary herpes, or recurrent herpes, means that one is experiencing another outbreak of the disease in the same area of the body that the virus had attacked before. However, recurrent HSV sores do not always appear on the very same spot of previous infectious: just the generalized area of previous infection.

Primary HSV is uncommon during pregnancy because most men will notify the expectant mom if he is developing any HSV symptoms or sores. Further, couples are most likely to be faithful to each other while they are going through the pregnancy together.

Author Note: The reader is referred to the Tales portion at the end of the book regarding *My Red head Patient from Santa Maria* for a clinical case of HSV during late pregnancy.

Marital conflicts, military service, or excessive travel away from the home, predispose marital partners to stray and become exposed to herpes. Within two to ten days after exposure, the infection manifests itself by preliminary burning in the areas where the skin eruption is destined to appear. Within a day or two, the skin eruption appears and groups of tiny water blisters (the size of pinheads) form on the skin areas; usually on the vulva and vagina as well as the penis. These blisters may enlarge, break open or coalesce to form large ulcerated areas of skin. Consequently, urination over these eroded areas of skin becomes very painful. At times, patients must urinate in a tub of water or in the shower to dilute the acidic urine from flowing over these painful sores. With primary herpes infection, the virus enters, takes over, and destroys the skin cells of the vulva and vagina. Spreading deeper into the skin, it infects nerve tissues and causes the severe pain characteristic of the disease. Eventually the virus gains access to the bloodstream and travels throughout the body (generalized infections). Generalized myalgias and bone aching, headache, low-grade fever and malaise can ensue. It is while the virus is traveling in the bloodstream that the virus can spread to the placenta and, uncommonly, through the placenta to the developing fetus.

In Primary HSV infection the immune system of the mother takes time to learn how to fight this virus and, shortly, develops antibodies against the virus. Meanwhile, glands (lymph nodes) in the groin enlarge in order to prevent further spread of the virus to the pelvic area. Such glands are noticeably swollen and painful. Once the immune system develops the proper antibodies against the virus, these antibodies forever circulate in the blood to kill any virus from gaining access to the bloodstream again. Hence, primary herpes infection can invade the bloodstream, while recurrent attacks are prevented from becoming "systemic" by the circulating immune antibodies. The body's immune system may, or may not, kill the entire herpes virus during primary infection. The virus, however, may be held in check by special defense cells (lymphocytes) and antibodies. Although no further replication of the viral particles occurs in the body, the virus still may lie dormant in the skin near, or within, nerve tissues.

When a person's generalized resistance is lowered by severe stress, fatigue or disease, the immune mechanism may fail; such that the virus may no longer held in check. The virus starts reproducing itself and thousands of viral particles begin to form in those cells, leading to an outbreak of herpes again. Thus, recurrent herpes arises from dormant virus in the body cells and not from recurrent exposure of a contact from another person. Recurrent herpes is a local relapse of viral infection that had already infected and is still present in an area of the body. The virus does not enter the bloodstream (systemic infection) because of body defenses and experienced immune mechanisms or *immunity*. Prior immunity and exposure to the HSV virus prevents dissemination of the infection throughout the body (*systemic infection*). Accordingly, the placenta and fetus should be protected in these *recurrent* or secondary infections. There are two main pathways that your baby can be exposed to the virus as follows:

<u>Primary</u> Systemic infections with HSV: virus may enter the bloodstream (*viremia*) with the potential to travel to both the placenta, amniotic sac and possibly to the baby

<u>Secondary</u> or Recurrent Infections of the genital tract, i.e. when infectious sores or *lesions* are locally present on the vulvar areas and in the vagina during labor.

Two other points:

1. 5% of pregnant women carry the HSV-2 virus whether they know it or not. HSV-2 infections can be "silent" or non-clinical. Not all women will have significant or noticeable symptoms after they have been infected. If unsure, a woman can be tested for past infection of the virus.
2. If there are active HSV sores in the genital tract and the amniotic sac inadvertently ruptures, the baby should be delivered by C-section as soon as possible. There is a 4 hour window of time in which the baby has less risk of possible infection.

The treatment of recurrent herpes during pregnancy is directed toward the following goals:

1. Definitive diagnosis of herpetic infection by culture, DNA swab (or smear) in the doctor's office (or clinic).
2. Symptom relief by the use of anesthetic creams and sprays.
3. Prevention of secondary infection of the herpes sores by other bacteria by careful hygienic measures and cleanliness.
4. Prevention of the spread of the virus to other parts of the body and to other persons close to the patient.
5. Most importantly, the spread of the virus to the baby during birth.

It is the responsibility of the physician to question (and the patient to disclose) whether she or her husband has had herpes in the past. If only the husband has had a history of herpes, then both he and she must be instructed on hygienic techniques to avoid exposure and spread of the virus to his wife during pregnancy. Complete sexual abstinence during recurrent infection in the male is the rule. Furthermore, it may be even wiser that the husband wears a condom during any sexual activity throughout the pregnancy. If only the wife has herpes, then it is, likewise, important that she not expose her husband to the disease by precluding sexual intercourse until the sores have healed. If the patient (or physician) is uncertain whether or not she or her husband has had herpes in the past or has an active sore at the present time, the diagnosis of HSV infection can be made in the physician's office:

By culturing or DNA swabbing the visible sore itself
By antibody testing specifically for the HSV-2 virus

The main goal to the management of herpes during pregnancy is to be sure that herpes is not present during labor. It is generally an accepted fact that healed herpetical sores are not infectious. The herpes virus is no longer replicating and shedding viral particles in the genital tract if two-to-three weeks have passed since an attack. Accordingly, if no recurrent episodes of herpes occur in the last three weeks of pregnancy, then a vaginal birth may be anticipated.

However, each and every week in the last month of pregnancy, a careful examination of the vulva, vagina, cervix and anal areas of the body should be made by the physician. A swab of these same areas is taken and transported to the laboratory in a special culture medium or by DNA testing. A positive culture, a positive DNA test or recurrent visible sores would preclude a vaginal delivery.

It is evident by now that a Cesarean section is the safest mode of delivery if herpes is present in the genital tract during labor. Only in this way can the baby be delivered without coming into direct contact with the herpes virus. Furthermore, should the amniotic sac leak any water during the last weeks of pregnancy (regardless of any labor contractions) *in the presence of active sores or lesions,* it is best that the baby be delivered by Cesarean section within 4-6 hours after membrane rupture. After six hours, the virus has had the opportunity to spread through the opening in the cervix, up to the amniotic sac to infect the baby. After six hours, the baby has, presumptively, been exposed to HSV and a Cesarean section could be less effective in avoiding infection the baby.

During primary infection, it is theoretically possible that the virus can spread to the placenta and to the baby by the bloodstream, (as mentioned in the paragraphs above). Should primary infection occur during the first 20 weeks of pregnancy, amniocentesis could be performed to ascertain if the amniotic sac has been contaminated by the virus. Should the amniotic sac culture grow out the virus (or positive on DNA testing), then it must be assumed that the baby has been similarly affected. Accordingly, the physician would treat immediately the pregnant patient with acyclovir to treat the infection in the mother and also the baby. If the baby is known to be infected, the couple may be given the option of terminating the pregnancy (most babies would be severely affected or even succumb to the infection). Should amniotic cultures be positive for herpes, then there is little to be gained by Cesarean section delivery in these cases - the baby has been exposed and is likely to be infected. As noted above, a severely affected fetus might not survive the pregnancy or the neonatal period.

The treatment of herpes infection in pregnancy is geared to the diagnosis of the condition and the prevention of spread to the fetus. In Table below, the treatment of primary as well as recurrent herpes is summarized.

Treatment of Herpes in Pregnancy

Prevention: Acyclovir 400 mg orally 2 to 3 per day after 36 weeks of pregnancy
Adjunctive Prevention:
   Keep immune defenses up:
        sufficient rest
        minimize stress
        well balanced diet
        adequate working conditions
        regular bathing/showering
        avoidance of colds, flus
        prenatal vitamins

Symptomatic Pain if herpes recurs during pregnancy:

Use anesthetic or hemorrhoid-type preparations and creams on the painful sores as needed three to four times per day:
- Americaine®
- Nupercaine®
- Solarcaine®
- Dermoplast®

Hygiene and Prevention of Secondary Infection (spreading HSV to eyes, mouth, and rectum:

Avoid secondary bacterial infection of herpes sores by keeping areas clean with soap and water and dry by a sun lamp or blow dryer. Do not share towels, wash cloths, bedding sheets, soap toothbrushes, combs.

Avoid spreading the virus by touching other parts of your body after handling the infected area.

No kissing on any parts of the body if oral herpes ("cold sores") is present in either the male or female.

Do not have sexual intercourse if genital herpes is present until the sores have completely disappeared.

Keeping the areas clean, and applying anesthetic creams, are the main goals in treatment.

Unfortunately, there is no antibiotic that has been FDA-approved for the treatment of herpes during pregnancy. Antibiotics, such as Penicillin, kill bacteria. Since herpes is a virus, only antiviral medications will kill the virus. Acyclovir (or Zovirax®, Famvir® or Valtrex® brands) is a time-tested anti-herpes medication that has shown effectiveness in treating herpes infections in a non-pregnant state. It has been shown to shorten the duration of the disease and, indirectly, decrease swelling, pain and severity of the disease. Furthermore, the time of viral shedding is decreased. At this time, acyclovir has not been approved for routine HSV prophylaxis use during pregnancy. However, there are a multitude of studies in the medical literature that proved that acyclovir prophylaxis is effective is preventing recurrent infection in the pregnant mother while simultaneously reducing viral shedding and exposure to the unborn baby. The drug is considered very safe during pregnancy as acyclovir does not become incorporated into Human DNA: It only gets incorporated into HSV DNA and thereby kills the virus from replicating.

It must be remembered that exposure of the fetus to the herpes virus does not necessarily lead to the development of severe infection in the fetus. Contact does not equate with necessary disease and infection. In fact, vaginal delivery at term in the presence of herpes virus, may only affect 20% of such babies. As mentioned, it is estimated that 5% of pregnant women in the United States are shedding the virus at any given time. Accordingly, it is felt by most authorities on herpes that many babies are being exposed to herpes unbeknownst to the mother (who may have never known that she had the disease in the first place!).Thus HSV infection can be silent and the appearance of sores is not always recognized or appreciated as being HSV by the patient herself.

Full term healthy babies inadvertently exposed to herpes during labor, i.e., mother that never knew that had been exposed, have only a 5-10% risk of contracting the disease.

It is important for the patient to understand that "any" risk of exposing your baby to herpes is too much of a risk. HSV infection is highly contagious. 40% of fetuses developing HSV infection in the newborn period can succumb to the disease. At least 40% of the fetuses that survive are severely affected by brain damage, mental retardation, and other severe physical and mental handicaps. At the minimum 10 to 20% will not suffer permanent damage. HSV virus, as mentioned above, has a special predilection to attack the nerve tissue.

The brain and the spinal cord are targeted areas of the baby's body for the virus to attack. It is because of the significant 20% risk of infection of the fetus at the time of birth (HSV is highly contagious) as well as the severe complications and damage (even death to the baby), that herpes must be carefully managed during pregnancy.

Diagnosis of Herpes Infections

Symptoms: pain, burning, itching and numbness in the targeted areas of the body (mouth, genitals, anus, penis), fever, malaise, generalized aching, fatigue, headache.

Signs: groups of small blisters surrounded by red borders that eventually rupture to form small or large skin ulcers. Glands (lymph nodes) may swell and enlarge in the groin or neck causing discomfort in those areas.

Laboratory tests: Immunological assay tests for herpes DNA are now currently the standard. In the past physicians had to rely on actual "HSV viral culture of newly erupted HSV blisters. Culture methods still remain as an adjunctive definitive test confirming the presence of herpes virus. Culture results usually take 3 to 7 days.

For an immediate diagnosis when it is not clear there is an HSV sore a "Pap smear" (i.e. Tzanck smear) might be taken of the blister for microscopic evaluation: the preparation would show characteristic cell changes of HSV or other viruses.

Mode of Delivery with Herpes in Pregnancy

Vaginal birth criteria:
Physical Examinations negative for herpes.
No symptoms of herpes during the previous month.
Genital tract cultures are reported "negative" for herpes
Patient has been taking Acyclovir 400 mg during the last month or weeks of pregnancy

Amniotic sac membranes are not ruptured
In cases of primary infection during pregnancy, amniotic fluid cultures are negative for herpes virus.

<u>C-section birth:</u>
Physical Examination is positive for herpes infection.
Cultures previously done in the last 2 weeks of pregnancy are positive for herpes.
In primary HSV infections amniocentesis shows that amniotic fluid and/or vulvar cultures/preps are positive for herpes.
Amniotic sac has been ruptured for less than six to eight hours without objective documentation
Symptoms are definitely present during labor

Author Note: Just to make things even more interesting, there was a patient in labor with an active HSV sore on her pubic area: directly in between the vaginal area and the abdominal area where a C-section incision would be made. In this case the author put the patient on IV acyclovir, treated the area with anti-septic and acyclovir ointment, and further covered the area well with bandages. The patient delivered vaginally without the baby contracting any HSV infection.

Another patient presented with recurrent HSV in the vulvar area at 39 weeks gestation. She had no prior history of any outbreaks in the past few years and forgot to tell me that she had had HSV infection in the past. I treated her with acyclovir and hoped she would not go into labor in the ensuing week. A search of the medical literature showed that viral reproduction would cease immediately. Any previous virus that was present would be absent (i.e., would not be found on a swab) in 2-3 days after commencement of acyclovir treatment. She delivered vaginally one week later: the sore was absent and she had no symptoms at the time of labor.

4. HIV, Hepatitis and Pregnancy

Since these diseases share many common considerations, HIV and Hepatitis are discussed together. Both HIV and

Hepatitis are caused by viruses. Pregnancy can occur in patients with these viral infections. Similarly, patients who are pregnant can be exposed to these diseases.

Pregnant health care workers, such as physicians, nurses and laboratory personnel are exposed daily to patients with these contagious viruses.

Universal precautions and protocols have been formulated and adopted by the medical community to limit their exposure to these viruses.

There are patients who are pregnant with HIV and hepatitis. Viral particle counts are the main measurements of the severity of these diseases and their capability of being contagious to others.

The compromise of liver function by hepatitis is measured by liver function testing.

Studies have shown that pregnant HIV patients can successfully prevent the spread of HIV to their unborn baby by taking antiviral (retro-viral) therapy.

Primary prevention of these viral infections is the mainstay of medical practice.

HIV disease is caused by a virus that attacks the human immune system. The virus is present and alive in all body "fluids," such as semen, saliva, tears, blood, etc. "Viral load" or the amount of viral particles in the body fluid to which one is exposed is a very important part of the equation: the risk of being contaminated with HIV virus and possibly developing AIDS (Autoimmune Immune Deficiency Syndrome) later.

Risk factors for HIV/ Hepatitis Exposure:

1. Homosexual women who engage in oral and anal intercourse with an HIV or Hepatitis infected partner.

2. Hemophiliacs who receive repeated transfusions with HIV or Hepatitis-contaminated blood or blood products.*
3. Women who are IV drug abusers who share contaminated needles and drugs with HIV/Hepatitis positive persons.
4. Babies who are born from untreated HIV/Hepatitis mothers.
5. Prostitutes who have repeated anal-oral-genital contact with HIV/Hepatitis-infected clients.

*Hospitals and blood banks have implemented procedures to eliminate this occurrence.

From this information, one can see that casual exposure to the HIV virus is unlikely to result in developing the disease. Going to school with HIV/Hepatitis patients or eating food prepared by an HIV victim, does not pose a significant health risk. A pregnant woman in a relationship with an HIV/Hepatitis male patient with sharing of body fluids can put her at increased risk of contracting the HIV/Hepatitis virus.

Nurses who take care of HIV patients on a daily basis do not have an increased risk of developing HIV/Hepatitis as long as the universal health precautions are adhered to:

1. Wearing of gloves and proper clothing when touching an H/H patient or handling their body fluids - sweat, tears, saliva, urine, etc.
2. Being careful not to puncture oneself with needles utilized by an H/H patient.
3. Proper handling and cleaning of soiled laundry, dishes and utensils of H/H patients.

To decrease the dangers of contracting H/H from blood transfusions in the heterosexual community, blood banks are screening all donated blood for these viruses. Blood donors can be tested for the HIV antibodies. Furthermore, should surgery become necessary, most blood banks have set up "designated donor" and "autologous" donation programs. Surgical patients can select their own blood donors and even bank their own blood for later use in surgery (within two weeks). Lastly, no cases of HIV have been reported from vaccines and immune globulin made from blood products.

Accordingly, the expectant mother has little to fear from these very serious diseases. With proper infection control measures, even medical, dental, nursing and other allied health professionals can feel comfortable in caring for the H/H patients. For further basic information about HIV, Hepatitis A, B, and C as well as the full blown HIV Syndrome, i.e. AIDS, you may access the CDC website or call the CDC (Center for Disease Control) for a four-minute tape presentation at 800-342-AIDS.

5. **Infectious Diseases during Pregnancy That Cause Serious Birth Defects:**

Rubella Virus: Cataracts, hearing deficits

Toxoplasmosis: Mental retardation (from raw meat, cats)

CMV Virus: Hearing loss, brain damage

Herpes Virus: Severe damage to nervous system

Parvovirus B19 ("5th Disease or "Slap Cheek Syndrome"): anemia in the fetus

6. **Medical Diseases during Pregnancy that cause serious Birth Defects:**

Diabetes: Heart, skull, cleft lip and palate, other defects

Seizure Disorders (mainly due to medications used to control convulsions) cleft lip and palate

CHAPTER 20
Obstetrical Tragedies

The author has to confess that loss of pregnancy by a patient is the worst, the really worst, part of the professional specialty. It is very, very difficult for him to have to inform a patient that she does not have a "normal pregnancy." The author has to tell patients about every other week that their pregnancy is not going to be a viable one, i.e. not going to further grow into the baby that they have hoped and wished for.

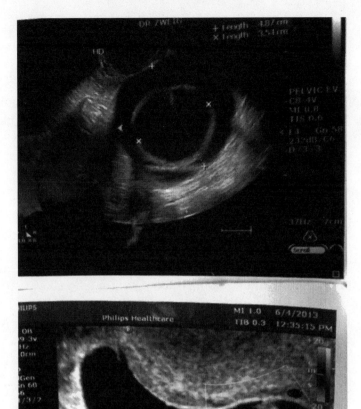

Figure 20-1 and Figure 20-2 Blighted Ovum.
Ultrasound pictures showing intrauterine pregnancies but no fetal heart beats (no color flow). Fetal poles or embryos may or may not be seen (none in upper photo but are seen as small irregular bodies (see lower photo)

The above photographs illustrate pregnancies with amniotic fluid but very small mass (fetal body without any heart beat or circulation to baby (there is no color- flow to fetal body).

Miscarriage (Spontaneous Abortion)

Unfortunately the joy of pregnancy and the expectation of baby and motherhood can be shattered by the sudden bleeding and cramping of miscarriage. Approximately 16% of all known pregnancies are lost. After the circulation to the pregnancy is lost, the uterus starts contracting to expel the pregnancy tissue. The *common* language term "abortion" means to most people the deliberate desire of a woman wanting to terminate her pregnancy. Medical terminology defines the word "abortion" to cover broadly <u>all</u> losses of pregnancy depending on (1) when they occur and (2) what caused them.

Types of Abortions (Important <u>Definitions</u>)

Spontaneous abortion: abortion occurring by itself.

Threatened abortion: bleeding and cramping in early pregnancy with uncertainty about continuation.

Inevitable abortion: bleeding, cramping associated with cervical dilation with certainty about loss

Imminent abortion: pregnancy tissue is seen in the open cervix with uterus ready to expel pregnancy

Incomplete abortion: passage of some, but not all pregnancy tissue.

Septic abortion: an infected (first or second trimester) pregnancy regardless of fetus alive or dead.

Legal or Therapeutic abortion: viable pregnancy that is terminated by patient because of:

1) Exposure to teratogenic viral infection, drugs, radiation
2) Psychiatric, medical or mental health conditions that may cause significant harm to the patient
3) Socio-economic circumstances (teenager at age 12), or
4) Rape, incest or other reason

Spontaneous abortion (or miscarriage) is the main topic of this section. Most miscarriages (95%) occur in the first 12 weeks of pregnancy and, accordingly, the first trimester is the most crucial period of time for pregnancy. Once the fetal heart beat is heard (or seen on ultrasonography), the chance of miscarriage becomes remote, i.e. less than 2% in most studies. The fetal heart is one of the most complex organ systems to form. Therefore, if the fetus has the genetic material to form a heart, it can be assumed that it has the "right stuff" (or chromosomes) to form a normal baby. Birth defects, including that of the heart, do occur despite the normal appearance and sound of a fetal heartbeat. Fortunately, such heart deformities are uncommon. However, at least 5% of all children are born with some type of birth defect or congenital anomaly that may manifest itself at the time of birth or later in life.

Examples of Congenital Anomalies:

Hydrocephalus or anencephaly
Cardiac abnormalities such as transposition or septal defect
Strawberry "mark" or hemangiomas
Extra fingers, toes, arms, legs
Pyloric stenosis (narrowed stomach outlet)
Cleft lip and/or palate
Dislocated hip
Bladder and kidney abnormalities

Spontaneous Abortions, or miscarriages, can and do occur in the second trimester of pregnancy. These losses are usually a result of the following causes:

- Severe infection affecting the normally developing fetus (Parvovirus B19, chlamydiae, Listeria monocytogenes, etc.).
- Cord accidents (knots, cord anomalies, cord tightening, etc.,
- Placental separations (perhaps due to an auto accident, methamphetamine abuse or other trauma)
- Severe other congenital birth defects that manifest later in pregnancy
- ABO, RH or other antibody iso-immunization

The first sign of miscarriage is vaginal bleeding. Initially "spotting" or a brown discharge is noticed by the pregnant woman. If a pelvic examination reveals an enlarged uterus and a mild amount of blood in the vagina, bed rest and restriction of activity is the standard treatment recommended. Either the bleeding stops or the bleeding becomes heavier. Severe uterine cramping, along with heavy bleeding usually signifies that the loss of pregnancy is inevitable or imminent.

Miscarriage is the result of the uterus trying to spontaneously pass or "contract out" an abnormal pregnancy. Approximately 16% of all confirmed pregnancies miscarry. Many more miscarriages probably occur, but are neither noticed by the patient nor documented by medical evaluation. A slightly late, or heavy menstrual period accompanied by increased breast sensitivity may, in fact, be an unsuspected, early miscarriage.

The most common cause of a miscarriage is a "blighted ovum." Genetic or chromosomal abnormalities account for the early demise of a severely defective embryo. The miscarriage (or abortion) is predetermined at the time of conception. Implantation of this conception occurs, but the pregnancy only advances to the point in which an immature placenta and small amniotic sac develop. Occasionally, a small mass of fetal tissue ("fetal pole") is seen. No heart beat can be visualized on the ultrasound screen because, usually, so much genetic information and material are absent that this complex organ, the heart, cannot be formed. The most common chromosomal defects found are single X (or deletions), triploidies (additional chromosomes), and polyploidies (extra sets of chromosomes).

Miscarriage can occur later in the first trimester despite having already seen an embryo with a heartbeat earlier. In these cases separation of the placenta, cord problems, drugs, infectious diseases and medical conditions in the pregnant mother (out of control diabetes) can be causes of these later losses.

The modern obstetrical approach to first trimester bleeding involves simple diagnostic evaluation:

> Ultrasound (exam for fetal embryo and heart beat).
> Physical examination (cervix open or closed, size and position of uterus).

Hormone levels (quantitative levels of Beta HCG that are plateauing or falling and progesterone levels).

Ultrasound reveals the presence of an embryo (or embryos!), detection of fetal heartbeat, and location of the pregnancy in the uterus. A patient with a positive pregnancy test but has no visualization of a gestational sac in the uterus on the ultrasound can point to a pregnancy in the tube; i.e., tubal ectopic pregnancy. If the fetal heart beat is seen on ultrasound with the gestational sac implanted high in the uterine cavity, then, most likely, the pregnancy is viable and risk of miscarriage is slim. If no fetal heart beat is seen, then a repeat ultrasound examination is recommended because the fetal heart does not form until at least 4 weeks from the time of conception. If examination is done too early, an early, but viable, pregnancy may be misdiagnosed as being "blighted" and incorrectly presumed to be doomed to miscarriage. Physical examination either reveals an open or closed cervix. Dilation of the cervical canal is not a poor prognostic sign; whereas, a closed cervical canal associated with minimal bleeding, points to a much more favorable prognosis. Increasing pregnancy hormone levels (Beta HCG and progesterone) are also presumptive evidence of a normally developing pregnancy. Other hormone evaluations are available but are not widely utilized: their significance may not be reliable.

Should repeat ultrasound or physical examination show that the pregnancy is "blighted" (i.e., no embryo present or no sign of a heart beat in a non-growing fetal mass), then the pregnancy is a most likely a non-viable one.

When the gestational sac measures 15 mm in all dimensions (width, height and depth) and there is no fetal heartbeat visible by color-flow, then the diagnosis of a blighted ovum or non-viable pregnancy is fairly well secured.

The patient has several options at this point:

1. Schedule a D&C to remove the "non-viable" pregnancy.
2. Wait until bleeding and cramping becomes more severe and hope that the uterus by itself will successfully pass all of the pregnancy tissue.

3. Schedule a D&C when the bleeding and cramps ensues and is severe.

If the patient has a spontaneous miscarriage the tissue at home, it is very important that she bring that tissue to the office (or hospital) for laboratory evaluation. An examination should be performed to be sure no more pregnancy tissue is left inside the uterus. Retained pregnancy can separate later with resultant delayed bleeding (sometimes severe or hemorrhage). Furthermore, such tissue is a perfect culture median for bacteria. A uterine infection (endometritis) may ensue. Accordingly, many gynecologists recommend a D&C, or uterine vacuum cleaning," to be sure all the pregnancy tissue has been removed. If, during examination, the cervix is closed and the bleeding and cramping have stopped, it can be assumed that the abortion is complete: all the tissue out. A repeat ultrasound exam may be performed at this time or during a checkup appointment to be sure all the pregnancy tissue is out.

Still, the patient should be told to watch for any signs of retained tissue:

1. Bleeding to the point where one saturates a pad per hour
2. Fever greater than 101 F
3. Severe cramping, not alleviated with Tylenol or aspirin
4. Continued irregular, heavy gushes of bleeding
5. Pelvic Pain that may signal the presence of a pregnancy in the tube (or other ectopic site)

Lastly, the patient's Rh factor should be checked. If she is Rh negative and her husband is Rh positive, a mini-dose of Rh immunoglobin (RhGgam,® i.e. MicroGgam®) should be given to her to prevent possible sensitization.

After a miscarriage, the bleeding (or "period") may last longer, one-to-three weeks but the bleeding is greatly curtailed if a D&C is performed. As long as the bleeding is gradually tapering down and stopping, there should be little concern. The next menstrual flow usually occurs within four-to-six weeks. It is advised that intercourse not be resumed until the bleeding has completely stopped: within one-to-two weeks.

Most physicians recommend that the couple wait one (or two) periods before attempting pregnancy again. Condoms, foam or suppositories may be safely utilized. Also, it has been shown that a daily prenatal vitamin tablet with additional folic acid be taken several months before conception. It has been associated with a reduction in the incidence of birth defects significantly. Lastly, the chance of miscarriage occurring again is 16%: no greater chances just because of a previous miscarriage.

In summary, a miscarriage is a "mixed blessing." It is nature's way in most cases of ridding itself of an abnormal pregnancy and an affected baby.

Ectopic Pregnancies

Pregnancies can implant in other areas of the reproductive tract other than the uterus. The most common abnormal area to implant is in the tube (>95%). An embryo can become "stuck" in any area of the tube, the ovary and the pelvis. The most common predisposing factor appears to be a previous pelvic infection due to chlamydiae. Endometriosis, previous abdominal surgery, or previous tubal ligation or sterilization are all other predisposing factors. The treatment of an ectopic pregnancy depends on its size and location: surgery or chemotherapy.

Stillborn

Any baby without a heartbeat after 24 weeks gestation is, by definition, is by definition a "fetal demise." Unfortunately, the most common cause is placental separation due to substance abuse, i.e. cocaine, methamphetamine, etc. Further causes of such losses are cord accidents and anomalies, ABO/Rh/antibody incompatibilities, infectious agents, etc.

After the diagnosis of an intrauterine fetal death is made most OB's will induce labor in order to evacuate the pregnancy as soon as possible. This horrible tragedy should be dealt with expeditiously so that the couple can grieve and move on psychologically.

CHAPTER 21

Postpartum Instructions

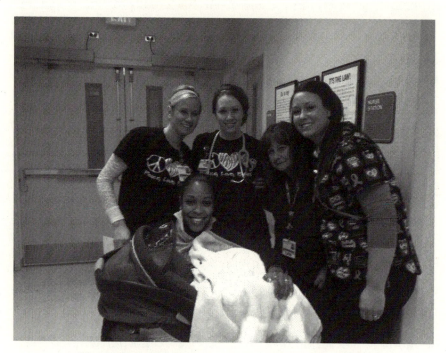

Figure 21-1 Our friendly (and beautiful) OB nurses congratulating you on your baby's birth

Congratulations on the birth of your beautiful newborn baby! If you thought your "labor" was over, now you are in for a real surprise: the work of raising your little "bundle of joy" has just begun. This chapter is a guide to some of the most common questions and problems that occur after having your baby.

How long will I stay in the hospital?

Most patients will stay in the hospital for at least 2 nights after a normal delivery and 2-3 nights after a C-section Birth. Each patient recovers differently from childbirth. If you have delivered early in the day, you may be able to go home sooner. Those patients who have undegone a postpartum tubal ligation may want to stay an extra day: even though the incision may be only 2 inches in size, it may feel more uncomfortable than you might think.

Average Length of Hospital Stays
First time mothers (Primipara): 2 to 3 days
Second baby or more (Secundagravidas and Multiparas): 2 days
C-section Mothers: 3 to 5 days

Baby Identification and Security bracelet

Your baby and you (as well as your husband or designated support person) will be banded with a security bracelet after the baby is born in the delivery room. It is extremely important that this band is stays on your wrist. Be careful that this band does not accidentally slips off while you and your baby are in the hospital. Your baby will also be banded on the wrist and leg. The baby's band is critically important for the safety of your baby: your baby's band will sound an alarm if you or anyone else carrying your baby attempts to leave the postpartum floor.

<u>Author anecdote</u>. When the author was practicing in California, he learned to appreciate the significant security aspects of the baby hand bands:

There was this story about a Chinese patient, Mrs. Wong. Apparently, the nursery nurse brought a *Caucasian* baby into her room for her to nurse. The RN checked the ID bracelets of the baby and Mrs. Wong. They matched and the nurse identified the baby as hers. Mrs. Wong looked at the baby and said to the nurse," this is not my baby!" The nurse then re-checked Mrs. Wong's security band and then the baby's security bracelet. Both bands matched again! The nurse told Mrs.

Wong that the bands were correct and that this baby was hers! Mrs. Wong replied, "No, this is not my baby." The nurse again replied that the bands matched and that this was indeed her baby. Mrs. Wong then stated, "No, this is not my baby. Two "Wong's" don't make a "White."

Before discharge from the hospital (or birth center), many questions frequently arise regarding the various aspects of postpartum care. We shall address these issues now.

Bathing and Showering

In the hospital or at home, you are permitted to take a bath or a shower. You may shampoo your hair at any time. Be careful to avoid getting soap into the vaginal area or vagina as it may burn or sting. Because of the increased, but normal, amount of bleeding after delivery, you may prefer to shower. If you had a C-section delivery, you should cover your incision during the first 24 hours in order to prevent too much moisture/water from soaking into the suture line: simply tape plastic wrap over the incision area. It is okay if the incision gets a little wet. After 24 hours the incision is sealed well and water cannot permeate it.

Bleeding, discharge and Infection after Delivery

After delivery, the lochial flow of blood is much more extensive than during a menstrual period. You will continue to bleed for at least four (4) to five (5) weeks after your delivery. Keep the area free of blood by changing your pads frequently. The hospital will supply pads and panties for you.

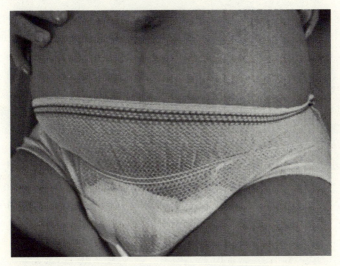

Figure 21-2 Genuine Hospital-issue "Secrets" panties

If dried blood, mucus or stool adheres to the hair or skin, rinse the areas with a squeeze bottle of dilute antiseptic soap solution (Betadine, pHisoderm, Hibiclens). Use of a baby wipes (any cleansing tissue) or soapy washcloth may also be helpful. The bleeding gradually gets less and less each day. During the first few days it is possible to pass large dark purple clots. These clots form in the uterine cavity after delivery. As the uterus contracts and becomes smaller in the first few days after delivery, these uterine contractions (*the after-pains*) squeeze these clots out from the uterine cavity and into the vagina. Typically, the bleeding becomes lighter with each day: the *lochia*, i.e., the blood after delivery becomes bright red, and then turns to a dark red, then pink and finally becomes a brown to black discharge.

Occasionally there can be excessive bleeding after delivery (**immediate** postpartum bleeding). While in the hospital your postpartum nurse will alert your physician of any abnormal bleeding. This bleeding can treated with uterine massage. Occasionally a pelvic exam is necessary at which time clots can be swept out of the cervix. Further, various medications may be utilized:

1. Pitocin in the IV fluid infusion
2. Methergine®
3. Prostaglandins such as Hemabate® and Cytotec®

Delayed postpartum bleeding usually manifests itself 2 to 4 weeks *after* delivery. It is caused by sub involution of the uterus, infection or retention of small placental fragments.

Uterine Sub involution is the postpartum diagnosis when the uterus does not completely shrink down to its normal size is caused by either a low grade infection (endometritis) of the uterine lining or retention of amniotic membranes and placenta fragments. Profuse bleeding can ensue. Initially subinvolution can be treated by antibiotics and uterine muscle stimulants (such as methergine). If bleeding continues to be heavy, a D & C may be necessary to remove infected tissue and membranes.

As stated before, the lochial flow changes in color and amount in a characteristic pattern; from a bright red to pink flow, then brown, and eventually a white discharge continues. Intermittent spotting and dark blood are not uncommon up until your six week checkup. Lastly, because of the risk of infection, it is recommended that you do not insert anything in the vagina for at least 2 weeks following delivery. Accordingly, douching, tampons and sex are not recommended during this period of time.

Warning Signs:

1. At any time the bleeding becomes heavy such that you soak through more than one pad per hour or you experience severe abdominal cramping or fever, you should immediately call the Hospital OB unit or the Hospital Switchboard and report these problems to your OB and/or the nurses..

2. Fever >101 degrees, especially with chills and shakiness

Physician Rounds and Hospital Visits after Delivery

Physicians normally make "Rounds" or hospital visits in the mornings but each physician has their own schedule. Further, other surgeries and deliveries as well as office emergencies may delay the physician from the morning schedule. Rounds at noon or even after-office hours may be the time your OB will be seeing you.

When the author makes rounds on my patients, He will check the firmness and position of the fundus. He will also check the perineum (the vaginal opening area and the rectum). The episiotomy (if one was done) will be inspected as well as a check for any hemorrhoid swelling or thrombosis. The legs will be checked for any swelling of the feet and tenderness of the calves.

The hospital will supply pads for the bleeding (lochial flow) that occur after delivery. The pads are held in place with some stretchy underwear (the hospital-issue "Secrets" but are certainly not as sexy as the "Victoria" kind).

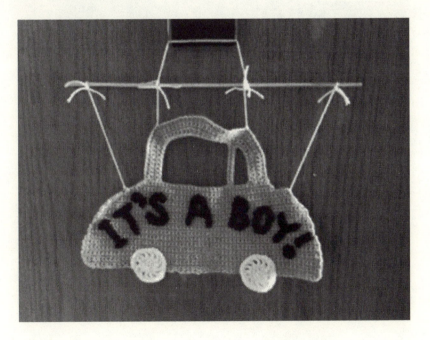

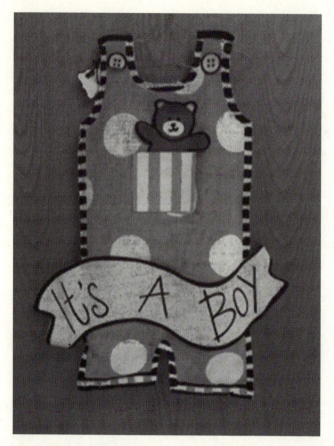

Figure 21-3 Door Signs on your hospital room. Photos of hospital door signs that patients have made or purchased for the door on their room while they are on the Postpartum Floor. (see the two door signs for a boy above and a girl below)

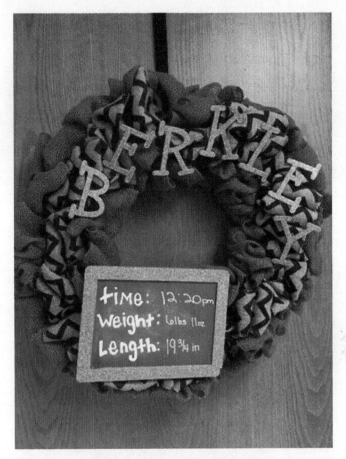

Figure 21-3 Door Art for a Girl

"New Father Sleeping Sickness"

When the author does make his usual rounds at about 9 am, he has noticed that most of the time the "new fathers" are completely asleep on the empty bed next to his patient.

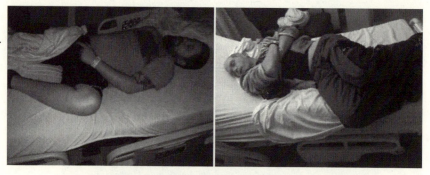

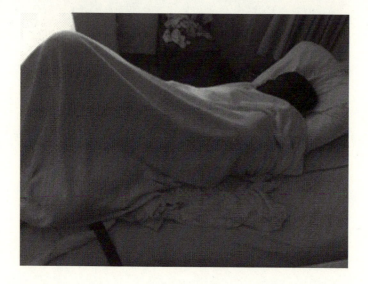

Figures 21-4a-c "New Fathers' Sleeping Sickness."

The new mom and baby are usually up, eating breakfast or watching the news on the TV. The new mom may be nursing or changing the diaper.

The author is uncertain as to the cause of this phenomenon. There have been no reports in the medical literature describing this syndrome despite its very common occurrence. The author has questioned many experienced postpartum nurses to see what they thought about this manifestation. The following explanations have been proposed:

1. The new father has a night job and just came to the hospital and "crashed."

2. The new father has been so overwhelmed emotionally, physically and mentally by the birth of his child that he has gone into an unconscious state.

3. The new father has been up all night tending to the baby: feeding his newborn, changing diapers, talking to his baby, etc. so that "mom" can sleep soundly all night without being disturbed. Now it is the new father's turn can go to sleep.

4. The new father has been up all night playing video games either at the hospital or at home.

5. The new father celebrated the birth of the baby by spending time at the bar that just closed at 2 am.

6. The new father does not have a job, sleeps all day and all night and, as Arlene Purvis, RN says, "they are just a bunch of lazy –sses!"

The author will leave it up to the reader as to which of the above explanations could account for "New Father's Sleeping Syndrome."

Perineal Care after Delivery

The vaginal area is going to be sore after your baby just delivered through it. Your vaginal and vulvar (outside) area may become swollen and hurt. Sometimes the swelling is such that you cannot void (pee) after the delivery. Tell your nurse if you are unable to urinate: we do not want your bladder to get over distended. Over distention can stretch out the muscles and nerve fibers of your bladder that further prevent urination. A catheter occasionally may need to be placed into the bladder for at least twenty four hours until bladder muscle tone can be re-established. Thereafter, the catheter can be removed and usually normal urination resumes.

She told me I needed to purchase the overnight Maxi pads for her on my way home from the office. I purchased the generic pads at the local grocery store. But, after she saw them, she told me that the generic brands do not have the "wings" on them. I said, "I didn't know your pads needed "to fly." She gave me a very mean look and was not amused. So a word to the wise for husbands, when it comes to pads (and peanut butter), you need to purchase the name brand pads such as Always®etc. – and don't skimp on the prices. The name brands are also more absorbent and keep the lochia away from your body: she said they last longer and are more comfortable.

--*Author*

After-pains

The uterus will contract even after the baby is born, so-called *after-pains*. These uterine contractions, though, uncomfortable, are part of the natural process of the uterus shrinking down to its normal size. These contractions further curtail your postpartum bleeding. Your bleeding will gradually taper off over the next 3-4 weeks (some patients have some spotting for a few more weeks).

Breastfeeding accentuates the pain. Therefore, it is recommended that you consider taking a "pain pill," or analgesic prior to breastfeeding. These after-pains usually respond well to ibuprofen.

Remember to NOT allow your pain pill to wear off completely: call the RN sooner than later because there may be a delay due to her working with other patients!

If you had an episiotomy

Your physician will tell you prior to the delivery if you need more room, i.e. a larger opening, in the vagina in order for the baby to be born without "tearing your tissues apart." A small cut is made at the opening to the vagina. A clean straight cut heals faster and there is less incisional pain.

Authors Note: I (and most OB's) always try NOT to cut or to do an episiotomy. But there have been many times that I had wished I had done one. I have seen scattered tears all the way around the vaginal opening. The next day, despite ice packs, the entire vulvar outside area is swollen. This scenario is much more uncomfortable that a straight "small" cut. Prior to a delivery the vaginal opening is routinely massaged with mineral oil and is gently stretched. Despite these best efforts the baby's head may just be too large for the vaginal opening: in this situation tearing (and bleeding) in all possible directions is possible.

After the placenta is delivered the episiotomy is closed with absorbable sutures. These stitches do not need to be removed later. These absorbing sutures dissolve in two to three weeks' time.

It is a small surgical "wound," and accordingly it is important to keep the episiotomy as clean and dry as possible. After going to the bathroom to urinate or have a bowel movement, or after changing a saturated pad of lochia flow, cleanse the area by rinsing the area off with a squeeze bottle of an antiseptic solution. Sitting in a regular bathtub or a sitz bath that fits over your toilet (available at your local pharmacy) can also keep the area clean and dry. To keep the area dry (moisture promotes the growth of bacteria) many hospitals may also provide heat lamps after your sitz bath or shower. Be careful to avoid getting burned with the heat lamp! At home you can use a blow drier (or reading lamp with incandescent bulb) to keep the area dry after cleansing.

The episiotomy is most sore during the first few days after delivery. Swelling and pain are best treated by an ice pack or, if at home, a "baggie" full of crushed ice. Heat by a heat lamp may also be soothing. Ice packs, heat lamps, soaking in the bathtub - whatever brings you relief - is the key to treatment. Also anesthetic sprays, such as Dermaplast® or Americaine® can be helpful.

Episiotomies are graded to their depth and length:

First degree: superficial break in the skin, i.e. skin "cut"
Second degree: skin and some deeper skin tissue (subcutaneous)

Third degree: outer rectal sphincter muscle affected
Fourth degree: incision affects external sphincter muscles as well as into the rectal area (mucosa torn)

Obviously, the deeper third and fourth degree tears are more painful. Stool softeners for three weeks are recommended to prevent hard bowel movements that can put more pressure on the suture line. However, it is very rare that any of these stitches can be broken by bowel movements or other physical activities. Softer bowel movements should help decrease any pressure or pain.

TREATMENT OF SORE EPISIOTOMIES

1) Sitz baths
2) Ice packs
3) Anesthetic sprays
4) Perineal lamp
5) Cleansing with antibacterial solutions

SIGNS OF EPISIOTOMY INFECTION (very uncommon, more frequent with bigger incisions)

1) Fever
2) Continued pain, swelling and redness
3) Drainage of pus, blood or fluid from suture area

Constipation

You may experience some difficulties with elimination following delivery. Constipation is already a problem during pregnancy because of the hormonal effects of progesterone. After your baby is born you are more immobilized and housebound with the care of your baby. The following measures are recommended to help you:

1. Drink more water

2. Eat more fruit and vegetables and other roughage, such as dried apricots, dates, raisins, or bran (either as a cereal, whole wheat bread or muffins). Eat at least 5-6 servings a day.
3. Be more physically active (especially walking)

If these measures are not effective, you can buy the following products over-the-counter at your pharmacy or supermarket:

a. Stool softeners such as generic DSS (Diocytl sodium succinate), Surfak®, Metamucil®, etc. Be sure that you drink a full 8 oz glass of water with these.
b. Laxatives such as Miralax®, Milk of Magnesia®, Senekot®, Dulcolax®, or Correctol®

Hemorrhoids

If you were fortunate not to develop hemorrhoids during pregnancy, you may be bothered with them *after* you deliver. When the baby's head completely occupies the pelvis during the second stage of labor, blood flow out of the pelvic veins is impaired. The veins inside the rectum will bulge and swell. The bearing down and pushing during the end of labor further aggravates this venous engorgement.

To help decrease the swelling, the following measures may provide relief:

a. Ice pack (plastic bag with crushed ice) may be applied to the area.
b. Over the counter acetaminophen (Tylenol®), ibuprofen (Motrin®), etc. for pain.
c. Try to stay off your feel and rest on your side as much as possible. Avoid prolonged standing.
d. Stool softeners are particularly useful if your bowel movements are hard. There is a general constipation during and after pregnancy. Tending to your newborn's care there is even less time for walking and exercise: constipation is the natural result. Diocytl sodium succinate (DSS) is a stool softener that is available over the counter. Brand names are Surfak®, Colace®, etc.

e. Lubricating the anal canal with Vaseline® and 1% hydrocortisone mixed together with help reduce the trauma and swelling with bowel movements. Commercial products available are Anusol HC, Preparation H, Proctofoam®, etc. Keeping the anal area clean is also important: sitting in a bowl of lukewarm water, i.e., "sitz bath", may provide a lot of immediate comfort.
f. For the acute pain of hemorrhoids, use local anesthetic creams/sprays such as Dermoplast®, Nupercaine®, Benzocaine®, etc. Apply at least three (3) times per day (and re-apply after each BM)
g. If a hard lump or mass forms inside the swollen hemorrhoid, such *thrombosed* hemorrhoids may need enucleated surgically.

Bladder problems

It is quite common not to be able to urinate as easily after both vaginal or C-section deliveries. Occasionally a bladder catheter may be needed for a few days until your bladder (and the stretched out muscles fibers and nerves) may return to normal.

Patients may also "leak" urine in the few weeks after delivery. With *Kegels* exercises bladder control should return to normal with a few weeks. *Kegel exercises* are the contraction of the pelvic muscles: similar to what most people due when they have to stop "peeing" or stop their urine flow half way through in order get up and help your child or answer the phone or doorbell. Squeeze as if you are trying to stop peeing and hold for at least 16 seconds. Try to do these sixteen (16) "crunches" (holding for 16 seconds): 6 or more times per day. It can be done while you are driving or shopping: nobody can see or tell what you are doing.

Leg Swelling and Pain

It is quite common to experience swelling of your feet after delivery. Such edema is due to the amount of IV fluids that are given during your labor. If you had an epidural, most patients will experience some edema: it is due to the excess amount of IV fluids given to you to prevent the potential of lowered blood pressure (Hypotension) that typically can occur with an epidural.

If only one leg is swollen and it is painful to walk on that leg, you could have formed a blood clot in that leg (see section on phlebitis below). Most OB units place compression hose or mechanical compression devices (Sequential Compression Devices, i.e. SCD's) prior to an epidural during labor or a C-section in order to prevent this problem.

Back and pelvic pain after delivery

Many patients will complain of low back pain after delivery. Sometimes the pain is localized to the area where the epidural was placed. The epidural site will remain uncomfortable for weeks just as any other deep injection would be expected to cause.

Patient may also notice low back pain or "tail bone" pain (coccyx) after delivery. With the passage of the baby's head through the pelvis the tail bone or coccyx (occasional the sacrum) can be placed under extrinsic pressure with resulting soreness. Uncommonly, the coccyx can be fractured or displaced during delivery.

Eye Changes

Many times the patient's eyes may become blood-shot after delivery. Because of the tremendous straining that attends pushing your baby out, the blood vessels in the white part of the eye will bleed. Such *petechial hemorrhages* will heal in a matter of days.

Nutrition and Dieting

Eating a well-balanced diet is just as important after pregnancy as it was while you were pregnant. A well-balanced diet consists of high protein foods (such as milk products, chicken, beans, fish and lean meats), fresh fruits and vegetables, as well as starches such as baked potatoes, rice, etc. Avoid fried foods due to absorbed saturated fats. Grill, bake or steam your foods. Try to stay away from "fast foods" (such as McDonalds's, Kentucky Fried Chicken, and Pizza Hut) as well as "junk foods" (such as potato chips, candies, etc.).

You may diet by reducing the amount of food you eat. Do not forget that it took you nine (9) months to put on the weight. It can take at least that amount of time to get back to your normal body weight and muscle tone. Drink at least eight full glasses of water a day. Avoid sodas which are high in sodium and sugar. Remember that "if you're not hungry, don't eat." Similarly, "if you are no longer hungry, stop eating!"

If you are nursing, your calorie requirements are different. In order to support your milk supply for your baby, you will need to increase your calorie intake by 300-500 a day. Your water intake should be *at least* eight glasses a day. Drink a glass of with each nursing.

An added bonus for breast feeding moms is that your weight loss is significantly faster than non-breastfeeding moms!

General Physical Activity

Rest.

With your baby waking up every three to four hours according to your baby's® schedule, it is important to get as much rest as possible. Preferably, rest whenever the baby goes down for a nap. You may feel like a "zombie", "always tired" and irritable in the first few weeks after delivery. Everyone wants to see you and your new baby. You must realize that many visitors will tire you even more. Therefore, try to limit your visitors, friends and relatives during the immediate postpartum weeks (unless, of course, they are coming over to cook you dinners, vacuum your home, clean your bathrooms, and mow the grass!) Carefully screen any visitors for any infectious diseases such as colds, flu, and diarrhea. Make sure your guests wash their hands before they hold your baby.

Author's Note: The author requests that family and friends NOT kiss the baby. Siblings and children that attend school and daycare centers bring home viruses and bacteria that could infect your newborn.

Do not allow people, particularly sick people, to kiss your baby in the first few months of the newborn period. Babies could care less but they do hate being sick!

Exercise

It is best to limit your activities to just walking during the first few weeks after delivery. Your uterus ("womb") is still enlarged and will wobble around if you jog or do any other bouncing activities. Further, your bleeding will increase and such increased flows will aggravate any anemia that may have resulted from your delivery. Muscle toning with light weights, stretching, as well as use of specifically-designed low impact equipment such as an Elliptical, TredClimber®, Treadmill, StairMaster®, etc. may be begun gradually.

C-section Deliveries

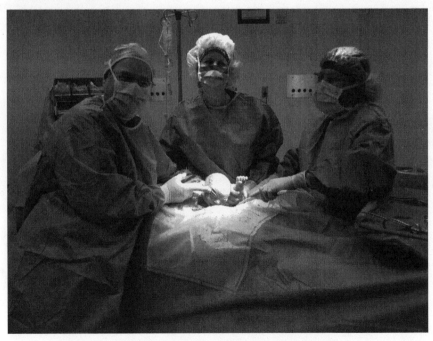

Figure 21-5 Baby already waving to everyone in the OR

1. C-section Incision care.

If you have had a C-section delivery, it is best to avoid putting tension on the incision line, i.e., bending over, heavy lifting, or any type of abdominal "crunches." Keep the incision line clean. You may wash the incision gently with soap and water. Clean off any collection of discolored "filmy stuff" with hydrogen peroxide. It is best to keep the area dry and exposed to the air. When your incision is under a fold of your "tummy," It is particularly important to wash the incision with soap and water – even "blow-dry" the area to keep it as dry as possible.

The area just above the incision and below the belly button will be "numb" for at least 3-4 months after the surgery. You may go up and down stairs carefully. If you feel any strain on the incision, you should limit your trips as much as possible. If your incision was closed with "under the skin" (*sub-cuticular*) stitches, you can expect your incision line to weep a little fluid (starting about 5 weeks after delivery).

A small amount of ooze may occur as the stitches are dissolving by themselves. To avoid tape burns or marks, I recommend that you cover your incision with a panty-liner: just place it over your incision and then pull your underwear up over it. Occasionally the incision will cut through a hair gland follicle: as the gland heals, a small abscess or pimple may form. It may ooze a small amount of pus but heal with keep the area clean with peroxide or antibiotic cream.

Patients having a C-section will have their urinary catheter removed on the 1st postoperative day. It is important that the patient be able to empty their bladder *completely* after it is removed. The nurses will chart your "I and O's," your input of fluids and your measured output of fluids. They will check your fundus and your bladder. Incomplete bladder emptying does occur from time to time due to medications and the surgery itself.

Author's Anecdote: On rounds in the hospital the author usually relates the following *silly* humor regarding the ability to urinate after surgery:

"If you are *French* going into the bathroom and you are *Italian* coming out of the bathroom, what are you *while you are in* the bathroom?

You ready for this?

Answer: *European*! (You're a peeing!)

2. **Anemia**. C-Section patients lose twice as much blood as vaginally delivered patients - approximately one third to one half of a quart of blood. Consequently, in addition to having major surgery, patients are further drained by the extra blood loss. Fatigue, dizziness and lightheadedness, and shortness of breath, characterize such patients with anemia. If anemia is severe, bed rest may have to be prescribed for two to three weeks until your bone marrow (along with oral Iron pills and Vitamin C!) can reproduce enough new red blood cells to replenish your previously depleted supply.

Anemia Precautions

> Get up slowly from bed, holding onto the side rails of the bed.
>
> Sit for a while.
>
> Get up slowly, holding onto your spouse, nurse or the side rails of your bed.
>
> If lightheadedness or faintness is felt, immediately lie back down in bed.

Be careful during a bath or shower. Blood is diverted to your skin surfaces, further aggravating a low central blood volume. Sit on a stool in the shower and have someone, such as a nurse, husband or relative, nearby in case faintness should occur.

3. ***Driving***. Driving should be resumed when you are able to move about comfortably. In general, you may resume driving when you feel comfortable enough to get in and out of your vehicle as well as turn your body around (to look in your rear view mirror and to check on your baby in the back seat). In order to check out your abilities and do a "test drive," try getting in and out of your car while it is parked in the driveway. Push on the gas and brake pedals. Turn around and look into the back seat. If you are anemic (and you should be taking your iron supplement twice a day!), you should wait at least three weeks before you resume driving.

4. ***Swimming***. When your bleeding has subsided (usually within 2 to 4 weeks), swimming may be resumed.

5. ***Stairs***. For the first few weeks after delivery, going up and down stairs may be difficult. Limit your trips during the day. It is rare that any stitches are broken or affected.

6. ***Breastfeeding***. Nursing your baby may be more difficult because of the discomfort when lifting and moving the baby from one side to another. Suckling also causes release of oxytocin from the pituitary gland. Oxytocin further contracts the uterine muscle and pulls on the suture line across the uterine muscle. After-pains that usually occur postpartum are further aggravated and heightened by the incision in the uterus itself. However, medications used to control postoperative pain (Demerol, Codeine, etc.)

7. S*ex*

I am always asked this question (usually by the new fathers).

My response is, "wait until you get home! It upsets the nurses! Just because you have "a room" here at the hospital does not mean you have to use it!"

In general, most women are not interested in sexual relations for several weeks after delivery (perhaps months and even years!). Bottom line: You can "be romantic" whenever you are in the mood and feel comfortable with trying. Most couples usually wait when the bleeding subsides and the vaginal opening has become less sensitive: usually in 3 to 6 weeks.

Constant caring for the baby, maintenance of the home, shopping, visitors, etc., result in overwhelming fatigue for the new mother. The vaginal opening is very sensitive after delivery (particularly when nursing). Further, If you have had stitches at the vaginal opening (*episiotomy*), it will take at least 5 to 6 weeks for that area to heal sufficiently to allow intercourse safely and comfortably. When relations are resumed, it is recommended that the couple use plenty (like a lot!) of lubricant (such as KY liquid and Astroglide©) to prevent "tearing" of the delicate tissues. Most husbands and partners are sympathetic to these circumstances and are able to divert their "energies" to help "mom with the care of their newborn, shopping, cleaning, etc." Alternately new fathers may just go to Hooters or Buffalo Wild Wings to watch the game! Hugging, kissing and other physical touching can provide the emotional satisfaction that each partner desires.

A "life cycle" event happens when a "couple" becomes instantly transformed into "parents" immediately after the baby is born. Both men and women look at themselves in a different way. Men change from being a husband (SO or FOB) and now become a father. A woman changes from the role of a wife (SO) and metamorphoses into becoming mother to a baby. New parents may not have "seen this coming" or understand these psychological changes in their own attitudes and feelings. Somehow sex is "different" as parents now: they no longer perceive themselves as the "hot couple" they used to be!

With no stitches in the vaginal area C-Section patients may be able to attempt sexual intercourse sooner. It is unlikely that any abdominal stitches can be broken during such activities.

Anecdote: One of my patients, Candice, called me 7 days after her C-section. She weighed close to 300lbs when she delivered. Her complaint was, "my rear end is asleep! Could I have a bedsore? What can I do about it? I told her that if her buttocks were asleep, she could wake them up by shaking them. If that didn't work, she could pour cold water on them. That usually wakes most things up! (I am sorry to be so facetious but really!)

Postpartum Depression

With the delivery of the placenta your pregnancy is finally at an end. The "hormonal high" that you have been riding for the past 9 months "bottoms out." Hormone levels go into a "free fall." Hormones "bathe" your entire brain: your moods, your emotions, your energy levels, etc. Further, you are no longer the focus of everyone's attention: the baby has now taken the center stage. Everyone is enamored with baby.

Many new moms will experience the feeling of depression to certain degree. However, some new moms may experience deeper "lows." Most new dads and family members as well as friends will observe your "baby blues" and step up to provide the needed emotional and physical support to the new mom that she needs.

Occasionally, despite the loving support of family and friends, the new mom still may not be able to function and becomes down casted as well as lethargic. When these symptoms, especially hopelessness and even suicidal thoughts, become evident, the family needs to alert her physician. Professional psychological or psychiatric counseling and occasionally, an anti-depressant medication can be helpful for a limited time until the new mom improves: usually within a month or two.

Birth Control.

As Jeff Foxworthy comically said, *"you might be a redneck if you have had 3 pregnancy tests before you ever took your first driving test!" Or, you might be a redneck if you have taken a pregnancy test and a sobriety test on the very same day!*

Although you have not had to worry about birth control for the past 9 months, you do need to think about an effective method ***now*** (unless, of course, you want to have another child very soon!). It is best to wait at least 6 months for your body to recover before planning another pregnancy. The commonly available forms of birth control are as follows:

- ♥ Barrier methods: condoms ("rubbers"), diaphragm, contraceptive jellies and foam, vaginal suppositories and vaginal film

- ♥ Hormonal methods: birth control pills, Nexplanon®, NuvaRing, Depo-Provera® or the birth control patches Evra®
- ♥ IUD (intrauterine devices) such as the Mirena or Paraguard
- ♥ Sterilization such as vasectomy or tubal ligation
- ♥ Abstinence (which really is not much fun!)

Very Important Point: Nexplanon© and Paraguard© IUD inserts may require *pre-authorization* (pre-certification) from your insurance company. They may also require a "referral form" from your Primary care physician. If you are serious about using one of these methods, be sure to check with your insurance company. If needed, contact your primary care physician during your pregnancy *before* you deliver for your referral: many primary MD's are booked up weeks in advance and they may require an appointment with them prior to approving any referral. Further, because of the poor reimbursement from third party payors (they many not cover the physician cost of the insertion and the supply of these devices), many OBs may not place them: you may need to seek out other community resources that may provide them.

Second Very Important Point: Sterilization is a ***permanent*** form of birth control. Most physicians discourage sterilization if a patient is less than 30 years of age. There is not a week that does not go by in which a patient comes to the office requesting that her "tubes be untied." Reversal of sterilization can be expensive: frequently greater than $15000.

Third Very Important Point: Breastfeeding patients can use the IUD (both Mirena and Paraguard), the Nexplanon implant, the mini-pill (progesterone only pill) as well as barrier methods.

Patient No. 1

The author had a patient in California who was age 39. She had had 4 C-sections. She became divorced and remarried a younger man in his early 30's: he did not have any children yet. She wanted me to put her tubes back together.

Patient No. 2

Another patient of mine in California wanted *only one* child. She wanted a tubal ligation. Two (2) years later she came back to me and asked that her tubal ligation be reversed: she had changed her mind and wanted another child!

I can go on and on about many other patients wanting reversals of their tubal ligations or vasectomies. The points that need to be stressed are as follows:

a. Life changes, circumstances change and you change from decade to decade. You may get the desire to have another child later in life.

b. Relationships change and people get divorced or God forbid, your mate is killed or dies from some horrible medical condition. You may re-marry and the new marriage may be perfect for another child.

c. Tragic Events occur such as the accidental death of your child or children. You can never "replace" that beautiful child with another, but the couple may still feel so much emptiness that another child may be desired in their lives.

If you are considering but not sure of sterilization, I highly recommend that you consider the IUD (Paraguard© or Mirena©): it is about the closest method akin to sterilization that there is but *it is reversible*. The Paraguard© is effective for at least 12 years (and probably longer) yet is can be easily removed in seconds and you instantly regain the ability to become pregnant again! Tubal reversals are not usually covered by your insurance carrier.

Other Special Postpartum Situations you want to know about after delivery

i) **Nursing.**

If you are nursing you should *not* choose the *standard* birth control pills: the estrogen in the pill will affect the quality and quantity of your milk. You still can use the "mini" pill because it contains only progesterone and will not affect your milk supply.

ii) **When to start Birth Control Pills.**

Birth control pills or the mini-pill can be started on the third Sunday after you deliver. DepoProvera® can be given before you leave the hospital or at your physician's office in 4 to 6 weeks.

iii) **IUD.**

Because the uterus should return to its natural size before it can retain an IUD, the IUD is usually inserted at your 6-week checkup appointment. Do not forget to get your <u>insurance authorization</u> or referral from your primary MD prior to you appointment!

iv) **Tubal Ligation.**

Although the incision is very small, patients do experience pain after the surgery. Analgesics ("pain pills") will be prescribed and will afford relief of your soreness. There may be some redness and some swelling around the incision. There also may be some bruising or dark discoloration. The stitches will dissolve by themselves. Some amount of discharge can be expected from the incision. Heavy lifting (over 25 pounds) should not be done for at least 8 weeks. As far as protection is concerned, the tubal ligation is effective immediately.

v) ***Anesthesia Side Effects***.

You can expect some soreness in your back for several weeks (the pain is at the site the epidural or spinal needle punctured your skin). If you had a general anesthetic ("went to sleep") for your baby's birth, you can expect a sore throat for a few days.

vi) ***IV site***. After your IV catheter is removed from your arm or hand, you can expect a little swelling and redness for several days. Occasionally a firm area or "cord" can be felt for several weeks. Hot compresses or a moist heating pad will provide relief.

Rh factor

If your blood type is Rh negative and your baby's blood type is Rh positive, you will receive an injection (**RhoGam**®) after your delivery. This injection prevents your body from developing antibodies to the Rh factor. Accordingly, future pregnancies with Rh negative babies will not be affected or compromised.

Rubella Vaccine

Because most people receive their immunizations during childhood, it is uncommon for anyone to be susceptible to this viral infection as an adult. However, some of us may still miss these vaccinations or the immunization is lost over the years. It is standard practice to check for Rubella susceptibility during pregnancy. If you are not immune or your test resulted in "intermediate immunity," you will receive the vaccination postpartum.

Smoking

Smoking is never healthy for anyone. Smoking from other people's cigarettes, cigars or pipes ("Second Hand Smoke) is also harmful and can be directly inhaled by the baby.

Smoking is an extremely unhealthy addiction. Smoking increases your risk of developing most types of cancer and progressively affects the circulation to **al**l your vital organs (brain with stroke, heart attacks, and lungs with COPD and legs with DVT). If you have stopped smoking during your pregnancy, ask your physician for additional help (if needed) to maintain your cessation. If your husband or partner smokes, it is a good time for him to quit as well. Second hand smoke affects the baby and can predispose the baby to various breathing problems including asthma, etc.

Smoking is the main cause of fires in homes across the country: it is one of the most frequent causes of death in very young children (and adults!) If visiting relatives or friends drop by and need to smoke, please ask them to leave the home and smoke outside.

Consult your physician's office regarding the various smoking cessation therapies that are available:

1. Quitting "cold turkey."
2. Nicorette or similar chewing medications
3. Medications such as Chantix, patches and Zyban/Wellbutrin.

If you or your spouse has not completely quit smoking during the pregnancy, *now is another "best opportunity" to Quit!*

Bladder Infections (UTI's)

UTI's are quite common after birth. Frequently urinary catheters are inserted after epidurals and prior to C-sections: catheters insertion can increase the chance of a UTI (Catheter associated UTI or "CAUTI)". The main symptoms are painful frequent voiding of small amounts of urine. The appearance of blood in your urine is another sign of infection. If flank pain and fever occur along with these symptoms, a kidney infection may have developed. Treatment consists of antibiotic medication, Vitamin C, cranberry juice and increased fluid intake to flush out the infection from the urinary tract.

Phlebitis (Blood Clot in your leg)

Infrequently a clot may form in a leg after delivery. Blood becomes quite "thick" (or hyper-coagulable) in the immediate postpartum period. Phlebitis (or inflammation of a vein secondary to clotting) occurs four times more frequently postpartum than during pregnancy. Symptoms that signal the onset of phlebitis are as follows:

1. Pain in a localized area of your leg, usually the calf, that is aggravating by walking or further weight-bearing on that extremity.
2. Pain in your calf when you bend your toes up toward your head.
3. Swelling and edema in only one of your ankles or calves.
4. A red, painful, thickened "cord" or vein in back part your leg.
5. Painful breathing and shortness of breath resulting from one of these clots breaking off from a leg or pelvic vein and traveling to your lungs (PE).

Should any of the above symptoms occur, call your physician immediately.

If a DVT is detected early and treated promptly other complications such as a PE (pulmonary embolism) can be avoided.

Breast Feeding Postpartum

If you are nursing, it is very common to have "sore nipples." First, it is important to be sure that you get as much of the areola into the baby's mouth as possible. To help "toughen" your nipples, leave the flaps of your nursing bra open under your blouse. Also, leaving your breasts exposed to the open air will help. **The first two weeks are the hardest but, if you can "tough it out," breastfeeding can be one of the most rewarding and beneficial things you can do for your baby.**

Breast crème (Masse® or lanolin) is usually not necessary but can be helpful. The areola contains "Montgomery glands" that secrete a lubricant that is natural and encourages the baby to nurse. However, if your nipples are becoming chapped or dry, breast cream may be helpful. Apply after nursing. It is not necessary to rinse off before the next feeding.

You can expect the glands in your axilla (your "armpit") to swell and become uncomfortable for several days during and after you milk comes in. No special treatment is necessary.

If you are breastfeeding and develop "red streaking" on one of you breasts along with a fever, you may have a breast infection. Infections can be treated quickly with antibiotics. Please call your physician if you think you have a breast infection. Further, the hospital has a "lactation specialist" that can be called as an additional resource of information and help.

Lactation Suppression

Unfortunately there are no approved medications to prevent your milk from "coming in." You should wear a clean and comfortable (but tight) bra for support at all times during this time (24 hours). Your milk will come in three to four days postpartum. Do not try to "squeeze out" your breast milk – it will only stimulate more milk to form. Your breasts will become engorged and swollen. Frozen bags of peas, placed on the breasts plus Tylenol, will afford some pain relief. You may also want to try cabbage leaves, which are placed in the bra, for milk suppression. Many new moms have sworn by this method. Usually the swelling will subside in a few days and the engorgement will subside. Redness around the areola or in the skin around the nipple is the first sign of a breast infection. Call your physician's office immediately if such redness, pain or fever develops.

Stitches

If you have had an episiotomy ("vaginal stitches") or a C-section, the suture material used to close the skin "dissolves" automatically in 3 weeks: unless otherwise instructed, these sutures do **not** need to be removed later. Some pain and tenderness is expected. The pain should diminish every day. To ease the pain from an episiotomy, it is recommended that you soak your bottom in warm water (with or without Epsom salts) either in the bathtub or in a basin that fits over your toilet ("sitz bath"). For more convenience, uses a squirt bottle filled with warm water and gently pour the water over your bottom while on the toilet. Also, you can apply anesthetic creams or sprays (Americaine®, Benzocaine, etc.) on the stitches. Occasionally, as some of the vaginal stitches dissolve, you will notice some threads coming out from your vaginal area. These sutures are usually blue or brown in color. Do not be alarmed. No special attention is needed or action required. Do not pull on the strands: they will continue to dissolves or fall out by themselves.

Medications

After your delivery you will need medication for the following reasons: these medications are safe and effective and will not interfere with breastfeeding.

Uterine Cramps (*afterpains*). Analgesics such as ibuprofen (Nuprin®, Advil®, Motrin®, etc.) as well as acetaminophen (Tylenol ®) are very helpful in relieving these pains. Usually 600 to 800 mg is needed to provide effective relief and should be taken every 6 to 8 hours. Breastfeeding moms will notice even more cramping during and after nursing. If you can, it is best to ask or take your medication 20 minutes before nursing.

Episiotomy or Postoperative C-section Pain. Ibuprofen (listed above) as well as hydrocodone products (Lortab®, Percocet®, etc), Tylenol®, can provide relief. Percocet®, Demerol®, and other analgesics may also be prescribed as indicated for certain patients.

Anemia. Iron is usually prescribed and recommended to all patients after delivery. The average blood loss during a normal vaginal delivery is a pint of blood. A patient loses a quart of blood after a C-section. Iron supplements should be taken 2 to 3 times per day. Vitamin C facilitates the absorption of Iron: take Iron (Ferrous Gluconate or Ferrous Sulfate 5 grains or 32 mg of elemental Iron) with Vitamin C 500 mg two (2) to three (3) times per day. Iron will cause your bowel movement to become black. Constipation is also a side effect: use stool softeners such as Colace®, Surfak®, Metamucil®, Doxidan®, Milk of Magnesia®, or other generics (DSS, diocyt sulfosuccinate) to help soften the stools. Drink plenty of water.

Prenatal Vitamins. In order to replenish your stores of vitamins and minerals that are siphoned off by the newborn during your pregnancy, it is recommended that you continue on prenatal vitamins for at least 1 to 3 months after your delivery. You should continue vitamin and Iron supplements while you are nursing.

Traveling with Baby

Of course, you will need an approved car seat in which to take your baby home. Please follow the instructions (which can be difficult) on how to attach the car seat properly to your vehicle.

Babies do NOT travel well (unless you lucked out with a great baby that likes to travel!). You will need to be sure your diaper bag is filled with diapers, wipes, extra clothes, binkies, bottles, nipples, cloths, etc.

Author's Note: To date, there is no diaper so designed as to contain the explosive poop coming from your baby's intestines.

Recently, however, I was walking through Wal-Mart and went through the baby department. I looked up at the diapers on the wall. Suddenly, it occurred to me that they have made significant technological breakthroughs in diaper construction. I saw on the side of the diaper box, "6 to12 pounds" so I guess these new diapers can now really hold a large load!

I do not recommend taking your baby (or your toddler) on a long road trip. It completely messes up their known daily routine. They get fussy. Then you and everyone else become irritable. The best solution is to find a family member or good friend for the days you are going to be gone. Believe, you and your baby will be happier!

Babies do not like changes in their schedule. You and your baby will settle into a daily routine of active time, nap time, feeding times and sleep time very quickly. An example of a baby that does not tolerate "routine change" is the so called the "fussy" baby on the airplane. The baby cries the entire flight. Finally as the plane lands, the baby is asleep. If you have to travel, bring everything that the baby is accustomed to having: same baby blanket, same toys, same clothes, etc. I even had to bring the same mattress and bedding so that my child would sleep in peace and be comfortable in secure the environment to which he was accustomed.

Warning Signs

If you experience any of the following situations after you are home, please call the Hospital Switchboard immediately (580-531-4700) and they will put you in touch with the office or hospital:

1. Bleeding. Any bleeding to the degree where you are soaking a napkin (pad) in less than one hour with bright red blood

2. Fever. Any fever over 101°

3. Painful Breathing or Difficulty in Breathing

4. Walking on one leg is extremely painful. Clots can form in your legs after delivery. Usually there is swelling of just one foot. There is a painful area or "cord' in your calf area.

5. Red and painful area in your breast. Mastitis is signaled by a reddish coloration near the nipple that is very sensitive. You may experience a severe "chill" which is usually followed by a high fever.

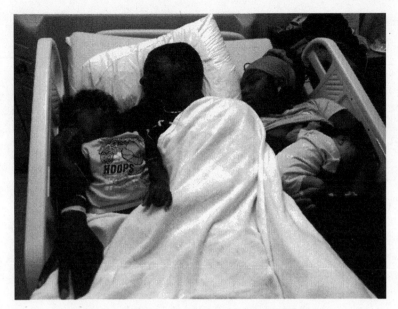

Figure 21-6 Postpartum family asleep.

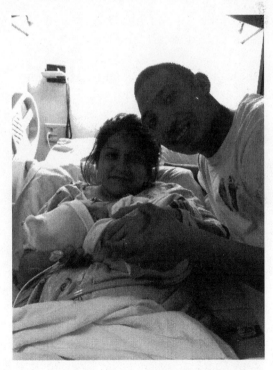

Figure 21-7 New Parents just about ready to take their newborn home.

The 6 Week Check-up Appointment

Unless otherwise directed, most patients should be re-examined six weeks postpartum. It is preferred that you make this checkup visit with the same doctor who delivered your baby or your regular OB if he/she was not on call when you delivered. Schedule your 6-week follow-up appointment during the first week after you are discharge from the hospital. At that time an examination and, if needed, a Pap smear, will be performed. Furthermore, it is a time to ask and discuss any questions or problems that may have been experiencing. Also, it is a good time to discuss birth control.

Remember that you may need to have a referral or a pre-authorization from your primary care physician or insurance company if you want an IUD or Nexplanon for birth control.

Some comments the author has heard during the 6 week checkup:

"My husband has done all the housework and chores. He goes shopping at the store. He does all the cooking."

"I finally cooked for the first time last night after 2 months. I cooked a roast. Husband was very happy with the food. Of course, I'm not sure if you consider it *cooking* when you use the crockpot!"

"The house is starting to look normal again."

Breasts and Breastfeeding

If you are nursing, the nipple area should be cleaned at least once a day. It is best to avoid using soap because the soap residue taste on the nipple may discourage the baby from suckling. If crusting and oils have built up on the nipples, use a mild soap followed by thorough rinsing to cleanse the areola and nipple. Usually, use of breast creams may not be necessary because self-lubricating glands (Montgomery's glands) are present in the areola. These glands produce and secrete a natural lubricant that encourages the baby to nurse. If scaling and dryness still occur, then a thin layer of breast cream (Masse or lanolin) can be rubbed gently into the nipple, areola and body of the breast. Be sure to rinse such creams off with water prior to the next breastfeeding if they have not already evaporated on the breast.

Some tenderness of the nipples is normal and usually disappears in about five to seven days. At the same time, you may note the appearance of chapped lips around the baby's mouth. These chapped lips are a result of the intense suckling by the baby and no treatment is necessary. Should your nipples crack or bleed "air-drying" or "sun tanning" by leaving your bra flaps down may be helpful and soothing. Always place the baby on the breast with the least sore nipple first, and then on the affected side. Nipple shields are rubber nipples placed over your nipple, and may also be helpful. Dry heat in the form of a light bulb, direct sunlight or a blow dryer promotes healing. Should any fever or areas of redness and pain occur, a breast infection may be developing. Contact your physician so that an antibiotic may be prescribed. Breastfeeding does not have to be discontinued.

Discharge Medications

Many obstetrical patients will be given medication for pain. Motrin 800 mg is the most preferred discharge medication. Occasionally, Lortab 5 mg, Norco 5 mg or Tylenol with codeine (Tylenol #3) may be needed. These medications provide comfort for *after pains*, swollen hemorrhoids, episiotomy and C-Section incision pain. If the patient is allergic or sensitive to codeine, another analgesic can be prescribed. These medications can be safely used while nursing. Lastly, it is recommended that patients continue to use their prenatal vitamins and iron postpartum. Other medications to treat thyroid, heart, lung and diabetic conditions should be continued as directed by your physician.

Supply Checklist for Baby

Baby Blanket: It is EXTREMELY IMPORTANT that parents chose a cozy soothing blanket for their baby. Babies become particularly attached to their blankets: it is their one consistent possession in their lives. *Blankies* provide them "security" wherever they go (for years!).

Also, just like their *blankies*, you should invest in a few soft animal toys: many babies and toddlers can't leave home without them! Buy 4 of the exact same soft toys because, as with *blankies*, they need to be washed, replaced, etc.

Diapers
Cleansing Wipes (and wipe warmer?)
Baby soap and Shampoo (J&J, Aveeno, Castile, etc.)
Receiving Blankets
Clothes for appropriate season of birth
Crib (with mattress, sheets, etc.) or Combo Pack'n Paly, Bassinet, etc.
Plastic Bath
Car seat
Stroller
Portable Seat for inside

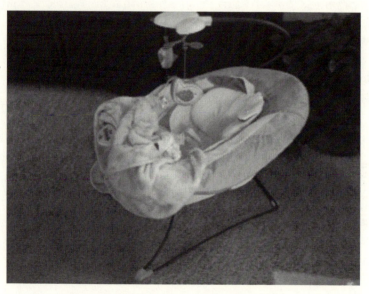

Figure 21-8 Baby musical cradle-bouncer

Blankies
Stuffed Animals (for 0 age group)
Nail clipper and Emory boards
Formula, bottles, bottle brush, nipples (if not breastfeeding)
Burping towels
Bulb syringes (mouth and nose)

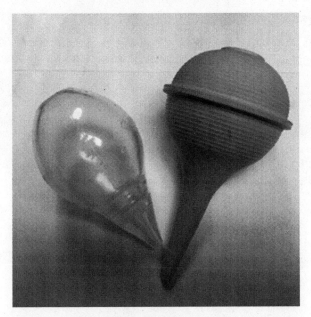

Figure 21-0-10 Bulb Syringe

Author's Anecdote: The author's child, Jessica, would not leave the house or go to sleep without her "Blankie." By the time she was 3 years old, the "Blankie" had been torn and shredded to the point that only a 10 inch square was left.

Another child would not part with his "Blankie" at any time whatsoever. The parent could not even wash the blanket until the child was fast asleep.

The OB nurses tell me that babies prefer the silky bordered blankets as they love the feel of the satin against their hands and bodies.

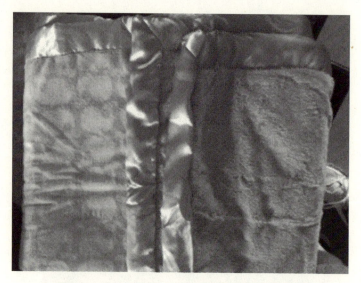

Figure 21-11 Silky bordered Baby Blankets

The author recommends that parents purchase <u>at least 4 blankets that are all the same</u>. In case a "blankie" needs to be washed, is left at home or another person's home, gets lost, gets torn to shreds, there are replacements available. Furthermore, one "Blankie" can be framed and kept for memorabilia for your child when he/she get older.

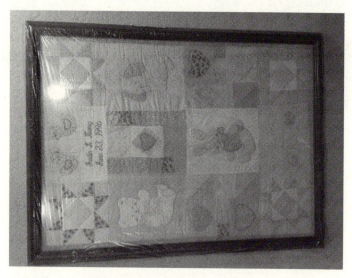

Figure 21-12 Blankie Dr. Zweig's son's Justin "Blankie framed and hanging in the hallway."

Car Seat: The reader is referred to current Consumer Reports

http://www.consumerreports.org/cro/babies-kids/baby-toddler/car-seats/car-seat-recommendations/convertible-car-seat.htm,

EvenFlo® Momentum 65®, Graco My Ride 65® and Cosco® brands car seats were on the "Recommended List."

Diapers: The reader is referred to the Consumer Reports website for up-to-date information regarding diapers

(http://consumerreports.org/cro/diapers/buying-guide.htm).

There is a very good discussion regarding the debate of "cloth versus disposables." In the past a major consumer magazine had recommended Pampers as the most cost-effective brand. Best bargains are at:

1. Walmart or Sams Club
2. Toys-R-Us
3. Target and K-Mart
4. Costco

Generic brands at Wal-Mart or Target (or your local Supermarket store) frequently are made by the major manufacturers such as Pampers, Huggies, etc.

Strollers: There are many types of strollers: umbrella, carriage, jogging, etc and the reader must decide which type will fit their needs (and their trunk space!)

Again the reader is referred to a very in depth discussion at Consumer Reports:

http://consumerreports.org/cro/babies-kids/baby-toddler/strollers/traditional-stroller-ratings/ratings-overview.htm

From the author's experience there are two major sources of weakness in a stroller:

a. The strength of the wheels and
b. the quality of the fabric

> Purchase a stroller with strong braided fabric or canvas. Vinyl tears apart. Also avoid plastic spoke-type wheels that tend to break. Steel spokes or solid hubs with rubber wheels will last through several children.

Umbrella-type strollers are easiest to use. Large "buggies" that carry baby (as well as older sister and a week's supply of groceries!) tend to be too heavy and bulky. They are a pain to set up or collapse. Any stroller that takes more than one to two minutes to set up just seems to be a little too long. Mothers are really moving at a rapid pace these days!

<u>Cuticle Scissors</u>: Cut baby's fingernails and toenails, and smooth off with emery board. We cannot have baby's face scratched up for the numerous photo sessions! Nurses at the hospital do not provide this service for you.

<u>Formula</u>: Discuss formula brands with your pediatrician. Further, there are many internet sites that provide information on the right selection for your baby:

http://www.consumerreports.org/cro/babies-kids/index.htm

www.**baby**center.com/choosing-and-using-**baby-formula**

Consumer Reports web site above has reviewed most baby products from formulas to strollers to cribs. Similac, Enfamil, Gerber, Naturesone, Prolacta, etc. are the most common brands of formula at most stores. Most retail chains also provide generic brand formula that is made by one of the major formula companies are much cheaper than the name brands. Hospitals may use certain brands, such as Similac because they are supplied to the hospital for a discounted price (sometimes without charge) by the company. The fact that your hospital supplies a certain brand formula does not mean hospitals endorse or recommend them. Reputable brands include Gerber, Enfamil and Similac. Powders that require preparation and mixing with water are cheapest, but ready-to-feed are more convenient, expensive, as well as weigh more in your diaper bag.

Baby's Clothing: Be sure that baby's clothes are fire retardant. A high percentage of polyester fabric may make baby sweat, overheat and predispose to diaper rash. Many national and local department stores have excellent baby and toddler sections:

>Target, Wal-Mart, TJ Max Homegoods™, Sears, Ross, Marshalls, JC Penny, Kohl's, Dillard's and Macy's.

Soaps: Mild soaps without deodorants, antiseptics or other chemicals to irritate baby's delicate skin are recommended. Dove, Ivory, or castile soap (available at health food stores) are some of the available brands.

Losing weight after your birth

Most patients will have a net weight gain of about 20 lbs. after they leave the hospital. Of course, it is more difficult to lose weight because your physical activities are curtailed due to your postpartum uterine "bulge" as well as fatigue from taking care of your baby. Further, weight loss during nursing may affect the nourishment of your baby. Breastfeeding does help weight loss. When possible, you may go back to the Gym to start re-toning your muscles. Stairmaster, Ellipticals, weights, treadmill walking etc. may be utilized. Wait at least two weeks after birth prior to running as your uterus is still shrinking and may be wobbly inside your abdomen.

Dieting is also important. Again, a "South Beach Diet" type of diet plan may be helpful. The following advice sums up some of the more significant points:

Weight Loss Counseling

1. Do not eat if you are not hungry: stop eating when you are no longer hungry
2. Exercise regularly to tone muscles
3. Drink 6-8 glasses of water or other fluids

4. Lipton diet green tea or other natural herbs prior to meals may help decrease your "hunger"

5. Do not eat after 7 PM

6. High protein, low CHO, i.e. carbohydrate diet (South Beach, Atkins or other low carbohydrate diet)

7. Simple weight loss formula: burn up more calories than calories that you eat!

8. Multivitamins should be taken daily

9. Food diary: write down everything you eat

10. Chew your food very slowly

11. Chew gum if you feel hungry. If you need a snack, celery, carrots, cucumbers, etc. may be eaten (preferably without the ranch dressing)

CHAPTER 22

Breast And Bottle Feeding

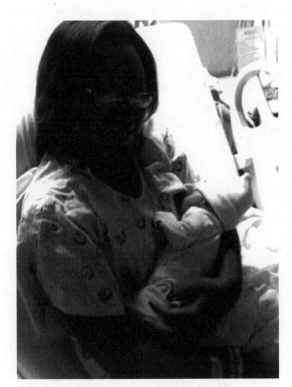

Figure 22-1 Food for Your Baby

Feeding your baby gives both the new mother and father a special and unique satisfaction. Physicians and nurses categorically recommend breastfeeding to their patients (unless the patient has pre-existing breast condition that precludes such). The second best recommendations is to both breastfeed and bottle-feed as needed. They consider bottle feeding and dad's involvement as a third best alternative. Truly, what is best for each family (and for the baby) depends on the personal abilities, desires and needs of the new parents. A third party or book should not pre-judge any one method as superior. This section of the book explains the advantages and disadvantages of breastfeeding and bottle feeding. The mother herself must make her own personal decision.

Breastfeeding

Breastfeeding is enjoying renewed popularity and enthusiasm. The 20th century of yesteryear believed that advances in science would allow Americans to perfect a "formula" better than that which nature had made by herself. Expectations of giving their newborns advanced enriched formulas, coupled with confused sexual implications of breastfeeding, had swung the pendulum toward bottle feeding. However, that pendulum has again swung back toward breastfeeding, as the generations of the 1960's and 1970's have "come back to nature."

No health professional or formula-producing company can dispute the superiority of breast milk over any man-made formula. Breast milk has exactly the right balance of human protein, lactose, fat, vitamins and minerals to nourish a newborn. Formulas such as Similac or Prosoybee are respectively cow-based or soybean-based protein mixtures. They are absolutely perfect for baby cows or baby soybeans, but not as good for baby humans. More importantly, some newborns are allergic to cow proteins or cannot digest the milk carbohydrate, i.e., lactose, which is contained in most formulas. Blacks in particular, are frequently lactose-intolerant. Bottle feeding newborn Black babies may not be possible if they are lactose intolerant.

TMI Historically, it was reported that one formula-manufacturing company began promoting and exalting the great benefits of bottle feeding to third world nations (in order to sell more formula and dry milk powders). They began their great pitch in Africa without realizing that many African Black newborns were lactose-intolerant.

Unable to digest these formulas, many Black newborns suffered until breast milk could be restored into their mother's breasts.

Besides being nutritionally perfect, breast milk is the original *convenience food*. No preparation is required. It is readily at hand. It requires no heating or defrosting. It goes wherever you go. Better yet, there is no clean up!

Breast milk also has important medical advantages: it contains antibodies against many of the diseases that the mother herself has experienced during her lifetime. When she is nursing, her newborn receives this passive "immunization" against these diseases. Accordingly, her baby immediately becomes protected from many of the bacterial, viral and fungal infection that the mother had ever experienced in all her years of life. The baby receives the benefits of a mother's lifetime ordeals with previous infectious disease.

It is well known that breastfed babies are thinner than their bottle-fed counterparts. There is no bottle to empty when nursing. Therefore, when the breasts are empty or the baby stops feeding, nature has decided when *enough is enough*. No over-feeding occurs. Lastly, breastfed babies are less likely to contract diarrhea due to maternal antibody presence in breast milk. Also, there are much greater chances of microbiological contamination of formula during preparation, cleaning and storage of bottles, nipples and formula itself.

Advantages of Breastfeeding

- Natural nutritional composition
- Original convenience and "fast food"
- Passive immunization from microbiological diseases due to secretion and presence of maternal antibodies in breast milk
- Decreased risks of diarrhea
- Decreased risk of over -fed and subsequent fat babies (and possibly fat adults!)

Disadvantages of breastfeeding almost entirely affect the mother, and uncommonly the baby. Breastfeeding can be quite messy (and embarrassing) with milk leaking through breast pads and dresses. If the nursing mother is not careful, nipples may crack, causing pain and occasionally leading to breast infection. If baby sleeps through a feeding or mom and dad go out for the evening, breasts can become engorged (swollen with milk) and become very uncomfortable. Awakening the baby and nursing before such a night out may solve this problem.

After nursing is stopped and the baby is weaned, stretch marks (*striae*) and decreased support (sagging) may irreversibly affect the beauty of the mother's breasts as they may have existed prior to the pregnancy. Ways to decrease such effects are discussed later in this chapter. Of course, nursing necessarily means that all feedings must be given by the mother: dad is left to sleep uninterrupted through the night. Actually, many a supportive dad will go to the nursery, soothe the crying baby, change the diaper, and bring the baby to the nursing mother while she rests a little longer in bed. Some women may also be too shy to nurse in locations outside the home (such as restaurants, swimming pools, supermarkets). A receiving blanket or other covering can shield the breast in such public settings.

Disadvantages of Breastfeeding

- Sore and painful nipples
- Breast engorgement
- Breast infection (mastitis)
- Messiness and social embarrassment
- Impediment to early return to work

Lastly, many women may not desire to nurse because their occupation or economic circumstances demand that they return to work within six weeks of delivery. To them, the establishment of a good nursing routine that is slowly or abruptly halted by weaning may not be worth the bother. There are many ways to solve such problems so that she can return to work and yet continue breastfeeding full time. Consult a lactation specialist that is affiliated with your physician's office or call the La Leche League or Nursing Council for assistance. Parenthetically, it is the author's experience that less than five percent of women continue to nurse full or part-time after they go back to work.

Preparation for Breastfeeding

After delivery the entire nipple is placed into the baby's mouth and, in effect, stretches the nipple out. The baby sucks on the areola, or the brown pigmented thick skin surrounding the nipple itself. By sucking on the areola, the baby compresses the milk reservoirs located directly underneath the areola. The nipple is only a pipeline, a conduit so that milk flows from the milk reservoirs in the areola through the nipple channels into the back of the baby's mouth. Should the baby suck only on the nipple, both mom and baby become upset. The baby obtains little or no milk, and the mother gets sore nipples.

Preparation for nursing can begin before delivery (however, there are some authorities are no longer recommending "nipple preparation" during late pregnancy). During the last four weeks of pregnancy the expectant mother could start "toughening" her nipples. There are techniques that may help to prepare the nipples for the rough treatment they are about to receive from the strong jaws of the baby Pulling the nipple out with two fingers and letting it snap back simulates the same action that occurs when the baby latches onto the breast itself. This pulling or teasing out exercise should be done *gently* fifteen times about four times during the day. Also brushing the breast lightly with a towel may thicken the skin covering the nipple and areola. Cutting out holes in an old bra so that the tops of the breasts protrude and rub up against your blouse or shirt promotes skin thickening and prepares the breasts for the future trauma they are about to receive.

At certain time lanolin-based creams may need to be applied to the breasts either before or after delivery. Many expectant mothers are particularly concerned about the appearance of acne-looking areas appearing on the areola during pregnancy. These raised skin pore-like areas are Montgomery's Glands. They secrete a special lubricating liquid that not only keeps the breast moisturized but also protects the breast from infection because of its antibiotic properties. Should the breast become dry or chapped, lanolin or other moisturizing creams may be applied lightly to the skin.

During pregnancy, the breast may leak or the expectant mother may be able to express a liquid from the nipples. Such a leakage is normal. It is not actually milk, but *colostrum*. Colostrum is a high protein-containing liquid secreted by the breasts during pregnancy and the first few days after delivery. There is no need to express or squeeze the colostrum out during pregnancy. Should a small residue or dried sweat be left on the breast at the end of the day, there is no need to scrub or otherwise harshly rub the nipple and areola. Gentle cleansing with small amounts of soap and water is all that is necessary.

Technique of Breastfeeding

Putting the baby to breast as soon as possible after delivery is the first big step toward successful nursing. If the baby is interested, he/she latches on easily. Automatically the nipple goes to the back of the baby's mouth and the baby sucks on the areola. Colostrum flows. On the other hand, the baby may not be hungry or interested (possibly from the effects of a long labor or certain medications). Do not be disappointed. Most babies are less inclined to any type of feedings for the first 24 to 48 hours after birth.

When nursing, there are several positions in which to hold the baby. Traditionally, the first position is to cradle the baby in your arms with the head of the baby supported in the angle of your elbow and upper arm. The baby's stomach should be approximated and touching your stomach. The baby can lay parallel to you while you are on your side (use pillows behind your back and behind the baby's back for support and positioning).

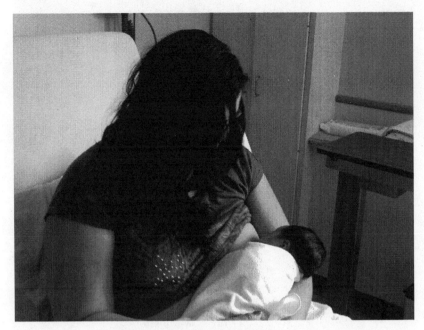

Figure 22-2 Classic Cradle Position

The baby can be held in the "football hold" with the baby's head emerging from under the arm pit. When lying down in bed, you can have the baby lying alongside of you but with the baby's feet above your head and the baby's head propped up against your breast (see illustrations).

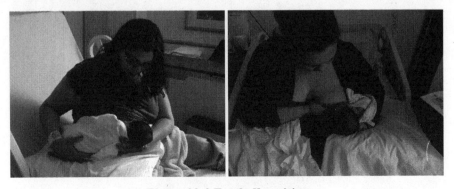

Figure 22-3 Football position

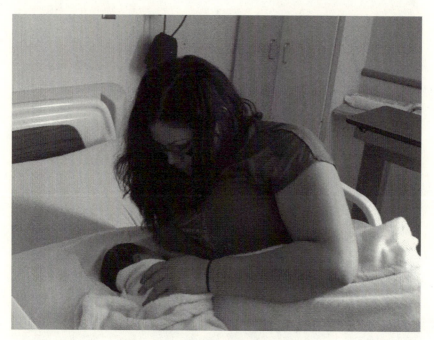

Figure 22-4 Lying down position

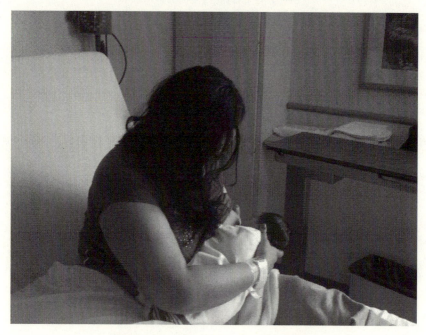

Figure 22-5 Modified Straddle holds

There are probably many other positions possible. Whatever position satisfies you and your baby is perfectly acceptable. The bottom line is that several positions of the baby on the breast provides some change of pace or position for the baby, and allows different sides of the breast to be subjected to the powerful suctioning jaws of the baby. Thus, all portions of the nipple and areola participate and reduce the possibility that only one small area of the breast be continuously suckled.

There is a very succinct guide for the first time "Nursing Mom" to Breast feeding techniques (reference: *American Baby*, to speak, to your baby. The rest of the + *app* on your phone to download videos that demonstrate these techniques) and is summarized as follows:

1. Getting ready for feeding.

Baby should be hungry (he is squirming or putting his fingers or hands in his mouth. Your breasts should be full. Place your thumb and index finger on the outer sides of the nipple, press backward into the breast and express some milk.

2. Putting his mouth on your breast.

Place your thumb on the upper part of your breast at 12 o'clock and your index finger at 6 o'clock and make your nipple "oval shaped." Rub your nipple along his upper lip and the baby will automatically open his mouth. Make sure your baby can breathe: you might need to press down on your breast above his nose with your left hand to help create a small depression or air space so your baby can breathe. Make sure the baby's head is tilted back and supported. Make sure you are comfortable sitting or lying down. A pillow or towel may be necessary to provide support your arm or head.

3. It will feel right for you and your baby.

If your breast does not hurt while nursing and the baby is relaxed, then nursing is proceeding normally. You can always break the baby's suction by placing a finger gently into the baby's mouth and then start again with repositioning the baby's mouth on your breast. The baby's mouth is like a "suction cup" on the breast and the baby uses his tongue to compress the milk out of your breast.

Breast feeding Key Points

1. **Nursing should be initiated as soon as possible after birth (even if by C-section).**

2. **Babies will generally lose about 10% of their birth weight in the first week of life but quickly regain their weight and more quickly.** You should not be discouraged from nursing "because the baby is losing weight and no, "you are not starving your baby!"

3. **Your baby's bowel movements will become lighter in color signifying that you are another "nursing success story."**

4. **Frequently, despite the best efforts by the mother and the baby, you may not be able to breastfeed your baby completely or at all.**

Two more important points in positioning:

- Be sure the baby's head is well supported either by your hand, elbow or pillow. Dad too, may be helpful in this regard. Do not allow the baby's head to hang from your nipple. Sore and painful nipples ensue as a consequence.
- Rotate the baby's place around the breast by utilizing all the above positions. As mentioned above, all areas of the nipple and areola can share in the wear and tear mutually. Furthermore, as described previously, do not allow the baby to suck on the nipple alone. Whether hungry or not, babies love to suck.

Suckling is extremely pleasurable to them. The mouth, jaws and face of the baby become the "center of the universe," so to speak, to your baby. The rest of the baby's anatomy takes a back seat. When the baby's teeth come in (from four to fourteen months of age) do not permit the baby to bite down on your nipple. Immediately take the baby off the breast, talk firmly to the baby with perhaps a light tap across the face so that a definitely negative signal is communicated to your baby. Repeat again and again, if necessary, so that baby learns that biting on the nipple is not permitted at any time. Lastly, when the baby is nursing on the breast, push down on the breast itself with a finger so that the baby's nose is free to breathe. Indenting the breast creates an air pocket so that baby's nostrils are not flush with the breast. Holding your nipple with your second and third fingers pushing in on the breast (the so-called "v" sign) accomplishes the same goal.

Initiation of Breastfeeding

It is important to put the baby to the breast whenever he/she is hungry in the first few days after birth. Even though the baby is receiving only colostrum, it is the suckling that stimulates the production of milk. The more suckling, the faster your milk comes in! Do not get the wrong impression. Colostrum is a very nutritious liquid that is composed of high quality protein. It is important that the baby first breastfeed before offering the baby glucose water, water or formula. Make the baby expend most of his energies suckling. In so doing, this stimulates the formation of more milk. In the first three or four days of life, allow the baby to nurse for about three to five minutes on each breast. The milk usually starts to be produced (*comes in*) within 72 hours after birth. The breasts become full, sometimes overly engorged. With some suckling or with the baby's cries by themselves, "let down" occurs and milk starts to flow.

The baby empties most of the breast within the first 7 minutes. Nursing 10 minutes on each side is more than enough. After 10 minutes the baby is suckling just for the pure pleasure and exercise of suckling in itself. As long as the baby is wetting its diapers (usually every hour or two) and having three or more bowel movements per day, the baby is getting enough.

The baby may be put to the breast every two to six hours as he desires to be fed. This is called *demand feeding*. Scheduled feedings have fallen into some disfavor, but with a little coaxing, most babies can develop a routine so that breastfeeding does not interfere with the rest of the family's daily schedule. For instance, when mom wants to go to sleep around 10 o'clock in the evening, it is quite permissible to wake the baby, give the baby a bath, stimulate and play with the baby, and lastly give the baby two "breast-fulls" of milk. The play activity, the bath and a full stomach tire the baby and allow for a long sleep for both the baby and mom. Also, if desired, a glass of beer or a small amount of other alcoholic beverage allows more milk to flow. Small amounts of alcohol diffuse into the milk (as well as mom) and both sleep longer. Furthermore, alcohol helps to stimulate a greater flow of milk to the baby; baby obtains more nourishment and can sleep longer. Also, mom's breasts are emptied further so that engorgement with new milk is delayed until later in the morning. Within a short duration of time a routine can be established. Should the baby awake in the middle of the night, nursing should be short and matter of fact. The middle of the night is no time for play. Seven (7) minutes on each side in a dimly lighted room and back to bed. A negative attitude toward the middle of the night feedings is quickly sensed by the baby, who avoids such trends in the future.

Sustaining Milk Production

At about three weeks of age (or ten to twelve pounds) the baby's caloric requirements increase. The baby cannot be totally satisfied even with both breasts. The trick is to put the baby to the breast more frequently—even every two hours for more than ten minutes if necessary. The increased suckling naturally stimulated more milk, and in a few days the baby becomes satisfied once again. Your milk is not poor or not rich enough for your baby. Similarly, your baby does not dislike your milk or becomes allergic to it. Pediatricians too easily encourage supplementing your breast milk with formula when they discover your baby had not gained (or even lost) weight from the two week visit compared to the six week visit. Hang in there, baby! Relax, drink more fluids, and understand what is happening. A growth spurt has caused a burst in your baby's appetite. Forewarned is forearmed. It is the author's experience that only one-half of the mothers who attempt nursing at the start are still nursing at their six week postpartum examination. It is because of the frustration of the growth spurts and temporarily low milk supply that causes most mothers to give up prematurely. Many physicians prescribe Reglan to help stimulate milk production during these periods of time: it is available by prescription by your OB and is taken 4 times per day.

Breast Engorgement

The risk of painful breast engorgement is probably lessened by demand type feeding. The hospital environment is not usually conducive to demand feedings. It is difficult for the mother to respond to her baby's sounds and cries of hunger if the nursery is located 35 yards away from her bed. The separation of the maternity beds from that of the nursery is not natural or medically desirable. Some enlightened hospital architects build the maternity beds around the nursery so that the mother's bed and the baby's crib are separated by only a wall—the top half of which is a glass window, so that mom can always see and hear her baby at any time. For more accessibility in some hospitals, all mom has to do in order to feed her baby is to slide out the drawer in the common window wall and the baby is instantly there in mom's arms.

Should engorgement or over swelling of the breast occur, there are several remedies are at hand. First, take a hot shower, or place a warm towel across your breasts. Massage your breasts, pushing down toward your rib cage while at the same time milking your breast and colostrum toward the nipple. Never squeeze or crush your breast tissue. Express a small amount of milk so that the baby can have a taste. Allow your baby to feed as frequently as necessary to relieve the engorgement. If you are still in the hospital, inform the nursery personnel in no uncertain terms that you want to be called or the baby brought to you whenever it is hungry. Above all, do not allow the nurses to give your baby any formula. If your baby's appetite is quenched then it is likely that the next feeding will be a poor one: further aggravating the engorgement problem. Only after the baby has nursed on each side should glucose water or plain water be used to relieve the baby's thirst (not his/her appetite).

Alternatively, if heat is not helpful, an ice pack (or a baggie full of crushed ice, supplied by an ever helpful husband), placed on both breasts may provide relief. In many women, coldness decreases circulation to the breast and allows swelling to dissipate. As in all situations, whatever works best for you is the best solution to your problem. The bottom line again is to avoid engorgement in the first place by

1) Demand feedings;

2) Correct positioning of the baby's mouth onto the areola—not the nipple;

3) Early initiation of nursing in the delivery and recovery rooms and,

4) Rooming in and early discharge from the hospital so that mother and baby can respond to each other's signals and needs.

Should engorgement occur despite your best efforts, breast massage, application of heat or cold as well as more frequent nursing usually alleviates the engorgement. A breast pump, whether manual, battery-operated or electric, may also be helpful in engorgement situations and is more fully discussed later in this section.

The Actual Nursing Process

When the baby cries is a normal signal that the baby is hungry. You should go to the baby's room and pick up the baby. Usually the diaper is wet or dirty (or both). Change the diaper and wash your hands (and hope that the baby doe not poop again after the feeding). Drink some fluid because nursing makes you very thirsty. If the baby is in a bassinet next to your bed, use the bedroom or other quiet room to nurse the baby. A living room with other adults or children is not very conducive for the relaxation and quiet required to effectively breastfeed. Soothing music may be played. Other children in the family can be given crayons and coloring books, or may be directed to watch TV, or read (Millennial children usually get turned on with their touch pads or DVD players). Teach other members of the family that breastfeeding time is a special time for all of you, the baby, mother and the other children (doing a favorite play activity).

Requirements for Effective Breastfeeding

A quiet room
A large glass of water or other desired beverage
A comfortable chair
A relaxed atmosphere with soothing music playing in the background

The nursing mother should find a comfortable position in her favorite chair. Many prefer a well-padded rocking chair so she may nurse and rock her baby simultaneously. This rocking motion may become ingrained into the baby's peace of mind so that gliding to and fro in a rocking chair remains an intensely pleasurable experience going into later life as an adult. (Maybe this is the explanation the author loves to rock in his oak rocking chair or delights going on the swing in the playground.) The baby should be placed in a comfortable position with the head well supported. Do not allow the baby to hang the weight of his head from your nipple or breast.

Stroking the side of the baby's face closest to your breast will cause baby to automatically turn its head toward the breast (the "rooting reflex"). Gently rub the baby's upper lip and its mouth automatically opens: another inborn reflex. Guide the nipple way back into the baby's mouth so that the mouth comes down and latches onto the areolar portion of your breast. Sucking commences almost immediately. Remember to create an air pocket by pushing your breast inward just above where the baby's nose comes in contact against the breast itself.

Breastfeeding is one of the most relaxing and pleasurable moments to be experienced by a woman. The closeness felt, the nurturing of another life, the love that is mutually shared, as well as the other deep emotions that are stirred up. Breastfeeding is a very personal and moving experience. Bottle-feeding can capture similar feelings, but some of that "peaceful easy feeling" that occurs as the milk flows through the breast into your baby is compromised.

After about five minutes on the breast, it is best to "burp" the baby. Be sure to break the suction of the baby's mouth on the nipple first. Otherwise sore nipples may ensue (or you will be minus a nipple or two!) Place your finger into the baby's mouth and the large suction hold is broken. Place the baby's head over your shoulder or place the baby square on your lap sitting up. Rub or tap gently on the lower part of the baby's back. Soon the bubble is raised and a large burp may be heard. Be sure that you have a "burping towel" or cloth to protect your clothes.

After one breast is emptied, burp the baby and switch to the other side. If the baby does not finish off the second breast, then start the next feeding session with the second, partially emptied breast. Again burp the baby and check the diaper to see if it needs to be changed. Babies frequently have bowel movements during or shortly after nursing. Depending on the time of day, the baby may be placed back into the crib, played with, or so situated so the rest of the family may function in their usual day-to-day activities.

It is crucial that the nursing mother wear a comfortable bra. Use cotton (never plastic or polyester) breast pad liners to absorb any milk leakage or other moisture. Bras should be accommodating, yet well-designed, to provide comfortable support for the increasing weight of the breasts. In the 60's and 70's many women went braless. The supporting ligaments of the breast became stretched out and weakened. Their breasts lost their round contours and sagged. Bras should be purchased on the large size to make room for further growth and more milk capacity. Bras also may shrink from frequent washing and drying. In reality, the nursing mother should buy several bras during her breastfeeding career. She should also purchase nursing bras designed so that the nursing flaps unbuckle or unsnap from above the breast. It is too hard to see over the breast if such snaps hinge on the bottom side of the cup.

There are some governmental programs that have been promulgated to encourage women to breastfeed. There is no doubt that breastfeeding your baby is the ideal method. *Baby-friendly Hospitals* is such a program. The maternity unit has to pass stringent measures to achieve this acclaimed status. No commercial formula is dispensed or supplied by the hospital in this program. Patients who choose not to breastfeed must purchase and provide the formula for their baby while it is still in the hospital nursery. In the author's opinion, It is truly unfortunate that political agendas and healthcare payments dictate the correct behavior to which patients and physicians must abide.

Lactation Specialist Deanna Price, RN, Has Some Special Advice

Breasts and Breastfeeding

Choosing not to breastfeed

If you choose not to breastfeed, it is recommended that you bind your breast with a tight fitting bra. No stimulation of the breasts is recommended: it is to your benefit. This suppression of stimulation may need to be done for 3-7 days up to a week. Every woman's response is different. It is important that you sleep in your bra and avoid sleeping on your side or stomach. Do not stand in the shower and allow the water to run over the breasts as this too can cause stimulation and encourage milk to come in. Cabbage leaves are especially useful for the drying up of milk. Essentially, you need a large head of green leaf cabbage. Pull off the leaves so that they are large and freeze them separately. Once they are frozen, drape them around the breasts leaving the nipple exposed. Then bind yourself with a tight fitting bra (or ace wraps). As the cabbage leaves become soggy, throw them away and replace them with fresh ones. The smell during this time may be undesirable. However, 24 hours of using the cabbage can result in a drastic reduction in your supply with minimal discomfort. Cabbage leaves can be used for this purpose for 24 to 48 hours. You must understand that no method is a guarantee. Some women will have milk despite their best efforts. Remember to wear a tight-fitting bra and the use of ice packs to reduce soft tissue swelling is also a great help. Ice should be used every two hours for 20 minutes at a time. Medications such as ibuprofen and Tylenol can assist with the discomfort as well. Check with your Health Care Provider (HCP) on how often to take these analgesics.

Breastfeeding

If you decide to nurse, the nipple and areola should be washed with warm water only. The areolas are supplied with Montgomery glands" These glands secrete a natural lubricant that cleanses and helps to toughen the nipple in preparation for nursing as well as encouraging the infant to nurse. There is no need to attempt to toughen the nipple ahead of time. Do not attempt to toughen them by using a washcloth and rubbing them. Excess stimulation of the nipple can cause oxytocin to be released from the hypothalamus that could cause and contribute to preterm labor. Care of the nipples and areolas is as simple as rinsing them with warm water only. Does not use soap on the nipple or areola as soaps have drying agents in them and can cause the Montgomery glands to dry and interfere with their physiologic function.

Unless dry or cracking, do not use lotions, oils, or creams on the nipples as these can clog the Montgomery glands, and again, they will not work as they are designed.

Whenever possible, it is recommended that you allow the nipples to air dry after showering, breastfeeding, etc. Air drying can assist in the preparation as well as healing of sore nipples. This technique will also allow the nipple to become erect when exposed to cool air. It is important that the nipples protrude to accomplish a good latch with minimal difficulty. If your nipples are flat or inverted (or they do not become erect with cold air), it is imperative that you seek assistance from a Lactation Consultant at least a week prior to delivery. There are "shields" that can be worn to assist with this problem. It is to your benefit that you seek assistance *prior* to delivery to avoid any unnecessary frustration for both you and your baby. If you have any concerns on whether you need shields, you can contact your Lactation Consultant for a consultation and she can determine if you need shields or not.

Once lactation has begun, the use of lanolin can be used to assist with dryness, cracking, soreness, and bleeding of the nipples. Nipple soreness is a normal process associated with breastfeeding in the first week postpartum. It generally peaks on the 4th day and should subside by the 7th. However, every woman is different: the time frame can vary with each nursing mom.

There may be excruciating pain with initial latch on but that pain should subside with 30 seconds of suckling. If the pain is excruciating throughout the feeding, there may be other problems that require immediate evaluation by a Lactation Consultant. Most of the time, it is simply a positioning of baby problem that is causing this discomfort. If you choose to use lanolin on the breast, there is no need to wipe that lanolin off prior to latching your baby on. It is completely safe for your baby. The process of trying to clean it off usually leads to increased trauma to the nipple which only complicates the situation. You may note the appearance of a blister on the baby's lip. This is completely normal and is as result of the intense suckling by the baby and no treatment is necessary.

If your breast develop a hard swollen, reddened area that becomes warm to the touch and accompanied by flu like symptoms, it is important to contact your HCP as mastitis can develop. Mastitis usually requires antibiotic therapy to cure. If you should develop mastitis, DO NOT *discontinue* breastfeeding. Mastitis is not an infection of the milk, it is a breast infection and breastfeeding should continue. It is recommended that breastfeeding begin on the side with the mastitis at each feeding until the mastitis clears up.

As for medication use during pregnancy, many medications are compatible with breastfeeding. If you are taking a medication and nursing, please check with your HCP (Health Care Provider) or your Lactation Consultant to ensure that your meds are compatible with nursing. It is not recommended that you take anything with an antihistamine in it. Antihistamines include medications such as Benadryl, Claritan, Zyrtec and Chlor-Tri-Metron. Antihistamines are used to dry up our sinuses and they will also dry up our milk. Please avoid other medications with antihistamines in them as well. Be sure to check the labels of OTC meds to ascertain whether they might contain antihistamine ingredients.

Breastfeeding is a 24 hour job. Normally infants will feed every 2-4 hours to include throughout the night. It is very important to maintain an adequate milk supply. Remember if you do not feed often enough or omit or delay any feedings, such inactivity can affect your milk supply. If you feel your milk supply is diminishing, your infant is not being satisfied and he may be at risk of losing weight. Please contact your HCP. They can help you augment your milk supply by prescribing a mediation (Reglan 10 mg) that can help boost your milk supply.

Engorgement is another problem you will most likely encounter in the first 10 days postpartum. As your milk comes in, soft tissue swelling usually ensues. Soft tissue swelling can cause engorgement, which in turn, can produce breast pain. The use of ice packs can assist with the reduction of the soft tissue swelling. Frequent feedings, not skipping or delaying feedings, is also a sure way to assist with the engorgement. If you feel your infant is not completely emptying the breasts with each feeding, it may become necessary to pump the breasts after feedings to remove the remaining breast milk. A complete or close to complete removal of breast milk helps to keep your milk supply up to capacity. When breast milk is left in the breasts, it signals our bodies that we have too much. Leaving milk in the breast with can cause a reduction in the hormone stimulation necessary to sustain lactation. Incomplete emptying of the breast can, In turn, cause a resultant reduction in your milk supply.

Positioning of the infant at the breast is essential for a good latch and proper transfer of milk from the breast to the infant. It is important to remember that whatever position you choose to use, belly to belly or chest to breast should be used in positioning. Remember, that you and I do not sit down to dinner and eat our meals with our heads turned to the side; infants also do not want to eat in this manner. Try to look at your infant and ensure he is in a proper body alignment. He should be against your chest with his head in a perfect alignment with his body. It is also important to support the breast with your hand during feedings. Once the infant latches on, do not let go of the breast. Remember gravity takes over when we do not support our breasts. If this happens, your infant is now playing tug of war with gravity. Lack of support of your breast leads to the following: increased soreness, cracking, and bleeding of the nipples. Remember, your nipples are delicate objects and suckling is new and traumatic to them.

Lastly, if you experience problems with breastfeeding that you feel require attention, please do not hesitate to contact your PCP or LC for assistance. Breastfeeding is the most nutritious start you can give your baby. It is perfectly matched nutrition and your success is important to your baby, to you and your medical support team. Remember, breastfeeding may be natural but it is a "learned art." And just as we have to practice dancing to get good at it, breastfeeding has to be practiced by you and your infant to get good at mastering it. Not all babies come out of the womb knowing how to nurse. Most of the time, they have to be taught. Do not expect miracles. Patience is the key.

Breast Infection (Mastitis)

Infection of the breast is a fairly common occurrence. Bacteria, usually of the staphylococcal or streptococcal variety, enter the breast through a crack in the skin. The skin and tissues of the breast provide a great culture media for those bacteria to grow and rapidly proliferate. Pain, redness and swelling of a small area of the breast usually herald the beginnings of a breast infection. Fever, incredibly out of proportion to the extent of the infection, may rapidly reach 103 degrees Fahrenheit. As if she were struck the mighty flu, the nursing mother feels greatly weakened and tired. Chills, headache, body flushing and muscle aching occur as well.

The nursing mother should not hesitate to call her physician immediately. He may have her come to the office for an examination. Alternatively, after several careful questions over the phone, she may be prescribed an antibiotic medication to combat the infection. An antibiotic such as penicillin or erythromycin is usually quite effective in killing the offending bacterial organisms. The mastitis patient should, at the same time, remind her physician of any drug allergies she has or of other medications she is simultaneously taking. Any medication that she is given does enter the breast milk in small amounts. However, such prescribed antibiotics are safe to take. Even though such medication can diffuse into your milk in trace amounts, it is safe for your newborn. An antibiotic is a valuable therapy in order to fight off the breast infection.

Mastitis will not alter significantly your breastfeeding regimen. Do not stop nursing on the breast on which the infection is located. Start nursing on the unaffected breast first. Then proceed, if necessary, to the affected side. Most breast infections take the form of a superficial cellulitis of the external breast skin that is away from the areola and nipple. Consequently, there is little risk that bacteria spreading from the infection can affect the milk. Even a breast abscess within the breast itself is walled-off and separated from the ducts carrying the milk toward the nipple. Any bacteria or pus that inadvertently does contaminate the milk and is swallowed by the baby is rapidly digested and sterilized by the strong peptic acids in the baby's stomach.

Clogged Ducts

Occasionally a lump or bulge may be felt or observed in the breast. Milk ducts may become plugged and give rise to a milk cyst. Breast massage, as described previously, may open and relieve the obstruction. Should swelling occur, an ice pack (a plastic bag of crushed ice) may be applied to the cyst. Swelling and edema around the duct is relieved and the compressed passageway opens up. Sometimes a physician may have to aspirate the milk cyst with a small needle in order to treat the problem. A special type of medication can be given to contract the glands and ducts so milk is pushed against the blocked passageway. The obstructed or narrowed duct is thus forced open and the blockage relieved.

Swollen Glands under your Arms

The glands, or lymph nodes, in your arm pit or at the top side of your breast may become swollen and painful at any time after the inception of lactation. More likely, these glands react during the initiation of breastfeeding, mastitis, plugged ducts and weaning of the baby. No treatment is necessary. However, Tylenol® (generic name is acetaminophen) and heat may alleviate any discomfort. These glands shrink and disappear within one to two weeks after lactation initiation. Any swelling or lump that persists beyond this time warrants an examination by your physician.

Embarrassing Let-Down

At various times and under certain selected conditions, breastfeeding mothers may experience an accidental "let down." In such a situation, try to prevent the let-down by concentrating on some other thought while simultaneously pressing your hands firmly against your breasts. Alternatively, hold your arms and hands in the praying position, hopefully preventing the let-down.

Inverted Nipples

Women with inverted nipples can breastfeed as well as those with extroverted ones. The nipples can be teased out and women can learn how to bring them out in the latter part of pregnancy. Nipple shields that hold the nipple out are available at your local drug store or from your local breastfeeding support groups or lactation consultant (other resources are The Nursing Council and the Le Leche League).

A cube of ice may be applied to the inverted nipple. The muscles around the nipple contract and make the nipple become erect. The nipple comes out from its inverted position so the baby can latch on and breastfeed very satisfactorily.

Previous Breast Surgery

Mothers with breast augmentation, whether under the breast or under the muscle, retain the ability to nurse normally. However, almost 90% of mothers with breast reduction surgery in which the nipples were surgically circumscribed and re-implanted higher the chest cannot nurse. Breast *lift* surgery has a variable effect. If you desire to nurse, you should obtain a copy of your operative report from your plastic surgeon so that your physician or lactation consultant can review the findings

Baby Favoring Only One Breast

Occasionally the baby desires to nurse on one breast and not the other. Physiologically and physically, both breasts are usually the same. Breasts in most women are not exactly the same size: it seems one side may be a little larger than the other. The nursing mother should try to get baby to feed on the "undesirable" breast first. Before putting the baby to that breast, however, perform manual breast massage. "Milking the milk" toward the milk reservoirs under the areola may make breastfeeding easier on this breast. Express some milk through the nipple so that baby obtains immediate gratification for very little work. Repeating this sequence feeding after feeding hopefully makes this breast just as desirable as the other one. Lastly, you can place a thin layer of corn syrup, honey or other sweet liquid on that nipple to make that breast taste better.

Nutrition for Breastfeeding

How much fluid do I need to drink when breastfeeding? Almost all women can breastfeed; yet, some women complain they are not making enough milk. A review of these mother's diets usually shows they are not drinking enough fluids. Your body will be unable to make enough milk if you do not provide it with the right materials. You should drink 12 to 16 eight-ounce glasses of water each day. You can substitute milk, juice, tea or other liquids for some of the fluids. A good rule of thumb is to sit down with a large glass of water each time you nurse. In this way, you will be replacing the fluids baby will be drinking in preparation for the next feeding. Thus, you will be staying one step ahead of the game.

Can I start a weight loss diet when breastfeeding?

Your body will burn up approximately 1,000 calories each day in making breast milk. Your body has made preparations for some of your caloric needs by storing up extra fat during your pregnancy. To make good quality milk and yet allow your body to use some of that stored fat, we recommend you use 500 calories from your fat store and eat an additional 500 calories in your diet. This means if you usually are consuming 1,800 calories per day before you were pregnant, you would require 2,300 calories while you are breastfeeding (losing 500 calories per day). In this way, you should lose around four to five pounds of stored fat each month. If you gained an excessive amount of weight during your pregnancy and have difficulty fitting in light exercise like walking, an additional 300 calories in your diet would be sufficient.

More important than calories you ingest, you should enough protein in your diet to make quality milk. As previously discussed, protein rich foods include fish, chicken, eggs, dairy products and meat. Your body requires extra 20 grams of protein per day. This protein will go into your breast milk. Your baby will use this protein to make muscle, blood, hormones, enzymes and as well as antibodies to help fight infections. To increase your diet by 300 calories and 20 grams of protein, you should eat an extra two ounces extra of a protein rich food (such as eggs, meat, chicken, fish or cheese) and one extra glass of milk.

Continue to take your prenatal vitamins as long as you are breastfeeding. You will need vitamins and minerals for your body as well as for the baby's. Also, eat a balanced diet with whole grain breads and cereals, fruits and vegetables, and milk.

Try to drink five glasses of milk (low-fat or nonfat) each day. You can substitute one glass of milk with other foods from the dairy group, such as cheese, yogurt, puddings or even ice cream. Milk provides the most utilizable source of calcium. If you are unable to drink milk or eat dairy products, you will need to take a calcium supplement (only those women who have a history of kidney stones should be wary of calcium supplements). Calcium is used primarily in the development of bones and teeth in your infant. If you do not obtain adequate calcium in your diet, calcium will be mobilized out from your bones. This will leave mom's bones more porous and can lead to osteoporosis (fragile bones that break easily) in your later years of life. Therefore, you need to take your diet seriously and monitor what you eat while you are breastfeeding. As they say, "make your calories count."

How do I know when there is enough milk?

You will know that you are making enough milk if your baby gains weight (approximately three to seven ounces per week). Another indicator is to monitor the baby's diapers. He/she should soak his/her diapers and have about six to ten (or more) wet diapers a day. If your baby had less than six wet diapers, you may want to nurse more often by waking your baby if he/she sleeps for long periods of time.

How often should I feed?

Breastfed babies may feed more frequently than formula fed infants since breast milk is easier to digest than formula. Physicians and nurses recommend feeding *on demand*, i.e. whenever baby is hungry. Usually a newborn will want to eat every two to three hours around the clock. As your baby grows, he will nurse less often. Your baby will need only breast milk (or formula) for the first four to six months of life. Do not begin feeding cereals or baby food until your baby is in this age range. His stomach and intestines are not mature enough. Large particles such as bacteria can more easily pass through the gut wall into his body. Solid food feedings can lead to more gastrointestinal infections or distress such as diarrhea and flu symptoms. Your pediatrician or dietician will be able to give you a more detailed feeding schedule upon request. A good reference book for feeding is *Child of Mine: Feeding with Love and Good Sense* by Ellyn Satter, R.D., Bull Publishing Company.

Milk Expression

The majority of breastfeeding women, at one time or another will need to express milk. Whether you are going to be a working mother or not, it is to your advantage to know and understand milk expression. For some women, the success of breastfeeding depends upon the amount of anxiety produced during all of these new experiences. Hopefully, you will find your questions answered here; if not, be reassured that your doctor will be able to advise you.

Most women are fortunate enough to begin breastfeeding shortly after childbirth. Putting your baby to your breast immediately is beneficial to all: baby obtains immediate valuable nutrition. Further, prompt nursing helps your uterus contract which, in turn, helps to minimize postpartum bleeding. The uterus more quickly shrinks down, or *involutes*, and stimulates the uterus to more promptly return to its pre-pregnancy size. Mother-infant bonding is facilitated. Breastfed babies are usually fed on demand. The baby's milk supply is secured by these frequent feedings. Mother and infant soon return home where the nursing and the nurturing experience continues with each feeding. Eventually though, the breastfeeding mother will find it necessary to be apart from her infant. She is then faced with two options. She may supplement with formula, which may cause the baby confusion and/or decrease her milk supply. Or, she may decide to express breast milk and leave it for bottle use. The latter is preferable for two reasons:

1) The baby has consistency and is used to the same milk, and

2) The mother's milk supply is maintained.

Facilitating Milk Expression

In order to facilitate the expression of milk, it is desirable for you to be able to stimulate the "let-down" or flow of milk. Normally, "let down" is done by the baby sucking. Stimulation of the nipple causes various hormonal responses causing the milk to flow. Once you are able to accomplish this let down, the work of pumping is virtually eliminated. Since it can take anywhere from one to several minutes of sucking for the baby to stimulate a "let-down," you should allow yourself this amount of time also for your milk to come in.

How to Express

Prior to expressing your milk when nursing, you should first carefully wash your hands. Hand washing should be done before handling the breasts while breastfeeding. The "let-down" reflex may be accomplished by continuous, gentle rolling of the nipples with your thumb and forefinger. Concentrate on the image of your baby sucking and visualize your milk flowing, and you should achieve success. Once the "let-down" reflex begins, you are ready to simply let the suction of your breast pump withdraw your milk. Amazingly, psychological and emotional influences have a direct effect on milk production. After expressing several times, you should become proficient at it. With such experience in milk expression you may now find extra time for reading, eating a snack or just taking this opportunity to relax!

Emphasis has been on the "let-down" reflex in order simply to point out that, by stimulating milk flow, pumping is made easier. It is not essential to do *express* in order to pump. If you are unable to stimulate milk flow, you will still be able to express your milk. Application of warm compresses, as well as gentle massage of the breasts prior to pumping, will facilitate the removal of milk.

Milk Supply

When expressing milk, it is important to remember that building your milk supply is a gradual process. Pay particular attention to maintaining a good fluid intake, proper nutrition, and adequate rest. You will eventually be able to recognize subtle changes that will clue you to the need for more rest or fluids. Intake of adequate fluids has a direct effect on milk production. If you are planning on going back to work, begin building your milk supply one to two months before your planned return. Building an adequate milk supply or surplus will enable you to store milk in the freezer. By building an adequate milk supply from the start, you can be assured that you will have enough supply at the end. Remember, unnecessary anxieties about going back to work can hinder milk production. So it is better to prepare yourself mentally for your return as well.

When to Express

Since all babies have different appetites and eating times, you will have to be the judge of when it is a good time for you to express. At first, you might try expressing milk either a couple of hours before baby's next feeding (or at least one hour after the last feeding). Don not be discouraged at getting only small amounts in the beginning; Remember, the more milk you express, the more milk you will produce. If you've recently fed the baby, then plan on getting little milk if any—babies are great at completely emptying the breasts! After establishing an adequate milk supply, some women are able to pump one breast while nursing the baby on the other. Of course, use of an easy to handle pump is essential for this pumping.

Breast Pumps

<u>Manual Pumps</u>: These are difficult to handle, time consuming, and require constant effort on your part (you are the energy source).

<u>Electric Pumps</u>: Although effective, they may be expensive and inconvenient (most are battery powered and effective or, if you rent a commercial type, a source of electricity is required to operate them). Reference: http://www.medela.us/

<u>Battery-Operated Pumps</u>: These pumps seem to be the answer for today's on-the-go mother. They are lightweight (approximately 8 ounces), easy to clean (dishwasher safe, boilable, and only three parts require cleaning), easy to handle (requires only one hand to use), fits easily into your purse and operates on two AA batteries. This pump provides the suction power of an electric pump, yet allows the ease of operation and portability that none of the others offer. It is priced only slightly higher than the manual pump.

Storing Breast Milk

After expressing breast milk, it should be placed into a sterile container (plastic bottle liners are convenient) and into the refrigerator. If you do choose to use plastic liners, be sure to secure the top with a bag tie or rubber band, and keep the bag upright in a cup to avoid spillage. Breast milk should be kept in the refrigerator no longer than 48 hours. It may then be placed in the freezer for further storage. Once frozen, in a conventional refrigerator-freezer, breast milk can be stored for approximately six weeks. In a deep-freezer breast milk can be stored for approximately six months. If you need to add fresh milk to already frozen milk, first refrigerate the fresh milk for a couple of hours before adding it. Breast milk should never be reheated, reused or left at room temperature, as it is perfect media for bacterial growth.

Thawing Breast Milk

Breast milk should be thawed gradually by placing the container under cold running water that is eventually made warmer until the milk is defrosted. You may then place the milk in warm water until the desired temperature is reached.

Breastfeeding Sequence in Brief

1. Pick up your baby and change the diaper as necessary.

2. Wash your hands.

3. Drink a large glass of fluid. Have another glass handy just in case you become thirsty again while nursing.

4. Be sure baby is definitely awake and has an appetite.

5. As necessary, do breast massage so that milk is brought from the breast ducts to the milk reservoirs under the areola.

6. Place baby in a comfortable position for you and be sure to support the baby's head so that it does not hang from the nipple.

7. Remember that the baby obtains 90 percent of the milk from one breast in less than seven minutes.

8. Burp baby as needed so that air trapped in baby's stomach is released.

9. Nursing preferably should take place in a private room favorable for relaxation and peace. A comfortable rocking chair and soothing music promote such an atmosphere.

Bottle-feeding

At various selected times after childbirth, women elect to bottle-feed. As mentioned elsewhere in this book, it is recommended that even breastfed infants become familiar with a nipple and bottle—just in case mom and dad go out for an evening. Many ardent breastfeeding advocates may take issue with this last statement. They think it's almost sacrilegious to offer a breastfeeding baby an artificial nipple and bottle. After such an offer, the baby may refuse the bottle because of his unfamiliarity with it. Prepare and familiarize your baby with the bottle. You never know when it may be necessary to express, freeze and store breast milk not fully taken by the baby.

Many women decide to bottle-feed their baby right from birth. These women may have to return to work early or feel more comfortable with the advantages that bottle feeding has to offer. Specifically, such women avoid the discomforts of breastfeeding and allow other members of the family to share in the feeding of the baby. Feeding-sharing permits an equitable distribution of caring, bonding and sleeping. Women who decide to bottle-feed should inform their physician of their decision in the last few weeks of their pregnancy. Because milk usually comes in without nursing, their physician can prescribe medication so that milk production and subsequent breast engorgement does not result. A hormone injection of estrogen or estrogen-androgen combination given just prior to delivery suppresses the entire lactation process. Alternatively, pills can be given orally for the first two weeks after birth to prevent the breast milk from forming. Despite such medications and injections, some patients still experience milk production. No method is guaranteed and nature can be persistent. In such cases, a tight bra and ice packs may alleviate any uncomfortable engorgement. Above all, do not squeeze, massage or try to express such milk. It only stimulates the formation of more milk.

It is the author's opinion that it is the unique physical nature and personalities of both the baby and the mother that ultimately determines the success or failure of breastfeeding. Some babies have such an insatiable appetite that the mother may be breastfeeding every two hours for thirty minute sessions. If such a harsh schedule is maintained for any length of time, that mother is going to tire with the effort. She cannot keep up with that baby's lactation requirements. Possibly the mother's breast itself has milk glands that do not produce the proper quantity of milk to satisfy the baby's needs. Stress, lack of adequate fluids, confidence, living conditions and other demands may impact on the success of a proper milk supply. In past times and cultures in which breastfeeding was the only method of nourishing a newborn, babies probably became thinner if their pleas for more milk were not met. Yet they survived. In such situations a wet nurse, i.e., a mother who kept her breasts functioning after weaning her baby to other foods, could also be called in to help a mother who was having difficulties with breastfeeding. On the other hand, some women have more than enough milk. In fact, their baby's demand cannot keep up with mom's supply! In such cases women can donate their extra milk to local milk banks to be used for premature babies and babies with other special dietary needs.

It is true that any woman can breastfeed. However, the author does not believe that women should force the issue on themselves or be forced into breastfeeding by others. You should not continue to breastfeed no matter how difficult it becomes. A frustrated baby and mother is the usual result. No medical study has ever shown any differences in the mental or physical health of the infant based on whether the baby was breastfed, bottle-fed, or a combination of both. What is most important is whether the feeding is given in a caring, tender and loving manner to the baby.

A *common myth* is that women with large breasts can provide more milk for their babies. In fact, a woman with very large breasts does not have any better breastfeeding capabilities than one who is flat-cheste.! Each has the same number of milk glands and ducts. Large breasts are only large because of the extra amount of fat deposited between these milk glands.

If bottle-feeding is chosen initially or supplementation is started later, the new mother can be reassured that there are a number of excellent commercially-made formulas available. In fact, mom can make up her own formula from dried milk, water, syrup and other ingredients. Homemade formulas can be found in many books on baby care. Consult with your pediatrician or family physician to see if your formula meets the necessary growing needs of your baby.

Commercially Available Formulas	
Similac®	Cow-lactose based
SMA®	Cow-lactose based
Enfamil®	Cow-lactose based
Soylac®	Soybean-based protein
Isomil®	Similac® Soy Isomil®. Soy for fussiness and gas
Pro-soy-be®	Soybean-based protein

Some formulas are fortified with added iron. Such formulas with iron may make your baby's bowel movement harder and more difficult to pass. Constipation and colicky pain may ensue. Most babies do not need to be supplemented with extra iron until they are at least three months of age. One should discuss the use of iron-enriched formulas with the baby's doctor before giving it to baby.

There are limited advantages to buying formulas that are labeled "ready to feed." Ready-to-feed formulas mean just that. They can be poured from the can right into the baby's bottle. Such formulas are convenient and can be carried in the baby's bag when away from home. No preparation is necessary, although they are more expensive and weigh more when carried around. Unused portions can be stored in the refrigerator for up to 24 hours. Thereafter, the formula should be discarded. Dried concentrate formulas need to be reconstituted with water. They are cheaper, weigh less to carry, and can be stored longer in powder form. Once prepared, formula should be utilized within 24 hours and then discarded. Tap water is perfectly satisfactory to use in preparing such formulas from the concentrated powders.

Nipples and bottles may be washed in the same manner as your other dishes and utensils. In the past, physicians recommended that everything be sterilized. Bottles and water were boiled. Physicians thought at the time that a newborn's stomach and intestinal tract was sterile, completely clean and free of all bacteria. Doctors wanted all nipples, bottles and formula sterile too. It was felt that when bacteria got into the baby's intestines, various diarrheas would result. Diarrheas presented a formidable medical problem. Today, medical scientists know that the baby's intestinal tract becomes rapidly colonized with a layer of protective bacteria within twelve hours of birth. Accordingly, bottles and nipples can be washed in the sink or in the dishwasher without harm. Be careful that the dishwasher is not too hot. Otherwise the nipples will melt!

Advantages of Bottle-feeding

1. allows other members of the family to feed baby (particularly in the middle of the night).

2. Avoids damage to breast skin (stretch marks) and supporting ligaments.

3. Avoids complications of nursing, such as mastitis.

4. Avoids engorgement, leakage and embarrassing let-down between feedings.

Lactation Suppression:

If you are going to bottle-feed only and want to prevent your milk from coming in, most experts are recommending *physical* methods of lactation suppression. A tight bra, ice packs, and care not to express milk from your breasts are the key methods. Your breasts will enlarge, perhaps become engorged with milk ("almost like a large rock") but after 3-4 days, your breasts will become less swollen and painful. Milk production will be shut down.

<u>Historical Note</u>: In the past there were medications available for lactation suppression, but they are no longer currently advised. The most common medication in the past was Parlodel® but its use was curtailed due to a reported increased associated risk of a stroke. This medication as well as estrogens can be utilized in some cases when breast engorgement must be completely avoided.

Weight Loss and getting back into Shape

As the author tells his patients prior to their discharge from the hospital, "you will still look pregnant for the next 4 weeks." Your abdominal wall muscles and skin have been stretched out for nearly 9 months and it will take weeks to get your figure back.

You can start a fitness program whenever you are physically able. In the first few weeks walking and using weights may be done. Usually most new moms are too tired to work out in the first 6 weeks after childbirth. After 4-6 weeks patients may go back to their usual physical routine: walking, biking or cycling, swimming, running, stair climber, elliptical, etc.

Weight loss is only accomplished by burning up more calories than you are consuming. Either eat less or exercise more or both!

Weight Management Discussion

1. Food Diary: write down everything you eat (I mean everything!)

2. Water: Drink 8 full 8 ounce glasses per day

3. Do NOT eat if you are not hungry, especially at noon and dinner times

4. Stop eating if you are full and no LONGER hungry

5. Low Carbohydrate diet: South Beach/Atkins diet

6. Muscle toning: treadmill, stepper, NordicTrack work up to 1 hours per day (in front of TV or a video program makes the time go by faster)

7. Good shoes, sweats, water, towels, music, wrist and head sweat bands.

8. Muscles burn calories! Toning and working out is key to long-term success.

9. Calories in minus Calories burned = Net weight loss (or gain!)

10. Avoid processed foods, food additives and preservatives, etc. (according to *Beyond Diet* Nutritionist, Isabel De Los Rios, reference, Beyond Diet.com)

CHAPTER 23

The Newborn

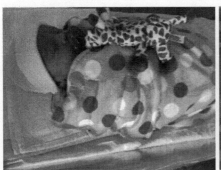 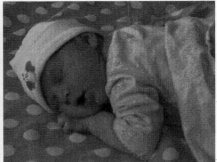

Figure 23-1 Your Newborn baby

Prenatal Visit with Your Pediatrician

It is prudent to set up an appointment with the physician who will be providing your baby his medical care. It makes litte difference whether this physician is a pediatrician or a family physician. The most important issues are (1) whether you feel very comfortable talking with this physician (2) whether he/she is up-to-date with all well-baby and infant care. It is perhaps helpful to know other information about the physician:

1. Board certification or eligibility, experience and years of practice (and does she/he have children?)

2. Office hours (availability during the day or Call Group Arrangements)

3. Phone Number to call at any time

4. The names of other physicians with which he is associated or to whom he has on-call for him when he is off-call or on vacation

5. Office hours (as well as after-hours coverage and emergency care)

It behooves you and your husband (or your significant other, SO) to set up an appointment while you are still pregnant. In this way you both can meet and approve of a physician that has your mutual confidence to take care of your new baby. It is helpful to ask common questions just to "break the ice" at this visit perhaps as follows:

1. Recommendations regarding infant car seats
2. Recommendations regarding positioning of baby at nights and after feeding
3. Vaccination schedule
4. Bathing frequency of baby (type of soap, shampoo)
5. Type of clothing to be worn
6. Treatment of "cradle cap"
7. When to call physician if your baby develops the following: fever, cold, diarrhea, rash, etc.

Hopefully, after such an interview appointment (usually at no cost to the patient), a new relationship between your family and this new physician will have been established.

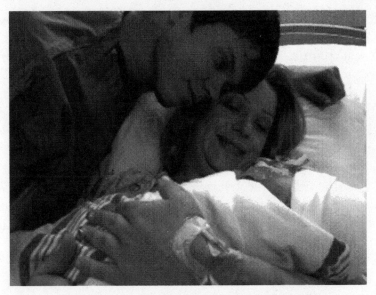

Figure 23-1 Mother, Dad and baby bonding

The Newborn

Now that the baby is born, it is hoped that you have selected a physician for your baby. The baby's physician can be a family physician or a Pediatrician. A Pediatrician is a specialist in Newborn and Child Care extending all the way through the teenage years (until age eighteen is reached). However, many family physicians have special interest and experience in newborn and child care. Though they may be a Board Certified Family Practitioner, they devote much of their attention to the care of children of all ages.

Concept of Parenting

There are many good books and other resources to learn how to become a good parent. Besides providing food, shelter and a warm environment for the newborn, there are many other aspects that go into becoming a "good parent." The background of becoming a good parent stems from the experiences you have had as a child. Your concept of parenthood develops from how your parents, brothers and sisters, relatives, close neighbors and friends have interacted with you. They have all influenced your growth and development as an adult. Many parents have recognized the positive aspects of their upbringing that they would also like to similarly cultivate in their own children. Adults can also recognize the deficits they may have engendered during their upbringing. Parents equally see the "negative role model" their parent portrayed and to which they would like to correct. Parents want to instill more positive behaviors and directions into their own children. Parenting is a very individual phenomenon. Every parent has their own viewpoint on parenting. Each parent may have important quality standards or skills that he would like the child to meet. It is very personal and individual in each couple. The mother and father should discuss their thoughts and goals for their baby and decide on the parenting styles they expect to follow and how they parenting methods should evolve.

The importance of giving your baby a proper name

Naming your baby is a very important obligation of the parents. Your baby will bear this name for the rest of her/his life (unless the name is so upsetting that the child legally changes the name at age 18!). Most couples name their baby after a deceased (or living) relative. Biblical names are always popular: Jesus, John, Mary, Joshua, Mathew, etc. Many fathers will names their child after themselves with the same first name but place a "junior" or the II or III after it. Many times a baby is named after a famous actor or actress at the time. There are many resources for baby names: books, internet sites, family, friends, etc. Many studies have proven how a person's *name* significantly influences the interaction that child will have with regard to acceptance, self-esteem, job opportunities, etc.

Parents feel that their child is unique want to give their baby a name that has never been used. I caution parents to be *very careful* when providing a name for your baby: the name sticks to the child and the name itself can have profound effects on the child and the child's self-image. It may affect or influence tremendously all her/his personal and occupational interactions for the rest of her/his life. Here are some examples of what I call imprudent "naming:"

Family Last names:

>Ball, they named their girl "Crystal"
>
>Register, they named their boy "Cash" Later in life, he married a woman named Carolyn or as she liked to be called, "Carrie" so the couple was always introduced as "Cash and Carrie"
>
>Wood, they named their girl "Holly"
>
>Green, they named their boy, "John Deere"
>
>Daniels, they named their boy, "Jack"
>
>Poole, they thought the girl's name could be "Cess" but they decided otherwise (maybe "Liver")
>
>Lloyd, he wanted to name their boy," Mongo" but she said no!
>
>The Pieces family, naming their baby girl "Reese"

Other names:

>Kanye West and Kim Kardashian named their child "North" (so she is called North West)
>
>Starr: they were not naming their Baby "North" or even "Porno!" How about "Shining?"
>
>Le-ah (from Georgia) pronounced "Ledasha," the dash is pronounced!
>
>Toshiba (from Tennessee), guess she glanced up at the TV screen in the room when she was asked by the Birth Certificate person what she was going to name her baby!
>
>Author anecdote: When the author asks his pregnant patients late in pregnancy what name they are considering for their child, the most frequent name he hears is "Donotknowyet!"

Lastly, the author tells his patients that if their baby boy does not have a name within one minute after birth, the boy's name automatically defaults to "Jeffrey!"

Newborn Health Screening and Testing

In the nursery the nurses will order a standard number of screening tests to diagnose conditions that may not be evident on previous ultrasounds and on the newborn physical exam.

Laboratory Testing

Blood Cell Disorders and Hemoglobinopathies (such Sickle Cell, Thalassemia)

Blood Type and Rh factor (mandatory if mother is RH Positive)

Thyroid Tests (TSH, etc.)

Inborn Errors of Amino Acid Metabolism Panel (such as PKU)

Inborn Errors of Organic Metabolism Panel

Inborn Errors of Fat Metabolism Panel

Cystic Fibrosis (if mother's screen during pregnancy was positive)

HIV

Substance Abuse Panel

Other Newborn Health Screening

Congenital Heart Disease by Pulse Oxygen

Congenital Deafness by a screening Hearing Exam

A detailed list of the newborn screens and their panels are listed in Appendix D (Courtesy of Wikepedia).

Preparing for your baby's arrival at home

There are many excellent resources that are available that you will need to take care of your baby when you bring the little "prince or princess" back to your home. The following is a brief list:

> Car Seat (see Consumer Reports for recommendations)
>
> Crib and/or bassinette (mattress, sheets, blankets, mobile toy, etc.)
>
> Changing Table (straps to hold baby down, storage for diapers, wipes, clothes, etc.)
>
> Diapers, cleansing wipes (cleansing wipe warmer), tissues, towels)
>
> Baby Bath (Baby shampoo, Castile or other mild soap, drying towels)
>
> Clothes (shirt, panties, socks, hand covers (prevent scratching of face with fingernails)
>
> Formula (unless breastfeeding) and baby bottles and nipples with brushes
>
> Diaper bag (with diapers, bottles, formula if bottle feeding, cleansing wipes, change of clothes, binkies, stuffed animals or other toys)
>
> Bulb syringe, Petroleum jelly, hydrocortisone cream (1% Hydrocortisone cream)
>
> Stroller (see Consumer Reports for best advice)
>
> ****Thermometer** (skin, ear, oral or rectal: essential to determine if your baby has a fever)
>
> Pacifiers (at least a dozen because you baby will drop them at anytime and anywhere!)

Newborn Physical Examination

Unfortunately, not every baby that comes out in the Delivery Room looks exactly like the smiling, round headed baby that is on the Gerber's food jar. When a baby is born, there is much blood around the head and arms. Furthermore, there is a white, cheesy cream ("vernix") that covers the baby's arms, hands, face and head.

Immediately after birth and first few days of life the baby's toes and fingers will be blue due to decreased circulation. The temperature control centers in the baby's brain try to preserve body heat and, therefore, purposely decrease blood flow to these areas of the body. *Acrocyanosis* is the medical term for blue fingers, toes, lips and ears in the first few days.

As stated above, the baby, in its attempt to conserve heat, decreases the circulation to the extremities and, accordingly, the fingers and toes are blue. Furthermore, the head is quite swollen from the compression forces that exist in the birth canal. The head will mold and become quite long and narrow. There may be a swelling of the back of the head (known as "caput"). Furthermore, there may be "molding" of the head during delivery so that the baby fits through the pelvic passageway: various shapes can result (occasionally called "cone-heads). The swelling of the scalp and the molding of the head will usually slowly decrease and become almost nonexistent in a few days.

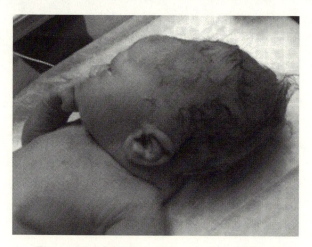

Figure 23-2 Molding of the newborn's head

Occasionally a blood vessel will break in the scalp on the head, usually on one side of the baby's head. This golf ball type lump is called a *cephalo-hematoma*. It may take as long as three months for such a lump to go away. The baby's head is quite malleable or pliable. It is built of soft bony tissue known as cartilage. This type of bone is very elastic so that the baby's head can mold and be quite bendable as it comes through the birth canal. In addition, these soft separated bony plates will allow the head to grow as the baby becomes bigger. Furthermore, these plates are loosely held together: there are defined areas of separation called *suture lines*. These spaces between the bony plates are the areas from which the skull plates can grow and expand. There are *soft spots* on the baby's head, both in front and in back. The front soft spot or *fontanel* is present until approximately 24 months. The posterior fontanel is less defined: I is not as easily detected and is located in the top back part of the head. This posterior fontanel usually will close in 2 months. Furthermore, it is surprising to note that the head is not fully developed until approximately age 2 (although it may seem to never fully develop in some folks).

As we further examine the newborn, we notice that the eyes are quite swollen. Again this is due to the pressures and compression forces during the labor. Quite commonly the baby will open one eye and keep the other eye shut. It is almost like the baby is trying to spy on you without you knowing it. If one looks into the mouth, one can see a couple of whitish pimples or cysts, known as Epstein's pearls, on the top part of the mouth. Occasionally the baby will be born with a tooth. If it happens to be loose, it should be removed: it could detach completely with the danger of the baby breathing the tooth into its lungs. The baby is covered with a fine coat of hair that can be either dark or light. This *lanugo* hair tends to disappear in the first few months of life.

The Baby's Skin

It is quite surprising, but the baby's skin will show many types of reactions. One of the more common reactions in the newborn is called *erythema toxicum*. These are reddish, raised, pimple-like areas on the chest and face, which resemble flea bites. This reaction be caused by some type of hypersensitivity or allergic reaction. These spots are quite temporary and occasionally disappear in hours or days. As you look further at the baby, there may be a dark blue-black discoloration or patch on the baby's buttocks. These "Mongolian spots" are more commonly seen in Asian and in Black babies. They subside anytime from within a few months, but occasionally can last up to 10 years. Small reddish spots can be seen on the back or the nape of the neck. These are called "stork bites." They, too, usually will vanish again within a few years. More commonly parents will note small, whitish type pimples on the nose, cheeks and chin. These little teeny spots are called "milia" and are really small cysts of the skin.

Another type of reaction that appears on the face is distended sweat glands: these skin "pimples" are called "miliaria crystallina." Other kinds of skin spots include "strawberry marks" or hemangiomas, which tend to disappear as the baby goes into early childhood. Rarely, a baby can have "harlequin syndrome," a condition in which the baby will turn half white on the right side of the body and half blue on the other. Harlequin Syndrome is caused by an immature nervous system. The nervous system controls the circulation to the body by increasing or decreasing the caliber of blood flow to these areas. When the body is half white, there is decreased circulation and this part of the body becomes white or anemic. On the other side, the vessels are dilated and, accordingly, because of the generous blood supply in the blood vessels, this part of the body appears blue. This Harlequin phenomenon usually will cease sometime in the first ten years of life.

The baby's chest usually will show enlarged nipples regardless whether the gender of the baby is a boy or a girl. Occasionally a bit of milk will be secreted from the breasts. This milk, called "witches milk" is due to the growth, development and function of the breast glands in the baby. This development of the breasts and milk is directly due from maternal hormones that transfer across the placenta into the baby's circulation. As soon as the baby becomes separated from the mother (i.e. birth), these hormones will cease diffusing into the baby's circulation. Hormones that have crossed over are eventually destroyed (metabolized). The previous development of the breasts will stop and the baby's breast will return to its normal quiescent state.

Benign enlargement of the nipples and breasts will subside by eighteen to twenty-four months.

As one looks at the baby's abdomen, one will see the clamped umbilical cord. The type of belly button that the baby will eventually form is already genetically predetermined. The way the umbilical cord is clamped, tied off or treated has no bearing on the future appearance of the belly button. There have been many attempts in many countries and cultures to try to "customize" the appearance of the belly button. Many such efforts, such as placing Band-Aids, coins, or marbles inside the belly button (or against the cord) simply do not work. Such manipulations will in no way affect the predetermined genetic appearance. In fact, it is discouraged from a medical standpoint that any foreign objects, such as marbles or gauze, be placed or pushed into the belly button for fear of causing infection or other problems. When one looks at the shriveling cord, there are three vessels, two arteries and one vein. There are no nerves in the umbilical cord and, accordingly, one does not need to be worried that touching the shriveling cord will in any way may hurt your baby. It is recommended that the cord be kept clean and dry. Using rubbing alcohol or hydrogen peroxide with cotton balls to keep the area dry and clean is all that is necessary for the cord to shrink and heal. Dryness is the key and the dried cord "stem" will fall off in 10 to 14 days.

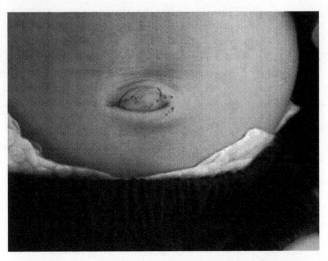

Figure 23-3Umbilical Cord Appearance healed

Author's Note: *no matter what the parent does to keep the cord clean and dry, it may still become moist, green- black and have an odor.*

Usually the shriveled, greenish-blackish, sometimes moist cord will fall off in approximately two weeks. It resembles the stem on an apple.

Furthermore, all babies have "pot bellies" until three to four years of age. There is no need to prevent your baby from crying in order to avoid a pot belly or an umbilical hernia. A hernia is a pooching out of the belly button and many babies have slight umbilical hernias at birth and into early infancy. There really is no need to be any concerned about such hernias; ninety percent disappear by age three. Hernias do not form and become larger by the baby's crying efforts.

The Baby's Genitalia ("Sexual anatomy")

Usually the testes will have descended into the scrotum by birth. If not, they may descend in the first few weeks after birth. Parent and physicians become concerned when there is delayed descent of the testicle. If not descended by one year of age, most experts recommend that they be surgically brought down into the scrotal sac at this time. The tip of the penis is covered with skin much like a flower is covered with its petals. To remove this skin covering of the penis, *circumcision* is done. There is much controversy in today's medical and general community about the advantages and disadvantages of a circumcision. The decision to circumcise your baby should be based on personal, cultural, religious and occasional medical reasons. If you decide to have your baby circumcised, the operation is really quite simple and takes only approximately five minutes. The operation involves minimal discomfort to the baby and, even though the baby does feel the discomfort, it does not cause any permanent mental scars or traumatic memories to the baby. There are two common surgical methods of removing the foreskin in use today in the US. One, *the plastibell method,* involves placing a plastic collar around the penis, which is secured to the penis by a single suture. The foreskin beyond the suture is then trimmed off. Using a different surgical technique, the *Gomco method,* a metal "helmet" is placed over the tip of the penis and, after a clamp seals off the blood and nerve tissue, then the foreskin can be cut safely without bleeding or injury to the penis. The collar does not have to remain on the penis for any extensive period of time.

Care after circumcision

In order to take care of the *Plastibell*-type circumcision, all you need to do is keep the penis clean with plain soap and water. The plastic collar will usually fall off in approximately seven to ten days.

If your baby has the metal type or *Gomco*-type circumcision, then it is recommended that you clean the penis by gently brushing with soapy gauze and then rinse with water. You can apply a little Vaseline around the tip of the penis so it does not stick to the baby's diapers. You should report any bleeding or signs of infection, that is, pus or swelling or redness of the penis, to your physician.

Author's Note: The Gomco or *Mogen*-clamp techniques of circumcision immediately trim the foreskin from the tip of the penis and there is no collar left on it. Almost always a little "discharge" forms around the tip of the penis and looks like pus. Such an icky appearance may look like an infection but this is how the penis looks after the *Gomco* circumcision. The *Plastibell* method keeps the penile "shaft" skin separate from the softer skin of the tip of the penis, the *prepuce*. When the author performs the *Plastibell* method, he tells the parents "that the plastic collar or ring around the tip of the penis will fall off in about 7-10 days (and, in jest, that the penis itself will fall off in another 3 weeks!)""

If one does not choose to circumcise your infant boy, then the care of the uncircumcised penis is really quite simple. One only needs to keep the penis clean with mild soap and water. Push back the foreskin to clean inside the penis. However, if it does not retract, then there is no need to force the issue. As the baby gets bigger, the adhesions between the foreskin and the penis will dissolve which, in turn, allows easier retraction and cleaning inside the penis.

In the newborn females, the baby may have some bleeding noted from the vagina. Because the reproductive hormones from the maternal system during pregnancy will cross over from the placenta, a lining may form inside the female newborn uterus. After separation at birth from the mother, these hormones will be metabolized and destroyed in the baby's liver. When these passively transferred *maternal* hormones are completely eliminated, then a "period" may occur in the newborn female. *Such bleeding can be expected to stop within the first two weeks after birth.*

The Babies Digestive System

Babies do spit up quite frequently in the newborn period. Their stomach is quite sensitive and, after feeding, it is important that the baby be placed in a sitting position so that the baby will not regurgitate its food. Be sure to wipe the baby's mouth of any formula or breast milk so that no irritation of the skin around the mouth will occur.

Author Note: Many babies will hiccup if they are laid horizontal after feeding: the milk lies against the top part of the stomach and close to the baby's diaphragm. The diaphragm may become "irritated" and causes the baby "to hiccup." Therefore, to help prevent these hiccups, keep your baby vertical for about 20 minutes after feedings.

Breastfeeding

The question of breastfeeding versus bottle feeding is a personal choice the mother has to make herself. People in the medical and general community should not over-advocate one method of another. It is true that breast milk is the best "natural" formula for your baby. Further, breast milk contains antibodies which have developed in your immune system during your lifetime. These antibodies are passively transferred to the baby during nursing. Furthermore, the breast milk that is formed has the proper composition of protein, carbohydrate, sugar, fat, temperature and consistency that is most desirable for a newborn. Commercial formulas use milk products from cows and soybeans. These commercial formulas try to replicate the same consistency and nutritional composition that exists in breast milk. Though formulas provide adequate nourishment for the growth of a newborn, they are not exactly the same: most formulas do not contain the same composition of vitamins, minerals and antibodies that exist in human breast milk.

The question of demand versus scheduled feeding is also difficult to answer. When the baby is born, the baby is usually placed on a schedule in the Newborn Nursery: usually a four hour schedule. It is recommended, however, in the first few weeks of life that the baby be placed on a baby demand schedule. Accordingly, you will be nursing your baby every two to six hours: depending on the baby's weight and his appetite. Furthermore, it is important in the first few days of life that the baby be placed to the breast whenever it does want to nurse. It is this sucking that stimulates the formation of milk and the eventual development of breast milk. In the first two or three weeks, it is recommended that the baby have a "push demand" type of schedule. In an attempt to put some order in her own personal life, it is important that, even though the baby has breast fed two or three hours ago, the mother should try to play with her baby, bathe the baby, or pursue other activities in order to try to extend the interval between feedings to a convenient time of four to six hours. Some mothers will try to nurse as completely as possible during the ten or eleven o'clock feeding so that she and the baby may sleep longer during the night. It is not uncommon for many mothers to drink a little beer at this time. The alcohol will encourage the further let-down and emptying of the breasts. The increased amount of milk, plus a little bit of the alcohol, will fill the baby's stomach and make the baby sleep longer.

Because babies have not had to use their lips in order to feed prior to birth, babies who breastfeed will usually develop small whitish callouses on their lips in the 1st week of life.

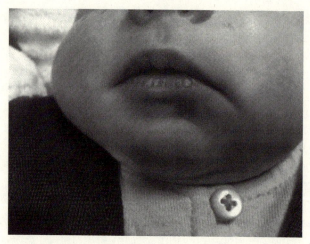

Figure 23-4 Thickened Lips on breastfeeding baby on 6th day after birth

There are no golden rules as far as supplementing the baby. No matter how perfect the mother tries to totally breast feed the baby, some babies will demand more. The amount of fluids, the amount of stress, time and other personal and family needs may decrease the amount of breast milk the mother has. At this point, the pediatrician or your family doctor may suggest supplementing the baby. Commercial formulas may be used for supplementation. Furthermore, by using such supplements, it is possible for the father or other family members to participate in the nourishment of your newborn. Usually the baby will be breast fed up to four months, and occasionally, clear up to two and one-half years of age. The length of time that one breast feeds their infant is basically a personal decision. It will depend on obligations at work and at home. For the most part, most babies are weaned at four months of age. It is usually at this time the baby's teeth will start coming in and, after one or two severe bites, the mother usually loses her interest to continue to breastfeed anymore. Supplements are also important so that the baby may get used to the nipple or the bottle. Babies are basically "creatures of habit." They do not like any changes in their diet or nourishment. It is difficult for a breast fed baby to know what a nipple or bottle is after two or three months of age. Accordingly, if the baby is offered such method of feeding, it will usually decline the nipple. Furthermore, if formula is present in the bottle, the baby has two new situations to deal with. First, it has not seen the nipple or bottle (which may be faster or slower than the flow he/she is used to). Second, the taste of the formula as opposed to breast milk may be completely different. No matter how hungry the baby is, it will not take the bottle. Even stored breast milk may be rejected by the baby: it is not accustomed to the plastic nipple and bottle. Situations do come up in the parent's life, such as a social engagement or even just a night out of the town. A relative or babysitter will be feeding the baby. It is at this point that the babysitter may want to offer the baby a bottle. The baby will not take the bottle and, accordingly, you will have an angry babysitter and baby when you do arrive back at home. Therefore, it is suggested that the baby be given a nipple and a bottle to get used to it for future situations. It might be best to start by placing breast milk in the bottle so that the baby gets sued to the nipple and the bottle. Later the parent may mix half the breast milk and half formula until the entire feeding session can be accomplished with formula in the bottle. It is with this technique that the baby is also weaned to a bottle. The baby is best weaned with such a schedule over a period of days to weeks: the baby needs to become accustomed to the gradual change in schedule.

Your Temperature Settings at home

It is recommended that the temperature in the home be regulated at approximately 72 degrees. It is not uncommon for newborn parents to experience a large rise in their electric or gas bills because of trying to keep the home temperature warmer. If the temperature is too high, the babies may experience an increased risk of respiratory infections. Such infections can occur, because at higher temperatures, the house becomes usually drier, warmer and dustier. These warmer conditions cause the mucus in the baby's nose and mouth to dry out. The babies start having stuffy noses; they start snorting and coughing. These are natural responses to high temperatures in the home. If the baby starts experiencing these symptoms, it is important that the baby's nose be suctioned. If the mucus becomes too thick, the baby may need application of saline nose drops. Do not use decongestants, such as Sudafed or other over-the-counter preparations. This will only further dry out the baby's mucous membranes and aggravate the problem. Humidifiers are useful for a limited period of time. However, if the humidifiers are kept on for extensive periods of time, they may grow mold. The baby can develop allergic reactions to the growth of mold in the house. Therefore, you should keep your home at approximately 68 to 72 degrees. As long as the baby is appropriately dressed and blanketed, you need not worry about the baby's warmth

It has been said that "you spend half of your adult life trying to teach your children how to walk and how to talk, and the remainder of your adult life telling them to sit down and shut up!"

--Anonymous

"Why yes, I love babies! In fact, I had one for breakfast!"

---W.C Fields

I guess you heard why grandparents and grandchildren get along so well: it is because they share a common enemy (it is YOU!)

Motherhood: the only place you can experience heaven and hell at the same time!!

--Misty Witten

I hope you have children that are just like you!

--Author's Mother

However, Mom didn't realize that one day she would have to be babysitting them! ---Author

Diapers

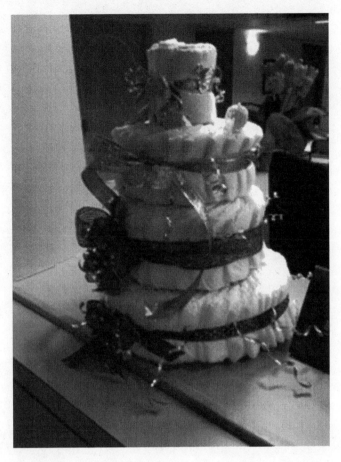

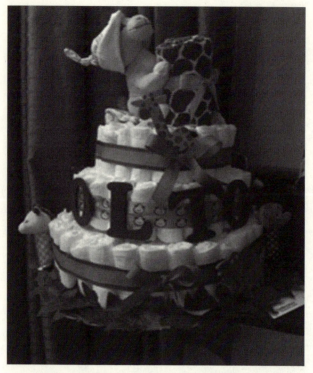

**Figure 23-5 Diaper "Cake" that OB nurses give
Diaper Cakes to recently delivered patients**

<u>Cloth Diaper Service</u>. Many authorities recommend that the newborn parent retain the services of a diaper service. The baby will go through approximately twenty diapers a day. In fact, as the baby goes through so many diapers, one begins to wonder whether changing the diaper actually stimulates the baby to naturally go to the bathroom! If you plan to launder the diapers yourself, it is recommended that you use a very low suds detergent. Use the exact amount of soap recommended on the box. Do not try to increase the amount of soap in order to get a cleaner diaper. It is also recommended that the diapers be doubly rinsed. Most American commercial washing machines have too short a rinse cycle. Too much detergent retained in the diaper can burn the baby's skin. For the most part, a diaper service with the diaper pail in the garage will suffice. In the diaper pail, it is recommended that you put Clorox and water so that the diapers will be cleansed. Many studies agree that cloth diapers are better and there is, accordingly, a decrease in the incidence of infections and diaper rash.

It is the "urine diapers" that are the main cause of diaper rash. If you rinse the baby's bottom with plain lukewarm water after removing the soaked diaper, your baby is unlikely to suffer from diaper rash.

<u>Disposable Paper Diapers</u>. Disposable diapers are probably the most commonly used type of diaper. Most parents agree that no diaper has yet been designed to contain the explosive bowel movements of a baby. Disposables are convenient and easier to put on. It is extremely difficult to put on cloth diapers when your baby is older and, as one parent said, "It is like trying to wrestle an alligator to the ground and trying to pin the diaper on at the same time."

Julie was totally amazed as she was feeding her newborn girl one morning, "My baby girl is a Superstar, I didn't know she could eat and poop all at the very same time without breaking stride."

A recent *Consumer's Report* has evaluated the various commercially available disposable diapers. The testing results showed that a "leading brand" came out on top with regard to the parameters of absorbency, cost, ease of changing along with the lower risk of diaper rash (please see Consumer Reports or other consumer magazines for the results of their testing). If your baby gets a diaper rash, it may take a week or so to heal completely.

<u>Author's anecdote</u>: When the author was shopping at one of the large national chain stores, he inadvertently took a short-cut through the Baby section. He noticed the various types and colors of diaper boxes all stacked up on the wall. On the side of one of the diaper boxes, he read, "5 to 10 lbs." He said to himself, "I guess they must have really improved the absorbency of diapers. I didn't know they can hold that much weight now!"

Lastly, for the stupid quip of the day regarding diapers,

"What do you say to a baby that wears *"Designer"* Diapers?

Answer (if are ready for this) Gucci, Gucci! (Goo Chee, Goo Chee!)

Circumcision

To circumcise or not to circumcise has been "The Question" over the past decades. It is a question that not only parents but also physicians have been debating. The crux of this issue is that a surgical procedure (on a sexual organ) may be painful to their innocent newborn male: to a certain extent a "guilt trip" laid upon new parents. If God created a covering for the penis, then why do need to remove it? In the author opinion, this issue is being scrutinized a little bit too seriously. Parents and medical personnel are giving circumcision more significance than it really deserves. This section hopes to give the reader sufficient information so that you may make that decision for your newborn boy.

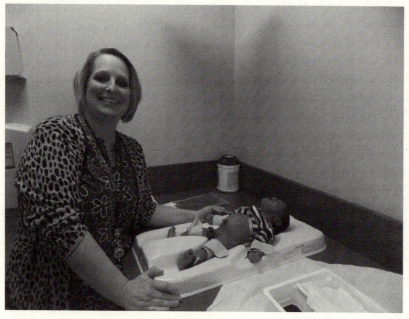

Figure 23-6 Circumcision Procedure. Deana Price RN preparing a baby for circumcision.

Circumcision is a very minor surgical procedure that involves removing the small amount of skin that covers the tip of the newborn's penis.

Parents really need to just listen to their gut feelings regarding circumcision and go with it. Languishing about the decision is not worth the emotional cost or your time—the Author.

A Little Historical and Religious Perspective

The practice of circumcision began back in Biblical times. According to the Bible, God commanded Abraham to have all the newborn males circumcised as part of his covenant with Him. In those times, tribal people wandered from place to place in order to find enough food, shelter and water for themselves and their herds of animals. They did not have the modern day conveniences of baths and showers in order to keep up their personal hygiene. Because dirt, bacteria, old skin and oil would collect under the foreskin of the penis, the men in these nomadic tribes would frequently get an infection of the foreskin. Because of these frequent penile infections, people in Biblical times started the practice of circumcising their newborn boys. Certainly hygienic conditions in the U. S. and Western World today are much improved. Still, in the Third World, conditions may have not changed very much from those Biblical times. What is relevant is that, regardless of modern day conveniences, proper care and cleanliness of the penis and foreskin has utmost importance in preventing penile infection.

Author's Note: Once after a tennis game the author and a friend were discussing the primitive conditions that our soldiers had to endure during the Vietnam War. This friend told me about his times in the jungles. Frequently, platoons would go out for maneuvers for weeks at a time. There was little opportunity or chance that they could shower or change their underwear. He remarked how many uncircumcised males in their troop suffered from severe infection of the penis, i.e., Balantitis. He described their pain and discomfort. Perhaps our Armed Forces today are at risk for penile infections if they are deployed to the Middle East and Africa. I am sure our troops have cleaner facilities available to them today. However, there may be some use for circumcision even in today's world: certainly in third 3rd world areas. How about climbers, hikers and campers? Usually they are afforded modern day conveniences situated along the trail or portable devices they can backpack.

Circumcision is performed on 70% or more of newborn males in the United States. Parents in Europe, Asia and Africa, as a rule, do not circumcise their babies. In the author's experience it appears that when other nationalities and ethnic groups assimilate into the American culture, these parents start circumcising their newborns as well. Most fathers in the US are most likely to circumcise their sons if they themselves have been circumcised.

> Anesthesia for Circumcision
>
> 1. Application of Emla® or other anesthetic cream to the foreskin for 30 minutes prior to the procedure
>
> 2. Local anesthesia block prior to procedure
>
> 3. Oral Medication as described below

Anesthesia is utilized in most cases. The nursery RN can apply an anesthetic cream to the entire penis 30 minutes prior to the procedure. Alternatively, a physician can inject with a very tiny needle a small amount of anesthetic into the nerves located at the base of the penis. During a traditional Jewish circumcision (called a *"Bris"*) the *Mohel,* i.e., one trained in doing the circumcision, moistens a small cotton gauze with sweet red wine and places it partially into the baby's mouth: the baby readily sucks on the gauze. The baby's cheeks absorbed the wine. The baby is comforted and may feel its soothing effects. In reality, the more important factors implicated in the pain experienced by the baby is first, the circumcision technique and second, how long it takes the physician to do it. If performed delicately, carefully and gently, the baby experiences only slight discomfort. As most physicians and nurses observe, most of the crying the baby displays is when it is the baby is placed onto the circumcision board.

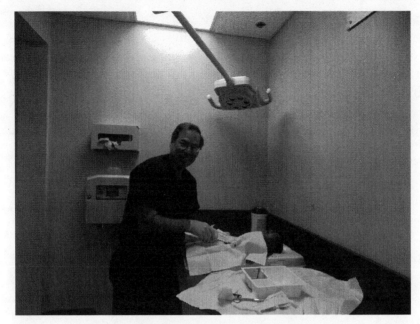

Figure 23-7 Circumcision Preparation. The author performing a circumcision

Circumcision is usually performed in the hospital (or birth center) prior to discharge of the newborn. However, the procedure can be performed elsewhere such as in the doctor's office or even at your own home anytime during the first six to eight weeks of life. Premature babies or small babies may have to postpone their circumcision until they weigh more. Larger babies may need the procedure sooner. It is best to ask your physician for his advice about timing and location.

According to Jewish law, newborn boys shall be circumcised on the eight day of life.

In Biblical times newborn males would bleed if the circumcision was done in the first few days of life. With experience and education it was discovered that the baby would not develop sufficient clotting ability until the 8th day of life. Today all newborns are given Vitamin K right after birth so that the baby's clotting ability would be stimulated immediately (coagulation factors are produced mainly in the liver).

In the Jewish religion, a Rabbi officiates at the circumcision or *Bris*. It is a formal religious ceremony: it celebrates Abraham's Covenant with God. There must be a *"minion,"* a defined number of Jewish members in attendance. Usually the Rabbi does not do the circumcision himself.

Circumcisions are usually performed by an obstetrician, a pediatrician, or the family physician.

The actual procedure itself does not take long—under ten minutes. The baby is placed in a molded bed. Its arms and legs are placed out of the way of the sterile field. The penis is prepped with an antiseptic solution and sterile drapes are placed around the penis. Two small clamps grasp the edges of the foreskin. The foreskin is gently freed from the head of the penis. It should be noted that the gentleness and slowness in doing the procedure makes the procedure more tolerable for the baby.

Most babies complain and are "more vocal" about being picked up and moved to the circumcision board than anything else.

GOMCO or MOGEN CLAMP METHOD. After the foreskin is separated from the penis itself, a clamp is placed over the penis. A metal cap (Gomco technique) is placed over the head of the penis to shield it out of the way. The tip of the penis is placed through the round circle portion of the clamp. The metal cap protects the penis but the edges of the cap come up snugly with the circle portion of the clamp. The base of the foreskin becomes trapped between the metal cap and the circular area. Slowly the circular device is tightened. A crease is thus formed and a blood-free cut can be made. The foreskin is placed in the clamp for at least five minutes. Thereafter, the blood vessels are sealed and the nerves are completely made numb. The foreskin can now be safely and painlessly removed with a scalpel.

PLASTIBELL METHOD. The Plastibell technique is utilized by most physicians today. It is very similar to the Gomco technique, but a plastic cap is substituted for the metal one. Instead of using the metal helmet and circular clamp, a suture is tied around the base of the plastic cap. The foreskin is trimmed and the top of the plastic cap is left opened through which the baby can pee. What remains around the end of the penis is a plastic collar which falls off after seven to ten days.

In order to make a more informed decision about circumcision, the reader may obtain further information about the procedure. For medical reasons alone, neither the American Academy of Pediatrics nor the American College of Obstetrics and Gynecologists recommend the *routine* circumcision of every newborn male. In the past, the medical community favored circumcision because the opinions at the time were that circumcision:

1) Absolutely prevented cancer of the penis, a very rare disease

2) Significantly reduced the risk of penile infections

3) Eliminate the possibility of "priapism" unlikely (that is, a scar that forms a tight band around the head of the penis, preventing erection or even urination

4) Usually results in easier care and cleaning of the penis

5) Circumcision as a newborn avoids the much greater risks of surgery should circumcision become necessary later in life.

Today, the problem is that physicians cannot predict and select which newborn males are likely to develop infections, cancer or foreskin scars. Yes, it does not seem reasonable to circumcise one hundred babies if only one or two will develop future foreskin problems. It is also not very difficult for parents to learn the proper care and cleaning of the foreskin.

On the other hand, there are compelling *non-medical* reasons for circumcision:

1) Husband, brother or other males in the family are circumcised. "He should not look different."

2) The Bible, religious faith or religious beliefs require circumcision.

3) Most American males are circumcised.

Statistically, approximately 70 percent of newborn males are circumcised today. Yet, the 30 percent of uncircumcised males are a large enough minority today to make the observed anatomical difference become viewed as more of a variation of normal rather than as "abnormal" or "unusual."

<u>Care of the Penis after circumcision</u>. As the author tells his patients, "Keep it clean and Vaseline!" These are the simple instructions given to new parents about the home care of the newly circumcised newborn. The baby will poop all over the penis within hours! The penis should be washed with soapy water and rinsed with water. If a Gomco/Mogen circumcision was performed, then parents should lightly coat the penis with Vaseline so that the penis does not stick to the diaper. Plastibell circumcisions should be kept dry so that the skin shrivels and the plastic ring falls off.

Newborn Monitoring Systems

Purchase a Newborn baby monitor? That is the most ridiculous thing to ever use if you want to get any sleep!

--Kelly Ripa (paraphrased from episode of Regis and Kelly)

There are a number of newborn monitoring systems available in order to remotely hear and see your baby via a camera to your bedroom, your smartphone or computer. Even daycare facilities now have sophisticated surveillance systems that can be transmitted so that you can watch your baby when you are at work.

Babies do cry frequently but such CRYING is not necessarily mean that the baby is in pain, is hungry or has a diaper emergency.

Utilizing a monitor at night is going to make it very difficult for you to sleep. If you baby has been recently fed and changed (and has been otherwise well), then being awaken each time your baby cries is going to drive you and your husband "crazy."

On the other hand, there are many other couples who may feel differently about this issue: seeing your baby on camera from your bedroom or kitchen can inform you whether the baby is crying because an arm got caught between the crib slats, is in an uncomfortable position, etc. Seeing and hearing your baby can give you the reassurance that the baby is just a little "fussy" or has a small bubble in their stomach.

Crying Babies

There is no question that babies cry. In the newborn period babies cry because they are hungry, have a wet or poopy diaper or otherwise uncomfortable. New moms and dads will quickly learn to distinguish a painful cry from an irritable one. Most babies' cries will be attenuated just by picking them up. If it has been awhile since their last feeding, then feeding the baby will solve the problem. Not all babies will cry with a soiled diaper. However, babies do cry when they are constipated. Only after they get that serious look in their face and poop will their distress leave.

Of course, the parents need to be sure that *no serious medical condition* is present by the major parameters of new born health: fever, nausea, baby will not feed or take the bottle, baby is not wetting diapers, baby is not pooping, baby is hot, baby is lethargic or cannot be easily awaken, etc. Bring your baby to your physician or local emergency room immediately.

Colic is another cited reason why babies may cry without being able to console them. Colic makes its appearance at about 2-3 months. The crying starts in the late afternoon to early evening. It is believed that gas bubbles form in the baby's intestines. Such gas causes intestinal cramping and pain. Holding and swaddling your baby as well as talking to your baby may be helpful. Uncommonly, remedies may be needed for the gas.

References:

http://en.wikipedia.org/wiki/Baby_colic
www.babycenter.com› Home› Crying & Colic› Why Babies Cry
www.webmd.com/parenting/**baby**/what-is-**colic**
www.mayoclinic.org/diseases-conditions/**colic**/.../con-20019091

Other reasons for babies to cry:

    Temperature conditions are too hot or too cold

    Clothing is uncomfortable

    Their position in the crib or in your arms in just not comfortable

    Your baby is tired and needs to go to sleep

    Your baby is cutting teeth (from 4-9 months of age)

    Your baby has "cabin fever" and needs a change of place and atmosphere: take your baby for a stroll outside (in the mall if it is winter time)

There are other times when you just cannot figure it out why your baby is crying: the baby was just fed, just had a new diaper and everything seems otherwise normal. Their crying is making you and/or the baby's dad really stressed out.

When you cannot relieve your baby's crying, then the best thing to do is put your baby back in their crib and close the door. Do not shake, scream at or spank your baby.

If you are still worried or stressed out, call your family and friends. You can always drive your baby to the hospital Emergency Room for help. Most of the time, just by driving to the hospital, the baby will be soothe by the ride and their crying will cease (and they will probably fall asleep).

A new program has been set up for parents to be educated about the baby's crying episode. This program has labeled the baby's inconsolable crying spells, *the Period of Purple*. Hospitals give each delivered mom and dad a DVD to see on this program. On this DVD is a 10 minute video on *Purple Crying* and a 17 min video on ways to soothe your baby. Included in the program is a 10-page booklet.

www.mayoclinic.org/diseases-conditions/colic/.../con-20019091

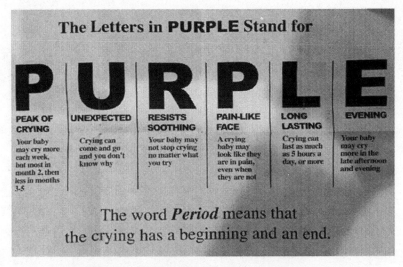

Figure 23-8 PURPLE Crying Pneumonic

Visit **www.PURPLEcrying.info** or call the NCSBS (National Center on Shaken Baby Syndrome) at (801) 447-9360

Sudden Infant Death Syndrome (SIDS)

SIDS is the No. 1 cause of deaths in babies aged 1 month to the 12th month. Fortunately, unexplained death in the first year of life, i.e. "Crib death," has been decreasing in frequency over the past two decades. There have been several significant changes in current guidelines that have led to these better outcomes:

First, babies should be put into their cribs so that they lie on their backs. Prior to 1990, most Pediatricians recommended that babies be put down on their stomach: if they spit up or vomited it was felt that such fluids would flow outward to the side of the face. Currently, experts believe that the baby's head has more mobility to either side (180 degrees) should they spit up, cough or vomit their formula or food. Consequently, there is less risk of aspiration of food contents into the stomach. Babies can have "tummy time" when she is awake with an adult close by and watching the baby.

Second, babies should not have their crib cluttered with blankets, bumpers or toys which could wrap around their necks or otherwise block their breathing abilities.

Third, babies should not sleep in bed with adults (or other children. Babies should not sleep in a chair, couch or other soft surface where they can be caught between the cushions.

Fourth, babies should not be exposed to smoke, i.e. tobacco or marijuana.

Lastly, do not give a baby a pacifier attached to strings. Contrary to popular misconception, pacifiers do not cause dental or other orthodontic problems.

Author's Note: My newborn girl at 4 months of age almost always turned automatically over onto her stomach immediately after being placed on her back in her crib. I guess she did not read the Guidelines!

For further information, the reader is directed to www.nicchd.nih.gov or www.ok.gov for more in-depth information.

Newborn Baby carriers

There are many types of baby carriers as there are strollers. Each type is designed for your style of parenting as well as weight capacities. Some mothers do not want to fuss with straps while other mothers want carriers to be solid and stable in order carry out more vigorous and athletic activities.

Author Note: As a father trying to carry out my usual "to do list" as well as care for the baby, I wanted to put my baby on a back carrier that was tough and supportive. Yes, Dad and baby were going to be close together: we were going to be physically connected. We were going to vacuum, wash the car, mow the grass, shop for Craftsmen tools at Sears while the "Lil Critter" was strapped to my back. My "baby backpack" needed a metal frame and good straps because I did not want him/her falling out when I bent over. Also, I did not want my baby to crawl out of the backpack when he/she got bored. Yes, we were attached to each other: I could even hear when he/she was pooping!

The reader is referred to Pregnancy & Newborn, PNMAG.COM, and April 2014. In this issue are illustrated the types of baby carriers:

Lillebaby COMPLETE All season (7-45 pounds) $135
Chicco Coda (7.5 to 25 pounds) $90
Beco Soleil (7 to 45 pounds) $140 (BECCOBABYCARRIER.COM)
Boba Carrier 4G (7 to 45 pounds) $130:
Lucky Baby Word SUPPORI Baby Carrier (15-33 pounds) $55: Hip Holder type
Earthy Bliss Kenzie Shoulder Ring Sling (7 to 45 pounds) $115: Sling type
Ergobaby Wrap (6.6 to 31 pounds) $80
Moby Wrap MLB Edition (birth to 35 pounds) $55: this model can place you MLB team logo on it!
Baby K'tan Baby Carrier (8-35 pounds) $50

AUTHOR'S NOTE: Justin, my own son, was in a room way over on the other side of the home when he was a newborn. Because we did not think we would be able to hear him when he cried, we purchased a baby monitor. When he did cry at nights, we would rush over to his room to see what he was crying about. Most of the time Justin s would have topped crying by the time we got to his room! Even Kelly Ripa, during her show Regis and *Kelly (*now *Kelly and Michael),* stated she stopped using her monitor system altogether!

Keeping Your Marriage Alive After the Baby Arrives

During the pregnancy your whole concentration was focused on becoming prepared for the event of childbirth itself. Your goal was to be sure that your baby arrived safely into this world. In this last chapter, you have become better acquainted with the many aspects of the newborn's personality and care. It may become a surprise as well to learn that your marriage had undergone a metamorphosis as well: a man and woman "couple" has been transformed into a "family."

Most parents blindly stumble through the first years of child-rearing. They learn by trial and error how to cope with the needs of the child and themselves. There has been very little in literature which explores in any depth the new parents' altered married relationship with their new roles as parents and a family. Becoming parents is a major social and emotional event in a marriage. The better prepared the couple is for dealing with the inevitable changes in their relationship, the better off the whole family will be.

This phase of nurturing a baby and young child can be one of the calmest as well as the stormiest in your lives. You are changing from lovers to parents. That transformation impacts every aspect of your relationship. The postpartum year is a period of time not only to redefine marital roles but also to begin building a new kind of relationship. Just as feeding your baby is crucial, so is learning to nurture yourselves as individuals and as partners. The greatest gift you can give your child is a caring, loving relationship between you and your spouse. Such a gift is further fortified by your own solid sense of self.

As parents face each child-care task, they are forced again and again to realize how different their anticipation of a task differed from the actual accomplishment of it. It is important to identify your expectations ahead of time and be prepared to alter them if reality proves to not match up for what you prepared. For instance, ask your spouse and yourself the following questions:

1) Do you assume that your sexual relationship will pick up where it left off? Erotic feelings, particularly on the part of

the female, diminish during the early nurturing months. Six weeks may be the time period necessary for proper healing of the vaginal area and the episiotomy (if performed). It takes time for a couple to establish a new intimate relationship.

2) How will your morning routine change now that they baby requires feeding and attention?

3) Who is going to watch the baby while dinner is being prepared?

4) Who is going to get up with the baby in the middle of the night when one or both of you has to work the next day?

5) Who is going to feed the baby? Babies require 8 to 10 feedings a day. Nursing is a full-time job!

6) Who is going to work outside the home so there will be money to support the family?

7) How will do the family care for the baby while each of you are performing other household tasks, like shopping, laundry, cooking, cleaning and home repairs? Babies sleep a great amount of time only during the first few weeks of life!

8) Who is going to get the diaper bag ready when you both go out for family trips and visits?

9) What if you have a cranky, colicky baby instead of one who is calm and contented?

10) Which part of the parenting job will you do together? What will be delegated to a specific parent and why? Which tasks will you take turns doing?

These are just some of the nitty-gritty issues you both will face from the first day you bring the baby home from the hospital. You cannot expect to have all your solutions ready before you actually experience some of the problems. What most parents are unprepared for are the feelings that accompany these adjustments. It is most important to remember that your feelings of occasional frustration, isolation, doubt, exhaustion and disappointment are as normal as the pride and joy that each parent experiences.

After decades of long extensive research medical scientists finally reported out in 2014 the significant breakthrough finding that <u>insanity</u> should now be considered an <u>inherited</u> disease: Yes, You get in from your children!

You may now be thinking, "What did we get ourselves into? Why are we having a baby?" If you anticipate the adjustments and admit your feelings while you are in the process of "becoming a family," you are adjusting in a healthy, constructive fashion. Remember the following concepts:

1) The difficulties related to this period of childbirth and newborn care do end—not quickly, but eventually!

2) It is crucial to continue talking with one another. Both of you are adjusting to new responsibilities. Be reassured that it is normal to find yourselves arguing and resenting new obligations. It takes time to work out viable solutions for you. Much frustration and anger comes from unrealistic expectations and exhaustion.

3) Share your experiences with other new parents. You are not alone. Other new parents are having the same experiences. Parents should discuss with other new parents their differing approaches and solutions to the same problems. Develop a good support system: parents, in-laws, brothers, sisters and good friends with children. If you need professional help, then do yourself and your baby a favor and get it. Your doctor can refer you to a qualified marriage and family counselor who specializes in helping couples through these transitions.

Lastly, it is important for couples to decide ahead of time and discuss how they want to bring up their children. Husband and wife may have completely different set of expectations and desires for their child. Each parent should answer the following questions and discuss their answers with each other:

1) What things did my own parents do for me that I would like to do for my own child? What activities, sports, trips, and skills did my parents give to me that I would like to give to my children?

2) What mannerisms, habits or teachings did my parents have that I do not want to pass along to my child?

Compare notes with your spouse and see if you can arrange a child development plan that will develop in your child the best personality traits, skills and habits of each parent. Remember, the child needs consistent signals and support from both parents. Above all, enjoy being a parent! It's a very rewarding experience (and an expensive proposition!)

Getting your baby to go to sleep

It's 2 am......Jaxon has been up 5 times already......maybe I'll just stay awake tonight, again...my little man never gets to rest...if he slept 4 solid hours I'd be shocked! ---Robin Spencer Whetzel

All babies are different. Some are great sleepers. Some are not. Books have been written on just this topic alone: *"How to get your Baby to Sleep at Night."*

It is extremely important to set a schedule *immediately* from the time your baby comes home...and you have to stick to it (unless you want to become a zombie and go crazy!). Babies need 12 hours of sleep. Prior to sleep time it is important to cut out the intense environmental stimuli, like the TV, and background sounds such as talking and music. Most babies relax in their baths. After their bath time comes sleep time. After laying your baby in the crib, dim the lighting. Then comes story time: your soothing voice while telling a story prepares your baby for the calmness and restfulness of sleep. The softness of their baby blanket tells them that everything is stable, secure and safe. The baby's eyes will close and your baby will be off to sleep.

"A Mother holds her children's hand for a while, but their hearts forever."
--Author Unknown

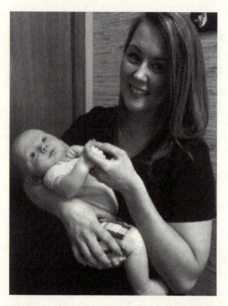

Figure 23-9 Mother holding her Baby's Hand

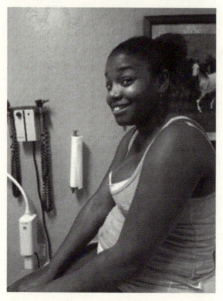

Figure 23-10 Shannon Badue "wisdom"

Babies are like pancakes: the 1ˢᵗ one you make you usually mess up, then the more you make, the better they get!"—Shannon Badue

If you want to teach your children how income taxes work, just eat 30% of their ice cream!

(Or take away 30% of their Halloween candy!)

Author's Experiences with his young children

1. *"Colic" pains by your newborn during the early months.*

    "Colic" is a very common discomfort experienced by babies in the early months of the newborn period. The baby becomes irritable and starts having crying spells in the late afternoon to the early evening hours. Physicians have postulated that the pain emanates from the baby's intestines: the muscle spasms of the intestinal tube are basically "cramping the baby's style." It is very difficult to console your baby and there seems nothing you can do to stop the crying and pain. Feeding the baby breast milk, formula or water does not help. Holding your baby and rubbing your baby's back to try to get out a "bubble" or gas does not work. In the author's first born girl, Jennifer, he would put her in the car seat in the back of his car and drive her to the nearest ice cream store (Baskin Robbins). By the time he came back home she was fast asleep in her car seat. The author gained 10 lbs. that year!

    With his 2ⁿᵈ girl, Jessica, he put her in the stroller and walked her around the neighborhood. After 5-10 minutes she would stop crying and her head would fall to the side as she slid into a deep sleep. But, you have to be very careful and slowly unfasten her from the stroller. Then gently and very cautiously lift her up. You had to be very careful in lowering her oh so slowly down onto her mattress in her crib. If you disturb her in the slightest manner during these very meticulous maneuvers, she would wake up instantly and start bawling all over again. "Now I have to back to square one, put her into the stroller and go for another trip around the block!

2. *Don't buy your toddler a The Hobby Horse*.

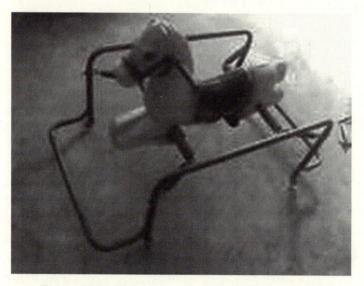

Figure 23-11 The Famous Children's Hobby Horse

My oldest son, Ben, fell in love with a Hobby Horse. We had to buy one at the local toy store. He would love to ride his Hobby Horse while we watched TV in the family room.

However, Ben, like most children, did not want to go to sleep at the usual time of 7:30 PM. He would ride up and down on his Hobby Horse no matter how sleepy he was.

From time to time we would try to remove him away from the Hobby Horse and tell him he needed to go upstairs to his bed to go to sleep. He would cry and fight. He would grip the Hobby Horse such that you could not pry him loose.

While we watched the TV Ben would continue to ride his "horsey." As he rode the horse, the springs attached to the horse would go creek-creek, cleek-cleek, etc. at a regular rate. However, when the sounds started becoming less frequent, we knew he was falling asleep. We could see him starting to close his eyes. At that point, we would again try to lift him up gently off the horse, but he would suddenly wake up and fight to stay on his horse.

We would go back to watching TV and the same sequence would ensue. Cleek-cleek, cleek-cleek etc. and the motions again would slow down. Unfortunately, it was at that sudden point in time that we heard a "big thud." Ben fell of the Hobby Horse onto the carpeted floor below.

Many a night the same scenario would play out. There was always the all too familiar sound of Ben hitting the floor! After a few times, we had to pad the floor with pillows to be sure he would not be injured in any way.. I guess we were all surprised that he actually finished Arizona State University with his Degree in Interior Design.

3. **Don't teach your children to swat flies.**

When Ben was about 3-4 years old, he would observe us swatting flies with the fly swatter. During the summer months when flies were most numerous and pesky, we would be swatting these insects right and left. One day, when we were busy somewhere else in the house, Ben noticed the flies buzzing around on the front picture window in the living room. So, Ben rushed into the kitchen to seek out the fly swatter and perform the task of killing flies like he learned from observing his parents. Ben searched for the fly swatter but he could not find it. So, he found the "very best next thing" that he could use to kill the flies: the ice cream scoop! Well, needless to say, Ben took a big swipe at the flies in the picture window. He missed the fly but he did a really great job on the window. The window people were out the next day and handed me a bill for $500.

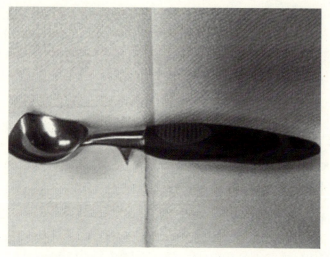

Figure 23-12 The Famous "ice cream scoop"

Moral to this story: If you have young children and flies, please invest in an electrical fly killer or other inexpensive device to rid your house of flies.

Addendum: Ben was my only child that could actually break Tonka toys. And, do not take your eyes off your child for any length of time: Ben also crawled up onto my vehicle in the garage and bent the windshield wiper blades!

4. *"Ben is dead."*

Per the usual daily routine in our family and many other families across the country, both my children take their baths at about 7 PM. My wife (Barbara at that time) would put both my young children (Jennifer age 3 and Benjamin age 1) into the bathtub together. She then went down the hallway, fluffed up the pillows and finally lay down in the bed. She picked up her book to read. As soon as she started reading, Jennifer called out from the bathtub, "Mommy, come here." As there was no crying going on and both kids were playing with their toys in the water, my wife said, "you children just need to play in the water." Jennifer persisted, "Mommy, come here." My wife knew that there were really no problems and did not want to get up after finally getting some rest at the end of the day. Again, Jennifer said, "Mommy, come here." At this point my wife just ignored her and kept on reading her book.

A long interval of time passes, perhaps 10 minutes. Suddenly, Jennifer cries out," Mommy, Mommy come here! Ben is dead!" My wife sprang up and rushed to the bathroom and peered into the bathtub. Both kids look up innocently at her simultaneously and smiled as if there was nothing wrong! You see, children do have a way of getting your attention and doing what you want them to do!

Moral to this Story: Kids get to know how to push your buttons!

5. **Health conscious mother nurtures a health conscious child.**

Courtney RN at the hospital relayed me the following conversation with her child at bedtime.

Courtney said to her baby girl, "Bella, good night. I love you!" Bella replied, "I love you, too, mommy like a granola bar." Courtney told her sister this "good night conversation." Her sister then retorted to Courtney, "Bella is definitely your child. If it were my kid, she would have said, "I love you like a *chocolate* bar!"

Author's Advice to his own Children

My advice to my oldest daughter:

The author instructed his oldest child, Jennifer, with the following advice with regard to her key to "The Good Life":

Learn to play tennis well. If you can be a great player, you can make a lot of money and be financially secure. Tennis is not just a game with necessary immense physical attributes. It is also a game requiring great mental skills. You have to outsmart your opponent. It is a game of wits and finesse. You can tell a lot about a person when you play tennis with them. You can tell how much they want to win. You can tell how honest they are (depending on who is calling the line shots). You can assess their physical abilities, their courage and tenacity, as well as their strategy in placing the ball. The game of tennis will allow you to assess your opponent's aggressiveness and energy when they are frequently rushing the net. You do not even have to speak the same language and you will get to know your opponent well.

If you are successful in playing the sport well, you will be able to travel around the world and play tournaments everywhere. You will become famous and be "a role model." You will be asked, and *be paid*, to make product endorsements: sunglasses, tennis clothes, and tennis rackets as well as breakfast cereals.

Unfortunately, my daughter did not take my advice! She presently is a territorial manager of a national clothing chain and is very happy being a mom and wife in the San Francisco Bay Area.

Author's advice to his two sons:

You only have to do one thing in life. I took each one of them out to the football field when they were 7 years old. I put the football down onto the football tee. I pointed to the field goal uprights about 20 feet away. I said to each of them, "All you have to do in life is kick this football through those uprights." If you are very good and consistent at performing this ability, you will be recruited to a professional football team. You will travel all around the United States. You may even travel to Great Britain and Japan to play exhibition football. They will pay you a great amount of money. You will be independently wealthy. You only have to play a few seconds during each of the games. Many times your field goal will be the deciding factor in winning the game. You will become a "hero." And the best part, no one can ever hit you!

Lastly, unlike me, you won't have to get up in the middle of the night to deliver a baby! You can sleep late every morning.

But they did not take my advice either.

For further information the reader is also advised to read the classic book, *Baby and Child Care*, by the original and most influential pediatrician of the 20th century, Dr. Benjamin Spock. The author read this book prior to having his first child and, accordingly, was able to pass the exam section on baby care on his National Medical Board.

Songs and Lyrics to inspire parents to persevere

1. I Hope You Dance, by Leann Womack, 1999

> **I hope you still feel small when you stand beside the ocean,
> Whenever one door closes I hope one more opens,
> Promise me that you'll give faith a fighting chance,
> And when you get the choice to sit it out or dance.**
>
> **Dance....I hope you dance.**

--- Songwriters
SANDERS, MARK DANIEL / SILLERS, TIA M

Published by
Lyrics © Universal Music Publishing Group, Sony/ATV Music Publishing LLC

2. *I Wish*, by Rascal Flatts

**I hope you never look back but you never forget
All the ones who love you and the place you left
I hope you always forgive and you never regret
And you help somebody every chance you get**

Songwriters

STEELE/ROBSON

Published by

Lyrics © Sony/ATV Music Publishing LLC

The reader will find the entire lyrics to each song helpful as they raise their children

Section 3. The "Tales" Section

CHAPTER 24

Old Wives Tales

1. **How you "carry" your baby.**

   As the old tales say, if you carry you baby "low," I.e. your bump is very low at the bottom of your abdomen, you're carrying a boy. A high "bump" means you are having a girl. Also, if you carry "in front," you are carrying a boy. If you are growing side to side, you are having a girl. None of this is stuff is true: your baby bump shape is determined by your height, weight, abdominal muscle tone and whether you are short or have a long waist. It also is dependent on the baby's weight and position in the uterus.

2. **"The Drano test"**

   This test goes as follows: mix your urine with Drano (the pipe un-clogger) and you will be able to determine the sex of your child. No one knows what color (green, blue or brown) signifies a particular sex. No one knows even the amount of urine and Drano® you are supposed to use! However, Drano is a dangerous substance and may cause body harm. If you spill some on your hands, your hands will change color immediately! So don't do this stupid test!

3. **Your baby's heart rate can determine its sex**.

   This tale goes as follows: if your baby's heart rate is above 140 beats per minute you are having a girl while heart rate slower than 140 means it is a boy. In reality, your baby's heart rate depends on what the baby is doing at the moment you listen for it: the baby could be moving around and thus the heart rate would be high just like your heart rate when you are moving or exercising. If your baby is sleeping then the heart rate could be the low side of normal at 120 beats per minute.

4. **Food Cravings**.

If you are craving sweets, then the baby is a girl. If you are craving salt, sour things or pickles you are having a boy. If you are eating ice cream and pickles together, then I do not want to know what kind of baby you are having!

5. **"Avoid taking baths."**

Not commonly heard these days, but there may be a worry that the bath water may seep into the vagina and into the uterus and affect your baby. The vagina is a closed and collapsed space and water does not normally enter the vagina (even when swimming or having sex in the hot tub). Furthermore, the cervix plugs the uterus like a cork in a wine bottle. Forget this stupid tale!

6. **Your body changes reveal the baby's sex.**

"A girl steals her mother's beauty" or a baby girl causes acne. On the other hand, a boy causes dry hands, "cold feet," etc. If your left breast gets bigger than your right, then you are having a boy and vice versa.

7. **Umbilical Cord Strangulation by raising your hands up above the shoulders.**

This tale goes as follows: if you raise your hands above your head, you can strangle your baby's umbilical cord around its neck. Again, whatever you do with your hands or feet does not cause any corresponding physical motions onto your baby. Your baby basically "sits in a water tank" with the cord floating at all times. The umbilical cord is similar to a *coiled* insulated telephone cord and the Almighty has designed it so that blood flow to the baby will not be compromised. Furthermore, in 25% of all deliveries the cord is wound loosely around the neck and *rarely* causes any problems!

8. **Drinking a lot of water keeps your baby clean**.

   It is said that if your drink 8 glasses of water per day that the amniotic fluid will stay clean and clear. The amniotic fluids always stay clean and clear (unless the baby is "stressed" by other abnormal conditions of the pregnancy). It is important to drink a lot of fluids and water during pregnancy anyway: especially during the hot humid summer months.

9. **The Ring Test.**

   Tie a string to your wedding ring. Hang your wedding ring over your tummy. If it swings back and forth, expect a girl. If it swings in a circle, you are having a boy. If you hold a necklace over your hand, the opposite is true: back and forth means a boy.

10. **Severe Heartburn means your baby will have lots of hair**.

    Again, the amount of hair your baby will have is determined by the baby's inheritance, its genes and the combination of the DNA from mom and dad.

11. **Husband's "Sympathy Weight Gain."**

    While the moms-to-be are craving chocolate, sweets, French fries and ice cream, it is quite common for the dads-to-be to eating the same junk right alongside of her: just "to be there for her!" The tales says that dad's excess weight gain is an indication of a girl. But, the extra weight gain by Dad only means that he is spending "quality time" with mom as well as with *Ben and Jerry!*

The photo below illustrates the sympathy weight gain in one of our patients (I am sure you can tell which one is pregnant, right?)

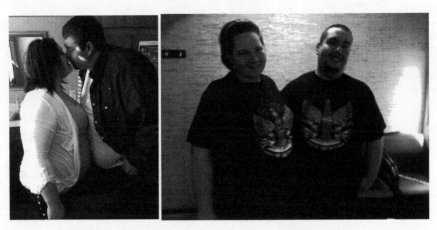

Figures 24-1 and Figure 24-2 "Love bird" patients: they were so cute together. Great Personalities!

12. My baby is posterior (OP-facing upwards) and my back is killing me!

When the baby is coming down with the back of the head pointed to the mother's back (or facing upwards), the baby is in the posterior position. Labor is typically longer in duration and the second stage is more difficult because it takes longer to push the baby through the vaginal canal. Most labor pain is referred to the back regardless of the position of the baby's head. 90 per cent of OP babies "turn on the perineum" just before they are born. So, there is some truth to the fact that OP babies might cause more discomfort in labor. But, then again, that is why doctors invented epidurals!

13. I passed my mucus plug! I need to go to the hospital!

As mentioned previously, passing of a "mucus plug" does not necessarily mean that you are about to go into labor or that you are in labor. It is the most frequent call to the OB nurses at the hospital. The patient should wait until there are other definitive signs of labor:

a. Regular uterine contractions that are 3-4 minutes apart
b. Loss of amniotic sac fluid
c. Bleeding
d. Increased pelvic pressure

14. Wearing a key around your neck will protect you from the Lunar eclipse (according to Mexican legend)

The patient seen below is wearing a key around her neck in order to protect her from the Lunar Eclipse. The key symbolizes a way to protect the eclipse from "damaging the baby." Specifically it is said, that direct exposure to a lunar eclipse will cause from the cleft lip/palate abnormality. Of course, the lunar eclipse has no effect on your developing baby.

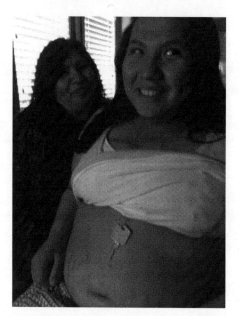

Figure 24-3 Key Protection from Moon rays.
My Puerto Rican girl who almost had a C-section due to a temporary fetal heart deceleration and a -3 station when 8 cm: baby came down just in time to deliver in the C-section OR.

However, it is very important to wear your house key because it is a sure way that you will never get locked out of your home again!

15. More babies are born when there is a full moon (A "Lunatic's "Theory?").

It is really "OLD OB Nurses Tale" that more babies are born during a full moon. Because of this myth, some OB nurses have actually rearranged their work schedule so that their nursing shifts do not coincide with the full moon days!

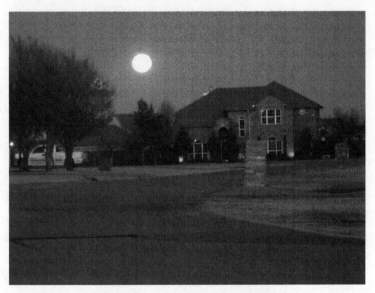

Figure 24-4 Full Moon for babies

The following is author's *synopsis* of a past Report from FOX 40 in Sacramento, CA:

> The OB nursing staff is always "on guard" when there's a full moon.
>
> When there was a full moon one weekend in Sacramento, California 45 babies entered the world. The Report stated that it was a possible record for the two-day period.
>
> Was it caused by a full moon and its gravitational force? Menstrual cycles and ovulation are influenced by the "lunar cycle." Then, so why childbirth can't be affected, similarly?

According to *Discovery Health*, the *theory* of the lunar effect on increased births during a full moon (complete moon surface exposed to the earth) causes an increased gravitational pull on water, i.e., the ocean high tides). Since the human body is made up of 80 percent water, the increased pull (when the moon is full) is believed to initiate labor and perhaps speed the childbirth process.

However, many studies have looked at larger data bases and have shown that there really is "no full moon effect" on increased number of births.

In 2005, researchers analyzed almost 600,000 births across 62 lunar cycles retrieved from birth certificates from 1997 to 2001. They found no significant differences in the frequency of births across the eight stages of the moon (Source: Mountain Area Health Education Center in North Carolina)

Scientific data does not erase this longstanding "myth." Hospital staffs and particularly the OB nurses are especially aware when there is a full moon: many nurses mark their calendars to avoid being on call those days!

"I think if you talk to anybody on the front lines of the hospital, emergency room doctors, labor and delivery, etc. it's always like that on the full moon, everyone for some reason is really busy," Matthew Guile, a doctor at Sutter Memorial, told Fox 40.

16. Your baby can "see the light!"

Adapted from American Baby (americanbaby.com May 2013)

The author had never heard of this Tale until he read the above article.

In your last trimester supposedly if you shine a flashlight on you baby bump, your baby "will see the light" and start moving. Further, you may feel your baby move toward (or, depending on the baby's attitude, gravitate away from) the beam of light. From a medical basis, the baby's eyes are developed and can open in the last weeks of pregnancy. The article states that "she'll react to the light."

Medical and anatomically evidence there is no way that light can penetrate the woman's abdominal wall as well as the uterine muscular wall. Even if the baby's eyes were open, light cannot penetrate these "walls" so that the baby will see any light. The amniotic cavity is pitch-black and the baby usually keeps their eyes closed.

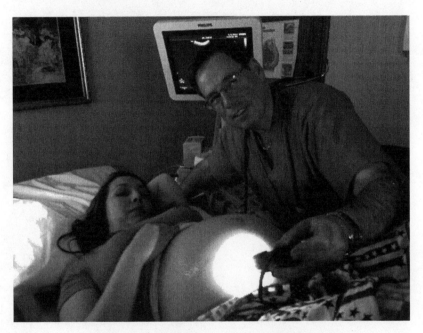

Figure 24-5 Baby sees the light? Does your baby react to the light?

We have checked this particular experimented with many patients and the results actually show the baby really cannot see any light while in the uterus: who would have known!

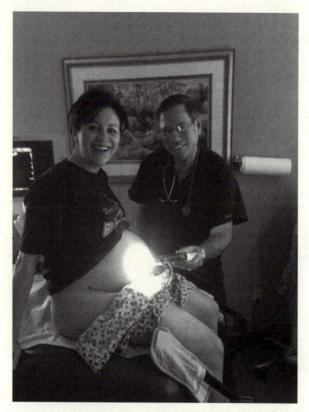

Figure 24-6 Babies seeing light. She said, "I think I felt the baby move!" Author said, "Maybe something else was moving!"."

More Old Wives Tales that try to predict the sex of your baby

The following are more or less similar "tales" (some reiterated differently from the last section) that have no truth or medical basis. These "sayings" or "myths" have been perpetuated for generations. They are presented here only for your amusement.

Your baby's heart rate

Whenever the author listens to the heartbeat of a baby during an office visit, the patient or a family member always ask me the baby's heart rate. According to "old wives tale," 140+ beats per minute indicates a girl, and below 140 a boy.

Drano Test-Revised

This "old wives tale" is fairly new and the author has been hearing it just from the past 20 years. It is the Drano test. You take mix a cup of urine (3 to 4 ounces) with a tablespoon of Drano.® In this test, the urine changes color. According to this test, your urine turns a certain color with the added drano as follows:

Green: you are having a girl

Blue: you are having a boy.

"Old Mayan Wives' Tale: Even and Odd numbers

This Tale is based on looking at two significant numbers: the age of the mother at the time of conception and the Mayan "year" of conception. If both numbers are even, it's supposed to be a girl. If one's even and one is odd, it's a boy. A variation of this tale is if the Mayan year is an even number, then if the mother's age is an even number, it is a girl. If the age of conception is an odd number, it is a boy. If the Mayan "year number" is odd, then the converse is still true.

The Key Test

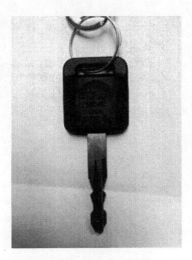

Figure 24-7 Key Test

Have a friend place a large key in front of the pregnant subject. According to this test, if the pregnant patient reaches for the key by the end of the key (or narrow part), it is a girl. If she tries to grab it by the head or rounded end of the key, it is a boy.

The Acne Test

This Tale is based on the old saying, "A baby girl steals all of her mother's beauty." Accordingly if you are experiencing more acne and blemishes than ever before, you are carrying a girl. If your complexion stays fairly normal, you are having a boy.

The Ring Test

This test is performed by taking off your wedding ring and tying it to a string of about 12 inches long. Hold the string in front of your baby bump. If the motion of the ring is "back and forth," then you are having a girl. If the motion of the ring makes a circular motion, you are having a boy.

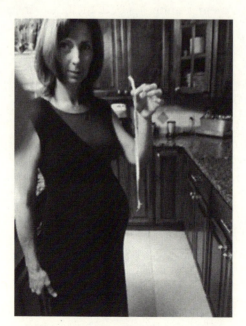

Figure 24-8 Morning Sickness Test

If you are experiencing rather severe morning sickness, then supposedly you are having a girl. If you are having very little nausea, you are having a boy.

The Linea Nigra Test

The "linea nigra" is a term translated from the Latin words meaning "black line. "There is a natural concentration of melanin producing cells ("melanocytes") in the body's midline area. Whether you form a "linea nigra" during your pregnancy depends on your race and ethnicity: it forms in darker skinned women such as Blacks and Hispanics. Caucasian women tend not to form them. If they do, it is a very faint line. This dark brownish line (about ½ inch in width) extends down the midline of your abdomen from the base of your sternum to your pubic area. Accordingly, you can tell the sex of your baby by the length of this line: If the line just runs from your pubic area to your belly button only, it is a girl. If the line runs all the way from your pubic area to the area just below your rib cage, then it is a boy.

THE "BLACK LINE," TAN NIPPLES AND OTHER COLOR CHANGES ON YOUR BODY

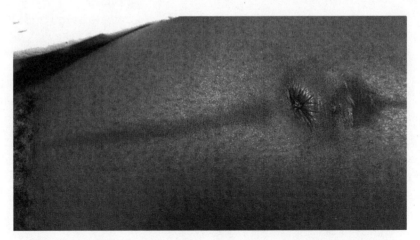

Figure 24-9 Linea Nigra. Photo of Black Line during Pregnancy

Similarly there also is a higher concentration melanocytes in your nipples and areola. As your pregnancy advances in weeks (particularly in the last half), your areola and nipples of your breasts, as well as your linea nigra, will darken progressively. The darkness of your nipples and the "black line" will fade in time only to come back again in future pregnancies. No treatment is necessary.

Mayan" Numbers Variation"

This Tale is a variation of the Mayan numbers calculation but uses your numerical age and the number of the month you conceived (January equals the number 1 and December gives you the number 12). You add your numerical age at the time of conception with the number of the month you conceived: if the resulting sum is an odd number, then you are having girl. Conversely, if the sum is an even number, then you are having a boy.

Cold Feet Tale

If your are complaining more of experiencing cold feet during your pregnancy, then supposedly you are having a boy. Conversely, if you notice that the temperature of feet has not really changed, then you are having a girl! Of course, this theory is based on the fact that you are wearing your shoes and socks when you go outside in the middle of winter!

Pillow Test

The direction or the position of your pillow when you sleep is the basis of this old tale. You probably will not know until you wake up.

If it is north or horizontal, then you may be having a boy. If the pillow lies vertical or lies below your head, it points to a girl gender. The bottom line: you are most likely to have gotten pregnant if you can't find your pillow or it fell off the bed!

How are you sleeping in your bed?

If you sleep on your left side while you are pregnant, then you are having a boy. Conversely, then if you are sleeping mostly on your right side, it is a girl.

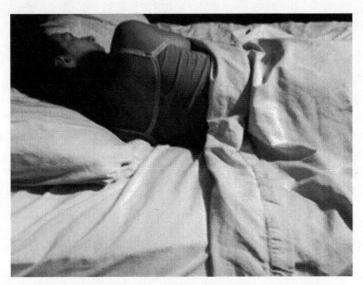

Figure 24-10 Sleeping position and the sex of a baby

Urine Color Test

From a medical standpoint the color of urine depends on primarily your water intake and the foods you eat. Apparently some "old wives" say that if you have bright yellow urine, you are supposedly having a boy. However, if your urine is either dull or even clear, then you are having a girl.

There is really no medical foundation for this Tale. It is important to keep hydrated during pregnancy to the point that your urine is clear and slightly colored. Some foods like asparagus which are rich nitrogen, give the urine an "ammonia" smell.

Hair Growth Theory

Certainly a male baby produces more testosterone from its young testes than a girl baby. However, there are no significant differences of testosterone in the maternal blood stream to the point a blood test on the mother can reveal the baby's gender. It is a good theory but to date, it has not been scientifically verified.

However, that does not stop some "Old Wives" from telling their daughters that if you are experiencing faster growth of hair on your head, armpits, legs and other places, then you are more likely having a boy. Certainly hair (and everything in your body!) grows faster when you are pregnant. From a medical standpoint hormones, such as growth hormone (HGH)and other male hormones (androgens). are secreted in significant amounts to affect the mother's body and her organs.

Shape of Your Belly Test

Apparently if your "baby bump" resembles a basketball, then you are supposedly carrying a boy. If your "bump" looks more oblong like a watermelon, then conversely you are carrying a girl.

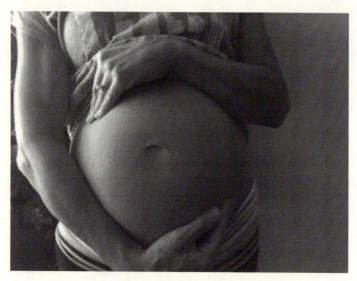

Figure 24-11 Bump Shape and sex

Nose Shape and Growth

This Tale is a corollary to the "Hair Growth" theory. Testosterone and other androgen hormone from a boy baby cause your nose to grow and change shape. However, as stated above, growth hormones and other hormones from the placenta can stimulate many maternal organs to grow and change.

Facial Changes

According to this Tale, the mother's face becomes rounder and fills out more if you are having a girl. If the shape of the face becomes longer and less round, conversely you supposedly are carrying a boy.

Demeanor and Agility

Apparently if a woman is coordinated and carries herself with grace, she is mostly like to have a girl. If she is not athletic and awkward or fumbling things, she is having a boy.

Show me your Hands

You can tell what a pregnant woman is having by the way she puts her hand out. If she puts her hands out and you see the back of her hands, then she is supposedly having a boy. If the hands come out with palms showing, she is having a girl.

Do you smell Garlic?

This Tale states that if a pregnant woman should eat garlic and she does not smell of the garlic thereafter, she is carrying a girl. If she does smell of garlic, she is having a boy. From a scientific basis, this Tale is dependent on the amount of garlic you eat (or can eat whole!). The more garlic you eat, the more likely your body is going to give off the garlic scent. It just makes commonsense, but who said these Tales are based on anything but coincidences.

Saving the best for Last? Skip this one if you are smart!

Since most of these "old wives tales" are usually directed to determining your baby's sex, I might as well throw in another bit of humor with regarding "how to tell the sex:"

Do you know how to tell "the sex" of a chromosome?

Are you ready for this? Are you sure?

Answer: "you pull down its genes!"

More Myths about Pregnancy

For 9 Myths about Pregnancy the reader is referred to the following link, **http://blogs.momaha.com/2014/03/9-pregnancy-myths-busted/**

CHAPTER 25

"Old Husband's Tales"

JUST TO BE FAIR:

(This space was intentionally left blank because there are no such things as "Old Husband's Tales!" Silly!

CHAPTER 26

Old Obstetrician Tales (Yes, there are such Tales!)

In this section the author would like to share some of his personal experiences with "Special Deliveries" during his career in Obstetrics.

<u>Author's Disclosure</u>: *These Stories may have been **enhanced** or changed* (author's discretion) in order to heighten the reader's interest.

The DaSilva Family

Anna DaSilva came to see me for her third pregnancy. She already had 2 boys. She desperately wanted a girl. If she had a girl, she stated that her family would have been completed. She would not want any more children. This girl would be her last baby. There was time before Ob doctors had routine ultrasound machines in the office. Anna and her husband, Alonso, were descendants from Portuguese roots as were many of patients in the East San Francisco Bay cities of Hayward and San Leandro. Her husband was a painter. He wanted a large family: he needed the boys to help him in his painting business. He wanted another boy!

Long story short: Anna went into labor in late evening one night. It was 2 o'clock in the morning when Anna was ready to deliver. I was sleepy and tired when I arrived at her room to deliver her. Anna had an epidural. The delivery was fairly normal. Anna delivered her baby girl! The husband was happy and sad at the same time. He knew he was not going to have another boy. After his girl delivered I cut the cord and gave Anna her baby girl. Then with my eyes barely open from lack of sleep, I looked up at Anna's tummy and it was still pretty large. By instinct I reached inside of Anna rechecked her: yes, I could feel another baby's head up there!

I then asked her to push some more and out came a beautiful baby boy! Everyone was happy and excited: Anna had her girl and Alonso had his boy! Yes, they had the family they wanted!

Anna had prayed for her girl and Alonso had wished for another boy. By some Grand Plan both had been blessed with the babies they had wanted at the very same time.

The Garabaldi Family

There was this large closely-knit Italian family named the Garibaldis. Most of the family had recently come over and emigrated from Italy. The grandson's wife was pregnant for the first time. Well, the day came that she was finally in labor. As what typically happens, the husband was right next to his wife in the delivery suite. His side of the family was there all cheering her on. The doctor was at the foot of the bed getting ready to deliver the baby. The doctor said to her, "push." With that effort a beautiful baby girl was born. The family went crazy and were screaming and crying.

The Ob doctor cut the cord. The Ob doctor then looked at the patient's abdomen and appeared very puzzled. He then placed his hand inside of her again. Suddenly the doctor yelled out to her, "to push hard again," and out came a beautiful baby boy! The family went crazy again and started shouting. Instantly the new father, the grandson, became very pale and white and quickly passed out onto the floor.

The next day the husband was going into the room to see his wife at the same time the doctor was making his rounds on her. The husband said to the Ob doctor apologetically, "I am so sorry I passed out. We were not expecting two babies! I just couldn't stand the unexpected surprise and, I guess, I fainted. Now I need to figure out a couple of names for the two babies.

The Ob doctor replied, "No, you don't.

The husband replied, "What do you mean?"

The Ob doctor said, "Well, your Uncle Garibaldi, he named the twins when you were passed out."

The husband asked the doctor, "He did? But, he just came over from Italy a month ago and he hardly speaks any English!

What did he name my baby girl?

The Ob doctor said, "Denise!"

The husband said, "Denise, huh! That's a very pretty name. Denise, I like it!"

Then he asked, "Well, what did he name my little baby boy?"

(Are you ready for this? Here it comes!)

The Ob doctor said, "De-nephew!"

Melanie, the Hairdresser Athlete

Melanie was a well-known and popular hairdresser in Fremont, CA. She was a beautiful lady. She worked out regularly at the Gym. Though she was 43 years of age, she still regularly turned guy's heads in the Gym. Melanie had two boys. She always longed to have a daughter.

Then one day she found out that her husband's ex-wife was pregnant. Not only was she pregnant but she was having a girl! This situation caused her great distress. She was now obsessed with the notion of getting pregnant and having her long desired daughter. She was my patient. I had seen me for regular annual pelvic exams.

Melanie made an appointment with me immediately after finding out that her ex-husband's wife was having a daughter. Now she wanted me to help her get pregnant at the age of 44. We tried months of fertility treatments in the office without success. I referred her to our IVF (In vitro Fertilization) r Reproductive Endocrinology physicians nearby. She finally became pregnant. Not only did she achieve pregnancy but she was pregnant with twins! Though she was now age 45 Melanie looked much younger and was a "knock out" in looks and figure. She had a "hard body." It compared better than that of most 25 year olds.

She continued to keep fit during her pregnancy. Her pregnancy was uncomplicated. She carried both those babies to near term. She never complained about anything during her pregnancy.

She had normal deliveries of both babies.

Yes, you guessed it.

She delivered two beautiful and healthy *boys*!

The City Councilman's Wife

I was taking care of our local city councilman's wife while she was in labor. Labor was not progressing and we had to deliver her by C-section. The C-section room was a room within the interior portion hospital and did not have any external access or windows to the outside. It was 5:30 PM and the C-section operation was underway. There was a thunderstorm passing over the region but it was not considered serious. The city councilman was at the head of the bed right next to the anesthesiologist and his wife. Just as we were ready to make the incision into the uterus and deliver the baby, the lights went out in the room. The Operating room was pitch black.

All hospitals are equipped with emergency generator backup systems. We waited for the emergency generator to kick in, but it did not. The nurses rushed to get the flashlights so that we could see dimly in the operating room. The fire station was just a mile away and within "eye sight" of the hospital. Very shortly, a group of fireman, carrying commercial portable lighting, burst into the OR. Apparently the backup generator was not functioning due to the fact a piece of wood had become stuck in the emergency switch. Nonetheless, while the fireman and the councilman held the flashlights for us to see, we finished the C-section and delivered a healthy baby boy!

I guess you can envision the probable TV commercial right now: Tall brave fireman in their fire repellant garbs holding up flashlights while the OB is doing the C-section. You can hear the commercial spokesman proclaiming,

"When the light goes out and you are charged with the duty to help bring new life into the world safely you know you can only trust and depend on these batteries in an emergency!

I can see the Energizer bunny and the *Copper Top* battery companies basking in their proud triumphal product success.

Zweig's Laws of Obstetrics

> The author was up in the middle of the night delivering a baby. It is okay to deliver a baby at 1 am or maybe at 5 am. But please, do not deliver a baby at 3am. This is the worst possible time of day for an obstetrician. You cannot get enough sleep prior to the birth or try to reclaim it after you get home at 5 am. It splits the night into two halves which never seem to ever get whole again. Consequently, I have promulgated my first two Laws of Obstetrics as follows:
>
> *First Law of Obstetrics*
> The time of a baby's birth is directly proportional to the time of conception.
>
> *Second Law of Obstetrics*
> The length or duration of a woman's time in labor is indirectly related to the frequency of sexual intercourse during pregnancy.

Corollary to the Second Law of Obstetrics (my fiancé is a Mathematics professor!)
What got you in this mess can get you out!

How to be sure your teen uses birth control (especially my teenager)

It was just another Saturday afternoon in Fremont, CA. I was spending "quality time" with my daughter, Jennifer. She was 14 years of age. As is custom in spending "quality time" with your daughter, you usually wind up at the mall buying clothes and other things that she "has to have." We were at Macy's in New Park Mall. She was trying on Guess jeans and jackets. Suddenly, my pager is going off (yes, this is a time before you could just carry around a cell phone). I ran over to the nearest pay phone in the store (there was such a thing as a pay phone in the US!). I called Labor and Delivery at Washington Hospital. The nurse told me that one of my young patients came into the hospital in active labor and "was going fast." She wanted me there ASAP. I went over to Jennifer and told her we had to go. I quickly paid for her clothes and drove off to the hospital about 2 miles east of the mall (but Mowry Blvd was always busy with traffic). As I was driving with her I realized that I could not get her home and still get back to the hospital in time: our home was 2 miles further east of the hospital. It then came to me: I would ask Jennifer if she would like to see her dad in action. Jennifer, I asked, "I can't take you home because this girl is going to deliver quickly. Would you like to see a baby born?" She said, "Sure, Dad."

Well, we quickly ran up the stairs to the Labor and Delivery Suite. I ran into the delivery room and asked the patient if my daughter could see her delivery. The patient yelled out at me (she laboring so quickly that she did not have time to get an epidural placed), "I don't care. Just get this baby out of me! She screamed out a few more words which I really don't think you would want to hear!

Jennifer was standing right next to me. Jennifer was frozen in action and watched in awe as the baby delivered through the tight vaginal opening. I cut the cord and gave the crying baby to the nursery nurse. I then proceeded to deliver the placenta. As the placenta started coming out, I heard Jennifer's voice behind me, say, "Dad, I'm leaving now!

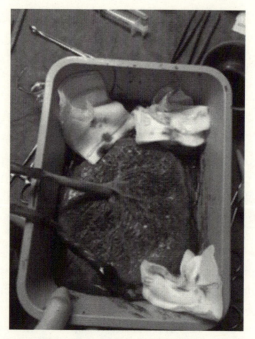

Figure 26-1 Placenta or "after-birth:" Placental Photo

It was a very fortuitous happening. From that moment on, Jennifer knew that she was never going to have a baby "anytime soon." I am happy to report than Jennifer became a very responsible teenager ("Hey Dad, I need the morning after pill"). She morphed into a very good Mom herself. After she first completed her B.A. degree, secured a promising career and had purchased her first home, she had my first grandchild when she was at age 34. I am so glad that I had the occasion to spend real *quality time* with my daughter *that* day!

The Story of Jennifer's Birth

I have to admit that Jennifer was a special child. It was a very unusual day when she was born at UCLA Medical Center. I was the ER (Emergency Room) Ob-Gyn. My shift as a 2nd year resident started at 7 am. I reported to the hospital and went down to ER. Usually there are about 1-2 patients waiting to be seen. The resident on the graveyard shift usually tries to sleep or procrastinate until 7 am and let the day Ob-Gyn see the patients that presented in the early morning hours.

I went down to the ER. Amazingly, there were no patients left over from the night shift. No one was waiting to be seen. Very strange, since the General Surgery residents loved to push the patients with "below the navel" abdominal pain to the Ob-Gyn residents. My Chairman of the Department was J. George Moore and he told us that, if the General Surgery residents didn't want to diagnose an appendicitis, that his Ob-Gyn Residents would! My chairman loved to tell the Chief of Surgery during the Chairman Meetings that his Ob-Gyn residents did 3 or 4 appendicitis surgeries during the previous month!

It was quite an unusual and eerie day. I decided to go over to the UCLA Hospital cafeteria and get some coffee and snack on whatever else they had left over from breakfast that might look good. While I was sipping my coffee and talking with some other residents, more than 35 minutes must have passed by. Then I did get paged to go to the ER. I quickly finished my coffee and hurried down to the ER.

When I arrived, I saw *my wife* being wheeled into the exam room. She had gone to work at California State Department of Highways as a civil engineer. While on her drafting stool, she had ruptured her membranes. She came in to the ER leaking amniotic fluid. She was 4 weeks from her due date. We were not expecting or anticipating an early arrival. I quickly verified that her membranes had ruptured and called her Ob-Gyn. I accompanied her to the Labor and Delivery suite. Janelle Goss, MD came and saw her in the labor room. She collected some of the amniotic fluid from the vagina with a syringe and submitted the specimen to the lab. Meanwhile my wife lay comfortable in her bed. It would take at least 24 hours to process the test results. She did not go into labor as could very well have happened (the further in days and weeks that you are distant from your due date, the less likely that you will go into labor and vice versa).

The next day the report came back: the amniotic fluid studies revealed that the Lecithin-Spingomyelin ratio (L/S ratio) was in the "mature" range and there would be a low chance that our baby would have respiratory problems if she were born at this time. After the positive test results were in, Induction of labor was started immediately.

At about 3-4 cm of dilatation, my wife had requested an epidural. I stood outside her labor room as the anesthesiologist put in her epidural. Suddenly, there was a ruckus in the labor room, the "code blue" emergency was called and nurses in her room rushed to bring the crash cart in. I was afraid for my wife and unborn baby's life. I didn't know what to do: I was not allowed to help and treat her. At this point, there really wasn't anything I could do. I was helpless in this situation. Everyone, all the physicians and nurses, was doing everything they could.

Apparently, there was an inadvertent intravascular injection of the anesthetic and my wife started "seeing spiders crawling all over the walls." Obviously she was frightened and feared for her life. She stabilized shortly thereafter and became quickly dilated. I coached her and I pushed with her with every contraction. I kept holding my breath with each of the pushes as she was doing. I was ready to pass out at any time!

The baby's heart beat was being monitored. When she was close to delivery, they brought her into the delivery room (at the time patients were moved from the labor room to a fully equipped delivery room but nowadays we do *both* labor and delivery in the "birthing rooms"). As my wife was close to deliver the fetal heart tones dropped down in the lows 70's and then bounced up into the 80's. Janelle Goss, MD was in the delivery room and immediately asked the nurse to get the forceps. The forceps were applied and within a two contractions, my baby girl was delivered at 4:23 pm April 19, 1975.

She was 4 weeks early but she did not have any respiratory problems. She had to be placed under the "Bili lights." Neonatal jaundice is a very common problem with premature babies. Her jaundice improved (Bilirubin=18.6) over the next 4 days and both Mom and Jennifer were finally coming home.

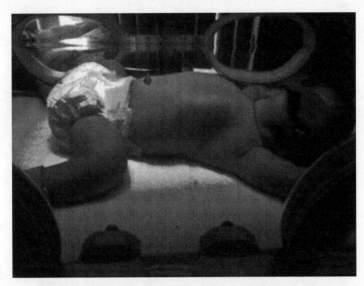

Figure 26-2 Jaundice Treatment Baby under the "Bili Lights" with sunglasses and "catching some rays"

The "moral" to this story is that Jennifer was a very special child. She delivered early and was always my "precocious child." She was just as precious as any child that is brought into this world. Jennifer overcame an anesthetic complication as well as obstetrical complications (premature rupture of membranes and a prolonged fetal heart bradycardia) prior to birth. Even an Ob-Gyn's wife can have serious problems with her pregnancy, labor and delivery. I don't think that Jennifer knows how many problems we negotiated prior to her entry into the world. So if there is anything you readily need to know about obstetrics is that a baby is a very important gift from God and you better do everything possible to protect her (or him).It is your responsibility to love and protect her for the rest of your life.

Seen below is a recent picture of my daughter, Jennifer and her two children, Emmy and Thomas.

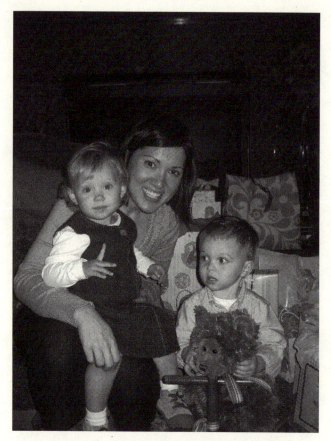

Figure 26-3 Dr. Zweig's daughter, Jennifer, with her daughter, Emerson, and son, Thomas

Four babies in 26 minutes

I was working my 12 hour shift at Kaiser Hospital in Hayward, CA. I went into Delivery room #1. The patient had been pushing for at least 2 hours and was getting pretty tired. She had an epidural. In fact, most patients at Kaiser received Epidurals.

I gowned and gloved and prepped the patient for delivery. The baby was fairly big: about 8-9 lbs. I asked for the Ob forceps. I greased them with betadine soap. I slid them around the baby's head. With each push I gently tugged downward and outward. The baby's head moved with each contraction. After 3 contractions the baby's head was crowning.

I slipped off the forceps. She was going to tear badly. I made a straight 2 inch incision (episiotomy) to make room for the large baby's head. The head and the rest of the baby came out. As I was clamping the cord, another OB nurse popped her head in the room and said that another patient was being moved into Delivery Room #2. As soon as the placenta delivered the Ob nurse stated I was now needed in Room #2. There was not a minute of time at this point to sew up my patient. I went in the second Delivery Room and put on new gown and gloves. The baby was already crowning. I lubricated the outer vaginal area and the baby came out. I clamped and cut the cord. I reached inside and felt another amniotic sac. She had twins, i.e., undiagnosed twins! The second twin was also coming "head first." I ruptured the second sac and within minutes the second twin's head was crowning. After the second twin delivered I waited and massaged the uterus. Shortly thereafter, the double "twins" placenta came out. I was cleaning her up when another OB nurse came into the room and said, "We need you in Delivery Room #3 immediately." Another "Prego" (short for pregnant patient in Obstetrical language) had come up from the ER and was pushing. As soon as she was wheeled into the delivery room, I could see another baby's head pushing out her vulvar area. The head was big and as the baby's head stretched and dilated the vaginal opening, I could see she was going to tear. I cut a small episiotomy. The baby delivered easily. I clamped and cut the cord, delivered the placenta, sewed her up and cleaned her off.

I went back to delivery room #1. The poor patient still had her legs up in the stirrups all during the aforementioned deliveries occurred. I finally got a chance to sew her up. Everything was fine. All of the above events occurred in the span of about 26 minutes!

The Isuzu Baby (Isuzu Trooper SUV)

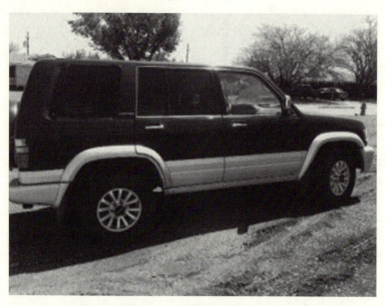

Figure 26-4 Picture of an Isuzu Trooper SUV

I was walking through the hospital corridor at San Ramon Regional Medical Center after finishing lunch in the hospital cafeteria. Suddenly over the overhead paging speaker came the loud urgent words of the Hospital Operator, "OB doctor stat to Hospital entrance. OB doctor needed immediately to report stat to the hospital entrance." I was about 20 feet from the hospital entrance and I had to go by it anyway in order to get back to my office. I said to myself, "the Hospital Operator must be wrong. She really meant OB doctor stat to the ER. Why would you need an OB doctor at the hospital entrance?"

As I hurried to the hospital entrance I saw this guy, the woman's husband frantically signally me to go to the front seat of his Isuzu vehicle. He opened the passenger door and there was his wife with her legs up on the dashboard.

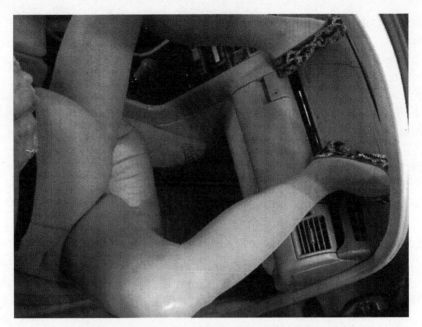

Figure 26-5 Image Reproduction of patient ready to deliver in front passenger seat.

The head was crowning: about ready to deliver. The husband told me that they had left Concord and driven at 80 miles per hour down I-680 in order to get to the hospital as fast as possible. He was now hysterical. The wife then said to me in a slow, calm and low voice, "please, doctor, don't let me tear."

It was her first baby. I could not believe how controlled and relaxed she was given the situation. I told her to push very gently and we very slowly allowed the vaginal opening to stretch over the head. The baby delivered easily and without any tears or laceration. As soon as I got the baby into my arms the OB staff had rushed down the hallways from Labor and Delivery. They brought the gurney and the BOA (Born out of Asepsis, i.e., the emergency quick delivery kit/sterile instruments) package. The OB nurse handed me the cord clamp and scissors and I handed the baby to the nursery nurses from inside the Isuzu door.

We put the new mom on the gurney and brought her to the Birthing Room. I delivered the placenta and cleaned her up. The baby had already been weighed and wrapped up like a burrito. As the nursery

RN gave her newly born baby to hold for the first time, instantly she became mother to the baby. You could see maternal smile and love on her face. Her arms embraced and protected her baby. A gentle and tender countenance beamed from all over her body.

I had nothing to do with it but somehow the local newspaper, *The San Ramon Valley Times*, got hold of this story. It was Front Page News in big bold type: BABY BORN IN FRONT SEAT OF ISUZU AND THE BABY IS A REALTROOPER!

I really can't make up these kinds of stories. It really happened. And, by the way, the woman's OB doctor never thanked me or extended the professional courtesy for delivering his patient.

April fool's Days

The OB nurses really get enthusiastic about this particular day: I am sure that this is the designated day on which they can play pranks on the doctors and get away with it.

I was starting my 24 hour shift on the 1st of April. I worked at Kaiser Hospital in Hayward, CA at that time.. Usually there may be one or two patients in labor. When I walked back to the Nurse's station, I looked on the OB blackboard (now a computer screen) and saw that all 6 of the labor rooms were full. There were names, status of cervical dilations, epidural placed, membranes ruptured, etc. There were the six charts on the desk with prenatal papers and other paperwork in the charts. I thought to myself, "this is already starting out a busy day and I just began my call. I asked the nurses which patients I needed to check or discuss with them. They all started laughing. Actually, there was no one in labor! They all said, "April Fools!" They got me!

In another incident I walked into the Labor suite at Washington Hospital in Fremont, CA. I usually check the Labor suite before making rounds on the postpartum floor. I looked up on the OB Board and saw the following information written: "Mrs. Wright delivered by ER doctor at 6:32 am." I immediately went over to the OB nurse. I asked her why I was not called sooner about my patient. First, I asked why I was not informed about my patient being in the hospital and second, why I was not called when she was ready for her delivery. I only lived 7 minutes from the hospital. The nurse looked at me very sternly and then said, "April Fool's Day!" Mrs. Wright was not there and she had not even delivered. They got me!

Lastly, the following year on April 1st at Washington Hospital, I asked the nursery RN that I needed to do a circumcision. It was to be performed on one of the baby boys I had delivered from the previous day. There are a series of procedures that need to be done prior to actually doing a circumcision: the nursery RN checks to see if the consents have been properly signed, verifies the baby band that it is the right baby, etc. She then puts the baby on a special restraint board, preps the area and opens up the sterile instruments package. Because these procedural steps take some amount of time, I usually go out to the postpartum floor and see one or two patients. I usually return in 5-10 minutes ready to do the circumcision. When I arrived in the nursery I saw that the baby had not even been placed on the board. The baby was still in his Isolette! I asked the nursery RN why the baby was not ready. She stated rather firmly to me, "you want to circumcise that baby?" I replied, "Yes, I do. I thought I had already asked you to do so 15 minutes ago!" She quickly went over to the Isolette, pulled the blanket down, picked up the baby and then suddenly threw *the baby* across the room at me! Completely flabbergasted and astonished, I desperately reach out and successfully caught the baby. At that instance I realize that "the baby" was just an imitation baby doll! I am sure you can hear the nurses telling everyone how well they fooled me that April 1st!

The Camper on Interstate 680

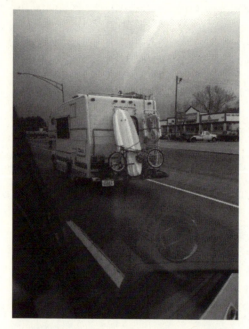

Figure 26-6 Interstate 680 Camper

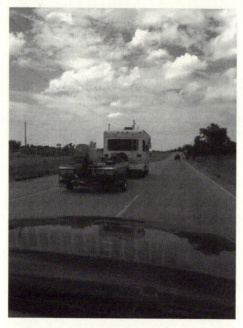

Figure 26-7 Camper on Interstate 680

I was called by a fellow Ob-Gyn colleague, Joel Klein, MD to help him with a C-section at John Muir Hospital at 5 o'clock. It was a Friday afternoon. California hospital staff rules required another MD physician assistant for all major surgeries including C-sections. I knew everyone was going to be headed out of town for the weekend. I tried to finish my office and get on the Interstate as fast as possible. It didn't work out like I wanted. The Interstate was crammed with back to back traffic. Vehicles were moving at a snail's pace. I knew all the exits and shortcuts on the Interstate in order to get to the hospital faster. I was traveling in the *fast* left lane, but it was not as fast as I wanted it to be given the set of my circumstances (my need to be helping with a C-section in 10 minutes time).

As I was moving slowly northward to the hospital, a camper truck was passing me by in the middle lane. He was towing a fishing boat. On the back of the camper were strapped bicycles and an outdoor grill. I even saw his fishing poles and his tackle boxes.

Here was the current state of affairs: I was rushing to help do a C-section on a Friday afternoon while this guy in the camper was head out for a great weekend of camping and fishing. I had a college degree from Johns Hopkins and a MD from UC San Francisco. I was even high school Valedictorian.

So I asked myself and I am asking you, "Who was the brightest guy on Interstate 680 at 5 PM this Friday at beginning of the weekend afternoon, the Ob-Gyn doctor or that happy guy rocking out in his camper and pulling his boat?"

Remembering Rita

I was really uncertain whether to share this story in this book. Rita came to me for her 4th pregnancy. The pregnancy and the delivery were routine and she delivered a healthy baby girl. Rita's husband was an electrician in Pleasanton, CA. He was in business by himself and had a few workers to help him out. He was quite busy and worked hard. He had a long day.

About 9 months after Rita delivered Rita went to her family physician for a skin mole to be removed. Apparently after her physician had injected the local anesthetic into her skin, Rita suffered a catastrophic reaction. She stopped breathing and collapsed. The physician office was less than 1 mile from the hospital. Resuscitation was begun at the office. Rita was transported to the hospital. Rita never regained consciousness and she died that same day. It was horrific and unbelievable. The entire community was shocked and stunned. Why do "bad things" happen to "good people?"

Rita's husband had 4 children to support. Family, friends and neighbors all came to help him out. He had to support his family and he could not be away from his business for any extended time.

About a month after the tragic death of Rita I had a new patient come to see me for an annual exam. She was, as I remember her telling me, a cousin of Rita. She had graduated college but had not found work. She was told about heart-rending loss of Rita. The family had gotten together and sought out solutions to help Rita's husband in his difficult situation. They asked her if she could help his family out on a temporary basis. She left Southern California and came to be "the nanny" for the children. She was there also to help him, the widower, with the household duties. It was a wonderful gesture and act of compassion.

After I saw her for the exam, I did not keep up with how she, the widowed father and the kids were doing. I know that her presence helped the family cope as well as they could. They were all trying to adjust to the loss of their mother.

The next time I saw the "Nanny" was at another office visit about one year later. Apparently the children, the nanny and the widowed husband had all "jived" together as a happy working family. The children were coping as best as possible without their mother and the widowed husband's business as an electrician was thriving. There were all happy together. So happy that the "Nanny" and the widowed husband fell in love and had married. She was now at my office for a special reason: she was seeing me for her first pregnancy!

I have reflected over the years about the sequence of catastrophic events that transpired in this family. I, however, consider this preceding story to have a "happy ending." From out of a horrible tragic happening, salvation, love and the rebirth of a new and perhaps, though not the same, rehabilitated family was made possible.

As Rascal Flatts sings in his beautiful ballad,

> "It's all part of a grander plan that is coming true
> But now I'm just rolling home into my lover's arms
> This much I know is true
> That God blessed the broken road that led me straight to you"

This story is dedicated to the memory of Rita who reminds all of us that we all do not travel down a smooth road. It is a "broken road" that we travel in life, in love and in our work. The "broken road" is the one that makes us "grow" as human beings and, in that process, makes each individual a better person. Each of us is transported as we become closer to being perfect in God's eyes (see Scott Peck, *The Road Less Traveled*).

As these classic musical groups, i.e. the Shirelles and the Mamas and Pappas, sang a long time ago, and as Rita would be saying to us today, in their song, *Dedicated to the One I* Love,

> Each night before you go to bed, my baby
> Whisper a little prayer for me, my baby,
> Yeah, and tell all the stars above, (All the stars)
> This is dedicated to the one I love

The Tennessee Trucker Woman

At a different time in my career, I moved from Northern California to Northwest Tennessee. Paris, Tennessee to be exact (I guess I was trying to get as far away as possible from my ex-wife)

In my office I was seeing a new patient who was pregnant. She was 41 years old, overweight (I'm being nice for not saying "obese"), was an insulin-dependent diabetic on high blood pressure medication (she had hypertension). For her livelihood she drove a truck, not just your average Silverado pickup truck, but a genuine 18-wheeler Big Rig Truck. Her job was hauling goods around the Southeast Interstates.

She also had a vertical scar from her first C-section. The first C-section was complicated by a wound infection. The incision on the uterus was "classic" type which means that her uterus could rupture anytime in late pregnancy without even being in labor. If she ruptured her uterus, she could lose the baby. She could even lose her very own life! She also had a thyroid problem. I was overwhelmed with the number of risk factors this patient had. She was early into her pregnancy when I first saw her. She was telling me how she was very careful in monitoring her blood sugars and her insulin. I went over all the risk factors (including her age with increased risk of Down's syndrome, diabetes with the increased risk of cleft palate and heart abnormalities, as well as the risk of uterine rupture, etc.) with her. She was not alarmed at all. Finally, as I was somewhat shaken with all these high risk factors, I blurted out to her, "You know, you could *die* from this pregnancy!" She calmly replied, "No, it is all in God's hands." I said to myself, "No, not exactly. It is really going to be "all in my hands" (with the help of God, I hope). I am not trying to espouse religious doctrine, but I believe God gives us some choice (in fact, a whole lot of decisions *we* make on our own) Please see the next story of Mr. Garcia from Alviso, CA that follows)

She was a good patient and was very compliant with controlling her diabetes and her blood pressure. In order to avoid risking rupture of her uterus, I delivered her 2 weeks early. The physicians at Vanderbilt University had recommended that I pull her abdominal roll down (her belly button was already at the level of her pubis, and make a vertical incision midline in her upper abdomen (above the belly button) and pull the baby out from the top of the uterus (a classic-type uterine incision in the thick muscular part of the uterus). I thought about that advice for weeks. When it came time to deliver her, I made a large elliptical incision all around the roll, took out the 15 lbs. wedge of fat, and then delivered the baby through the lower part of the uterus as is customarily done. I closed her up and she went home in 3 days without any infection!

So, the question is, was the Tennessee Trucker right all along, "It was in God's hands?"

When she was being wheeled chaired out of the hospital, I think even I heard a voice from above cheering her on "Keep on Trucking!"

Mr. Juan Garcia of Alviso, CA but it is a not a pregnancy story

This is not another pregnancy story. It is about free choice and God's providence. You have to think about it and decide for yourself whether you, as an individual, have self- determination or that your life is pre-destined or pre-determined.

Mr. Juan Garcia lived in Alviso; CA. Alviso is a small town on the southeast tip of the San Francisco Bay. The town lives in a flood plain. Whenever there is a very heavy rainy season, this area of the bay gets flooded. Well, this story occurs during one of those heavy rainy seasons.

Alviso is going to be flooded again and the police have called for a general evacuation of the area. The police cars arrive and knock on Mr. Garcia's door. The water level is already going through the front door. The police tell Mr. Garcia to come with them in order to avoid harm. Mr. Garcia says to them, "I go to Church every Sunday and pray to God. He will not let anything happen to me!" The police say "okay," but you better get out. Mr. Garcia goes up to his second floor. An hour later, the water rises higher. A Disaster Relief boat comes by his home and yells out to him, "You better get out now or you could be harmed." Mr. Garcia says to them, "I go to Church every Sunday and pray to God. He will not let anything happen to me!" The Disaster Boat leaves him. The water now rises to the second floor. Mr. Garcia goes up and stands on his roof. A rescue helicopter spots him and lowers the basket so he can climb in. "You better get out before you die." Mr. Garcia again say, "I go to Church every Sunday and pray to God. He will not let anything happen to me!" The helicopter leaves. Sure enough, Mr. Garcia is swept off the roof and dies. He now stands before the Pearly Gates of Heaven talking to St. Peter. Mr. Garcia is complaining to him. "I just don't understand how this could happen. I go to Church and pray to God every Sunday. I want to speak to God if I may." St Peter says he will ask God. Soon enough, Mr. Garcia gets his request for an audience with God. He is now standing before God.

Mr. Garcia says to God, "I cannot understand how I could die. I have been a faithful and religious soul and have always practiced your Word. I just can't believe that you would not help me and let me die!" God then leaned over to Mr. Garcia and said, "What do you mean I didn't try to help you. I sent out 3 rescue teams to save you and you didn't listen to any of them!

Do we all miss opportunities in life or do we do we just don't recognize them? There are many doors to open in life: life is all about picking the right ones. Or do we pick the doors chosen for us?

There is a time for everyone if they only learn, that the twisting kaleidoscope moves us all in turn
There's a rhyme and reason to the wild outdoors

From "Can you Feel the Love Tonight," Sir Elton John

We are all ordinary. We are all boring. We are all spectacular. We are all shy. We are all bold. We are all heroes. We are all helpless. It just depends on the day. –Brad Melzer

My Hispanic Newlywed

I was a second year resident at UCLA when this 19 year old newlywed Hispanic girl came to the ER for evaluation in the early morning hours. She had been married just the previous day. Her chief symptom was vaginal bleeding. The bleeding had ensued this past night after they had consummated their marriage. I thought, "He might have been a little rough with her" as she had admitted to being a virgin prior to their marriage. There probably is a little vaginal tear that may need a suture or two."

She was slight of build and thin. She had an average height. She did not appear to be in much pain. She had a concerned countenance upon her.

I placed the vaginal speculum (the duck bill metal instrument) inside her but I really didn't see anything except a little dark blood. Then I did a bimanual (placed two fingers inside to evaluate the uterus and ovaries). To my instant surprise I was directly feeling one ovary with my fingers: usually you only feel a portion of the ovary lying near or against the vaginal wall. She was a narrow framed young woman. "No," I said to myself; he could not have rammed his penis right through the back wall of the vagina into the abdominal cavity. I couldn't imagine how much this penetration must have hurt her. I had never heard of this event ever happening.

I immediately called my Chief Resident and told him the clinical situation. He said "I don't believe you. "Not possible," he said. He said he was coming straight down to the ER to check out this crazy story. He, too, gently examined the young woman. He could not believe what had happened. He called one of our attending professors. They, too, never recalled such a complication. We took the newlywed woman to the OR, put her asleep, and sewed up the rent in the back wall of her vagina.

But, the story does not end here. I saw this sweet woman again 8 weeks later in the clinic. She was pregnant! I wondered what route the sperm took to get to the egg: directly to the ovary or perhaps through the uterus as is the normal route. Her pregnancy proceeded to near term when she developed severe pre-eclampsia (high blood pressure, swelling and spilling protein in her urine). We had to induce her labor and get the baby delivered in order to treat the disease. As I said, she was a narrow framed girl with a small pelvis. After many hours of labor, we realized that the baby was too big for her pelvis. We took her to the OR for a C-section. I do not recall ever seeing or meeting her husband. I think he left her sometime in the middle of her pregnancy. She and the baby did well after surgery. I saw her two years later. She was pregnant again. I am not sure who fathered the baby because it was about this time in my career that I stopped asking these type of *social* questions: it just got too depressing for me. Sadly, this pregnancy ended in a miscarriage. I was the physician who had to do her D&C.

The Red Hair Girl from Santa Maria, CA

I was a second year resident at UCLA when we accepted this girl as a transfer from Santa Maria Community Hospital that was located about 125 miles up the coast. She was 36 weeks pregnant with her first child. She was transferred to UCLA Medical Center because of a severe kidney infection. I initially thought that the Ob's in Santa Maria could have easily managed to take care of this patient themselves: just start her on broad spectrum antibiotics and she will recover. Her fever was 103.5 degrees F. We admitted her to the Ob-Gyn ICU on the second floor. She did have a high fever and there was a significant risk of systemic spread of the infection. In other medical words, she was "septic." Her urine testing, however, did not suggest a severe kidney infection. Kidney infections in pregnancy can be quite serious: high fever, chills, rigors and overall prostration.

After 24 hours of admission this patient started developing small blisters on her vulvar area. "A little bit of herpes to go along with her kidney infection," I said to myself.

A routine chemistry panel revealed very abnormal liver function tests. We pursued the evaluation one step further and those tests revealed severe liver infection, i.e. hepatitis. Her specific liver enzymes, the SGOT and SGPT were 2500 (normal is <90). She became somnolent, almost semi-comatose. Her coagulation panel (ability to clot blood when bleeding) was severely abnormal and clotting factors was "going south" rapidly. This patient had a severe hepatitis and was slipping into hepatic coma. But what was the cause of the hepatitis? She was not a drug user. Her Hepatitis A test was negative. We did not have testing for Hepatitis B or C at this time.

The patient became non-responsive. Her liver enzymes went from 2500 to 20,000. She was now comatose. The next day her enzymes were 250. Her liver was in complete failure. There was no hope. She was going to die. We speculated that she could have Herpes Hepatitis.

Upjohn Pharmaceutical was in a drug trial for the treatment of herpes genitalis. There were only 3 known cases of systemic "Herpes Hepatitis" in the world medical literature. Upjohn Pharmaceutical Company could not release the experimental drug acyclovir unless there was biopsy-proven documentation of herpes hepatitis.

The Red-headed patient had blood drawn. Her coagulation panel was so horrible that she would not stop bleeding if any kind of bleeding were to occur (blood draw or even surgery). At this point the entire UCLA OB-GYN faculty was involved in this patient's case: all the professors in the departments fo Gynecologic oncology, Gynecologists and Obstetrics. We were huddled down in the ICU. Finally a plan was devised: we would do a liver biopsy at the time of C-section, confirm the diagnosis of herpes hepatitis and immediately obtain the acyclovir from Upjohn to save this patient.

I was charged with the job of transfusing this patient enough coagulation factors to normalize her coagulation ability in order to perform a C-section. I had been up the entire night: from 6 PM till 8 am the next day. I was up all night transfusing *every* clotting product we had in the blood bank: cryoprecipitate, Konine®, etc. and you name it. I was personally pumping clotting factor transfusions into this patient. It was now 8 am. I was Chief Resident of Obstetrics Department when this patient came in on my watch. However this patient could not clot blood. She still did not have sufficient clotting ability. The C-section was scheduled for 8 am. The Gynecologic Oncologists were planning to do the liver biopsy just after we obtained surgical access to her inner abdomen but before we performed the uterine incision to deliver the baby.

A needle biopsy of the liver was done by Dr. Watson Waters. We proceeded to deliver the baby. The baby came out screaming. It appeared to be un-affected by the hepatitis in the mother. Karen Branch MD, the 4th year chief resident was assigned the task to do the C-section despite the fact that I was the 3rd year Chief Resident of Obstetrics. I assisted her. Karen was closing the uterus as fast as she could. During the second layer closure of the uterus she lifted the needle holder and caught my hand. The needle which had been sewing up the uterus pierced my hand. I had no idea what kind of hepatitis this red head patient had. Whatever virus or bacteria that caused this rare kind of hepatitis, it was *deadly*.

I just got inoculated with a needle infected with this unknown form of deadly hepatitis. I had been up all night supervising the transfusion of blood products and coagulation factors into this patient. When I was struck by this contaminated needle, I knew that I was now going to die as quickly as my patient was dying. We had no diagnosis of the kind of hepatitis with which she was infected. Without a diagnosis, there was no hope of any cure. I was going to be dead in a day or two.

I saw my whole life pass before me. I said good bye to my wife, my mother and father and my brother. I passed out and was helped to a bed outside the Operating Room. Another resident came in to help Karen Branch MD to finish the C-section. I woke up in the resident's sleep room a few hours later.

I went home and told my wife that I was a "goner." After a good night's rest and night off I reported to the Gastroenterology clinic the next day for a work up for hepatitis exposure. I received immunizations for Hepatitis A and B (we had no treatment for Hepatitis C, etc. in those days). I received a huge injected dose of gamma globulin to help me possibly fight this exposure to this lethal form of unknown hepatitis.

The biopsy of the liver done at C-section on our red haired girl came back the next day. It revealed Herpes hepatitis. It was the 4th case known in the world. Upjohn released the new experimental drug, acyclovir, but it was too late. The red haired girl slipped into hepatic coma and died the very next day. The baby was unaffected. The baby was cradled in the husband's arms. I realized from that day forward how precious life was and how quickly your life's circumstances could drastically change. I did not suffer any hepatitis. I did not become infected with systemic herpes.

The problem was that no one involved in this girl's death really questioned what had happened. This beautiful red-haired girl was having her 1st baby. She died from a Primary Herpes Infection during her pregnancy. She had never been exposed or infected with the herpes virus.

***There is an "old doctors tale" that "red heads" seem to have the most complications in medicine.*--**Author Note.

Being redhead and being pregnant (compromised immunologic state), she did not have the immunologic ability to fight this herpes virus. She was gone. The baby survived and was unaffected. How did this patient get herpes?

The husband may have had herpes in the past: he had sex with her with an open and infectious sore. He did not tell her or he did not think it would cause any harm. Or, may he, too, became infected during her pregnancy by some other woman with active herpes. The "guy-view" may retort that the red haired pregnant girl had a one-night stand with an old boyfriend who transmitted the herpes to her at that time.

Regardless, the herpes virus was transmitted and my patient died. I never knew the underlying circumstances. Case closed?

<u>Take home message</u>: If either partner or spouse has a history or gets infected with herpes, you must tell your partner, especially if she is pregnant. Herpes is seldom fatal to adults but it can be fatal to newborns and to some susceptible pregnant women if infection is present during pregnancy.

Hamrell's line

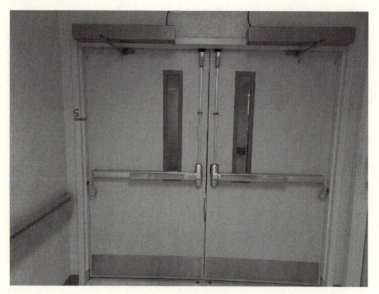

Figure 26-8 Hamrell's Line Photo reproduction of the doors to UCLA OB suite with Hamrell's line drawn at 5 foot mark.

Chuck Hamrell, MD was a fellow resident of mine at UCLA. I need to give him credit for an observation he made during his rotation on OB. He realized that most of the patients that were 5 foot in height or less had an increased risk (>50%)of a C-section. He correlated a woman's height with the dimensions of the birth passageway. I am not sure if it was a novel observation. However, prior to a C-section at UCLA every patient had to be typed and cross matched for 2 units of blood. Accordingly, Dr. Hamrell drew a line 5' (five feet) up from the floor at the entry doors to the OB suite at UCLA. Any patient that walked under that line was typed and cross matched for blood and was considered at higher risk for a probable C-section.

Buying "Protection" for my Ultrasound Probe.

Ultrasound images of a baby have technologically progressed considerably over the past decades. Initially, images could only be obtained with an "external" or abdominal probe on the lower part of the abdomen just over the area of the uterus and ovaries. One of the most important advances was the introduction of the "vaginal" probe transducer. This probe could be placed into the pelvis through the vagina and obtain direct and closer images of the pregnant uterus. In order to provide sanitized protection for patients, the ultrasound probe is covered with a condom sheath. Ultrasound gel (warmed lubricant) is deposited into the condom for conductivity as well as all over the outside of the condom for lubrication as it is inserted gently into the vagina.

Because ultrasound machines were not generally available for use in the OB office in the early days condoms were not yet supplied for purchase from the usual commercial medical suppliers to medical offices.

In order to obtain lubricated condoms the author had to go down to the local pharmacy and purchase them. Regardless whether you are male or female; it is still very embarrassing to buy condoms at the store when there are people (and maybe some of your own patients) in the line in front and in back of you where they could be eyeing what you are about to purchase.

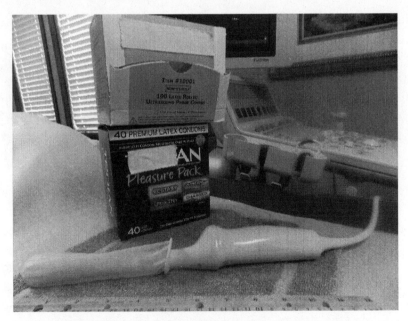

Figure 26-9 Condoms used to cover Ultrasound Probes

I had a plan to overcome this very awkward situation. I decided I would go down to the local pharmacy late on a week night just before closing time when there would be very few people in the store. I would swiftly grab as many condom boxes as I could (maybe 6 boxes of 40) and rush to the check-out stand before anyone would ever notice me or my purchase. I wanted to obtain as many boxes as I could so that I would not have to go through this uncomfortable scenario very frequently.

One Saturday night after a delivery I went down to the local Drug chain store and went inside. I scanned the store quickly and, to my delight, there was only one other customer in the store. She was way in the back: perhaps she was looking at the beauty products.

I quickly went to the "male merchandise" area, snatched 6 boxes of condoms off the shelf and scurried to the check-out stand. I also grabbed several tubes of lubricating gel for the office. Just as I was loading the boxes onto the conveyor belt, I noticed that the tissues were also "on sale." I swiftly piled on 10 boxes of tissues onto the stand.

Just at that exact moment two teenage couples came into the store to purchase ice cream cones. The ice cream counter area was right in the front area of the store with easy visibility to my check-out stand. The store clerk was initially headed in my direction to check me out but decided to help the teenagers first. At this point I was hoping that the teenager couples (who were really hanging on each other) would not turn their heads and notice me at the check stand and my planned purchases.

After one of the teenage girls received her double scooped ice cream cone, she turned away from the ice cream counter and looked around the store. Of course, she spotted me at the check-out stand and noticed my purchases. Instantly, she turns back to her boyfriend and jabbed at his shoulder. He turned to her. She went up to his ear and whispered into it. He immediately turned his full attention to look at me and the situation. He quickly nudged the other teen boy and told him to investigate "the situation" that is occurring on check stand number 1. All of the teens start cracking up.

Well, unfortunately there was no "hole available for me to crawl into" at this moment. I was caught red-handed. My plan to inconspicuously buy condoms (and other sex related products) had gone up in smoke.

Well, the teenagers had their "giggles" and they finally left the store while simultaneously licking their ice cream cones: perhaps in a rather obscene manner or maybe that was my interpretation at the time. The store clerk came back to the check stand to check me out. As the boxes of condoms, lubricant and tissues were being scanned and placed into bags, I just knew what the store clerk must have been going through his mind about my purchases and me on a Saturday night! I am sure he was thinking, "This guy really thinks he is going to get lucky this weekend!"

In order to try to "burst his on-going lewd thought bubble, "I knew had to say something to him about my items. I looked at the store clerk very seriously and I said nonchalantly, "These condoms are to protect my ultrasound probe at my medical office!"

I am very certain that the store clerk then chuckled to himself, "Right! It is just another crazy Saturday night in San Ramon, CA."

Runaway Teen travels down a hard road with metamorphosis into a Respected Physician

The author is writing this story because it demonstrates that personal drive and courage can prevail in one's life.

The author was completely unaware of the previous *life* this amazing female physician had experienced prior to becoming a physician. Dana was born in Boston, Massachusetts. Her parents had established a family. Soon there were four children. Her parents really never encouraged her in school. They did not appreciate her abilities or recognize the potential talents she possessed. Consequently, she herself did not aspire to any lofty career possibilities after high school. She had done well academically in school but, due to her parental lack of expectations and inspiration, she consequently had little motivation and perhaps self-worth to aspire and achieve. She did not need to apply herself any further.

> *"I figured I would get a job after high school
> and that is all that I needed to do."*

Dana was stuck many times after school and on weekends babysitting her three younger siblings. She had stated she wanted to be a cardiologist. She was a typical teenage trying to enjoy the times. Her parents got divorced: apparently her Dad was having an affair. Her mother picked up Dana and the other kids and moved them to Idaho: Dana's grandmother and the rest of the family were originally from this state. Most of the entire family was still living there.

Her father was an engineer. He had no formal college degree. He was now working back in Arizona where his family was had originally settled.

Dana had started one high school in Idaho, but within two years her mother moved to another home: Dana had to change high schools again in her senior year. She was said that being in a different high school was like taking her out of the United States and placing her in a "foreign country. She felt like "a foreigner in a new school." She did not know anybody and she was only going to be at that school for less than 8 months. Her grades were good and she was able to graduate school early at the age of 17. Her mother expected her to continue to watch over her younger siblings. She wanted to have more fun. When she was not watching her brothers and sisters, she wanted to hang out with friends and do the usual activities that other teens were doing. Out of school in the spring and age 17, she knew that she suddenly had a lot of time on her hands. Though she did not reveal to me the details (perhaps sex or alcohol), she was grounded shortly after graduation. Stuck at home with babysitting most of the time, she felt extremely frustrated and angry.

Although she did not tell me the reason (perhaps alcohol or sex), she was grounded after her early graduation in spring time. She decided she just had to leave this home situation. She asked her current boyfriend to drive her to Yellowstone National Park. He dropped her off and went back to Idaho. She did not tell her parents where she was. Her parents never called her boyfriend to ask where she had gone.

She easily obtained a job as a waitress in the restaurant in Yellowstone. Yellowstone was a beautiful park. She thrived in its immense splendor and magnificence: the mountains, the trees, the geysers, etc. She could easily take the van to work, but many times she enjoyed just walking the 1.5 mile trail through the forest from the restaurant to the cabin. ." The contract company managing the restaurant required employees to be over the age of 18. She was still 17 but told them she was 18. Her birthday was coming in a few months. She needed to stall the company's human resources department a little longer. She told them that she did not have her birth certificate but was in the process of obtaining an official copy from Massachusetts (she told me she did have the birth certificate on her but she did not want to reveal her true age. The paychecks kept coming to her for the next few months.

At Yellowstone she met and dated another worker from Montana. His family was in the auto body and fender collision repair business. He had worked with his father and easily became adept in these vehicle repairs. They fell in love.

Her boyfriend had "a lot of connections." He told Dana he found a job opportunity, an auto body job, in Vale, Colorado. Afraid she was going to be "found out" to be only 17 and lose her job, she told her boyfriend, she said, "She was going with him."

In Vale, Colorado she was able to get a job at CGI, a radar manufacturer. She enjoyed the work. The money was good. Times were exciting and they were having a wonderful time together. She had her independence from home and she was making it on her own.

He was doing well financially in the auto shop in Vale. However, he got into a dispute with the owners. He was fired. She was able to get him a job at CGI where she worked. They both were doing well and enjoying life. She advanced quickly and, as she stated, "I had a great paying job."

Several months later, they were driving the company car one Friday night. They were stopped at a police check point. He was driving. She was in the passenger seat. As many women do when they do not want to carry their purse, she had given him her driver's license to hold in his wallet. He did not have his wallet: not sure where he left it. It could have been at the bar. He gets busted. Not just by the police, but also by the company. They both get fired for their actions and behavior.

Fortunately, her boyfriend quickly found an even better job in a body shop near Fairfield, California. They left Colorado and settled in the city of Fairfield. She became pregnant. He was bringing in a good paycheck from his job. She delivered a baby girl shortly thereafter at the local hospital.

After the baby was born, she and her boyfriend became married. After the baby was born, she and her boyfriend became married. When the baby was still young, she obtained another part-time waitress job. Initially she obtained a job at Schlotsky's Deli restaurant. In the first few months of her job, her daughter, Beth, became very sick. Beth had pneumonia and, because of the severity, she had to be admitted to UC Medical Center. Of course, as all mothers do, she had to stop working and be with her daughter in the hospital. Dana was fired. Beth improved after spending a week in the hospital. Dana was emotionally and physically exhausted from this near-death situation with her daughter. However, after Beth fully recuperated, Dana easily obtained another job at an even better opportunity at another restaurant in Fairfield. She was a smart and attractive and her restaurant patrons loved her. She became pregnant again.

It seemed that her husband was not accepting the responsibility of being a husband and father to two children. He started drinking more and perhaps using drugs.

An oil field worker, named Robert, had started coming to her restaurant on a frequent basis. It was not too long that it seemed he only wanted Dana to wait on him. It was becoming clear to her that Robert had become attracted to her. There were occasions when Dana's husband would come into her restaurant. To her, he had seemed changed. He no longer had that "attractive twinkle" in his eyes. He seemed mean. She said, "You see evil in his eyes. I felt he was possessed by the devil." Even Robert noticed his unfriendly personality, "I am very concerned for you, Dana, "said Robert.

Robert knew that Dana was married: he was respectful of her difficult situation. He did not want to be a factor in their deteriorating marriage.

Not too much time thereafter, she suspected and it became evident to her that her husband was cheating on her. The second baby was born.

Shortly thereafter, he started getting verbally and physically abusive. At that point she feared for herself and the children. She left him. She worked more hours at the Fairfield restaurant until the baby boy was born.

She confided that she and Robert did go out together a few times. One day while she was waiting on Robert, he had asked her if she could do him a small favor. He had a favorite necklace but the clasp was broken. Because he worked long shifts during the daytime hours (8 am to 8 pm), he asked if she could find some time during the day to get it fixed for him. He gave her $20. Of course, she agreed to the favor.

When Dana left her husband, she left almost everything she had behind in the home they were renting. She was now living in a homeless shelter. However, her living and money circumstances were closing in on her quickly. She made a rare telephone call back to her mother in Idaho and relayed to her the difficult living situation she was in. In the next few hours she got a phone call from her father. He was arriving in Oakland in a few hours. He was coming to rescue her and the children.

Her father had relocated and lived in Southern California. He, too, had landed a great job at Northrup Grumman. He had re-married but the new wife, as expected, was not too keen on the new living situation. Her father had purchased a home close to the beach. It was the first time she had an opportunity to spend time with her two children. They enjoyed taking the bus to the beach and playing in the sand and water. With regard to financial support, Dana stated, "I could not tell Dad that Susan (his current wife) had enrolled me into Medi-Cal (the Medicaid health insurance program in California as well as food stamps and AFDC—Aid to Families with Dependent Children). The new wife did not to be monetarily affected by her new step daughter and step children.

She had left in such a hurry from Fairfield that she had no time to fix and return the necklace to Robert, the oil field worker. She did not have his address or phone number. She was resourceful and with a few inquiries (she read through the phone book!), she was finally able to contact him. She said, "I still have your necklace, but I spent your $20 dollars." Upon finding out that she had left Northern California, he asked her if he could come to Southern California to visit her. He had never been to beaches of Southern California but he wanted to see her even more.

Her father was working as a key engineer in the development of the Stealth bomber. His knowledge in stealth technology was so valued that the Northrup Grumman felt it necessary to put security measures in place. Accordingly, her father, his home and family were guarded by security teams. She recalls how the plains-clothes personnel would follow her and the children as they boarded the bus to the beach.

Dana and Robert remained in constant contact. He asked Dana again if he could to visit her. He said, "I never been to Southern California and I would like to see you." Robert came to visit her. He, too, noticed the security detail following them around. Finally, after a few days of being shadowed, he walked over to the security patrol car and asked to talk with them. He said, "Well, if you are going to trail us down to the beach and back again, why do we all just go in your car and forget the bus!"

They enjoyed the time they had together. Dana had received her final legal papers from the County Courthouse that she was finally divorced

A few weeks later after his visit, Robert called Dana. He asked her, "Will you marry me." She said, "Yes." She was going back to Fairfield with her two children.

Robert lived on the family farm near Woodland, California. Dana's two children were enrolled in school in Fairfield.

Dana made it a guiding principle in her role as a mother, "My children are not going to be moved from school to school like I was. They are going to be raised in a stable home and stay in the same school."

Further, Dana and Robert had made a special pledge to each other, "If either one of us feels the urge or the temptation to be unfaithful, we will first tell each other of the problem. We are not going to cheat on each other like our former spouses had done."

Robert was having greater difficulty working the oil fields. Over the years it was taking a toll physically on his body. He had completed 3 years of college, but never finished. He had been prosperous in the oil field work and financially he could afford to go back to college and get his teaching degree. His older brother had already become a teacher and now had advanced to the position of principle in Woodland, California.

Dana, too, was interested in going back to school: she too wanted to realize her dreams of becoming a physician. Both children were flourishing in the school: both kids were academically at the top of their classes.

Within a year Robert graduated with his teaching credential. His brother asked if he could teach in his school in Woodland. Robert had a new job, but Woodland was far enough in distance away from Dana and the kids. He commuted and would see them on the weekends. He was teaching physical education and history at the high school level.

Within four years Dana graduated Summa Cum Laude from the university. Her children were still in high school: she was not going to move the teens while in high school. For the next few years, Dana became a teacher at the high school in the same school district as the teens. She taught anatomy and physiology. She still had a medicine career in the back of her mind. Her gifted daughter, Beth, was now in her senior year.

Robert said to her, "Well, Dana, if you want to become a doctor, then you should become a doctor."

Robert was very much in love with Dana and would do anything in the world for her. At the age of 38 Dana applied and was accepted into the University Of California School Of Medicine at Davis. Now Dana and Robert could be back together: Davis was close enough to Woodland so that Robert could still teach in while living in Davis. At the very same time her exceptional daughter was accepted to California State University. She, too, wanted to become a physician.

Dana did well in medical school. However, she was so awe-struck with her rotation in Obstetrics that she decided she no longer wanted to be a cardiologist. She was going to be an Obstetrician and deliver babies. At the very same time Dana entered into the Ob-Gyn residency program in Davis, her daughter, Beth got accepted to the UC School of Medicine in San Francisco.

Dana struggles were just beginning. Her residency director was a difficult to work with. He reportedly had been through "20 Ob-Gyn Residency Programs" himself before he finally finished as a Chief Resident. He was now a Residency Program Director. She told me that at one point, the Residency Director completely fired the entire second year residency class. Dana and the others had to pick up the slack and extra work. Dana did say he showed greater leniency to the male residents and she considered him a male chauvinist." After she finished her Ob-Gyn residency Dana and Robert settled back to the family farm house in Woodland. Dana became an Ob-Gyn physician in the nearby city.

Still, Dana had to pass her Board Certification. I was certain that, given Dana's intelligence and her observed surgery skills, that she would not having any trouble passing on the first attempt. Dana studied hard each night. She took Board Review classes in Las Vegas and over the internet. When she took the oral exams, she received the horrible news that she did not pass. The Board would not tell her or anyone who did not pass what questions they had missed.

Dana studied again. She took more review courses. She received more personal tutoring. She took the exam for the second time. Again, sadly she did not pass. At this point and perhaps earlier, I wondered if her former residency director was behind the scenes in nixing her future career. The author believes that such an explanation is possible: the author received a phone call from a physician at the residency program about 6 months after she began her private practice. He asked me, "How is she performing at the hospital? "Of course, I stated that she was a very conscientious physician. It was unusual for a residency program to make such inquires after the residents graduate. I am certain that Board Examiners talk to the residency staff regarding their opinion of their resident prior to giving the oral Board Exam.

Undaunted, Dana prepared for the third attempt. Dana had sacrificed her life to pass the Board exam: no vacations, no fine dining, no trips to the city, and no time with her children and now grandchild. She had little time to spend with her husband. He took care of the cooking and household activities. She took the third Board exam and this time, without any question, she passed! Further, her daughter finished her radiology residency. Multiple practice opportunities were offered to her and a promising career shined in front of her. Her son graduated the university and was pursuing a career in Accounting/CPA.

Despite the fact that she spent 3 hard years trying to obtain her needed Board Certification, Dana had built up a respected and busy Ob-Gyn practice. I knew from the day I met her that she was going to be successful physician: she was attractive and had energy, enthusiasm, humility and a great and warm personality (the author believes that the American people pick their Presidents based on these qualities rather than their education or experience). Maybe more importantly, Dana still possessed an optimistic viewpoint of life and people. "To this day, Dana stated to me, my mother has never seen her grandchildren. The children's father has yet to see his first again and he never saw the second born son. The last I heard was that he had stolen the company car. His whereabouts are still unknown to me. When I asked the children if they wanted to see their biologic father, they both stated they would rather not bother." Robert has been and continues to be the real father in their lives.

One day during surgery the author asked Dana, "So what is the *moral* to *your story*?" She did not hesitate in her response, "Despite all previous situations and hurdles, anyone can overcome and succeed if they really put their mind to it."

I am reminded of a question that Diane Sawyer, as a young reported, once asked President Nixon just prior to his resignation from office. Diane Sawyer was at the end of her interview with the former President and she had basically run out of questions to ask him. Off the top of her mind, she asked Nixon, "Well, did you have fun being President?" He quickly fired back his response, "Having fun had never ever entered his mind during his presidency and his long embattled road to political in office." It was a very sad insight into the life of this man who had battled politically, both winning and failed campaigns, to finally achieve his goal of being President.

I am hoping that Dana and her family have arrived at the point in their lives that they all could now start enjoying life itself. "From pregnant teenager to respected physician, Dana is just another one of those many remarkable American heroes that make up the human fabric of the United States.

The author did not relate this story just to celebrate the successful journey of a distinguished colleague: there are lessons in this tale for new parents-to-be.

1. Children naturally are influenced by the expectations and hopes of their parents. Motivating children to be "the best they can be" is a basic responsibility of the parents (or unfortunately *a parent* as was the case with Dana and the same circumstances that play out of the United States is the more common).

2. Any man can be a biological father to children, but it takes *real* responsibility to follow through and be their *Real Dad*.

Children do not necessarily need material things, but they do crave the love, the time and attention you give them. They need stability of the home location. They need, as Dana accomplished, to reside in the same city, the same school and grow up with their friends. Parents in their behaviors and action profoundly influence the lives of their children. At least give them hope, raise their own expectations of themselves and feed their self-esteem.

3. Not everyone will get the opportunity of a *Second Chance*. When Dana met Robert she was on her way to getting a second chance: a second chance to succeed and a second marriage. With Robert's support, love and encouragement Dana was able to achieve her life goals and achieve happiness.

4. Children need role models and heroes. Children naturally imitate their parents (or other relatives or friends) and they want *to be like* them. Let them *dream*, as my father said more than once to me, "You can be anything you want to be. You could even become President of the United States if you wanted to. My job is to put a roof over your head, put food on the table to nourish you and give you the capacity to go to school so that you can succeed in whatever you want to do." As Dana stated, "There are no obstacles you cannot overcome." She should know. As Henry Ford said over 100 year ago,

"Life is a series of experiences, each of which makes us bigger, even though it is hard to realize this. For the world was built to develop character, and we must learn that the setbacks and griefs which we endure help us in our marching onward."

The author still has two lingering questions in his mind: did Dana ever get Robert's necklace fixed and, did Dana ever give Robert back his $20?

The Biggest Baby I ever delivered

I would have never guessed that the largest baby (in weight) would occur toward the twilight years of my career.

Michelle had initially made an appointment with me because of irregular menstrual periods. She was overweight. She had been overweight since high school. She would skip her periods: sometimes missing 4-6 months at a time. She was 26 years old now. Her exam revealed her endometrium, the lining inside her uterus, was abnormally thickened. She was treated with a hormone called progesterone: the hormone that she would normally be produced with regular menstrual cycles. However, her endometrium did not decrease in thickness. An endometrial biopsy was performed. The biopsy revealed that she had an early cancer of the uterus. It was unfortunate that a diagnosis of her gynecological condition was not made in her teenage years: polycystic ovarian syndrome (PCOS).

PCOS is a gynecological condition characterized by irregular menstrual periods, abnormal weight gain, excess hair, oily skin and relative infertility. PCOS is most likely represented in an inheritable gene sequence with an obvious predisposition to manifest itself after puberty. If recognized early in the teen years, excess weight gain and hair as well as acne can be vitiated. Birth control pills are the main course of therapy until children are desired.

By the time I first saw Michelle her gynecological condition progressed to an extreme point. Many gynecologists would have recommended that she undergo hysterectomy. Since Michelle had no children yet, I decided to try to reverse her early cancer with hormone chemotherapy. Within 3 months her repeat biopsy was negative for cancer. To be safe, I treated her for another 3 months.

I did not see Michelle for follow appointments for at least 2 years. The next time I saw Michelle she had become pregnant. Michelle had dropped some weight: from 290 down to 276 lbs. Michelle was still overweight (as was her husband). Because of weight and other inheritable factors Michelle was diagnosed with adult onset diabetes (AODM). She had been placed on metformin by her family physician.

Many patients who ordinarily have regular menstrual periods (due to infrequent ovulation) become pregnant in the first few months after being placed on metformin. Michelle was referred to the Diabetes Clinic for more careful control of her diabetes: glucose tolerance progressively worsens as the pregnancy advances. She attended just one session. Michelle offered up a number of issues:

1. She stated she had financial difficulty with the $50 copayments at the diabetes clinic.

2. She had trouble paying for the brand names insulins she was prescribed. Generic diabetic medications were substituted for her.

3. She did not follow the meal plans or physical activity that was prescribed.

She stated that she was self-monitoring her diabetes.

Her pregnancy progressed without any further problems. She and her husband were traveling out of state frequently with his business. It was difficult to keep track of her blood sugars.

As Michelle approached her due date, the baby just seemed to be exploding in size. Michelle had a normal, if not, large pelvis. Her birth canal could easily accommodate a 10 pound baby. Well controlled gestational diabetics are recommended to be delivered at least one week prior to their due date. Still, Michelle would not go into labor. Her cervix remained closed. The baby's head never *engaged* or dropped down into the pelvis. Ultrasound measurements continued to show the baby growing in size: from 4400 grams all the way up to an unbelievable 5400 grams. Obstetric guidelines recommend that all babies measuring over 4500 grams are more safely delivered by C-section: shoulders become wedged into the midpelvis and the delivery can be become greatly complicated.

We delivered Michelle by C-section at 39 weeks of gestation. The baby weighed in at 13 pounds and 12 ounces.

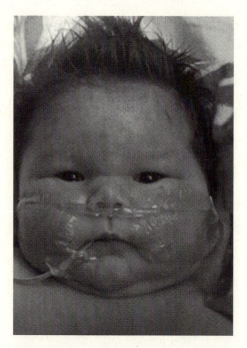

The baby's large size was a complicated problem in the nursery. Typically such large babies have blood sugar and heart problems. Michelle's baby had a very complicated course. The baby's heart was in congestive heart failure: it could not pump blood through the large circulatory system not typically found in a newborn. To treat the heart failure, the baby had to be placed on beta blockers and be transferred to the NICU (Neonatal Intensive Care Unit). The baby stayed 4 weeks in the NICU prior to being discharged. Fortunately, the baby's blood sugar was not a significant issue in the newborn period.

The lessons of Michelle's pregnancy are quite straight forward:

1. Maintain rigorous control of your blood sugars during pregnancy: it helps insure the birth of a healthy baby. Yes, it is difficult to stick your fingers and check your blood sugar four times per day.

2. If you choose to have a baby, "no expense or trouble" should be spared. Keep your appointments with the diabetic nurses.

Check your blood sugars 2 hours after each meal. Follow the diet you are prescribed. Keep physically active to burn calories.

3. In the very best scenario, plan your pregnancy ahead of time. Lose weight and become physically fit *prior* to conception. Make a pre-conceptual appointment with your Ob-Gyn.

Little Patient in San Ramon, CA

I was seeing patients one afternoon at my office in San Ramon, CA. A new OB patient was ushered into one of the exam room. I always like to talk to new patients prior to them getting undressed for physical examination.

This new OB patient was early in her pregnancy: about 8 weeks along. She was very short in height. When my nurse measured how tall she was, she found to be just 4'10". I took down her medical and family history. She related to me that she had a congenital abnormality, i.e., she was born with spinal bifida (an opening above the tail bone). Her height was affected. When I examined her, I found that her corresponding pelvic size was very small. I thought to myself, "I don't think even a grapefruit could pass through her pelvis."

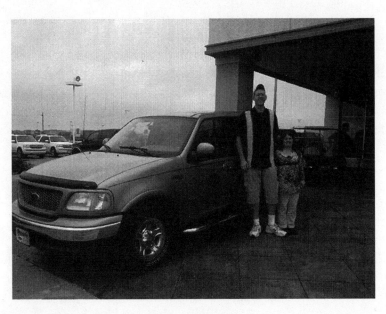

Indeed she was about 8 weeks pregnant. We could see the baby's outline as well as the baby's heartbeat on the ultrasound. After the examination was completed, I allowed her to get dressed. I would provide with more pregnancy information to her after she had put her clothes back on. It is uneasy for the patient as well as the physician to be talking when the patient is basically naked with a scanty exam gown over her. Everyone is uncomfortable in this situation.

After I re-entered the room, the patient stated to me, "Doctor, I have to tell you something. I don't want to have a C-section!" I said, "Well, we will wait and see how big a baby you will be having later in your pregnancy. I sure hope it will be small. Your pelvis is very small. It is related to your short height and the spina bifida. Hopefully your baby's head will fit." Then she said, "I want you to meet my husband. He is here in the waiting room." As I was finishing a few more medical notes in her chart, she went to the waiting room and brought him into the exam room. As I turned around to shake his hand, my head gazed up to greet him. My head kept extending straight up almost to the ceiling to see him: he was 6'6" tall!

Her pregnancy proceeded without any significant problems. When she was very close to her due date, I noted that the baby's head did not drop into the pelvis (engagement, which typically happens in most primigravidas two weeks prior to their due date). The baby's estimated fetal weight was 8 to 9 lbs. There was very little chance that that baby could deliver through her small pelvis. I knew she would require a C-section in order to safely deliver the baby. I did not want my patient to suffer 10 to 12 hours of labor just to prove an academic point. However in California, her HMO Insurance Plan required a Perinatology consultation and 2nd opinion prior to an elective *Primary* (or first C-section). Most insurance companies would not approve a C-section without the patient first "having a trial of labor."

After she was seen by the Perinatologist, with whom I have worked with many times in the past, the Perinatologist called me. She said that she recommended that she try to labor and see if the baby could delivery vaginally. I said to her, "I have checked her pelvic measurements and estimated the baby's size. If you believe in your professional experience that you would allow her to labor, then you can take over her care and be responsible for her obstetrical course of events. The Perinatologist then said, "Let me check her pelvic measurements and I will call you back." Within 10 minutes she called back and said, "Yes, I agree with you. There is no way that baby is going to fit and it would be cruel to let her needlessly labor with almost no chance of a vaginal birth." The patient was satisfied and understood the problem. We delivered her by C-section and had a very healthy 9 lb. baby boy without complication.

Now for the record, a patient's height does not necessarily mean that a person cannot deliver normal size or even big babies. My ex-mother-in-law was Chinese, was 4'11" and delivered nine pound babies. As I have stated in the section on labor and delivery, "it is not the size of the donut, but the donut hole."

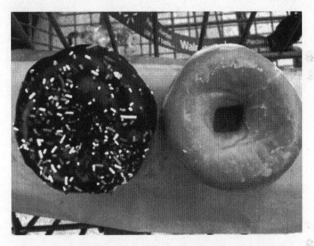

Figure 26-10 Donut Analogy to Birth Canal Size

However, there is a mathematical association with height and the size of the pelvic oval.

A more recent case was quite similar. A 15 year old Hispanic teen was seen for her pregnancy. She, too, was quite short: only 5 foot tall. The father of the baby was not as tall as the above case. He was much shorter: about 5 foot 6 inches. Myah's pelvis was about as small as the patient above. However, in this situation, I was planning on allowing her to go into labor and give her a chance to deliver vaginally. Well, she, too, went post term, i.e., 41 weeks. Ultrasound measurements of the baby showed that the baby weight 4065 grams, or more than 8.5 lbs. The amniotic fluid levels were adequate, but somewhat decreased. The umbilical artery Doppler blood flow to the baby was normal. The baby' head was "un-engaged" and floating above the pelvic brim. The cervix was uneffaced, long and closed.

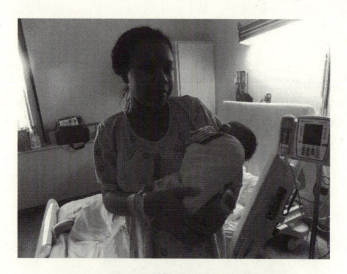

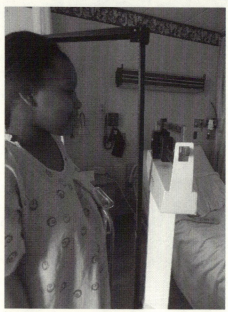

Figure 26-11 and Figure 26-12 Height and Pelvic Capacity Correlation

I counseled Myah's mom and Myah. I explained to both of them that I did not think there was a fair chance of her delivering her baby vaginally but I would try. I scheduled her for induction that night.

She came in to the OB suite at 12:15 midnight. She was admitted and placed on the fetal monitor. Just prior to being given her 1st dose of Cytotec, the baby's heart rate dipped significantly. I was called at 2:30 am and was informed of the clinical situation. I told the nurse to hold off the Cytotec and to continue to monitor the baby. The baby recovered but at about 6 am the baby's heart rate had another deceleration. At that point we called in the OR team to do an emergency C-section. We delivered the baby: as we open up the uterus, we noticed that the baby had "pooped "inside, i.e. had passed *meconium* (a sign of fetal stress). There is a protocol for treatment of the baby with meconium in the amniotic fluid. The baby's airway must be immediately suctioned even before the baby is allowed to take a first breath. Proper airway care was performed immediately upon birth. The baby did just fine.

OB's try their very best to avoid C-sections but unfortunately, for them and their patients, it seems the today's patients have too many high risk factors: weight, diabetes, poor nutrition, etc. Every pregnant couple is different and unique: physically, mentally and educationally. The "art of medicine," perhaps for the most part, is commonsense mixed with experience: it tells you that you cannot fit "a square peg through a circle!" Again, as stated in the Labor Section, the ability for a patient to deliver a baby vaginally depends on the 4 P's: the passageway, the passenger, the uterine powers, and the size of the pelvis. All of these objective measurements and data must be plugged into the OB's brain when he attending a patient's care during labor. Not everyone is a candidate for a trial of labor.

Dr. Karen Branch and the Male Medical Students

The UCLA Ob-Gyn Residents meeting was held on Saturday mornings at 9 am and continued, occasionally, all the way to noon. All the residents and all the faculty were required to be present. J. George Moore, MD was chairman of the Department. At this time in medicine, the "Woman's Movement" and "Women's Liberation" was just getting started (mid 1970's). Dr. Moore was, for all intents and purposes a "male chauvinist" in his views regarding women in medicine and probably in the workplace. Most people would probably call him just "old fashioned." I sometimes wonder if America is a better place now that women must be Breadwinners as well as wives, mothers and homemakers. I admire today's generation of women: they are accomplished in all venues of endeavor yet set aside the time and take weeks out of their jobs to have children and nurture them.

During this Saturday Department meeting the Chief Resident of Obstetrics and the Chief Resident on the Gynecology Service provided the statistics of the previous week and presented interesting clinical cases. Karen Branch MD was a second year resident who had just transferred her training from Johns Hopkins to UCLA. She had done her "tour of duty" taking care of the medical disasters emanating in the ghetto neighborhoods of Baltimore. She was a tough, sleeves rolled up, cigar smoking "John Wayne" feminist if there ever was one. She definitely was their *role* model. She came into the meeting and plop herself down on the couch in the back of the room. The Chief Resident of Gynecology was reporting on a case as follows,

"The following case is a 22 year old female medical student with secondary amenorrhea (medical term for cessation of menses/periods after having them for several years)." At that moment the Chief of the Department, Dr. Moore interrupted the Chief Resident and stated, "I *wonder* how many female medical students have secondary amenorrhea?"

At that point Karen, after just lighting up her Tiparillo® cigar (people could smoke in hospitals at that time) spoke up promptly and answered his question with a resounding voice from the back of the room. She said, "The answer to your question is that there are exactly as many *female* medical students with primary amenorrhea as there are *male* medical students with impotence!" There was a huge outburst of laughter and applause from everyone in the room: she brought the house down as they say.

Future Lawton Nurse says "Castor Oil does not work!"

Sheila was a teenager and strong headed. Sheila was 38 weeks pregnant. She was due on New Year's Day. That was two weeks too long to wait. She was impatient and wanted to have her baby now. She heard that you could cause labor if you drank castor oil.

Her Ob, Dr. Johns, was a faithful University of Oklahoma (OU) alumnus and attended every single OU football game he could. Sheila adored her OB. During her OB appointment on a Friday morning she told him that she was thinking about using Castor Oil to help induce labor. He admonished and scolded her not to even think about taking any castor oil. More importantly the last OU season football game was the next day on Saturday. He definitely planned on being at that game in Norman, OK.

That night she had eaten "take-out" for dinner from Hardy's in Lawton. She was determined and gung ho. She took double dose of castor oil, (according to the directions so stated on the back of the castor oil bottle).

She then decided to travel a little ways out of town to the Wichita Mountains Estates area just "to hang out with friends." Traveling the 8 miles north on Interstate 44, her car just so happen to run out of gas right at mile marker 18. It was about 1 mile from the off-ramp.

She put on her blinking lights and waited. She watched a total of three (3) OHP (OK Highway Patrol) cars go by. She already had the "cha chas" and had to go down to the grass area off the Interstate to poop. Two hours went by. She was having a "pity party." She had already gone 3 times on the grass down from the Interstate road side. When she was leaving the grassy area during her last poop there, she had heard a howling cry, perhaps a coyote or some other wild animal. It sounded the animal was *really* close by. Finally, she gave up and she, with pregnant belly and all, started to push the car to the off ramp that descended onto the Medicine Park Hwy. The car made to the off-ramp; she got in quickly and coasted down to the highway. At that point a guy in a pick-up truck stopped. He got out and said he would help her out. He then pushed her vehicle to the Love's Travel

Stop. She instantly got her vehicle "gassed up." She got to her friend's home and was, at last, safe. However, she still had diarrhea. She slept very little. That next morning she decided to go Christmas shopping. She hopped in her car and went to Central Mall. As it was now close to lunch time she went into the mall and decided to eat at the Chic-Fil-A. As soon as she got her meal, she suddenly started to experience a gushing fluid out of her vagina and onto her own shoes. She went directly to the hospital at about 1 pm. Dr. Johns was preparing to go to the game at 3 pm. He arrived in the Obstetrics unit well-dressed in an OU red flannel shirt. She hung her head down as she apologized to him for taking the castor oil against his wishes. She was 6 cm. The game started in 2 hours. She said to herself, "he hates me" for what she had done. Dr. Johns ordered her to put on the OU game on her TV in her labor room. He instructed her she could never change the game channel.

Her cervix stopped dilating at 7 cm and had to be stimulated with Pitocin. She never got an epidural. She finally got completely dilated. It is now about 10 PM on a Saturday night. Sheila had done some research during her pregnancy: she did not want an episiotomy. She had practiced labial massage and vaginal stretching during the last part of her pregnancy. She told Dr. Johns she did NOT want to be cut! I don't need an episiotomy. Dr. Johns threw up his hands in disgust. He stated, "I am not going to argue about it." She knew Dr. Johns really, really hated her now. Sheila pushed for 2 hours. With every push a little diarrhea leaked from her bottom.

> *Author's Note: If I ever get to Heaven, I need to talk to God regarding his design for the exit of body waste. As one might surmise, God must have always thought himself as a "City Planner." Why else would he put the "playground" between the sewer system and the garbage dump?" I am sure God said to Himself, "Those humans will never find it there!"*

Dr. Johns had missed his game. He sat there in the delivery room and was wiping her bottom off with each and every push. With each contraction and push the baby's heart rate decelerated. She finally delivered but her vaginal opening had torn irregularly with delivery of the head. Dr. Johns had obeyed her request not "to be cut" and have an episiotomy. Dr. Johns now had the task to "repair the puzzle that was formally known as Sheila's vagina!"

Baby and mom did well.

Most interesting was the story Sheila read in *The Lawton Constitution newspaper* one week later. A dead male body had been found right at Hwy Marker #18 where Sheila's car had run out of gas. According to the newspaper, the body had apparently had been there for a while given the state of the body at the time of coroner's examination. Sheila thought about the dead man and instantly reflected on the previous week when she delivered. She realized that she probably had been pooping within a dozen feet of that dead body. She was grateful she did not accidentally trip on the body when she was pooping off the roadside!

The Author Digs further into Sheila's Story

I have done further research on the veracity of Sheila's Story. I have contacted both Hardy's and Chic-Fil-A and they both these establishments have gone on public record stating that served any food they served was in any way contaminated and responsible for illness in their patrons. They rejected any responsibility for Sheila's diarrhea. I have gone down to City Hall and *The Lawton Constitution* newspaper archives. I have found that sometime after the newspaper report, the County Coroner had signed off that the death of that man was caused by the man slipped on a very large deposit of stool in the surrounding grass area. He took a severe fall: he either died from the resultinghead injury or perhaps, from inhaling the toxic fumes emanating from Sheila's poop. Just prior to his almost instant death, the man had made a howling cry (the one Sheila had heard in the distance). So the moral of this story is that you should never use castor oil to induce labor in late pregnancy because it can be lethal to *other people*! The Toxicology studies on a sample of the poop at the State Lab confirmed those results. For the good of the general public I have contacted the corporate headquarters of the company making castor oil. They have agreed to add this possible complication to their "Warning Label" on the back of their bottle: "not to be used in late pregnancy as this product can be associated with loose stools and uterine contractions."

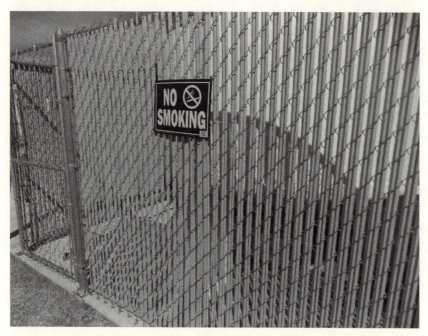

Figure 26-13 The official *"Sheila Toxic Dump Site"* (as seen from Interstate 44)

The Breech delivery with Dr. Bill Dignam

I was a 2nd year resident at UCLA when we attempting to deliver this patient with the breech presentation *vaginally*. There was a protocol at UCLA regarding the criteria that had to be met in order to allow a breech to deliver vaginally. This particular patient fit the protocol: average size baby in the *frank* breech position with normal size pelvis (as documented by clinical exam and x-ray pelvimetry measurements). The labor proceeded normally without the need for Pitocin stimulation.

Dr. Bill Dignam was a kind and gentle soul who had been blessed with 5 girls (at least you can't say he didn't try!). I remember one late afternoon when one of his patients came into the OB suite in active labor. The fetal heart beat was dropping with each contraction.

We called him to come as quickly as possible and we prepared for a possible C-section. The OB residents were frantic. Dr. Dignam makes his usual leisurely entrance into the OB suite, goes into the changing room and dons his scrubs He comes out and walks at his easy-going pace to the delivery room in which his patient had been transferred. He washes his hands. Calm and composed he walks into the delivery room, puts on his gown and gloves and asks the patient to push. Within a push or two the baby comes out screaming as if there was no drama had ensued prior to the baby's birth. Dr. Bill Dignam was man of dignity and stature: something of a cross between the Pope and Johnny Carson. No circumstances ever rattled him. He was a model to be emulated.

To continue with the story the patient with the breech was brought into the delivery room when she was completely dilated. Dr. Bill Dignam took a seat in the back of the delivery room to observe the delivery. The breech baby's bottom was presenting at the vaginal opening. We residents were prepared. We had seen other breech deliveries by the other residents. We had thoroughly studied the method of delivery. The baby's bottom came out first. I then delivered one leg and then the other. My intern held up the bottom of the baby with a towel. But the head would not come down. I quickly asked the nurses for the Piper forceps. I struggled to get the forceps around the baby's head that was higher upwards in the pelvis. The baby's head was not coming out. I thought it might be stuck. I looked at Dr. Dignam and was expecting him to start shouting out some instructions (or even come over to the delivery table to help). He sat calmly in the chair still observing the delivery. Finally, by some means the head came down further. The forceps could not be applied around the head correctly. With a gentle pull the baby's head delivered. The baby was screaming and vigorous. My scrub top was soaked with perspiration and I had to wipe my forehead off. I was really frazzled from the stress of this delayed breech birth.

After the delivery Dr. Dignam ushered me the intern and me into the resident's room. We sat down to hear what he had to say. Like the Reverend Mr. Black (in the Kingston Trio ballad, *The Reverend Mr. Black*) he started talking to me "in a voice that was as kind and gentle as could be. He then proceeded to cut me down like a big oak tree." He proceeded to tell me the following advice and passed onto me all of his "pearls of wisdom" from all his years of obstetrics on how to properly deliver a breech baby:

a. The delivery bed must be elevated to a height so that you can visualize the pelvis at the proper eye level into the vagina

b. The nurse or resident has to be standing over the abdomen of the patient from the side to keep constant pressure and flexion of the after coming head

c. Once the arms are delivered you must pull downward on the body and another physician must exert even more pressure from the top in order to bring the head down into the true pelvis.

d. If the head does not move easily through the vagina, then the Piper forceps can easily be applied to the head but only after the head is "in the true mid- pelvis and well engaged. Only At this point is the head now at the proper level (station) in the pelvis to easily see and apply the Piper forceps.

Dr. Dignam taught us by allowing us to struggle through situations first and then he would go over and review each point in time what was happening: what could have been done differently in the course of events so that you would learn from it. I guess his teaching method worked because I remember every detail he said to me to this very day! Every physician who has even known and been taught by Dr. Dignam will acknowledge the profound effect he has had on their education and character as an OB-GYN.

The Pregnant Teenager who was lost and Hurt

She wrote this story: these are her own words but annotated grammatically by the author.

I was just a teenage girl who was lost and hurt. I was hurt because my father gave up his rights to my sister and me "because he was angry." When I became a young teen, I turned to weed and alcohol to help deal with the pain and the anger that I was feeling. I loved the feeling I was getting from the drugs and alcohol that I used almost every weekend. I would give up my last five dollars just to get a sack of weed. I kept lying to myself and the lying started to get worse. I started sleeping around because I just didn't care about myself anymore. I lost all respect for myself. I also lost respect for my family: I did not care if I hurt them or not. I was worried about my feelings more than theirs.

My grades started slipping. I even popped pills in class. I did not even know what pills I was taking. I took sleeping pills and slept in all my classes. Further, I would then drive around town with the pill still in my system. I would even drive with my siblings in the car with me. I could hardly keep my eyes open when driving home. When I did arrive at home, an argument would ensue because my parents were contacted about my behavior at school. Of course, I would lie to my parents and deny it was true. I told them that I had asked for medicine because I didn't feel good. Months passed and I was still doing the drugs and the partying.

Then I met my current girlfriend. She was beyond amazing. She had a job. She never did drugs and was attending college. She knew what she wanted in life. She had "a purpose in life, "an attribute that I really loved about her. She helped change me. She was so patient with me during the time I was trying to change my behavior and life. She never gave up on me. She had faith that I could be a better person. I stopped the weed and my grades started to get better. I met her family and liked them. Shortly thereafter, she proposed to me. Of course, I said yes. However, there was a big problem: my family did not know about her. For the longest time I kept our relationship a secret. We were together for almost a year.

After that year, I decided to end our relationship. As an excuse to end it with her, I used the fact that "the whole secret situation" was too much for me to handle anymore. In actuality, I really started talking again to my ex-boyfriend. I was back with my old friends. I again started to smoke weed. I had been cheating on her. She did everything in her power to make our relationship work out: she was even giving me money for weed and letting me smoke whenever I felt. However, I was mentally finished with our relationship. Despite the facts that she was giving me money and letting me smoke, I did not really want us to get us back together.

Not even a month later I met another guy: I did not know it but he was going to be the father of my child. He was basically me but in male form. He sold weed and he smoked it as well. He stole things from people. He was the "bad boy" type: that kind of personality was what caught my eye. We would smoke and then have un-protected sex. We did not care if I got pregnant or not.

Not too much later in time, we were at the mall when I noticed something changing in my body. It was there at the mall that I started complaining that my breasts were hurting. The smell of the Chinese food that my boyfriend had ordered made me sick to my stomach. I told him that something was wrong. I told him that we should take a pregnancy test just to make sure. I took the test and my results were a big blue plus sign. I was excited because I always wanted to be a mommy.

I had stopped smoking and partying. I got a job. I enrolled in another school so I could finish early. I wanted to focus on my health and the health of my baby. We went to the pregnancy resource center to do another pregnancy test and it came out positive as well. They did an ultrasound. When I saw my little baby on the screen, I could not stop smiling: I was actually seeing "my little blessing." The father of my child looked at me and said, "That was two minutes wasted" because he had no clue what he was seeing on the ultrasound screen. I just let his toxic comment go through one ear and out the other (instead of saying something that would stir up an argument). I had my first doctor appointment with Dr. Zweig. I thought the pregnancy was doing well. However, a couple days later after my appointment I got a phone call from his office: they said I had a chlamydial infection. I called the father crying. I told him the news and asked why he didn't tell me about his disease. His response was "why are you making such a big deal out of it you act like you have herpes. Just get the pill!"

After that I called everything off with him. Furthermore, I found out he was still smoking (after he promised me he going to stop). Also it became obvious to me that he had probably been cheating on me the whole time we were together.

I started to work things out with my ex-girlfriend. I told her everything that had happened. She hugged me and told me everything was going to be okay. She said that she understood the situation I was in. She had my back: we could get back together. My family found out about her and, surprisingly they ended up loving her! We were now finally back together and the relationship was renewed. She supported me mentally and financially during my pregnancy. She took me to the hospital when I was sick. She drove me to and accompanied me to all my appointments. She started to work more hours in order to have extra money to purchase all the items for the nursery. She accepted the baby as if he was hers. She was there with me holding my hand during the special appointment when we found out that I was having a little boy. We both agreed on the name, "Bryant Hudson." As finances were getting tight, we were able to move in with her grandparents. We needed the extra help. We made the spare bedroom in grandpa's house into Bryant's room. My grandma went shopping and purchased everything my little man needed: she knew we could not afford all of it. My baby had everything he needed and more.

As the pregnancy progressed, we were getting more excited to meet our little man. However, I started to have complications with my pregnancy. I broke out into the pregnancy-related rash *called pruritic urticarial papules of pregnancy*, i.e. PUPPS. In addition, I also developed a heat rash. The rash became so severe that even taking a shower was painful. When I scratched, my skin would bleed. Dr. Zweig prescribed me medication to help with the itching. But, the rash did not go away. It spread all over my back and neck. It was further started to spread onto my stomach and chest. When I reached 38 weeks I could barely walk: my legs had become so swollen that they were starting to bruise. I had to request an earlier appointment with Dr. Zweig to tell him about my worsening rash. He checked the baby. He stated that the baby was perfectly fine. However, when he did a pelvic exam to see if my cervix had dilated, he told me that

I was barely one centimeter. I busted out crying because I was so disappointed. He told me that I could get dressed and that he would be back to discuss a treatment plan for me. Of course, I was scared because I was uncertain of what was going to happen. He came back in the exam room. He asked me, "Do you want to be induced?" I said, "Yes," without any hesitation. The pregnancy was really becoming too painful.

He told me to come in Thursday night after 12 midnight. At that time they would start inducing my labor. Thursday night came and we went to the OB unit at Southwestern Medical Center. The nurse placed a small pill in the back of my vagina under the cervix in order to thin my cervix out. Less than an hour later I was starting to feel some contractions in my back. They were just a little bit uncomfortable. At 8 am Friday morning the nurses started a Pitocin infusion to strengthen my contractions. By 12 noon I was dilated to 4 centimeters. My cervix dilated from a four to a seven within two hours. In another 2 hours my cervix dilated from a 7 to a 9. Suddenly, the nurses came into my labor in order to put an oxygen mask over my face. They had me turn on my left side: Bryant's heart rate was dropping. I did not have a clear mind at this point. Because of the medication I had taken earlier, I could not understand what was really happening. I started to feel a lot of pressure as if I had to use the restroom. I called the nurses and they checked me. The RN said that I was completely dilated. It was time "to push." Everyone was asked to leave the room. I wanted my mom, my grandma, my sister and, of course, my partner to stay in the room. I wanted them there with me through the whole birthing experience. With my sister and my partner at the head of the bed and my grandma and mom holding my feet I started to push at 4pm. After I had pushed for only 20 minutes, Dr. Zweig came in the room. Then the realization hit me that my little man was about to be born. Bryant was sunny side up and Dr. Zweig had to use the vacuum and turn him as I was pushing. I delivered my son at 4:59 pm. He weighed 6lb 3oz and was 19.5 in long. His umbilical cord was wrapped around his neck twice. He was not crying but I did hear him grunting. They let my partner hold him and take him back to the nursery. She did not leave his side.

Two hours later I finally got to meet my baby boy. He was beyond perfect. We stayed in the hospital for three days. I did need a few stitches. Prior to discharge Bryant was circumcised. We were released home within 36 hours. The entire family and Bryant came straight home. We carefully got Bryant to become familiar and comfortable in the new home environment. Bryant is a very good baby. I could not ask for a better son or even a better partner.

My son changed me into a better person. He has made my future brighter. I was so impressed with this birth experience that I have decided to go to nursing school. I am looking for a part time job to support my education and professional goal. If I had not become pregnant, I feel I would have either gone to jail or worse yet, be dead! Accordingly, I feel God allowed me to become pregnant and deliver a son for a reason. I have never questioned Him, "Why?"

My life is really complete and I would not have changed any of the life circumstances that have led me to this point in my existence: the beginning of my son's life was the sole cause of a beginning of a "new life" for me. I guess, God always tries to perform miracles through his Sons.

Dr. Gandhi and his Breech Girl

After trying standard fertility treatments at our office, Dr. Gandhi's wife became pregnant again by assisted reproductive technique in her hometown of Chicago. She had achieved her first pregnancy by the same technique and had stored several other embryos for possible future pregnancies. She was not very talkative and her husband, a Family practice physician made the effort to be with her for most of her appointments. Her pregnancy was relatively uncomplicated. During her last part of pregnancy we observed that the baby girl liked to stay in the Breech position (guess she didn't like being upside down). Two weeks out from her due date, the baby stayed in the breech position. At that point there are two options:

    a. Deliver by C-section

b. Attempt an external cephalic version (turn the breech around by externally manipulating the baby with your hands after the uterus has been relaxed with medication)

Dr. Gandhi was unaware of this second option. He had never heard of it. He consulted his family and other physicians even as far as those physicians in his native county of India. He said, "No physician in India has heard of this obstetrical maneuver. I told him that we perform the procedure in the OB suite with Operating Room open and prepared. Further the OR surgical crew would be present and ready to do a stat C-section if there are any problems with the baby during the version attempt. The baby is monitored at very frequent intervals during the procedure. In essence, by being successful with this intervention, you avoid the standard C-section option. You really do not have anything to lose in trying because safety has been brought into the equation by having the ability to get the baby out by C-section within minutes. He was still a little bit leery but finally acquiesced.

We scheduled her version at the hospital. Ultrasound was done prior to the attempt: you never know when the baby might have turned by itself in the meantime. The baby was still breech. I pushed up the breech vaginally into the right pelvic area, removed by hand and quickly moved by hand to catch the baby's bottom from going back into the pelvis. With my other hand I pushed the baby's head forward and downward in a forward somersault. The first attempt was not successful. I repeated the same maneuvers again except I pushed the baby's bottom to the left side and pushed the forehead backwards and down in a backward somersault. The baby turned with slow steady pressure and massaged the baby's head into the area of the pelvis. Ultrasound was repeated and the baby's heart beat was fine. We started her on Pitocin to induce labor now that the baby's head was pointed in the right position. Within a few hours Mrs. Gandhi was completely dilated. She started to push the baby through the pelvis. With each contraction the baby's heartbeat would drop down the 80's. The baby would not tolerate this stress for too long without being at risk for oxygen deprivation. I asked the nurse at that moment for the vacuum cup in order to rescue the baby from this impending compromise. The vacuum cup was applied to the baby's head (much like a plumber's plunger). With her pushing efforts and my gentle tugging we were able to guide the baby out of the birth canal and out of this distress. It seems there always has to be drama and a climax to a *doctor's wife's* pregnancy and delivery! A doctor's wife, doctors and nurses somehow turn out to be the most challenging patients to care for.

The Koerber Story

I first started seeing Samantha Koerber for her 4th pregnancy. She had a pulmonary embolism, a PE (a blood clot in her lung) within days after her last and 3rd delivery. She was on blood thinners for 3 months after this complication. Due to this high risk medical condition, she was told after her last pregnancy and PE that she should not have any more pregnancies. Samantha goofed up and, despite the medical advice to the contrary, she became pregnant. On her first OB visit Samantha was stunned when the ultrasound showed 2 gestational sacs. Samantha was having twins! The look on Samantha's face was "priceless." She was beyond shock and disbelief. Samantha was overweight (I am being nice, she was obese), had hypertension and was diabetic during pregnancies. With a previous PE and now twins Samantha (and I) were both apprehensive with regard to her care and survival. Samantha's husband was also obese and suffered medical conditions, too.

As is standard treatment for a patient with a previous PE or DVT history, Samantha was placed on a blood thinner, Lovenox, to avoid PE and DVT during her current pregnancy. Samantha was a "basket case" throughout her pregnancy as she worried about her own possible death and the lives of her twins.

Samantha went into labor at 37 weeks: 50% of twins typically deliver earlier than 36 weeks. For the past 2 weeks both babies were in the vertex positions: both head were down. Samantha was having a girl and boy. During her labor the second twin, boy, was found to be in the Breech position. Samantha had an epidural placed at 4-5 cm of dilatation.

When she was ready to deliver the first baby, we brought her into the C-section room. Anesthesia and the OR team was present and ready in case we had to do a stat C-section for the second Breech twin. The nursery team for both babies was present. Extra OB nurses were also needed to be present. The first twin's head came down quickly with a few pushes and delivered. The second twin was still in the feet first position: *a complete* breech by definition. I purposely did not rupture the 2nd sac so that I could turn or float the breech baby into the head down position again. The ultrasound was in the room. I tried to push up the breech to Samantha's right side of her pelvis and push clockwise down on the baby's head in a backwards flip-flop. The baby did not budge. I tried again and the baby would not move. Then I tried to push the breech and legs into Samantha's left pelvic side and push counterclockwise downward on the head to do a forward somersault. I was not successful. The baby was tolerating all of these external maneuvers very well.

The critical moment had now arrived: to do a C-section on the second breech twin or to try a complete breech extraction and accomplish a vaginal birth. The later maneuver always carried a risk of so-called "hanging" the head, i.e. the head getting stuck in the pelvis with the possibility of injury to the baby. I hoped that if the head did get stuck, I could immediately do a C-section and rescue the baby. I knew that a C-section (major abdominal surgery) would substantially increase Samantha's risks of PE, DVT, wound infection, etc. I really wanted to avoid this choice. I had performed several breech extractions in my residency training and early in my practice years. In fact, we never did a C-section for a second twin at UCLA (as I could recall). Times have changed: no OB doctor is going to risk a malpractice suit. This physician was caught in between the proverbial "rock and a hard place." You have to balance the risks of two patients: the mother and the baby. I knew that the second twin boy was not going to be much larger than 7lbs. I knew that Samantha could and had delivered larger babies in previous pregnancies. I had one of the OB nurses get scrubbed up and get gowned. I called for the Piper forceps so that I could extricate the baby's head should it get wedged into the pelvis during the attempted vaginal delivery. I had the OB nurse at my side to hold up the babies legs up in a towel upward so that I see into the vagina and apply the forceps to the baby's head and pull the baby out (gently, that is).

I made my decision. I put my sterile gloved hand up into the vagina. The epidural provided Samantha with sufficient anesthesia that she could not feel any discomfort. I grabbed hold of both of the baby's feet through the intact amniotic sac and pulled the baby down through the vagina. In the process the amniotic sac ruptured. I had another OB nurse following and pushing the baby's head on the abdomen (see preceding story, *Breech Birth with Dr. Dignam*). The baby slipped out of the uterus and out into the world without a hitch. It was the first time that many nurses had ever seen a breech deliver vaginally. I believe to this day that this decision was the correct *obstetrical* choice for both the baby and Samantha. Risk management and malpractice have stopped the medical profession from educating and training new obstetricians in breech and forceps deliveries to the detriment of patient care. On the other hand, the current risk decision would be to do a C-section on the 2nd twin and hope that Samantha's only complication will be a wound infection. She would be put on Lovenox shortly after delivery as well as SCD's (sequential compression devices) on both legs. Her risk of DVT (deep venous thrombosis) and PE (pulmonary embolus or clots that travel from legs/pelvis to lungs) doubled with a C-section delivery. I knew these facts and, as Robert Frost has written in his famous poem:

> I shall be telling this with sigh,
> Somewhere ages and ages hence:
> Two roads diverged in a wood, and I—I took the one less traveled by,
> And that has made all the difference."

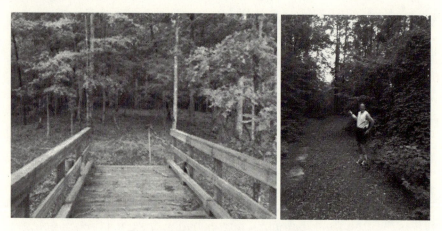

Figure 26-15 Road Less Traveled

Perhaps I may have saved Samantha's life that day but I chose to travel down that *other road* on that day. I know it made *a difference*.

P.S. Samantha is pregnant again!

Typhoon Yaling (was renamed later as Patsy by The Weather Service).

This story was given to the author by the mother, now age 65. The author has re-written wrote her story from her Notes).

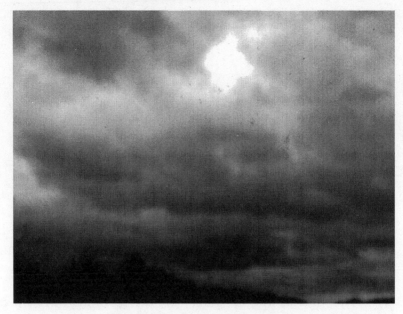

Figure 26-16 Image of storm front

This story is told to the author by the mother of one of his patients now expecting with her first child.

The afternoon of November 21, 1970 was the date of a raging typhoon bearing down on Manila Bay in the Philippines. The severity of typhoons was shown by the different colored flags being flown in various locations:

Black Flag was the worst category.

Typhoon Yaling/Typhoon Patsy

Statistical Data:

> Hit Luzon, Philippines on November 19, 1970 with winds of 139 mph
>
> Date: November 17-20, 1970
>
> Death and injuries:
> 	One of the deadliest to hit Philippines: 106 killed (with 351 missing) 135 killed at sea due to shipping communications
> Wind speed: highest recorded at 200 kph
> City of Manila: storm center with total of 241 deaths
> Losses: 80 million dollars
> Refugees: 31, 380
> Storm Area: 2917 miles over 8 days

Electricity was out in Manila. Roads were closed due to downed trees that lay strewn across them. There was every form of storm devastation. We lived in a home across the water from Manila Bay. Huge ships were already being tossed up on the beaches and roads. The name of this was tropical storm was "Typhoon Yoling." It was to be one of the worst typhoons known in Philippine weather history.

I knew my baby was coming soon. The roads were closed. We had to walk a few blocks inland and try to seek shelter. I was stubborn and I wanted a "San Miguel" and a grilled cheese sandwich.

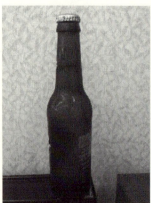 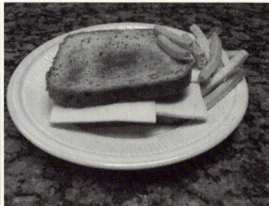

Figure 26-17 "San Miguel" Beer and a Grilled Cheese Sandwich

I was not going to the hospital until I got them. We stopped at "the Fish Pond" (a restaurant) while the storm started to pass through. When my labor pains got pretty close together, we hailed a taxi to take us (my husband and I) to the Manila Sanitarium and Hospital. It was about 4 miles away. A mile from the hospital there were downed trees in the road and the taxi could go no further. We had to get out and walk. I would walk for a small distance and then I had to stop for a while. But, the pains were coming closer. The wind was blowing us all around. He was tough fighting the winds in front of us.

Finally, we did make it to the hospital. However, the hospital had no power. A small generator was being used for only the most critical of patients. I was taken to the delivery room with the only light being provided by a Coleman lantern. The nurse held the lantern over the Doctor's shoulder (Dr. Jesse Umali). I was given something for the labor pain. The medication immediately started to have a strange and weird effect on me. I distinctly remember telling the nurse to "get my camel. I am leaving!"

I guess, I started recalling my times in Egypt where I had visited not too long ago in the past. I knew I said it, but I couldn't stop myself. Just as the baby was about to be born, the Lantern went out.

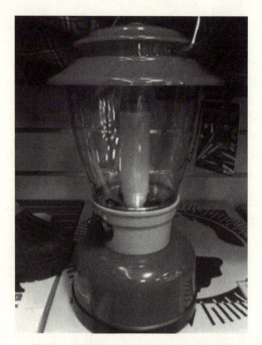

Figure 26-18 Classic Lantern Photo

It was very dark. No one, not even the Doctor, could see. No one could tell me whether it was a boy or a girl! The baby was healthy and was born without any other incident. About 10 minutes later, another lantern was brought in and I found out I had had a girl! We were going to name her "Yolanda" because she was born during this historic typhoon named Yoling. However, after we heard of the horrible damage and destruction, as well as the loss of so many people from that typhoon, we decided it would not be appropriate to name my child "Yolanda." I named her Marina who is now 42 years old. I remember the experience like it was yesterday.

This mother concludes with the following statement: I know my story sounds like one of those "it was a dark and stormy night" but it really was!

The moral to this story is as follows:

1. "San Miguel" beer and labor pain drugs do not mix very well together!

2. During a typhoon when all the roads are blocked by downed trees, you better have a *camel* handy and ready to go so it can get you safely to the hospital.
3. Before you go to a hospital during a horrific storm, it is best to pack a flashlight with batteries so you will be able to see the sex of your baby when it is born!
4. Do not order a grilled cheese sandwich from a restaurant named "The Fish Pond!" It is probably best to just order the fish!
5. Lastly, you should never be eating and drinking when you are in labor. You are lucky the lights were out so that the hospital staff did not see that mess you made when you up-chucked the cheese sandwich just prior to you giving birth!

"I want a Pepsi"

This story is about a patient who had a long and difficult labor. Jane had her amniotic sac start leaking at about 1:00 am in the early morning. Her cervix was only 1 cm dilated and 50% effaced. She was full term: 40 weeks pregnant. Her contractions were not regular. Per our usually "active management of labor" protocol, Pitocin augmentation of labor was begun. She progressed to 4 cm at 10 am. At that point she requested an epidural anesthesia. She had already received two doses of Stadol during the time her cervix dilated from 1 to 4 cm.

She became completely dilated at 3 pm. She started pushing in the 2nd stage of her labor. Her baby was relatively large. She pushed for over 2 hours. I remember to this very day the picture in my mind of what I saw when I entered the Labor Room. She was sitting up and had grabbed hold of the back of her legs. Her hair was a complete mess with locks of her hair in all directions. She was not just sweating but her gown and forehead were wet. She had purposely opened up her hospital gown and portions of her chest and abdomen were exposed. She had a mission: she was going to push this baby out no matter how tired or cranky she was.

She was the epitome of courage, determination and guts that a typical American woman emanates when she has a tough job to do.

Well, I pushed with her for another 30 minutes. At that point I offered the option of using a vacuum cup to help her deliver her baby. She consented. Within a few contractions the baby slid out and was born. The baby did not immediately cry but with stimulation and with drying the baby off, the baby perked up. The baby was now crying loudly. The nursery nurse was given the baby immediately so that the baby could be further dried off and suctioned. Within 5 minutes the baby was cleaned up and mummy wrapped in a new baby receiving blanket. The nursery nurse then went over to her bed with the baby in hand and asked Jane, "Do you want to hold your baby?"

After such a long labor and an arduous 3 hours of pushing, Jane was thirsty and dehydrated. Sweat was dripping from her forehead. Her gown was wet.

In response to the nurse's question, Jane cried out, "No, I do not want to hold the baby. No, No, I want a Pepsi!"

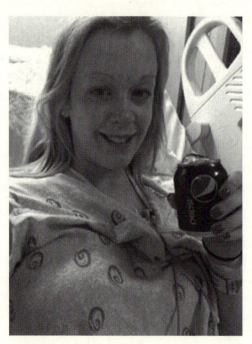

Figure 26-19 Reproduced Photo of "Jane with her Pepsi"

In the past the Pepsi soda company used to advertise, "Pepsi, for the Next Generation."

Pregnant 16 year old single Tennessee Teenager

Susan was a pregnant 16 year old teen in Paris, TN. As soon as her boyfriend found out she was pregnant, he immediately split up with her (was gone) and did not want anything to do with her (or as the soon-to-be-born child). For the record many teenage boys (and even older men in other age groups) are mostly into sex rather than relationships and starting families. I frequently comment to others that, "the fastest way to lose a guy is to tell him you are pregnant."

Midway into her pregnancy I noticed on an ultrasound an abnormal mass in the baby's abdomen. When I again looked at it several weeks later, the mass had grown. I referred her to the Perinatologist at Vanderbilt University for their evaluation. They diagnosed the mass to be originating from the kidney. They said that they would consult and team up with me on her OB care during her pregnancy. Vanderbilt was in Nashville and was 90 minutes from Paris, TN. At her subsequent visits I could see the kidney mass getting larger. At 36 weeks the mass took up half the space in the baby's abdomen.

During her 37 week visit to Vanderbilt the Perinatologist determined that the baby was "in distress." They performed an emergency C-section to save the baby. I was not notified about the situation or the C-section until a few days later and after the turn-of-events. I was not included as her referring OB to be in the decision making loop with regard to the clinical situation.

Biopsy of the baby's kidney mass after birth showed that the baby had a very rare congenital kidney *cancer*. The baby received not only chemotherapy but every therapy that was available to help save the baby. The baby died at 6 months of age at Vanderbilt Children's Center. The teen mom had traveled back and forth to Nashville many times during the weeks and was at her baby's side every day and night that she could. The father of the baby was "uninvolved" and never saw his baby.

Though this pregnancy story is remembered from the distant past, I bring it up because it illustrates some of the ethical dilemmas that physicians face on a day to day basis. The teen underwent a C-section for this baby. Due to most hospital protocols and liability concerns today, she will likely have to have future C-sections with her subsequent pregnancies. The baby did not survive. The C-section only left her with a surgical scar on her abdomen. Much worse are the scars on her emotional as well as her future psychological well-being. She was a courageous young teen who stepped up to the plate, accepted her responsibilities as the baby's mother and tended to her care until her baby died. It is just another example of what teen and most moms do all over the country every day. Mothers protect their young at all costs and hardships.

I think about the medical side of the story. What if the teen mom had asked the Perinatologist the question, "what is there was any chance of survival despite the C-section?" If there was so little hope for the baby, perhaps "letting the baby go naturally" without a C-section at that point in time might have been an option. It would have avoided or reduced the amount of physical and mental anguish that she and her doctors (and nurses) went through in the subsequent 6 months.

The same situations life and death ordeals occur at the opposite end of life, as it happened in the medical care of my best friend, Jude Lyons. He was diagnosed with Stage 4 Lung Cancer at the age of 58. If the chemotherapy does not have an immediate beneficial effect, then at what point does the medical team stop the therapy, face reality and alleviate the pain for both the patient and the family? As physicians and other health professionals, we have to question and think very carefully of what we are trying to accomplish for the long run for our patients.

Fast forward to 2014 and to another family, the Dolofts, who faced a similar difficult ethical situation.

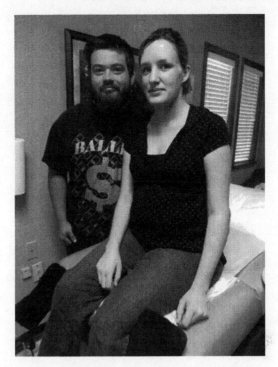

Figure 26-20 Teen Pregnancy: the Dolofts

Zoe was 19 years old and was pregnant for the first time. The first ultrasound at 8 weeks pregnant was not normal: the fetus took up more than 60% of the amniotic sac, i.e., there was much less amniotic fluid than normal. I assumed a genetic abnormality and was concerned that she would lose the pregnancy in the first trimester. The pregnancy progressed and the baby's heart rate was normal. We did the genetic marker screen which returned negative for most chromosomal abnormalities. I did the Panorama (NIPS, i.e. non-invasive prenatal testing) for Down's syndrome and other genetic abnormalities. These tests, too, were returned being surprisingly normal. The pregnancy progressed despite there was very little amniotic fluid around the baby. The baby was referred for further Level 3 ultrasounds at Southwestern, and later, OU Medical Center in OKC. The right kidney was absent. The left kidney was functioning minimally: little urine was being produced. The bladder could not be visualized. There are two important points here:

1. Amniotic fluid is formed *primarily* produced by the baby's kidney output and urine that flows into the cavity.

2. The baby's lungs need amniotic fluid in order to develop and grow properly. The baby's alveoli and bronchi need fluid in order to be distended in order to undergo the normal maturation process.

The placental circulation through the umbilical cord to the baby (umbilical Doppler flow) was normal. Zoe received Betamethasone (a steroid) at 32 weeks to help speed and assist with the development of the baby's lungs.

At 36 weeks the baby was delivered by C-section at University of Oklahoma Medical Center. The decision to deliver the baby and to do a C-section was a collaborative one by neonatologists, nephrologists, Perinatolgists, etc.

Immediately after birth the baby could not be ventilated due to pulmonary hypoplasia (lack of lung development and maturation). The baby lived 5 hours.

Similar to the 16 year old Tennessee teenager, Zoe underwent a primary C-section with a very grim hope that the baby could survive. Just another example how Americans will brave the toughest conditions and odds to undergo a C-section to save an unborn child with very few glimmers of hope

The Pyrimidalis Muscles

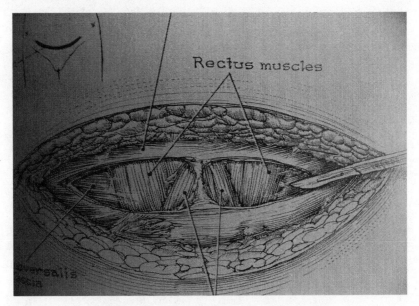

Figure 26-21 PYRIMIDALIS MUSCLES

J. George Moore, MD was the Chief of the Department of Ob-Gyn at UCLA Medical Center when I entered my residency there. Dr. Moore was the youngest Department Head of Service at Columbia University in New York City as well as at UCLA in his day: he was a young gifted bright scholar who took distinct pride in imparting his own "stamp" of training on his residents. Despite his academic achievements in his professional career, his personal life was horrifically scarred by the loss of his own son in a rafting accident in his early adulthood.

Dr. Moore was keenly interested (and entertained!) with the rhythmic motions of the female pelvis during a certain female dance: we are talking about *belly dancing* here. At the end of each year when the senior residents were graduating, Dr. Moore always made sure that there were belly dancers at the party held at his home in the hills overlooking Westwood Village located West Los Angeles. He was certain that the Pyrimidalis muscles were crucial in producing the sexual sway of the female figure during belly dancing. When Dr. Moore scrubbed in with your during an open abdominal surgery, it was absolutely prohibited that any resident would ever compromise or otherwise damage these most important muscles. These muscles were sacrosanct and to this very day, I am extremely careful that these muscles are preserved and never, in any way, damaged during a C-section or other abdominal wall surgery.

Cassandra, a Pregnant Runner who saved her Doctor's Life

I first met Cassandra when she was pregnant with her third child. Cassandra first child was affected by Rubella Syndrome ("German measles"). At this time almost everyone in the US receives their Rubella vaccine (MMR vaccination) during childhood. Hence, most Americans are protected from contracting this viral disease during pregnancy. However, not everyone obtains the vaccination during childhood. It still can affect un-vaccinated patients, whether pregnant or not, today. Rubella vaccination and its immunity may "wear off" after 20 years. Some patients, many of whom have recently emigrated from other countries (where they do not routinely perform routine vaccinations) can also be susceptible or become infected. Therefore, Rubella Syndrome can still affect unborn babies today. Ob-Gyns routinely screen for rubella immunity with the laboratory testing obtained after the first OB office visit. Again, most patients in the US will have received their vaccination as a baby.

Rubella syndrome occurs in a developing fetus of a pregnant woman who has contracted rubella during her *first trimester*. There is a 51% chance that the infant will be affected in the *first* 12 weeks of pregnancy.

CRS (Congenital Rubella Syndrome) can consist of some or all of the deficits listed below:

a. Deafness (sensor-neural) –50%
b. Eye abnormalities –43%
c. Congenital heart disease, mostly PDA (Patent Ductus Arteriosis)—50%
d. Mental Retardation

Cassandra was babysitting her older sister's child when she was pregnant in her first trimester. Cassandra niece was sick but her older sister attributed her sickness to just "the flu." Her niece was having the typical symptoms. Rubella is commonly accompanied by a low grade fever, swollen glands along the neck and back of the head, joint pains, headache and eye inflammation. The incubation period of time is 2-3 weeks after exposure. It is hard for patients and physicians to put the timing and the disease together. Rubella is a very uncommon viral infection and many physicians have never seen a case in their career.

Cassandra's baby had some hearing loss and some vision deficits. All in all, her child managed well.

Cassandra presented me with the challenging questions as to what extreme could exercise be performed during pregnancy. Cassandra was "a runner" and always had been. She was part Cherokee and maybe running was "in her roots." She was not about to let pregnancy get in her way of her running! I told her that her heart was already working 50% more than normal by just being pregnant. Running could put even more strain on her heart. Further, the jostling that goes on with running, i.e. the up and down bouncing of the pregnant uterus could potentially disrupt the placenta. Cassandra naturally slowed down as her pregnancy proceeded. She was cautious and the pregnancy was not disturbed.

Part of this story is about the limits of exercise one can perform during pregnancy. Another part of the story is about Cassandra next pregnancy and her normal delivery. The last part of the story illustrates the immunization issue and that she had a child with CRS.

This story really starts when Cassandra comes to this author for her 6 week postpartum checkup. As could be anticipated, Cassandra already had started running again: in fact, 2 weeks after she delivered. Cassandra had lost most of all the weight she had gained during pregnancy. To be honest, Cassandra was "in great physical shape" from a male point of view (some women would naturally be jealous of her!). The author performed her 6 week postpartum exam and her Pap smear. She got dressed and we discussed birth control. Just prior to leaving the exam room Cassandra remarked to me that I, her

Ob-Gyn, was "getting a little porky!" I was a little taken aback by her straight forward comment. In my mind I knew she was right: I had been gaining some weight. I was not watching my diet. Because of my busy practice, I was always tired and sleep-deprived. Having the time to exercise was almost non-existent. Then Cassandra said to me, "I want to see you down at Lake Elizabeth tomorrow morning at 6 am. We, my husband and I as well as *you,* are going to jog around Lake Elizabeth." Cassandra husband was an athletic handsome well-tanned guy that was quite affable fellow with a great personality. Further, he was a very successful car salesman.

I had sometimes in the past visited and strolled on the pathways of Lake Elizabeth (which was a man-made lake in the middle of Fremont's Central Park). It was, to be exact 2.7 miles in circumference. I told Cassandra, "I have been living here for over 5 years and," to tell you the truth, Cassandra, I have never even walked around Lake Elizabeth, let alone, jog it!"

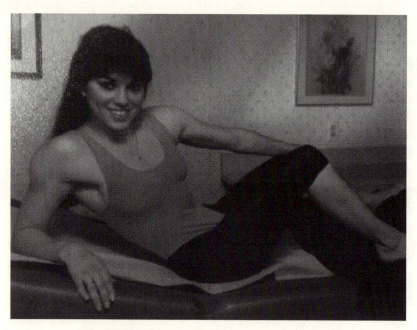

Figure 26-22 Photo Recreation, "Cassandra"

She replied back to me in a rather commanding voice, "you better be there!"

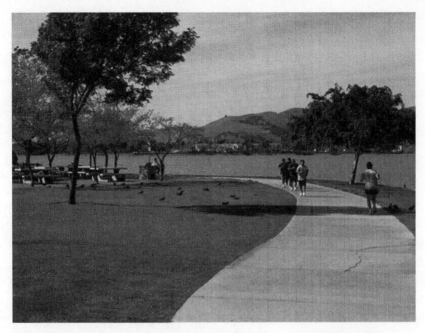

Figure 26-23 Photograph of Lake Elizabeth and jogging path.

I felt I needed to humor Cassandra and I needed to be a good sport. I knew that she was a good runner and she would leave me "in the dust." Quickly she and her husband, also a jogger, would be bored with such a slow poke and not bother to keep me to this running scheme of hers. Well, the next day I did show up at 6 am in the morning (no patients were in labor). I did start jogging around the lake but I also had to stop and walk many times to catch my breath. Cassandra and her husband would jog back and around me. By the end of the first week I was able to jog completely around Lake Elizabeth without stopping. I picked up speed with every week. I was almost able to keep up with Cassandra and her husband as well as with a few other couples that joined us in the mornings. At this point in this story, I have to confess a very important fact: Cassandra, as well as many of her girlfriends, looked pretty attractive from the backside (as well as from front side!) so there was plenty of *incentive* for me to keep jogging behind her!

I must admit now that I have not stopped jogging since Cassandra and her husband got me started on it. It has been over 25 years now.

I may not be running around Lake Elizabeth anymore because I had subsequently moved from Fremont, CA. I did purchase a treadmill for my work-out area in my bedroom. There is no excuse in the world for me not to get on my treadmill (cannot blame the outside weather, etc.). The flat screen TV mounted on the wall keeps me focused on the morning shows: particularly CNBC and the current economic news.

When I had a spiral CT scan at Comanche County Memorial Hospital a few years ago, the radiologist remarked that I had no calcium deposits in my coronary arteries. Coronary Heart disease, diabetes and hypertension were common medical conditions in my family (and particularly my parents). The author is free of all these serious medical conditions and is not taking any prescription medications. He has maintained his weight. I can say truthfully that Cassandra and her husband must have saved my life. I owe it all to her calling me out. Thank you, Cassandra and Andrew!

The moral to this story is four-fold:

1. Illnesses caused by viruses and other infectious diseases can cause serious birth defects prior to 6 weeks gestation. In fact, your baby's heart is completely formed even before you miss your next menstrual period. Therefore, when you are trying to get pregnant, it is important to avoid contact with people with obvious communicable diseases. Lastly, during your pregnancy it is still prudent to avoid any person with an infectious disease. Lastly, make sure your immunizations are up-to-date!
2. No matter what age you are or what you occupation may have there is always the opportunity to put regular exercise into your daily routine. Pregnancy is still a good time to start "becoming fit." Walking, swimming, biking, etc. can always be initiated. It makes no difference what kind of exercises you do and what equipment you use or prefer. Flexing your muscles is what is most important. As Nike says, "Just do it."
3. The third moral is that if you are going to start jogging with a group, in this instance a couple whose husbands is the sales manager at the most successful car dealership in your city, you most likely are able to get a great deal on a new car like I did!

4. The fourth moral (and maybe the most significant one) with regard to this story is this very point: if you are going to start jogging for the first time, make sure you start off by jogging behind a woman who looks like "Pocahontas" (or more directed to the women readers of this book, a Hugh Jackman, Channing Tatum or other good looking hunks as shown below.

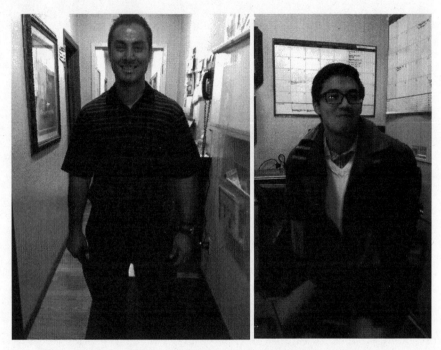

Left, Figure 26-24. An Example of some male "Eye Candy" to jog behind: Right, Figure 26-25 Jog behind him? (Author's son!)

The Story of Patty (on a winter's day)

Though I was never certain that I was real believer in the Almighty, my mind and my life had been changed forever.

Patty was a very sweet and kind person: she was working as one of our postpartum nurse at our local hospital. She was a wonderful nurse and she was very caring to all the new mothers on the floor. Unfortunately, Patty was born with an inherited metabolic problem that caused excess weight gain and relative infertility. Patty was 355 lbs. I am sure a lot of people made fun of Patty because of her weight during her lifetime. She was probably bullied and teased a lot about her weight. Patty managed to survive these negative circumstances. She was a great and caring nurse. Patty did not have a current boyfriend and had never been married. As Patty was getting into her mid 30's, Patty wanted to be a mother whether she was married or not. She came to see me for fertility. I have always had a special interest in fertility. I felt I had a unique calling to be able to assist patients with this need and desire for children and family.

Patty had irregular periods. She wanted me to get her pregnant. Since she was not married, she wanted to be artificially inseminated with donor sperm. We started her on fertility medications. During the second month of fertility treatment I saw a mature egg in her right ovary during her ultrasound evaluation. At that point I gave her an HCG (Human Chorionic Gonadotropin) injection to "trigger" ovulation at mid-cycle. HCG is given so that the egg can be released or ejected from egg follicle in the ovary. Artificial Insemination was required. Two weeks later Patty was pregnant!

I performed an ultrasound as part of her first Ob appointment. It was at that moment that I saw two (2) pregnancy sacs: I must have missed the other mature egg in her left ovary. During that office visit Patty asked me about her use of an inhaler for asthma during the pregnancy. I had forgotten that Patty had asthma. With her weight, the twins and her asthma the horrible thought ran straight through my brain that I may have "just killed" Patty by helping her get pregnant. I was having second thoughts about the treatment I had performed on her.

Patty's pregnancy progressed normally. He weight also increased a little. With her weight, age and the twins Patty needed to be treated for pregnancy-related diabetes. Patty was conscientious about controlling her blood sugars. She took her vitamins. Her iron, etc. Patty was very excited about having the twins. She started buying all the baby stuff that she was going to needing: double strollers, diapers, etc. She fixed up the room for the twins in her apartment just a couple of blocks down from the hospital.

It was a rainy afternoon when Patty came to Labor and Delivery for a labor check at 36 weeks. She thought she was in early labor. I came over from the office to check her. Her cervix was closed and was not effaced. I told her that we would monitor the twins and watch for any changes. I gave instructions to the nurses and headed home about 5:30 in the afternoon.

As I was turning the corner and seeing my house in the distance, my cell phone was buzzing with a call from Labor and Delivery. Patty's membranes had ruptured and the nurse felt a cord in the vagina. I told the nurses to call the OR staff and the anesthesiologist on-call for an emergency stat C-section. I rushed back to the hospital.

When I ran into the room I immediately checked Patty. One of the twin's umbilical cords had prolapsed into the vagina. I could not feel a pulse in the cord. Her cervix was still closed. I thought, "How could have the cord prolapsed through this cervix when it was closed?" I grabbed the ultrasound and searched for the heartbeats of the twins. I saw one twin and the heart was beating strong. But I could not even see the second twin: Patty's abdominal wall was too large and thick. The ultrasound machine could not penetrate her and I could do nothing more. It was at that moment that I had to tell Patty the very worst of news: that there was no pulse in one twin's cord and that one baby was dead. I told her, "It was going to be stillborn." I was feeling so sad for Patty and very upset with this complication. The entire OB staff was quiet and glum for the impending stillborn twin at this time.

The anesthesiologist, Tom Philbert MD, came into the Labor and Delivery suite. He stated that the OR table was not built for Patty's weight: now 375 lbs. The staff got a 2nd OR table out of the other OR. We both OR tables together side by side. There was no rush now: one baby was dead and the other twin's heart beat was normal and strong. We continued to monitor the live baby.

We moved Patty onto the OR table. Tom Philbert MD attempted to put in a spinal anesthetic. He tried several times trying to pass the needle through the fat pad overlying her spine. Because of her weight and thickness of the back, we could not even feel her spine and the spaces in between. He did not want to put her to sleep (General

Anesthesia) because if the increased medical risks due to her shorter neck (unable to intubate her), her weight and asthma. He said he could not even reach the spinal space with his needle: the needle was not long enough to penetrate her and the spinal space. At that moment I remembered that I had some *extended-length* epidermal needles in my changing locker. These longer epidural needles had been specially designed for overweight patients like Patty. They had been lying there for over 6 months. These longer needles were given to me to try out from a company representative that had come to office. I was not doing epidurals anymore: the anesthesia department was providing that service now. I brought them to the hospital and left them in my locker in the OB suite.

I went back to the locker and gave Tom Philbert the needles: he was surprised that I had them and yes, they were the long enough to do the anesthesia. I thought to myself that it was surely coincidence that I was given those needle samples, left them in my locker in Labor and Delivery and now they were needed, absolutely essential, for Patty's special case). Sure enough, Tom sank the spinal with the first attempt with the long needle. Patty was numb and we were preparing to drape her and make the incision.

I had called two other OB physicians (Sheldon Baroff MD and Judith Scott MD) just to help me with Patty: I needed two physicians just to retract away the large abdominal wall. I made the incision from side to side. Patty was the largest patient on whom I had ever operated. The abdominal wall fat was at least 10 inches in thickness. By the time I had entered the abdominal cavity I could barely see the uterus itself. It was at the bottom of deep, deep incision: at least 12 inches down. I could no longer bend over the OR tables. My back was aching and my shirt was wet with nervous perspiration. I crawled up onto the OR table and with my knees bent, actually knelling over into Patty's incision. There was only enough exposure to see a small part of the uterus: 3 inches side to side and 8 inches up and down. I knew that, if we did the usual side to side incision in the uterus that I could lacerate into the uterine arteries that entered through the sides of the uterus. If the incision extended into those arteries, the blood loss would be so swift and uncontrollable. We would definitely lose Patty. I had already lost one of the twins. I could not lose Patty.

I hesitated and deliberated carefully before I made my decision on which way I should make the incision into the uterus. The delay in surgery was nerve-racking to Sheldon Baroff MD and he was getting impatient. As stated above, he was one of the physicians assisting me. He started yelling at me, "Make a decision, you got to make a decision on how you are going to open up the uterus."

I told him I was going up and down on the uterus. I was not going to take the risk: I was going to avoid the uterine arteries altogether. It was a version of the "Classic C-section," not commonly performed for most C-sections today. I did a "low vertical" incision." It did involve cutting the "muscle part" of the uterus. It was also harder to close and stitch up afterwards. I opened up the uterus and got the first twin out. This twin started crying the instance I touched her. It was the live one., I thought, at least we have one healthy baby for Patty.

At this very moment, I felt an unusual sensation "a little wind or breeze" that one would typically feel as if someone had just walked quickly behind them. But, *no one* had walked behind me.

At that point I ruptured the membranes of the second sac to get the stillborn delivered. As I lifted this second twin girl out, she, too, started moving and crying. She was vigorous and alive! The entire Operating Room staff burst out into tears and started crying. Tom Philbert (who sang in his Church's Choir) told me he felt a "presence" in the room at that moment and during all of Patty's surgery. How could this twin girl be alive? I could not feel a pulse in her cord. "Did I not feel the cord properly?" "What was going on here?"

Yes, there was a different atmosphere and surreal feeling in the OR that night. Everyone felt it.

I remember all the circumstances of this special occurrence to this very day and I am certain that I will remember that day the rest of my life. One may never see a miracle happen in their lifetime, but I did. Everyone in the OR that night did. God was there for Patty and He was there for Patty's babies. Though I was never certain that I was real Believer, my mind and my life had changed forever. I think about the long epidural needles that were given to me 6 months prior to Patty's delivery: I did not recognize the name of the company that made them and I never saw that manufacturer's name (or representative) again in my life. I have always wondered *who* really gave them to me now.

To this very day, I think how Patty, Victoria and Valerie are doing and how an Angel (or God himself) had stepped in, intervened and blessed them that day. I cannot help but choke up, break down and cry whenever I tell anyone this very real true story. I have delivered thousands of babies during my career, but surely this was the most emotional and most powerful one of my life. I was touched because God had touched me and everyone in the OR that night. God was there for Patty and He was there for Patty's babies. Though I was never certain that I was real believer, my mind and my life had been changed forever.

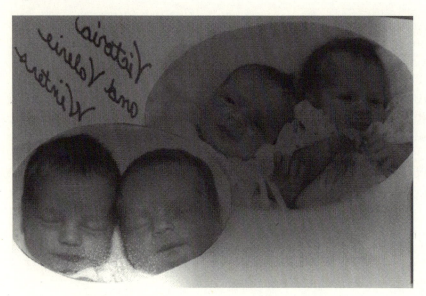

Figure 26-26 Patty's Twins: Victoria and Valerie

Match.com

She said," I thought we had a very good relationship. I didn't know we were having any problems." They were married for over 20 years. She was 41 and a college professor in Baltimore, Maryland. He was a Navy Seal in the US Navy but served now in the President's Special Security Detail in Washington DC about 75 miles away. Their story line is all too familiar and so typical in America today.

The beginning of the story starts in **Buffalo**, New York where she grows up and attends high school. She possesses musical talent and excels at playing the violin. She would play in her high school orchestra and would be asked to fill in at the local Philharmonic. She received a music scholarship to the Peabody in her senior year of high school. However, during her high school year, her mother endured a long battle with cancer. With the death of her mom, she becomes very depressed and discouraged.

Money was necessarily short at hand with the medical expenses incurred by her mother's illness. Similarly, jobs were scarce in Buffalo. She needed to get away and start a new, and perhaps, an adventurous life. She hears that there are opportunities for young women in the armed forces. After graduating from high school she leaves Buffalo and joins the Navy. Joining the Navy and leaving town was the best move she could make at this time.

He, her future husband, too, was a recent high school graduate from the Heartland, Oklahoma to be more specific. They meet for the first time in San Diego while she was in basic training. He, after graduating college, entered OCS (Officer's Candidate School). No different than millions of other young people: they start dating and begin falling in love. Accidents happen: One year later she finds she is pregnant. Not really planning to get married at any time soon, circumstances have forced them to make a decision. He was not ready. She was not ready. They both stepped up to their responsibilities as future parents and got married. They hoped it was part of God's plan or destiny. They would make a go of it and make it work.

She delivers her baby boy in San Diego. Shortly thereafter, her 2 years in the Navy are up. They move to Bethesda, Maryland. He continues his career in the Navy and becomes a Navy Seal. He rises quickly in the officer ranks. While raising the baby at home, she starts back to school and earns her bachelor degree in math and music education

I hate to tell you this truism but 20 years goes by pretty fast: especially when you are raising a family and studying toward a teaching degree in college. It was at the University that the professors recognized her special aptitude for mathematics. Calculus and advanced algebraic equations seem to be "a breeze" for her to understand and learn. Soon she starts teaching algebra at the high school algebra and calculus at the University. Time has passed quickly and their son was already in high school. He was playing Varsity football. Dad was now in the President's Security Detail in D.C. He would come home on the weekends or when he could. He had to share an apartment with other Navy personnel in D.C.

You could see it coming: 40's-something male beginning a midlife crisis in Nation's Capital. He meets another woman and they hook up. Meanwhile she is working and being a mother at home raising her teenage boy. After he comes home one weekend, she notices some irritation in her vaginal area. "Oh, she says to herself. I must have cut myself while shaving down there." But it heals slower than the usual razor burns. She says, "There is no way I could have an STD (sexually transmitted disease). She thinks nothing of the sore outside her vagina anymore.

It is a trite saying but "life is not really greener on the other side of the fence." As one reads in the newspapers and scandal magazines every day, many men leave their beautiful intelligent wife for a "younger and sexier model." Sometimes guys just do not appreciate what they already have. Couples need excitement, date nights, etc. to break up the monotony of day-to-day life of work and home. Over the years married folks start taking each other for granted. Perhaps, in her case, she was responsible for doing all the family banking and budgeting. He confesses to her that he felt "controlled" by her. People just do not know what really goes on in couples lives. However, men would flirt with her saying that she had an attractive figure and admired her long legs.

He filed for divorce. She was completely taken by surprise. She wanted to work it out. He said, "No, I know people who have gone to counseling and it never works out. It is just a waste of time and money." He moved out. Actually, there was not much more to take since he was already living in DC. She was devastated and felt she had failed. She started second guessing herself. "Do I look bad? Not pretty anymore? Did I talk down to him or was I too critical?" She was so distraught she could not eat. She rapidly dropped 30 pounds. She felt very insecure about herself and her physical being. At the advice of a co-teacher, she went to a professional photographer to take glamor photographs of her even more "slinkier" figure.

As Alabama had sung in their song, "Lady Down on Love," more than two decades ago (reader is referred to read all the lyrics of the song),

Now she's a lady, down on love
She needs someone to gently pick her up
She's got her freedom, but she rather be bound
To a man who would love her, and never let her down

----Written by Randy Owen and recorded by Alabama1983

About the Song (from Wikipedia, the Free Encyclopedia)

"Lady Down on Love" is a song about divorce – told first from her side and, in the second verse, his side.

Songwriter Randy Owen recalled to country music journalist Tom Roland that the idea for the song came about when, during a performance at a nightclub in Bowling Green, Kentucky, he learned that a group of women were celebrating a friend's divorce with a night out on the town. However, the divorcée was not having a good time, because she was mourning the end of her marriage and thinking about what should have been – that she should be at home with her husband.

In an effort to escape the devastating effects of the divorce, she decides to move to a small town near Lawton, OK. It is an area close to her ex-husband's parents with whom she enjoyed a good relationship. The Grandparents are happy to see the teenager more frequently and be more interactive with him.

She joins a new church and plays the violin there every Sunday. She was very congenial and easily made many good friends quickly. She starts teaching at the high school. She made friends with many of her fellow teacher colleagues. She starts to "network." She keeps herself busy. There were out of town church events, dancing, exercising, etc. These many activities keep her mind from missing her family in Buffalo and the life she had known for more than 20 years.

Now you, the reader, may be wondering about the title to this story and where is the author going with this story.

Her friend tells her she should start dating. Her friend suggests that she go on the internet dating site, Match. Com. So they both go on the website together. They pour through hundreds of possible matches. 2 matches seemed interesting: an Army officer at Ft. Sill was attractive and an engineer from Tinker Air Force Base. She initiates communication with both men through the dating website, Match.com. She starts emailing "conversations" with both men. She dated the engineer first. He was a really nice guy, but she feels no physical "vibrations" or attraction. As George Strait sings,

"You can't make a heart love somebody
You can tell it what to do but it won't listen at all
You can't make a heart love somebody,
You can lead a heart to love, but you can't make it fall."

--written by Johnny MacRae and Steve Clark, 1994

> About the Song (from Wikipedia):
>
> The song is about a man who proposes to his girlfriend, but she rejects it. In a play on the cliché, "You can lead a horse to water but you can't make him drink," the woman tearfully explains that—despite her best efforts—she is simply not in love with her boyfriend ("*You can lead a heart to love, but you can't make him fall*").

She continued talking to the Army officer over Match.Com and they enjoyed a couple dates together. The relationship was heating up quickly. After many phone conversations with this guy and a few dates she invited him to her place for dinner. However, during the dinner an "ice storm" blew in quickly. By the time they were done eating, the lights went out and the roads were not passable. He had to spend the night. They went to the bedroom. They made love. It had been awhile for her and she was naturally craving love and affection. Her self-esteem was low. They fell asleep. When they awoke in the morning, they made passionate love again. The temperature outside also warmed up. When the road conditions improved, he left back to the base.

He called her the next day. He made some comments that "maybe things were moving too fast." He said he was not planning on seeing her again.

The engineer wanted to see her again. They dated again but she realized that there was really no chemistry between them.

Within a few weeks she noticed that her body seemed to be feeling a little different. Her breasts were more full and sore. "I must have over-worked my **"pecs"** (pectoralis muscles) too much!" When she was late for her menstrual period, she suspected that she might be pregnant. She texted him, "I must talk to you about something very important." He called back immediately. She told him that her pregnancy test was positive. He was polite enough but he, of course, wanted a paternity test done.

A paternity test can be done but only after the baby's blood is tested. Normally paternity testing can only occur after the baby is born: basically 8 months hence forward.

Her ex-husband had had a vasectomy almost immediately after their only son was born. She was a little surprised that he didn't want any more children. They were both still young in their 20's but she didn't oppose the idea. After she had finished her divorce, she once had quipped to her girlfriends jokingly, "maybe I will meet someone and have another baby!"

Well, her prophesy came true.

As you probably guessed, this is where I, the author, come into the story. She had made an appointment with my office for obstetrical care. I was not supposed to see her for her first prenatal visit for another week. However, she started to have some bleeding and mild cramping. My office staff got her an appointment that day as soon as she could get off school. She came to the office with Marcy, a church friend. She was obviously stressed out and worried about the pregnancy. She had never entertained the option of terminating this "oops baby." I think that down to the heart of the matter she had always wanted another baby. Perhaps she had harbored a very long subconscious resentment and anger because her-now "ex" did not want any more children. "He was always good with kids," she stated on more than a number of occasions. Maybe the "baby" would provide her a new start, certainly another turn to her life. "Was God giving her a "new blessing" and a new mission he had planned out for her?"

I did her physical and pelvic exam. An ultrasound on her pregnancy was promptly performed. She was very early in her pregnancy: about 5 weeks. I could not visualize a fetal pole or the fetal heartbeat. The pregnancy "sac" looked normal enough. I saw no bleeding around the placental site. I told her I wanted to order some hormonal levels on her: a quantitative HCG and a serum progesterone level. Both tests came back within the normal range. I gave her a call and told her the "positive" results. I reassured her that I was optimistic about the pregnancy. I tried to reassure her. She sounded like she was somewhat comforted. As some say, "time will tell" if this pregnancy is going to be a normal one.

The pregnancy proceeded without any further problems. Of course, it had been 20 years since her first son was born. She was 41 years old. She did not think she could become pregnant at this age. She had purchased some condoms after her divorce but had left them in the night stand. The soldier on his part did not ask her about contraception. She was too embarrassed to ask him to use the condoms. It was the heat of the moment. Sometimes (maybe most times?) you become thoughtless at these moments: they both had a lapse of judgment. Or, was fate bearing down on their two lives that accidentally met in time?

At the next appointment I could make out the outline of the fetus on ultrasound as well as the fetal heartbeat. Everything was "growing nicely." Of course, because of her age, she underwent more extensive prenatal genetic evaluation. At 18 weeks the "anatomy" ultrasound combined with prenatal multiple marker testing was performed. The baby was normal as far as testing could predict.

She was scheduled for induction in the last week of her pregnancy. Of course, her friend Marcy was there as she had been for most of her appointments. Her due date was in late October: she would need to get a substitute teacher for her classes. She could stay longer on her pregnancy leave by taking advantage of the upcoming Christmas Holidays: she would have an extra 2 weeks off so she could bond and care for her new baby longer.

She did not have an epidural for her first delivery. She scarcely remembered her first labor. She thinks she just received some medications in her IV. She entered the labor suite at 2-3 cm. We started inducing her with Pitocin at 6 am. When I saw her at 8:30 she was close to 3-4 cm. I broke her water. She went into more active labor. She requested an epidural. She went quickly thereafter and was completely dilated by noon. She started pushing. The baby was pretty good size: approximately 8 lbs., I thought. The pushing stage, i.e., the 2nd stage of labor took a little while: close to an hour. The nurses put her legs up in the supporting stirrups. The opening was prepped and draped. I spread mineral oil generously all over the vulva and vaginal opening. It looked like the tissues would stretch enough so I would not have to do an episiotomy. I let the head slowly dilate the opening. The head was delivered slowly, but then the shoulders were stuck and did not come down. I asked the nurses to push her legs back further in the McRobert's position. The shoulders were still not budging. I asked the nurse to push suprapubically to her left side and I pulled a little further downward with the head. The shoulders rotated off the pubic bone and into the true pelvis. With further gentle outward pressure the shoulders started moving down. Finally the baby delivered. The baby was, as expected, a little slow to start crying. The baby had "pooped" a little bit. The baby was blue and the head was red from the blood temporarily trapped in the head. After suctioning the baby and stimulating him, the baby perked up. His head still remained a little purple from the very short delay in delivery. I told her "not to worry." The baby was going to be "just fine."

As I have told a lot of my patients in this slightly common "shoulder dystocia" problem (in order to reassure them), "Boys are blue and girls are pink!"

The nurses brought the scale in. The baby weighed 9 lbs. and 8 oz.! No wonder I had trouble getting those shoulders out!

Her sister had come in from out of town to help her with the baby. Her sister was retired from her career at General Motors in Buffalo.

Her postpartum recovery was uneventful. She went home on her 2nd postpartum day. Prior to her discharge I asked her what she was going to name her baby boy. I was delighted when she said she was naming him "Jeffrey."

Six weeks of time can pass quite quickly these days. She was back in the office for her 6 week check-up. She was nursing the baby and everything was going well. Another sister came from out of town to help her with the baby. Her brother and his wife lived close by in Oklahoma City. They would come down and do their "tour of duty," i.e. to help her with the house and the baby.

Genetic testing to check the paternity of the baby boy was done one month after birth. Sure enough, the genetic tests on the baby also came back showing that the baby's father was indeed the Ft. Sill soldier.

During one of the office visits, she and I had gotten on to the subject of food. Steak was the item of discussion. I chimed in saying that I always prefer to grill my steaks "the Bobby Flay Method."

Bobby's method is fairly simple: coat the steaks with olive oil, season with salt and pepper or "steak seasoning," and put them on a grill when the coals are just right (white but not falling apart). Put your timer on: 5 minutes on one side and 5 minutes on the other side. Take the steaks off the grill. DO NOT CUT them until they have rested at least 10-15 minutes. At that point the steaks are medium rare and perfect! She was not too familiar with a charcoal grill. She was used to the gas grill: just turn on the gas, push the button, and behold instant fire. Voila!

About 2 weeks later she called me. She said she had met a "new guy." She was pretty excited about him. She wanted to cook him dinner: specifically steaks. She wanted me to explain the "Bobbie Flay" recipe again. She purchased the Filet Mignon steaks and their "Grilling date" was set. Sure enough, after a few simple directions and she was ready to grill the steaks. Her date had already made a salad and baked potatoes. The grill was ready. The steaks were coated, seasoned and put on the grill. She said they came out perfectly!

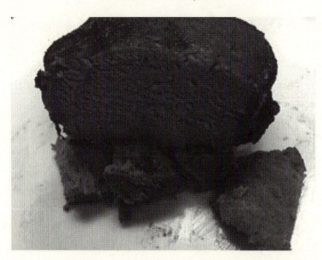

Figure 26-27 Filet Mignon grilled the "Bobby Flay" way

As she and her date sat on the bar stools, they both suddenly gazed into each other's eyes and at that epiphany moment they made an emotional connection. After that night their love began and a relationship started to bloom.

We are all part of God's creation. Is "The Book of Life" already totally written? How much "free will" are we given? What are the roles of *providence and grace*? Doors become closed right in front of you but other doors open up near you. You make choices or are you really choosing by yourself?

She and her boyfriend have been together going on over 5 years now. He did not plan on helping her raise another child. The child was part of the package. Knowing her, she was truly an "angel on earth." He could not ask for any other woman more perfect to be part of his life. They are "best friends" and "best roommates." They are even great tennis partners! When trying to solve everyday problems she always is there to help him solve them: she always has "his back" and she always can think of a solution when he cannot. He respects her brain (and her body). There are a lot of women who just become more beautiful and endearing with age. They cook together and "when the sun goes down, everything gets a little hotter." He always says, I have always wondered if her little sexy movements are done purposely or do they just come naturally. He said to her, "Do you think you have me *Buffaloed*?"

Some sage observations from my life's experiences:

If you can go on a long *road trip* with the "love of your life" and you do not get "on each other's nerves" or get into any major disagreements, then you have found the right person for you. Psychologists have always stated that compatibility is based on sameness: same work ethics, same values, same tastes and likes, same attitudes and mutual respect. If you are both each other's clones, there is still enough "stuff" in this world with which to disagree and "fight about!"

If you can paint (even wallpaper) together and not get on each other's nerves, then you have indeed found the right partner. Further, if you can take a long road trip together and get along, you may be compatible.

Doing these activities together are, in my opinion, a critical "acid test" of your future relationship success.

There are some relevant points to telling you this story.

1. This story is not unique. In fact, it is very common. The rise and fall of the American family: people meet; have children, time passes, midlife crises, and divorce. Sometimes the story is longer and sometimes it is shorter. I wish schools would mandate teaching "Marriage and the Family" in high school again. A course on relationships and communication skills would also help cut down the divorce rate and improve friendships as well as workplace happiness.

2. If you do not use birth control, you will most definitely get pregnant. As one patient stated to me, "you should not get angry with your baby's daddy, you picked him!"

3. Shoulder dystocia (shoulders stuck and hanging up on the pubic bone) is a very real problem in delivery rooms across the country. It is directly correlated with the size of the baby

(associated particularly with gestational diabetic pregnancies). OB doctors can be tipped off by the slow progress of labor in the first stage of labor, but mostly by the longer 2nd stage of pushing as in this story. However, it can manifest itself suddenly without any notice. A patient with a small pelvis can experience shoulder dystocia even with an average size baby.

4. One man's "ex" can be some another guy's "treasure." The reader is directed to the following youtube.com link:

http://www.youtube.com/watch?v=BuWEvVR8D2U&feature=player_embedded

Her boyfriend thanks God every night for having her in his life. She truly believes that they are "soul mates."

5. We all travel "down the broken road" and God bless, I hope you find yourself in life "on the mended side."

I know we've been friends forever
But now I think I'm feeling something totally new
And after all this time I opened up my eyes
Now I see you were always with me

Author Update: Unbelievably, she is pregnant again! The story will be continued (at least until the baby is born and be announced in the next edition to this book!)

The next story is purposely put at the end of the "Tales" section because not all pregnancy stories turn out with a "Happy Ending." The Reader can continue to read this story with the admission that these events very infrequently occur and are NOT representative. They are true stories that the author experienced early in his training at UCLA medical center some 40 years ago. Obstetrics and technology has advanced to such a degree that these events would not have occurred in today's modern practice of Obstetrics. The Reader is "on her own" should she decide to read them.

The Linda Castro Story

I was not sure whether I should be recounting this patient's OB story in this book. I met Mrs. Linda Castro when I was an Intern at UCLA: it was my first rotation on OB. Warren Fujimoto, MD was the 3rd year Chief OB Resident and he was in charge of the Obstetric Service. Dr. Fujimoto was a brilliant and caring physician: he had been in the Navy as a Flight Surgeon prior to beginning his residency at UCLA. He was well-liked by everyone and was voted the "Best Teacher of the Year" by all the residents and medical students at UCLA.

Linda Castro was admitted to the labor room one morning with contractions. I was not the intern taking care of her but all of the interns knew what was going on with all the patients in labor. Her labor was progressing slowly. Prior to beginning any stimulation of labor it was the protocol at UCLA that all patients had to undergo pelvimetry x-rays: basically x-rays of the bony pelvis so that objective measurements of the inlet and mid-pelvis could be taken (according to *Mengerts' rule*—you can Google his rule if you are interested). In this way we could assess the adequacy of the birth passageway. Her measurements were calculated and the pelvis was "average." Her membranes were ruptured. An internal uterine pressure catheter (IUPC) was placed: we needed objective measurement of the strength of her contractions. A fetal scalp electrode (FSE) was placed to directly monitor the baby's heart rate. Now the Pitocin augmentation of labor could be started. I left for home around 6 PM that day.

However when I came to Labor and Delivery the next morning, I saw with disbelief that Linda Castro was still on the Labor Board: Linda was still in labor. She was now close to laboring for over 24 hours. Her cervix was still only 8 centimeters. Her baby's head was not descending well into the pelvis. About 10 am that morning Linda spiked a fever to 102 degrees. In those days patients had to have a full "trial of labor" prior to undergoing a C-section. Dr. Fujimoto had been pressing the Attendings (the Departmental OB Staff Professors) to allow him to go ahead and get her delivered by C-section when she started becoming septic. The Attending wanted to wait and give her more time. Linda was cultured and placed on antibiotics. She finally got to complete cervical dilatation and started pushing.

The baby would not descend. Again, Dr. Fujimoto argued for her to be "sectioned." After several more hours without progress the Attendings at UCLA finally agreed. It was like going to the Supreme Court to get a final decision. Linda was finally taken to the C-section room and delivered. The baby came out fine.

Linda's post-operative course was complicated. She continued to spike fevers. After the 3rd day Linda was placed on heparin (Blood thinner) as well as "triple antibiotics" (ampicillin, cleocin and gentamycin). It was felt that she may now have progressed to septic pelvic thrombophlebitis (uterine infection with infection spreading to the blood vessels around the uterus). On her 4th post-operative day Linda suddenly had developed severe chest pains and significant breathing problems. She was immediately put into the ICU. Her oxygen saturation was 80% (normal =98%). A second pulmonary embolus struck Linda one hour later and she "coded," i.e., stopped breathing with no heartbeat. After a long and extensive resuscitation effort for over an hour she was brought back. Sadly, Linda was essentially "brain dead" from this moment on. She was eventually transferred from the UCLA Medical Center to a Nursing home where she died 2 months later.

Now why would I want to tell my patients this very, very tragic horrible story? It is because I want my readers to know that people *can die* when they decide to become pregnant. Linda died and the story of Linda Castro affected me and my practice of Obstetrics forever from then until this present day. The Attendings at UCLA Medical Center were so focused on objectivity, i.e., measurements and labor curves that they forgot "the art of medicine." They shunned the direct physical examination of the patient as well as the baby's size. They would not take into account the position and flexion of the baby's head: those were obsolete data points. They practiced *academic* Obstetrics.

Even back then, it was old *Obstetric saying* from many centuries ago that stated, "A woman shall not see two sunrises while she is in labor."

In 2012 the State of Oklahoma Medicaid Program (and perhaps other States) has promulgated a standard or "Primary C-section rate" of

18% for all OB patients without a previous C-section. If an OB's C-section rate is greater than 18% for over 12 month cycle all his OB records are reviewed by the State in order to see if a physician is *un-necessarily* doing too many C-sections. In order to avoid such "reviews" many physicians will allow labors to proceed for longer lengths of time. Hopefully, no so long that another "Linda Castro Story" occurs. Certainly C-section rates have risen in the last 2o years, but patients have drastically changed also. The average "weigh in" when patients arrive in labor has increased from 170 pounds to 239 lbs. The "obesity factor" today has caused a related increase in gestational diabetes and hypertension as well as fat deposits in the pelvis obstructing the baby from coming through the birth canal. Obese pregnant patients are more likely to suffer glucose intolerance, that is, Diabetes itself. They are more likely to develop high blood pressure. They have a higher C-section rate. Because of the large amount of fat on their back, spinal and epidural anesthesia is much more difficult to perform. Spinal headaches and local infections are more common. Wound infections of the C-sections scars occur more frequently.

I have read Emmanuel Friedman's classic text on Labor as well as *The Active Management of Labor* by the physicians at the University of Dublin in the Rotunda Birthing Hospital. Together with my many years of experience caring for patients in labor and the personal reports of my colleagues I know that a patient should deliver within approximately 12 hours of beginning "true labor." The cervix will dilate at a certain rate and the baby's head will descend into the pelvis with a direct mathematical relationship to the cervical dilatation. Estimated fetal weights by exam and objectively with ultrasound can give us a rather good calculation of fetal weight. We no longer obtain pelvic x-rays. Unfortunately many of today's clinicians are not taught "clinical pelvimetry" and the art of estimating pelvic shapes and measurements. I, and my patients, can thank Linda Castro for allowing this physician to be able to manage his labor patients efficiently such that not even an extra hour is spent in needless labor. If she is showing all the signs that she needs a C-section, the C-section shall be performed as swiftly and as promptly as it can be done.

Women make all the RULES

(See next section)

THE RULES

The **FEMAL**E always makes *the Rules*

The Rules are subject to change at any time without prior notification

No **MAL**E can possibly know all *the Rules*

If the **FEMALE** suspects that the **MALE** knows all the rules

She must immediately change some or all of *the Rules*

The **FEMALE** is never wrong

If the **FEMALE** is wrong, it is due to a misunderstanding

which is a direct result of the **MALE** did or said wrong

The **Male** must immediately apologize for causing said misunderstanding

The **FEMALE** may change her mind at any time

The **MALE** may never change his mind

without the expressed written consent of the **FEMALE**

The **FEMALE** has a right to be angry or upset at any time

The **MALE** must remain calm at all times

unless the **FEMALE** wants him to be angry and/or upset

The **FEMALE** must, under no circumstances, let the **MALE** know

whether or not she wants him to be angry and/or upset

The **MALE** is expected to mind read at all times

> The **FEMALE** is ready when she is ready
>
> The **MALE** must be ready at all times
>
> Any attempt to document the *Rules* can result in bodily harm
>
> The **MALE** who does not abide by *the Rul*es can't take the heat,
>
> lacks backbone and is a wimp.

This story has been voted "Women's Favorite E-mail of the Year:"

> A man was sick and tired of going to work every day while his wife stayed home.
>
> He wanted her to see what he went through so he prayed"
>
> "Dear Lord"
>
> I go to work every day and put in 8 hours while my wife merely stays at home.
>
> I want her to know what I go through, so please allow her body to switch with mine for a day."
>
> God, in his infinite wisdom, granted the man's wish.
>
> The next morning, sure enough, the man awoke as a woman...
>
> He arose, cooked breakfast for his mate, awaked the kids, set out their school clothes,
>
> Fed them breakfast, packed their lunches, drove them to school, came home and picked
>
> Up the dry cleaning, took it to the dry cleaners and stopped at the bank to make a deposit,
>
> Went grocery shopping, and then drove home to put away the groceries,
>
> Paid the bills and balanced the check book.

He cleaned the cat's litter box and bathed the dog.

And he hurried to make the beds, do the laundry, vacuum, dust,

And sweep and mop the kitchen floor.

Ran to the school to pick up the kids and got into an argument with them on the way home.

Set out milk and cookies and got the kids organized to do their homework.

Then, set up the ironing board and watched TV while he did the ironing.

At 4:30 he began peeling potatoes and washing vegetables for salad, breaded the pork chops and snapped fresh beans for supper.

After supper, he cleaned the kitchen, ran the dishwasher, folded laundry,

Bathe the kids and put them to bed.

At 9 P.M. he was exhausted and, though his daily chores weren't finished, he went to bed where he was expected to make love, which he managed to get through without complaint.

The next morning, he awoke and immediately knelt by the bed and said:

"Lord, I don't know what I was thinking. I was so wrong to envy my wife's being able to stay home all day. Please, Oh! Please, let us trade back. Amen!"

The Lord, in his infinite wisdom, replied:

My son, I feel you have learned your lesson and I will be happy to change you back

But you'll have to wait nine months. You got pregnant last night"

Figure 26-28. Women's Favorite Story of the Year

"Old Troubadour" as sung by George Strait

Sometime I feel like Jesse James, still trying to make a name,
Knowing nothings gonna change what I am,
I was a young troubadour when I rode in on a song,
And I'll be an old troubadour when I'm gone

----Writers: LESLIE SATCHER and MONTY HOLMES

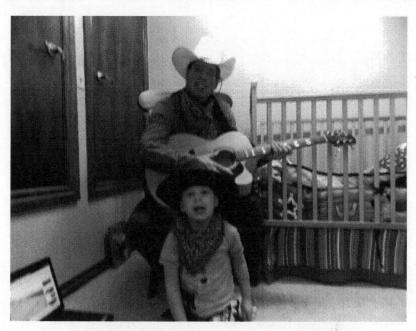

Figure 23-29 Old OB "Troubadour:" Author,
Old Obstetrician as an Old Troubadour in his own way

The Last Time

So while you are living in these times,
Remember there are only so many them
And when they are gone, you will yearn for just one more day of them.
For the last time.

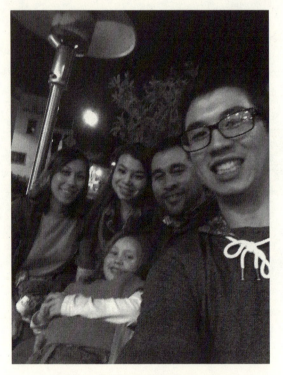

Figure 23-30 Authors' Family
(Jennifer, Jessica, Emma, Ben and Justin)

-----**Author Unknown** but attributed to Danniel J. Lennax, as the true author of this heartfelt poem

Credit Origination: http://embracinghomemaking.net/2014/09lasttime/

From www.embracinghomemaking.net

CHAPTER 27
Concluding Words: Footprints in the Sand and Winnie-the-Pooh

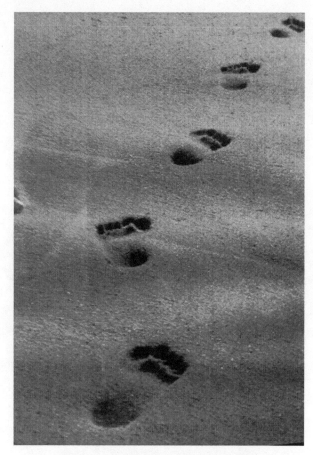

Figure 23-31 Footprints in the Sand

One night a man had a dream.
He dreamed he was walking along the beach with the Lord.
Across the sky flashed scenes from his life. For each scene,
He noticed two sets of footprints in the sand: one belonging to him and the other to the Lord.

When the last scene of his life flashed before him, he looked back at the footprints in the sand.
He noticed that many times along the path of his
Life there was only one set of footprints. He also
Noticed that it happened at the very lowest and
The Saddest times in his life.

This really bothered him and he questioned the
Lord about it. "Lord, you said that once I decided
To follow you, you'd walk with me all the way.
But I have noticed that during the most troublesome
Times in my life, there is only one set of footprints.
I don't understand why when I needed you most
You would leave me.

The Lord replied, "My child, my precious child, I
Love you and I would never leave you. During your
Times of trial and suffering when you see only one set of footprints,
It was then that I carried you.

--Author Unknown

> *"If ever there is tomorrow when we're not together... there is something you must always remember. You are braver than you believe, stronger than you seem, and smarter than you think. But the most important thing is, even if we're apart... I'll always be with you."*
>
> --A.A. Milne, Winnie-the-Pooh

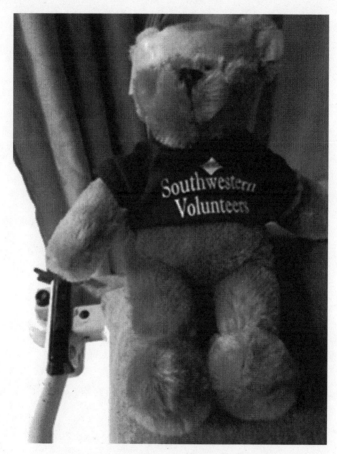

**Figure 23-32 Winnie-the-Pooh-like Bear
by Southwestern Volunteers**

APPENDIX A

Other questions asked by my pregnant patients.

Why did the Author write this Book?

I have been practicing OB for many decades (it seems like I just started yesterday!). I see a "New OB" patient almost every day. I provide information about nutrition, exercise, lab testing, etc. to each patient. Finally, I decided I needed to write down "my OB talk/instructions" onto paper (now actually electronically on computer).

When I first began my Ob-Gyn practice at Kaiser Hospital in Hayward, CA, I was the physician responsible for giving the "OB talks" to the patients. I gave 4 individual talks that rotated each month as follows:

Labor and Delivery,

Pain relief and anesthesia during labor

Breastfeeding and postpartum care

Nutrition during pregnancy.

About 15 years ago I started writing this book: I incorporated these 4 OB lectures into chapters of a book. I wanted to write a book about pregnancy that "tells it like it really is." But, I got busy with family and children (and I could not find a "catchy title"). Now with perhaps a catchy title, "Pregnancy is a REAL MOTHER!" I have resumed this project and, as Larry the cable guy says, "Get her done."

Why did you choose Obstetrics as a medical specialty?

When I was in medical school, I never would have thought that I would have chosen OB as a lifetime career: probably I would be a Family Practice physician or Internist. When I was a child I would watch Robert Young in the TV show Dr. Welby MD. Thereafter, I was soon watching other "Doctor Shows", such as *Dr. Kildare* and *Ben Casey MD*.

I felt strongly about Internal Medicine or Family Medicine: I prized the establishment of a relationship with patients and their family. Connections, getting to know your patients well over the years, and the continuity of care were most important for me: it is the true art of medicine (which is being lost today with the continuing fragmentation of care). At UC San Francisco (University of California) Internists were the "intellectual" physicians as opposed to the less brainy skilled workers called Surgeons. During my 3rd year rotation on the Medical Service at the renovated original UC Hospital, I admitted Mrs. Hahn for care. I had reviewed all three volumes of her chart. She was now in her 60's. Since the very beginnings of her disease and continuing care with her Rheumatologist at UC, she had received the highest level of care. She had RA (Rheumatoid Arthritis) since she was in her 20's. She was diagnosed with RA with a new test at that time, called the Rheumatoid Factor. She was one of the first patients to receive the new drug, cortisone, for therapy.

At the time I met her as a 3rd medical student she had already been through cortisone, had maxed out on gold therapy, had one knee and one hip replacement and her hands were mangled as badly as I had ever seen for a patient with RA. She was now being admitted for hydrotherapy. She could hardly walk.

It was at this point I realized that I could not really "make a difference" or "cure anyone" if I chose Internal Medicine as a career. I could only alleviate some of my patient's discomforts as they slowly progressed through the natural course of their medical conditions. I was basically an intermediary between the Radiology, Laboratory and Pharmacology Departments. I directed therapy but I, myself, was not making my patients better with my very own hands. I was very discouraged at this point.

Then I rotated onto Obstetrics at UC Moffitt Hospital in San Francisco. The delivery rooms were on the 16th Floor of hospital. The UC Moffitt Hospital was built on Parnassus Heights which was one of San Francisco's highest "hills." This "hill" was already 12 stories above ground level. The hospital was built on top of this" hill" and it went another 16 stories up into the sky. You could see the "white castle" of UC Hospital from anywhere in Golden Gate Park. It truly was "The Ivory Tower of Learning" in this very worldly city. The OB suite was on the top floor, i.e. the 16th Floor. The hospital towered so high into the sky that the delivery rooms were "above the fog" and blue sky was all that could be seen through the windows.

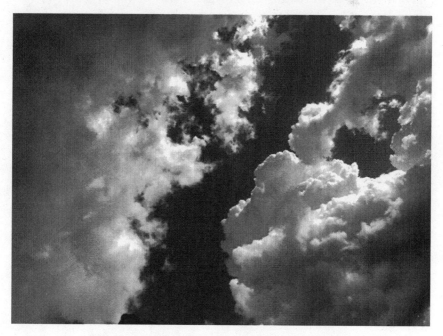

Figure A-1 Heavens around the Delivery Room

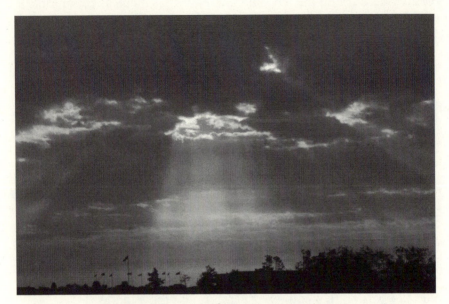

Figure A-2 Heavens Shining Light with the birth of our angelic babies

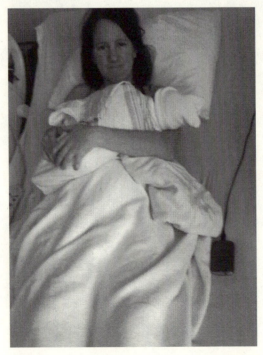

Figure A-3 White Linins and white baby blanket

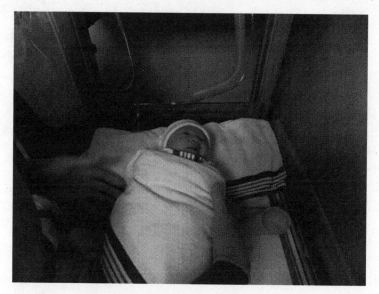

Figure A-4 Photo of a Newborn baby:
another perfect baby just having been delivered from
Heaven and all wrapped up in white (mostly!).

There were also a large "sky operatory windows" over the delivery tables that for the most part became the ceilings in the delivery rooms. The physicians and delivering mothers could see the blue sky and the clouds above. Further, there were large picture windows that comprised the sides of the delivery rooms that made up the external walls. You were, for the most part, "in the clouds." All the sheets covering the patients were *white*. All the scrubs we wore were *white*. Then, as the babies delivered, they were immediately wrapped into their *white* blankets.

Everything was white and pure: babies seem to be coming out of the skies around us and being delivered by the "OB shepherds" in white. This "White Phenomenon" in the OB Suite at UC San Francisco illustrated above is what inspired the author of the purity and heavenliness of the specialty of Obstetrics.

You "had to be there." You had to feel the air and the spiritual ambience: you were delivering babies "from Heaven." It was so clean and innocent. Every birth I saw was just an amazing miracle happening. I was struck with this awe-inspiring experience. From that very moment on, I knew I "had to do this!" It was truly an epiphany moment in my life. From that experience I started down the road I have been on for the past nearly 4 decades. 8500+ babies later, I am still excited about "delivering babies."

I had been intentionally put into the medical care of Mrs. Hahn so that that experience would guide me the specialty of Obstetrics and Gynecology.

Finally, I was doing providing medical care "with my own hands" and I had "to be there" to safeguard the passage of these unborn babies into this wonderful world. It was a personal or divine "Calling" that I needed to answer.

Dedication

This Book is dedicated to the Memory of two very special people that were in my life. I would like to start this dedication by first quoting the following poem:

If Tomorrow Never Comes

Posted by <u>Don Barnes</u>

If I knew it would be the last time
that I'd see you fall asleep,
I would tuck you in more tightly
and pray the Lord, your soul to keep.

This poem was quoted by Pastor Don Barnes on July 28, 2013 at Lawton First Assembly Bridges & Relationships

How to Make Love Last

The first person to whom this book is dedicated is Mrs. Deborah Kaplan.

She passed away from breast cancer at the age of 39. She was the Rabbi's wife at the synagogue in Fremont, CA. I was practicing in this city at this time. They had moved from Birmingham, AL to

Fremont, CA. I delivered two of her three daughters. I also was there when she miscarried two other pregnancies. It was shortly after the birth of Sharon that Debbie and I got together and she started reviewing some of the early writings for this book. Debbie, the Rabbi, and her family were always a community beacon that brought love, kindness and happiness to their entire congregation and to all other people in this world.

The second person for whom this book is dedicated is to Mr. Jude Lyons.

I met him in Greensboro, GA when I was in practice there. He initially was my insurance broker. He was a jack of all trades. In the later years of his life he would be fixing up churches, bathroom and kitchen renovations, etc. He could do anything that had to do with construction. He came from Pennsylvania and he was a "True Yankee." He always was spouting out old aphorisms and other practical advice. He recounted his colorful stories as an EMT, as a hospital maintenance person etc.

Jude was also a "Bread maker "enthusiast," like I am. He was quite a cook and baker. Unfortunately, Jude took up smoking at a young age and continued to smoke as an adult. Like his father and sister he, too, came down with lung cancer. When it was evident that he only had one more year to live, I requested that he write down (or dictate) all the important information and sage advice he would like to leave his family and friends. He knew all "the pearls of wisdom" when came to properly hanging sheetrock, plumbing, squaring off rafters, etc. His grandchildren and others would have a written documentary about his life, his witty sayings and his work. But, he didn't. He could be very stubborn at times. He didn't heed my advice.

However, since his untimely death I am now more inspired to take my own advice seriously. It is for these reasons, I have written this book. It is an effort to provide the information regarding pregnancy to my patients (and perhaps to many other expecting parents). I am hoping that all expecting moms can benefit from the knowledge and information so detailed in this book.

I have one last comment to make about Jude. He had an outstanding recipe for bran muffins. Again, Jude did not write his great recipe down so I did (he told me the recipe over the phone). So that others may also may have and enjoy his recipe, I am presenting *The Jude's Legacy Bran Muffin Recipe* as follows:

Jude Lyons Legacy Raisin Bran Muffin Recipe

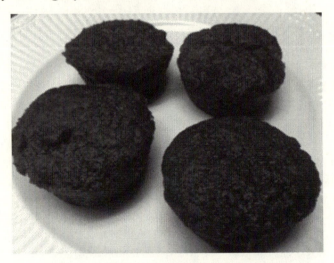

Figure A-5 Bran Muffins "Jude Legacy

Ingredients:

Raisin Bran cereal 20 ounces
Raisins 1 cup
Craisins® 1 cup
Pecans ¾ cup
Crisco 1 loaf
Sugar 3 1/2 cups
Whole wheat flour 5 cups
Baking soda 5 tsps.
Salt 1 ½ tsps.
Nutmeg 2 tsps.
Buttermilk 1 quart
Eggs 4

Large mixing bowl or "Pail" (see below)

Directions: Mix cereals, baking soda, nutmeg (freshly ground) salt and wheat bread flour together. Immerse the raisins and Craisins in 2 cups of warm water. Mix Crisco with sugar and then add the buttermilk. Lightly roast the Pecans on the oven in a small frying pan. Mix up the eggs in a separate bowl. Add the raisins and Craisins together with the cereal/flour mixture. Then stir in the dry ingredients, the flour/bread mixture into the wet ingredients, i.e. the Crisco buttermilk. Add in the eggs. Lastly stir in the pecan pieces. Jude says to mix all of the above in a "pail" so maybe you know how Jude would do things.

This recipe produces a large number of muffins:

If using 12-muffin pan: 60 muffins
If using a 9 muffin-pan: 36 muffins.

You can take half of the recipe and bag it for the freezer for another day.

"Toast" of the Town

In regard to eating healthy in the Diet and Nutrition section, the author has mentioned he has been making his own bread at home since 1994. So if you want to eat "The Toast of the Town," he is leaving you, the Reader, with his fool-proof recipe:

4lb Bread maker: spray the bottom and spatula with non-stick spray

In the following order place into the bread pail:

1 and ½ cups of Warm milk: 5 Tbsps. of dry milk or ¾ cup of half and half and ¾ cup of 2% milk

1 cup of white bread flour (King Arthur, Gold Medal, etc.)

1 cup of wheat bread flour (Gold Medal, Pillsbury, White Lily, etc.)

5 teaspoon of gluten (unless you are gluten sensitive)

1 large egg

2 cups of Bob's Red Mill Wheat flour (regular or organic)

¾ cup of honey (slightly warm)

4 Tbsps. (1/2 stick) butter (melted room temperature)

2 teaspoons of yeast (Red Star or Fleishmann's)

For extra healthiness, add ¼ cup of whole flaxseeds and or chia seeds

Mix all the ingredients together with a spatula prior to turning on the Breadmaker

Slice and place in toaster at medium. Lastly, Coat your toast with butter. Yum!

Dr. Zweig 2013 Commencement Speech to the graduating OU Medical Family Practice Residents in Lawton, OK.

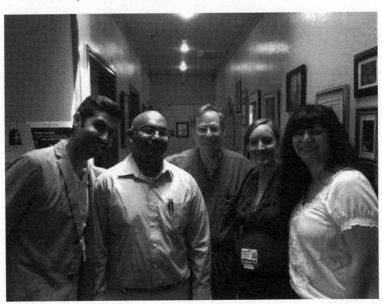

Figure A-6 Senior Graduating OU Family Residents Photograph of 2013

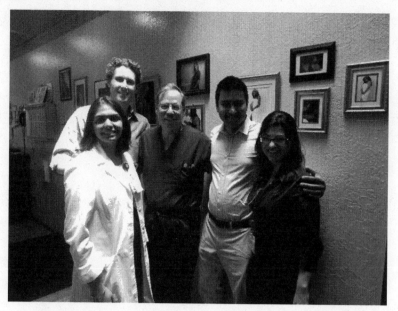

Figure A-7 OU Family Practice Graduating Class of 21014

Title: Everything I Really Needed to Know about Medicine I learned in my Residency (and a lot more even after my Residency!)

I say, Good Evening, Graduating Residents, Current and New residents, Faculty, Family and Friends and those at the NSA who may be listening in.

First, my sincere congratulations to our NEW Family Physicians!

I still freshly remember, and as you will too, the leaving of the Training Program to embark onto your new Career in Medicine. I have seen how previous Graduates have woven themselves into the fabric of the Lawton Medical Community: to mention a just a few of the illustrious physicians like Drs. Jarik Paszcowiack, Aryan Kadaver, Jeff Miller, Elena Shea, Francois Dutoit, Ivanka Vassileva, Leslie Aiku, and Mayank Dave.

As the "Most Interesting Physician in the World" told me yesterday (note: must be acquainted with Dos Equus® Beer commercial currently being advertised), "I may not always want to become a family physician, but if I did, I would choose the OU Family Residency Program!" Stay thirsty and alert my friends!

Well I didn't know he meant about the "thirsty part" of what he said, but after a little research, I found out. He was talking the following toast he had made in the past:

To my friends who enjoy a glass of wine, and

To those who don't and are always seen with a glass of water in their hand,

As Ben Franklin has said:

In Wine there is wisdom,

In Beer there is freedom

In Water there are Bacteria!

In a number of carefully controlled trials, scientists have demonstrated that if we drink 1 liter of water each day, that

At the end of the Year we would have absorbed more than 1 kilo of E. Coli--a bacteria found in feces

In other words, we are consuming 1 kilo of poop!

However we do NOT run that risk when drinking wine or beer (or tequila, gin, rum whiskey or other spirits),

Because alcohol has to go through a purification process: boiling, filtering and/or fermenting.

Remember: Water = Poop

Wine = Health

Therefore, it's better drink wine and talk Stupid,

Than to drink water and be Full of Sh**t!

At this point, I would like to borrow from Robert Fulgrum his format from his well-known book and call this speech,

Everything I Really Needed to Know about Medicine I learned in my Residency (and a lot more after my Residency!)"

My words of counsel are as follows

1. There are a "finite" number of patients and years that you will practice medicine. It is an "absolute" number.

I was told this "pearl of wisdom" by Dr. Beretta, an Italian General Surgeon in Fremont, CA. He caught me in the Doctor's lounge one morning just as was finishing my 1st year out in private practice. He stated to me, there that there are a *finite* number of patients you are going to deliver and see in your career. It is, to be exact, a concrete and an *absolute* number. He said, "You can reach that number of OB deliveries in the first 40 years of practice or worse, in the first 15!" (i.e. Sudden death from a heart attack by working too hard!).

So the bottom line is that you have to take your career in Medicine in stride: just like the runner doing a marathon.

2. Be Nice to your nurses and other hospital staff and they will be nice to you. They can make your life miserable by calling you and waking you up in the middle of the night for all kinds of questions and orders.

3. Never speak "ill" of other doctors, your colleagues or other hospital staff. You may be a better doctor but don't let your ego take hold of you. As Reagan stated you need to "Walk in their shoes" (Malpractice) Most malpractice suits are caused by off-handed comments by one doctor on another doctor's care. You do not want to spend days or weeks in a Court Room away from your practice and patients.

4. Love your partner and your family (Divorce). As I have looked around my medical colleagues, I have come to the conclusion that the long term *secret* to financial success is staying married to just one person. The physicians that are still struggling today are the ones that have been through one or two divorce battles. So remember these words for <u>guaranteed</u> <u>financial</u> success:

One car
One House
One Wife
Now you can throw that Wall Street Journal into the trash

Or, as a lot of my women patients tell me, "A Happy Wife gives you have a Happy Life."

Leo Tolstoy stated, "What counts in making a Happy Marriage is not so how compatible you are but how you <u>deal</u> with the incompatibilities." or as Henny Youngman stated, "The secret to a Happy marriage still remains .... "a secret."

And, as I have said to others previously, "I always tried to <u>drown</u> my problems, but I can't get my ex-wife, to go swimming!"

But, honestly, the best marital advice I have heard is from Dr. Phil (from his book, Relationship Rescue) He has a really good formula:

The Best Relationships Equal "Being Best Friends" and "Meeting Each other Needs."

The important part is that each partner has to know what their needs are and then communicate those needs to each other. I would add another aspect of that formula: that "Being best roommates." Therefore Best Friends, Best Roommates and Meeting each other's NEEDS is the key to the most successful Relationships.

As Groucho Marx has stated, "Marriage is a Wonderful Institution as long as you don't mind being in an Institution for the rest of your life!"

5th pearl. Exercise Regularly: the Greeks have always said a healthy mind depends on a healthy body.

I, like other physicians in this room, incorporated running into my life about half way through my career.

6th point. Get rid of "unhappy patients." 20% of your patients will give you 80% of your practice headaches."

As Billy Currington sings in his Country song,

God is Great

The Beer is Good

And, *Patients* are crazy!

7. Practice where you want to live. The grass is NOT much greener anywhere else. I, myself, have had 6 career moves.

8. Time is your most precious asset. As Kenny Chesney said in his popular song, "Don't Blink,"

Don't blink, just like that you're six years old
and you take a nap and you wake up and you're 25
then your high school sweetheart becomes your wife.
Trust me friend, 100 years goes faster than you think

Author recommends that the reader read all the written lyrics of the song in order to appreciate the awesome message of the song (www.azlyrics.com/lyrics/kennychesney/dontblink.html)

Point 9. Protect yourself, <u>please</u>. Wash your hands frequently, Use Gloves, masks and avoid contaminating circumstances, such as needles and body fluids.

Do not risk the same tragedy that befell Dr. Reid, Chairmen Department of Ob-Gyn at Harvard: He got stuck by a needle during surgery, came down with fulminant Hepatitis and died quickly at the very height of his esteemed career.

10. And, the Last point, I want to make, is tell all of you what has the Family Residency has <u>taught me</u>.

It has demonstrated to me personally how Immigration has been and will be one of the most important factors in making and continuing to make the United States "Great." For example,

1. Albert Einstein, emigrated from Germany, and he formulated the "Theory of Relativity"
2. Nicola Tesla, came from Serbia-Croatia. He proved that AC, not DC as Edison had discovered, was the only type of electricity that was going to be carried to every home safely.
3. Steve Jobs, Founder of Apple Computer. He had a Syrian biologic father but was adopted at birth by a father that was Armenian.

There are countless millions of others that have come to the US and <u>transformed</u> this country to what it has attained today.

The US has been a <u>magnet</u> for 10's of thousands of talented people from all over the world.

(I, myself, am a second generation Romanian-Russian)

As further examples, the graduating Residents that are here before us tonight:

1. Dr. Julide Akman-Carmichael is from Turkey
2. Dr. Teney John is from India
3. Dr. Salman Virani is from Pakistan via Miami
4. And, Dr. Kristi Mason is from a small country in SW Oklahoma called Lawton.

(Reader must understand that Dan Mullins Nissan in Lawton has car commercials on all the local TV channels that have blurted out on TV for years, "We are at 2nd and Gore, "The Center of the Universe" to understand the following sentence)

I always tell people and patients that I am so glad that I came to Lawton, because otherwise if I had not come to Lawton, I would have never found the "Center of the Universe." Well, Lawton sure does seem to be the "Center of the Universe" that has the power of gravity to pull so many exceptional people from all parts of the world to this wonderful city

By the way, do you think that Dan Mullins might have a self-esteem or ego problem??

I say to the Graduating Physicians now:

You have your entire life and careers before you. From a phone call last night, I want you to know right now that the US Gov't and the IRS are personally wishing you well and are counting on your practices to generate millions of dollars in tax revenues to help finance the Federal Budget.

Further, in jest, in order to stop annual IRS Tax audits, avoid becoming a member of the American Heritage Foundation and contribute regularly to the Democratic Party! (Reference to the IRS Scandal in which conservative groups applying for Tax Exempt status were reportedly treated differently than liberal groups)

Again, thank you for allowing me the privilege to speak to you tonight during this momentous achievement and life cycle event in your lives.

Congratulations again and best wishes to the graduating physicians, your families and friends, and the faculty that has guided your course.

And, as George Zimmerman formerly of The Men's Wearhouse would say, and I paraphrase, "You're going to like the way you Look" after receiving your Medical Training Here.

"I guarantee it!"

APPENDIX B

Additional Resources Prenatal Non-Invasive Testing (NIPS) Diagnosis

There are at least 3 new blood tests that have become available that can "screen," not diagnose the most common chromosomal abnormalities:

1. Trisomy 21 (Down's syndrome)
2. Trisomy 18 (Edward's Syndrome)
3. Trisomy 13 (Patau's Syndrome)

In addition, some of these new tests can detect other chromosomal abnormalities.

These tests use the cell-free "fetal" DNA in the mother's bloodstream to study the baby's chromosomes.

There are some "problems" with these new tests:

1. How well can a specific test differentiate between maternal and fetal cell free DNA (cfDNA)?

2. What is the methodology utilized by all of the involved biotechnical companies: SNF's, i.e. single nucleotide polymorphism technology?

3. What if the mother has a "balanced translocation" or carries other chromosomal abnormalities that may be attributed to the baby? Also, it is known that mother's own blood cells lose their "X chromosome" with age: after the age of 35 progressively just at the time these tests become important in prenatal diagnosis?

4. What if the "cfDNA fraction" is less than the necessary 3.5% amount of DNA needed to perform the test?

5. The weight of the mother, i.e. greater than 165 lbs. may eliminate some patient's from utilizing these tests.

6. Will your insurance carrier "cover" these new tests? Prior authorizations? What are the "out-of-pocket" costs to the patient?

At this time the author, as well as other OBs are still trying to deal with all of the above questions in order to guide our patients around the new technology. Most of the tests report 99% accuracy but what about the 1% that have "false positive" results?

Accordingly, the present chemical screening testing (Penta, Quad, Triple Screens, etc) will continue to be used with Level 3 ultrasound, the NIPS blood testing described below backed up by CVS and amniocentesis as recommended by the Perinatologist team.

Harmony Blood Test

Learn more about the Harmony test (http://www.ariosadx.com/expecting-parents/)

	False Positive Rate*	Detection Rate**
Harmony Prenatal Test	Less than 1 in 1,000	More than 99 in 100

	False Positive Rate*	Detection Rate**
Traditional Test	1 in 20	85 in 100

* Reports a high risk for Down syndrome when it is NOT actually present
** Correctly indicates a high risk for Down syndrome when it IS present

Figure B-1 Harmony™ Prenatal Test Summary

Materni21

From the Sequenom Corporate Website regarding Materni21 as follows:

THE ENHANCED SEQUENCING SERIES, EXCLUSIVELY FOR THE MATERNIT21 PLUS TEST

Meaningful answers. Clear results. The power of MPS.
Massively parallel sequencing (MPS) is uniquely positioned to realize the promise of delivering relevant, enhanced information. Other methods lack the adaptability to efficiently add meaningful content.

The MaterniT21 PLUS test delivers revolutionary content. This is merely a glimpse of all that it will offer you and your patients over time. You can count on the MaterniT21 PLUS test to provide you with clarity, allowing you to provide the most advanced information available to your patients, noninvasively.

INNOVATION TRANSLATING TO PREMIUM CONTENT

In addition to content that you have come to rely on (chromosomes 21, 18, 13, X and fetal gender), the Enhanced Sequencing Series includes:

- 22q deletion syndrome (**DiGeorge**)
- 5p (**Cri-du-chat syndrome**)
- 15q (**Prader-Willi/Angelman syndromes**)
- 1p36 deletion syndrome
- 4p (**Wolf-Hirschhorn syndrome**)
- 8q (**Langer-Giedion syndrome**)
- 11q (**Jacobsen syndrome**)
- Trisomy 16
- Trisomy 22

Source: http://laboratories.sequenom.com/maternit21plus/prenatal-test-information-for-providers?gclid=CPLvp_7X8MECFSMA7AodXn0AkA

Quest Diagnostics, one of the largest laboratories in the US, is now providing only one NIPS test : the QNATAL. Quest has been licensed by Sequenom to provide the Materni21 NIPS testing in-house under the name of QNATAL as of March 2015.

Panorama Test

About Panorama™

Below is information <u>directly</u> from the Panorama website, from which the reader can research for further information.

http://www.panoramatest.com/en/healthcare-provider/#about

Panorama is a non-invasive prenatal screening test (NIPT) for fetal chromosomal abnormalities. The test uses advanced bioinformatics technology to evaluate fetal (of placental origin) DNA in maternal blood.

Only Panorama can distinguish between fetal and maternal DNA in the mother's blood to give you and your patient vital information about the fetus. With a comprehensive panel of chromosomal aneuploidies and micro-deletions, Panorama delivers the most accurate results of any screening test, as early as 9 weeks of gestation, to help you manage your patient's pregnancy.

New sunscreen labels

Summarized from the following article, "New sunscreen labels: How to read the fine Print" by Kim Painter, Special for USA TODAY4:10 p.m. EDT April 26, 2013

The new FDA Labels help consumers understand how the products protects with regard with not just sunburn, but wrinkles and more important, skin cancer.

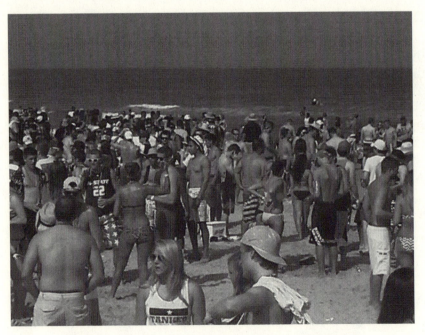

Figure B-2 Sunscreen required with sun at the beach

SUMMARY POINTS:

- Sunscreens have "new" FDA Labels: it is not just an SBF number, but about shielding from both UVA and UVB light, re-application timing, and limited protection against sunburn, wrinkles and skin cancer.
- All Sunscreen label s must conform to standard laboratory testing
- Sunscreens are not "foolproof:" with enough sun exposure you are "going to get burned!"

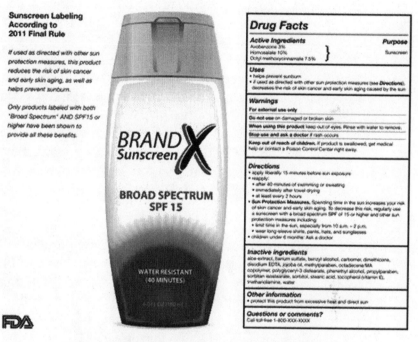

Figure B-3 New Sunscreen Labels. Labels inform consumers that sunscreens help reduce the risk of skin cancer, according to a 2011 final rule. (Photo: FDA)

Here's what you need to know:

- **SPF numbers are still important.** SPF numbers range from 2 to 100 and tell you how well the product protects you from the sun's ultraviolet B (UVB) rays. Further, these products may only be protective for a "window of time" such as 2 hours. Re-application is then needed: maybe sooner if you go into the water.

- **FDA now has "Warning Labels."** Products with SPFs below 15 protect only against sunburn, not skin aging or skin cancer." Still, many people mistakenly believe that they can "tan" better with low SBF number less than 15.

- **Broader spectrum Products Labels.** These products provide significant protection from both UVB and UVA rays because both these wavelengths can lead to wrinkles and skin cancer. Before companies can put this information on their label they must pass certain mandated testing.

- **There is a difference between "water-resistant" and "waterproof."** It is ambiguous to consumers to know the difference. All products can wash off, wear off or be "sweated off." Labels must now state how often quantitated in time intervals such as 30 to 90 minutes how often a product must be re-applied to be effective in preventing sunburn, wrinkles or skin cancer. Again, products must be tested to support their claims.

- **Sunscreen is "Not Totally" protective.** These products all have limitations: if you spend enough time in the sun on one day or during the year, you are still "at risk" for skin cancer, cataracts, wrinkles and sunburn. You still must limit your time to direct or indirect sun (or "tanning beds") UV light exposure. Sunglasses, shirts that provide UV protection, hats, pants, etc. are all part of the common sense approach to healthy skin and eyes.

The Obstetrical Forceps

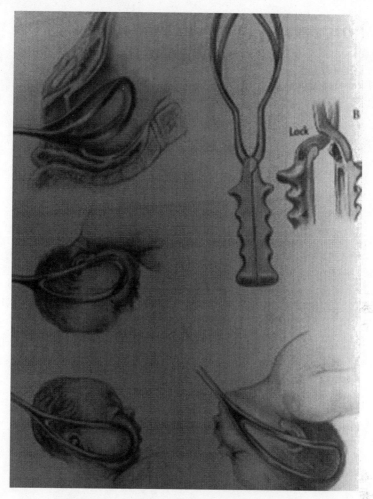

Figure B-4 Obstetrical Forceps Illustration

A "Doctors Note"

Jeffrey L. Zweig, MD, Inc
Jeffrey L. Zweig, M.D.
DEA AZ8231106 Lic 24890 NPI 1134155302
Wolf Creek Medical Center
4417 West Gore Blvd
Suite #3
Lawton, OK 73505
580-357-1002 Fax: 580-357-1004

Name Mary Smith DOB
Address Date

℞ (Please Print)

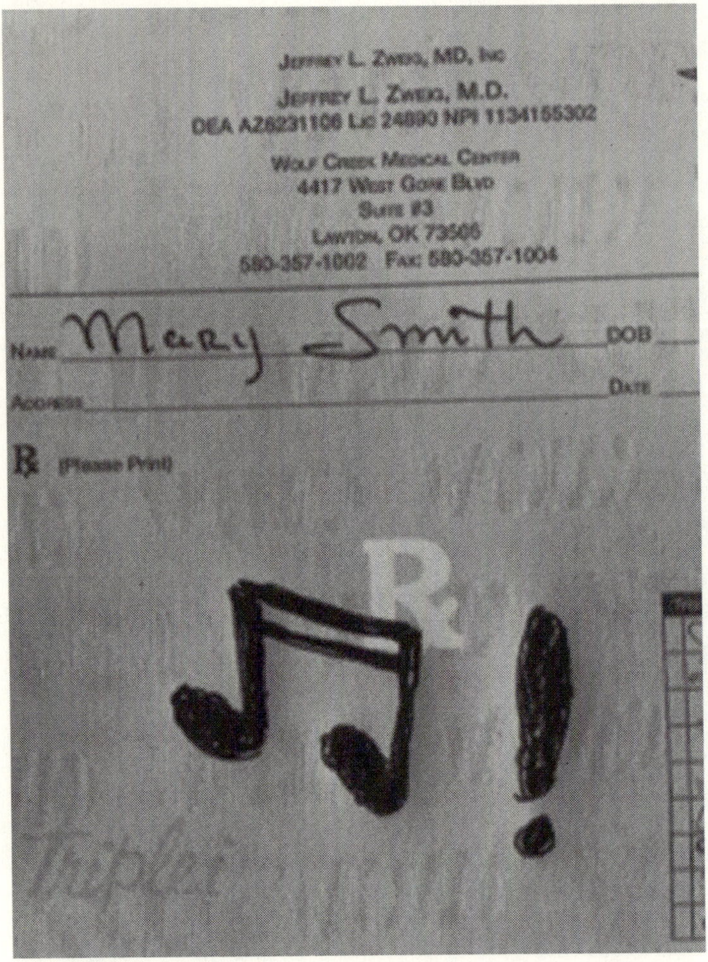

Figure B-6 A "Doctor's Note You need a "Doctor's Note?

APPENDIX C

How did I become Pregnant?

Yes, it was a girl in a red sundress …..

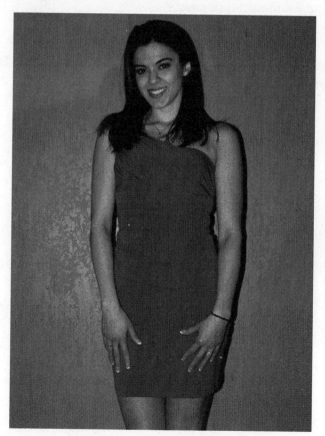

Figure C-1 The Girl in a Red Sundress

Something about a truck in a field and, a girl in a red sundress
with an ice cold beer to her lips, begging for another kiss
Something about you and me and the birds and the bees
And Lord have mercy it's a beautiful thing: Ain't nothing about it luck, something about a truck

--written and sung by Kip Moore, "Something about a Truck."

(TMI: You only need to read this section if you really want to know how your egg got to meet your husband's sperm!)

Let's start it with a goodnight kiss, my lips, your lips
Let's start it with a long goodbye, get wrapped up tight
Let's spend all night right here,
Let's start it with a goodnight kiss.

---Writers: JASON SELLERS, RANDY HOUSER AND BOB HATCH AS SUNG BY RANDY HOUSER

How do you become pregnant: the Reproductive Story down "Physiological Road"

There are many women (including mothers who have had several children!) who have never fully understood how they have become pregnant. This section intends to clarify the anatomy and physiology of human reproduction, so that any woman can gain a better understanding of her body, her menstrual cycles, and the miracle of life itself.

Fundamentally, an egg from the woman's ovary unites with a sperm from the male testicle. How, where, and when they meet is a different and complex story.

In each ovary, there are 10 to 50,000 eggs contained within the cortex or outer layer (envelop) of the ovary (basically an egg reservoir). An *egg follicle unit* consists of an egg surrounded by hundreds of granulosa cells that nourish and support this egg. *Granulosa* cells are chiefly responsible for producing the female hormone called estrogen. When a menstrual period starts, the amount of estrogen hormone falls to a very low level.

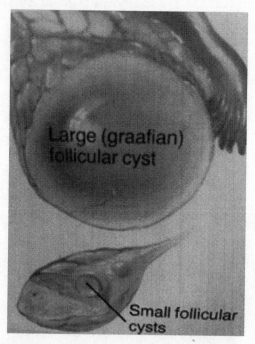

Figure C-2 Mature Egg Follicle unit about ready to be released or "ovulate."

The pituitary gland (which sits at the base of the brain right behind the nasal passageways) continuously monitors the blood levels of estrogen. When estrogen levels in the blood stream "bottom out," the pituitary becomes activated to bring estrogen levels back up. The pituitary gland releases into the blood a protein "messenger" or hormone, called FSH (Follicle Stimulating Hormone). The FSH hormone travels to the ovary and stimulates egg follicle growth. Stimulation of the egg follicle units causes the granulosa cells around the egg to multiply, increases in size, and produce more estrogen hormone. Actually several egg follicles respond to FSH, but for some reason only one follicle in one ovary becomes dominant: "the egg of the month." Occasionally when FSH levels are extraordinarily high, two or more egg follicles become stimulated to grow and become dominant. If eggs from one, or both, are released and subsequently fertilized, twins or triplet pregnancies may result. Fertility drugs, such as Clomiphene Citrate (Clomid©) or Gonadotropins (FSH or FSH/LH preparations), cause high levels of FSH in the bloodstream; hence, multiple births are associated with these medications. When there are no more eggs in the ovary, little or no estrogen is produced despite the stimulation from FSH. If all egg follicles from the ovaries are depleted, menopause ensues. Menopause is diagnosed by high blood levels of FSH, Inhibin B and low blood levels of estrogen.

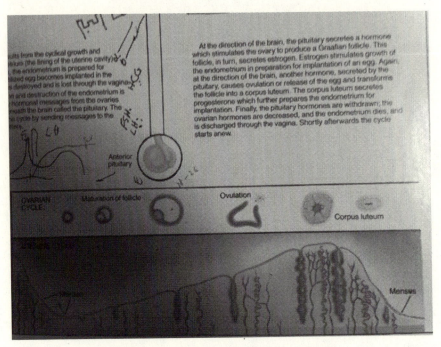

Figure C-3 Egg preparing its own bed
(or endometrium) it will "sleep" or grow in.

The developing "egg follicle" on top with the corresponding growth of the endometrium as the egg grows, ovulates and the formation of the corpus luteum after the "egg follicle unit" is disrupted.

The enlarging egg follicle is accompanied by an explosive growth in the number of surrounding granulosa cells. Increased production of estrogen from the multiplying and enlarging granulosa cells results in higher and higher levels of estrogen in the bloodstream.

The estrogen so generated by the egg follicle travels to two main places:

(1) Back to the pituitary gland, and
(2) To the uterus.

In the pituitary gland, estrogen attaches and binds itself to special receptor sites. In essence, estrogen feeds back and tells the pituitary gland that sufficient amounts of estrogen are being produced by the enlarging ovarian follicles (resulting from the previous rising FSH hormone produced by the pituitary gland).

What happens with too much FSH?

1. Too many egg follicles will develop (multiple births).
2. Ovarian cyst (s)

High levels FSH hormone can produce a "giant follicle" or "Ovarian Cyst. Most "Ovarian Cysts" are those of the "follicle"-type.

The ovarian follicle thus, modulates the amount of FSH activity: rising levels of estrogen have a negative feedback on the pituitary gland to curtail the production of FSH,

Estrogen levels will peak at a certain hormone level: a level of 1200 to 1600 units. A peak height of estrogen production causes the pituitary gland to release another hormone called LH (Luteinizing Hormone. The" LH Peak "is produced by the *positiv*e feedback of the" estrogen peak"-- a reaction in the pituitary gland. LH travels from the pituitary gland to the ovary. LH "triggers "the ovary to release the egg from its follicle (the follicle is the surface of the ovary itself and then the follicle, like a water balloon ruptures). Release of the egg from the ovary is called "ovulation." The "LH peak" can be detected by the popular "ovulation kits" available at your pharmacy (ClearBlue Easy, EPT, etc.). Couples trying to get pregnant can more accurately "time" their "fertility zone:" the egg ovulates about 24 hours after the LH surge or your positive ovulation test.

TMI (too much information) regarding sex selection

There is a popular book entitled, "How to choose the sex of your Baby," that gives folks a comprehensive review of the information available on how couples can improve "the odds" of conceiving a boy or girl during this "fertility zone."

Simultaneously with its effect on the pituitary, rising amounts of estrogen hormone travel to the uterus. Estrogen stimulates the production of a new inner lining layer (endometrium) inside the uterine cavity. It is essential for one to see that the egg follicle not only orchestrates its own release from the ovary, but also produces for itself the creation of a fertile "nesting ground." This nesting ground or "endometrium" lies further down the tube into the uterine cavity. The sperm fertilize the egg at the end of the tube. The fertilized egg will eventually travel, implant and grow. The estrogen stimulates the uterus to develop a new lining to replace the one shed during the previous menstrual period. Estrogen transforms a barren field into a fertile one by the middle of a menstrual cycle (mid-cycle): the usual time of ovulation. Plowed, watered, fertilized, and cultivated, the lining in the uterus becomes prepared so as to sustain the growth of the new embryo.

At mid-cycle, the egg follicle gravitates to the surface of the ovary. The "roof" over the egg follicle disintegrates so that the egg can be jettisoned into the open "mouth" of the fallopian tube. Prior to ovulation, the open end of the fallopian tube is sweeping methodically all over the surface of the ovary (much like a pool sweep!) in order to vacuum up the egg as it is released from the ovarian follicle. Mid-cycle intercourse climaxes with the ejaculation of millions of sperm into the back of the vagina. Semen normally contains 30 to 200 million sperm per milliliter with average ejaculate volume of 2 to 5 milliliters (about a teaspoon).

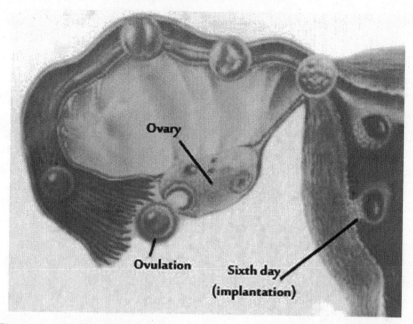

Figure C-4 Fertilization of egg, transport down the tube and implantation.

The sperm "attacking the egg" at the end of the tube and the egg's migration down the tube to eventually implant in the uterus.

The sperm swim up into the cervical opening. The mucus glands just inside the cervix provide a staging ground for the sperm. Over the next 24 to 48 hours, sperm are continually being launched from the cervical staging ground into the uterine cavity. At the top of the uterus, sperm swim into both the right and left tubes. In the tube, the sperm swim in mucus-type water. Cilia (or hairs) projecting from the surface of the cells within the tube, brush and sweep the sperm toward the distal end of the tube. Muscles within the wall of the tube contract rhythmically in an upward direction (essentially squeezing i.e. "peristalsis") like waves on the ocean. The tubal walls are and further propelling the sperm upward. At the end of the tube (the fimbriated end), the egg waits patiently for the "herd" of sperm to come for her. As a note, the peristalsis of the tubal smooth muscle along with the sweeping motion of the cilia propel and help accelerate the sperm transit time to the end of the tube: sperm can reach the end of the tube in 30 minutes or less (it's too late for birth control at this point!).

The egg is surrounded by a sticky coating (called the "zona pellucida"). Many sperm are required to digest away this covering. Thousands of sperm become mired or stuck in this coating, but eventually one succeeds and "mates" with the egg. Combination of the egg and sperm together forms a single cell. This cell grows and divides into two cells, then four, and a new human being begins to develop. Simultaneously with cell multiplication, the developing embryo travels down the tube toward the uterine cavity. The trip usually takes three to four days. When the embryo reaches the uterine cavity, it implants itself in the well-developed lining of the uterine cavity, the same lining that the egg diligently prepared for itself while in the egg follicle. This lush and fertile lining is precisely ready for implantation of the embryo. The embryo continues to develop and grow until it is finally "harvested" as a "baby" from the uterine cavity during childbirth.

The ovarian egg follicle, "unroofed" at the top, is not quite finished yet. A new roof forms and the follicle is sealed up. Cells within the follicle undergo a "transformation" as a result of an alteration of blood flow within the follicle. These so-called "granulosa" cells become converted into *"theca" cells*: the follicle is now termed a "corpus luteum." Theca cells produce mainly progesterone and small amounts of estrogen.

Author Note: Progesterone levels can be measured in the "luteal phase," the 14 days after ovulation as an indicator of a "quality ovulation" or luteal phase "adequacy." Further progesterone levels can be measured in early pregnancy to evaluate "the health" of a growing embryo.

Progesterone and estrogen together continue to nourish and support the endometrial lining and its new inhabitant, the embryo. The theca cells in this corpus luteum can only live 14 days and then they self-destruct. The embryo must implant and grow quickly. Cells from the embryo grow into the endometrial lining much like roots grow from a plant in the ground. The root system must develop and take hold within this 14-day time limit. Otherwise the corpus luteum dissolves and the ground "dries up." This root system (the developing placenta) produces a special hormone: HCG (Human Chorionic

Gonadotropin). HCG from the embryo's placenta travels into the mother's bloodstream and eventually reaches the corpus luteum. HCG apparently has a profound effect on the corpus luteum: it nourishes and sustains the corpus luteum so that it can survive past 14 days. Accordingly, HCG from the placenta sustains the corpus luteum's power to keep the endometrial ground "wet and fertile." Without HCG, the corpus luteum self-destructs: the endometrial lining "dries up" and disintegrates. Blood vessels in the lining also disintegrate and the menstrual period starts. The embryo and placenta in the lining is washed out of the uterus with the menstrual flow. Normally, however, HCG allows the corpus luteum to stay alive for two to three months, the critical amount of time necessary for the placenta to completely develop and grow to the point that it can provide the fetus with all its material needs: food, water and shelter.

It is the hormone HCG (Human Chorionic Gonadotropin) from the placenta that is the basis for the "pregnancy test." A "pregnancy test" detects circulating levels of HCG in the blood (serum pregnancy test) or HCG in the urine (urine pregnancy test). HCG in the blood is filtered by the mother's kidneys and becomes trapped in the urine.

Our developing fetus is now pretty well established and on its way!

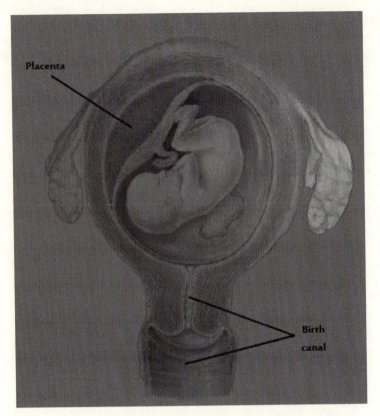

Figure 0-1 Figure C-5 Anatomy of Pregnancy and the 10-12 week size fetus in the uterus

Author's note:

I guess I have always been fascinated by how quickly the egg (and that future child!) seizes control of your body and your entire subsequent life. I thought that this domination of the family only began after birth!

The developing egg follicle sends estrogen up to the pituitary gland to curtail FSH levels. If FSH levels are not "turned down" by the estrogen, the pituitary gland increases the production of even higher FSH levels. Higher FSH levels may stimulate several follicles to grow. If multiple follicles grow and ovulate, multiple births could result. Could this be the time of the earliest manifestation of sibling rivalry? The egg also sends estrogen way down the road to the uterus so that the fertilized egg has a ready-built home to live in for the next nine months.

APPENDIX D

Vaccination Guidelines for Pregnant Women

GUIDELINES FOR VACCINATING PREGNANT WOMEN

Vaccination of pregnant women should be considered on the basis of risk vs. benefit. Risk to a developing fetus from vaccination of the mother during pregnancy is theoretical. No evidence exists of risk to the fetus from vaccinating pregnant women with inactivated virus or bacterial vaccines or toxoids. Live vaccines administered to a pregnant woman pose a theoretical risk to the fetus; therefore, live, attenuated virus and live bacterial vaccines generally are contraindicated during pregnancy. Benefits of vaccinating pregnant women usually outweigh potential risks when the likelihood of disease exposure is high, when infection would pose a risk to the mother or fetus, and when the vaccine is unlikely to cause harm. The following table may be used as a general guide.

	VACCINE	GENERAL RECOMMENDATION FOR USE IN PREGNANT WOMEN
ROUTINE	Hepatitis A[1]	Recommended if otherwise indicated
	Hepatitis B[2]	Recommended in some circumstances

GUIDELINES FOR VACCINATING PREGNANT WOMEN

Vaccination of pregnant women should be considered on the basis of risk vs. benefit. Risk to a developing fetus from vaccination of the mother during pregnancy is theoretical. No evidence exists of risk to the fetus from vaccinating pregnant women with inactivated virus or bacterial vaccines or toxoids. Live vaccines administered to a pregnant woman pose a theoretical risk to the fetus; therefore, live, attenuated virus and live bacterial vaccines generally are contraindicated during pregnancy. Benefits of vaccinating pregnant women usually outweigh potential risks when the likelihood of disease exposure is high, when infection would pose a risk to the mother or fetus, and when the vaccine is unlikely to cause harm. The following table may be used as a general guide.

VACCINE	GENERAL RECOMMENDATION FOR USE IN PREGNANT WOMEN
Human Papillomavirus (HPV)[3]	Not recommended
Influenza (Inactivated)	Recommended
Influenza (LAIV)*	Contraindicated
Measles, Mumps, Rubella (MMR)*	Contraindicated
Meningococcal (MCV4)[4]	May be used if otherwise indicated
Pneumococcal (PCV13)[5]	Inadequate data for specific recommendation
Pneumococcal (PPV23)[6]	Inadequate data for specific recommendation
Inactivated Poliovirus (IPV)[7]	May be used if needed

GUIDELINES FOR VACCINATING PREGNANT WOMEN

Vaccination of pregnant women should be considered on the basis of risk vs. benefit. Risk to a developing fetus from vaccination of the mother during pregnancy is theoretical. No evidence exists of risk to the fetus from vaccinating pregnant women with inactivated virus or bacterial vaccines or toxoids. Live vaccines administered to a pregnant woman pose a theoretical risk to the fetus; therefore, live, attenuated virus and live bacterial vaccines generally are contraindicated during pregnancy. Benefits of vaccinating pregnant women usually outweigh potential risks when the likelihood of disease exposure is high, when infection would pose a risk to the mother or fetus, and when the vaccine is unlikely to cause harm. The following table may be used as a general guide.

	VACCINE	GENERAL RECOMMENDATION FOR USE IN PREGNANT WOMEN
	Tetanus, Diphtheria (Td)	Should be used if otherwise indicated
	Tetanus, Diphtheria, Pertussis (Tdap)[8]	Recommended
	Varicella*	Contraindicated
	Zoster*	Contraindicated
TRAVEL & OTHER	Anthrax[9]	Low risk of exposure - not recommended. High risk of exposure - may be used.
	BCG*	Contraindicated
	Japanese Encephalitis (JE)[10]	Inadequate data for specific recommendation
	Meningococcal (MPSV4)	May be used if otherwise indicated
	Rabies	May be used if otherwise indicated

GUIDELINES FOR VACCINATING PREGNANT WOMEN

Vaccination of pregnant women should be considered on the basis of risk vs. benefit. Risk to a developing fetus from vaccination of the mother during pregnancy is theoretical. No evidence exists of risk to the fetus from vaccinating pregnant women with inactivated virus or bacterial vaccines or toxoids. Live vaccines administered to a pregnant woman pose a theoretical risk to the fetus; therefore, live, attenuated virus and live bacterial vaccines generally are contraindicated during pregnancy. Benefits of vaccinating pregnant women usually outweigh potential risks when the likelihood of disease exposure is high, when infection would pose a risk to the mother or fetus, and when the vaccine is unlikely to cause harm. The following table may be used as a general guide.

VACCINE	GENERAL RECOMMENDATION FOR USE IN PREGNANT WOMEN
Typhoid (Oral* & Parenteral)[11]	Inadequate data for specific recommendation
Vaccinia*[12]	Pre-exposure - contraindicated. Post-exposure - recommended.
Yellow Fever*[13]	May be used if benefit outweights risk

*Live attenuated vaccine

NOTES

GUIDELINES FOR VACCINATING PREGNANT WOMEN

Vaccination of pregnant women should be considered on the basis of risk vs. benefit. Risk to a developing fetus from vaccination of the mother during pregnancy is theoretical. No evidence exists of risk to the fetus from vaccinating pregnant women with inactivated virus or bacterial vaccines or toxoids. Live vaccines administered to a pregnant woman pose a theoretical risk to the fetus; therefore, live, attenuated virus and live bacterial vaccines generally are contraindicated during pregnancy. Benefits of vaccinating pregnant women usually outweigh potential risks when the likelihood of disease exposure is high, when infection would pose a risk to the mother or fetus, and when the vaccine is unlikely to cause harm. The following table may be used as a general guide.

VACCINE	GENERAL RECOMMENDATION FOR USE IN PREGNANT WOMEN

1. **Hepatitis A Vaccine:** Recommended if another high risk condition or other indication is present.

2. **Hepatitis B Vaccine:** Pregnant women who are identified as being at risk for HBV infection during pregnancy (eg, having more than one sex partner during the previous 6 months, been evaluated or treated for an STD, recent or current injection drug use, or having had an HBsAg-positive sex partner) should be vaccinated.

3. **Human Papillomavirus (HPV) Vaccine:** HPV vaccines are not recommended for use in pregnant women. If a woman is found to be pregnant after initiating the vaccination series, the remainder of the 3-dose series should be delayed until completion of pregnancy. Pregnancy testing is not needed before vaccination. If a vaccine dose has been administered during pregnancy, no intervention is needed.

GUIDELINES FOR VACCINATING PREGNANT WOMEN

Vaccination of pregnant women should be considered on the basis of risk vs. benefit. Risk to a developing fetus from vaccination of the mother during pregnancy is theoretical. No evidence exists of risk to the fetus from vaccinating pregnant women with inactivated virus or bacterial vaccines or toxoids. Live vaccines administered to a pregnant woman pose a theoretical risk to the fetus; therefore, live, attenuated virus and live bacterial vaccines generally are contraindicated during pregnancy. Benefits of vaccinating pregnant women usually outweigh potential risks when the likelihood of disease exposure is high, when infection would pose a risk to the mother or fetus, and when the vaccine is unlikely to cause harm. The following table may be used as a general guide.

VACCINE	GENERAL RECOMMENDATION FOR USE IN PREGNANT WOMEN

4. **Meningococcal Conjugate Vaccine (MCV4):** No data is available on the vaccination of pregnant women with MCV4. Women of childbearing age who become aware that they were pregnant at the time of MCV4 vaccination should contact their health-care provider or the vaccine manufacturer.

5. **Pneumococcal Conjugate Vaccine (PCV13):** Pregnancy recommendations have not been published at this time; use of PCV13 is limited among women of childbearing age.

6. **Pneumococcal Polysaccharide Vaccine (PPV23):** The safety of PPV23 during the first trimester of pregnancy has not been evaluated, although no adverse consequences have been reported among newborns whose mothers were inadvertently vaccinated during pregnancy.

GUIDELINES FOR VACCINATING PREGNANT WOMEN

Vaccination of pregnant women should be considered on the basis of risk vs. benefit. Risk to a developing fetus from vaccination of the mother during pregnancy is theoretical. No evidence exists of risk to the fetus from vaccinating pregnant women with inactivated virus or bacterial vaccines or toxoids. Live vaccines administered to a pregnant woman pose a theoretical risk to the fetus; therefore, live, attenuated virus and live bacterial vaccines generally are contraindicated during pregnancy. Benefits of vaccinating pregnant women usually outweigh potential risks when the likelihood of disease exposure is high, when infection would pose a risk to the mother or fetus, and when the vaccine is unlikely to cause harm. The following table may be used as a general guide.

VACCINE	GENERAL RECOMMENDATION FOR USE IN PREGNANT WOMEN

7. **Inactivated Polio Vaccine (IPV):** Vaccination of pregnant women should be avoided on theoretical grounds. However, if a pregnant woman is at increased risk for infection and requires immediate protection, IPV can be administered in accordance with the recommended schedules for adults.

8. **Tetanus, Diphtheria, acellular Pertussis (Tdap) Vaccine:** One dose of Tdap should be administered during each pregnancy irrespective of the patient's prior history of receiving Tdap. To maximize the maternal antibody response and passive antibody transfer to the infant, optimal timing for Tdap administration is between 27 and 36 weeks of gestation although Tdap may be given at any time during pregnancy. For women not previously vaccinated with Tdap, if Tdap is not administered during pregnancy, Tdap should be administered immediately postpartum.

GUIDELINES FOR VACCINATING PREGNANT WOMEN

Vaccination of pregnant women should be considered on the basis of risk vs. benefit. Risk to a developing fetus from vaccination of the mother during pregnancy is theoretical. No evidence exists of risk to the fetus from vaccinating pregnant women with inactivated virus or bacterial vaccines or toxoids. Live vaccines administered to a pregnant woman pose a theoretical risk to the fetus; therefore, live, attenuated virus and live bacterial vaccines generally are contraindicated during pregnancy. Benefits of vaccinating pregnant women usually outweigh potential risks when the likelihood of disease exposure is high, when infection would pose a risk to the mother or fetus, and when the vaccine is unlikely to cause harm. The following table may be used as a general guide.

VACCINE	GENERAL RECOMMENDATION FOR USE IN PREGNANT WOMEN

Wound Management: If a Td booster is indicated for a pregnant woman, Tdap should be administered. *Unknown or Incomplete Tetanus Vaccination*: Pregnant women who never have been vaccinated against tetanus should receive three doses containing tetanus and reduced diphtheria toxoids. The recommended schedule is 0, 4 weeks and 6 through 12 months. Tdap should replace 1 dose of Td, preferably between 27 and 36 weeks gestation.

9. **Anthrax Vaccine:** In a pre-event setting with low risk for exposure to aerosolized *B. anthracis* spores, vaccination of pregnant women is not recommended and should be deferred until after pregnancy. In a post-event setting with a high risk of exposure, pregnancy is neither a precaution nor a contraindication to PEP. Pregnant women at risk for inhalation anthrax should receive AVA and 60 days of antimicrobial therapy as described.

GUIDELINES FOR VACCINATING PREGNANT WOMEN

Vaccination of pregnant women should be considered on the basis of risk vs. benefit. Risk to a developing fetus from vaccination of the mother during pregnancy is theoretical. No evidence exists of risk to the fetus from vaccinating pregnant women with inactivated virus or bacterial vaccines or toxoids. Live vaccines administered to a pregnant woman pose a theoretical risk to the fetus; therefore, live, attenuated virus and live bacterial vaccines generally are contraindicated during pregnancy. Benefits of vaccinating pregnant women usually outweigh potential risks when the likelihood of disease exposure is high, when infection would pose a risk to the mother or fetus, and when the vaccine is unlikely to cause harm. The following table may be used as a general guide.

VACCINE	GENERAL RECOMMENDATION FOR USE IN PREGNANT WOMEN

10. **Japanese Encephalitis (JE) Vaccine:** No controlled studies have assessed the safety, immunogenicity, or efficacy of Ixiaro in pregnant women.

11. **Typhoid Vaccine:** No data have been reported on the use of any of the typhoid vaccines in pregnancy.

12. **Vaccinia (smallpox) Vaccine:** Should not be administered in a pre-event setting to pregnant women or to women who are trying to become pregnant. If a pregnant woman is inadvertently vaccinated or if she becomes pregnant within 4 weeks after smallpox vaccination, she should be counseled regarding concern for the fetus. Smallpox vaccination during pregnancy should not be a reason to terminate pregnancy. Pregnant women who have had a definite exposure to smallpox virus (ie, face-to-face, household, or close-proximity contact with a smallpox patient) and are, therefore, at high risk for contracting the disease, should be vaccinated.

GUIDELINES FOR VACCINATING PREGNANT WOMEN

Vaccination of pregnant women should be considered on the basis of risk vs. benefit. Risk to a developing fetus from vaccination of the mother during pregnancy is theoretical. No evidence exists of risk to the fetus from vaccinating pregnant women with inactivated virus or bacterial vaccines or toxoids. Live vaccines administered to a pregnant woman pose a theoretical risk to the fetus; therefore, live, attenuated virus and live bacterial vaccines generally are contraindicated during pregnancy. Benefits of vaccinating pregnant women usually outweigh potential risks when the likelihood of disease exposure is high, when infection would pose a risk to the mother or fetus, and when the vaccine is unlikely to cause harm. The following table may be used as a general guide.

VACCINE	GENERAL RECOMMENDATION FOR USE IN PREGNANT WOMEN

When the level of exposure risk is undetermined, the decision to vaccinate should be made after assessment by the clinician and the patient of the potential risks versus the benefits of smallpox vaccination.

13. **Yellow Fever Vaccine:** Pregnancy is a precaution for YF vaccine administration. If travel is unavoidable, and the risks for YFV exposure outweigh the vaccination risks, a pregnant woman should be vaccinated. If the risks for vaccination outweigh the risks for YFV exposure, pregnant women should be issued a medical waiver to fulfill health regulations. Although no specific data are available, a woman should wait 4 weeks after receiving YF vaccine before conceiving.

GUIDELINES FOR VACCINATING PREGNANT WOMEN

Vaccination of pregnant women should be considered on the basis of risk vs. benefit. Risk to a developing fetus from vaccination of the mother during pregnancy is theoretical. No evidence exists of risk to the fetus from vaccinating pregnant women with inactivated virus or bacterial vaccines or toxoids. Live vaccines administered to a pregnant woman pose a theoretical risk to the fetus; therefore, live, attenuated virus and live bacterial vaccines generally are contraindicated during pregnancy. Benefits of vaccinating pregnant women usually outweigh potential risks when the likelihood of disease exposure is high, when infection would pose a risk to the mother or fetus, and when the vaccine is unlikely to cause harm. The following table may be used as a general guide.

VACCINE	GENERAL RECOMMENDATION FOR USE IN PREGNANT WOMEN

REFERENCES

For information on individual vaccines, please see vaccine monograph at www.eMPR.com, contact company for labeling and/or call the National Immunization Hotline at 800-232-4636.

Source: Advisory Committee in Immunization Practices. *Guidelines for Vaccinating Pregnant Women.* April 2013. Available at: http://www.cdc.gov/vaccines/pubs/downloads/b_preg_guide.pdf.

(Rev. 12/2013)

List of disorders included in newborn screening programs

From Wikipedia, the free encyclopedia

This is a **list of disorders included in newborn screening programs** around the world, along with information on testing methodologies, disease incidence and rationale for being included in screening programs.

American College of Medical Genetics recommendations

Core panel

The following conditions and disorders were recommended as a "core panel" by the 2005 report of the American College of Medical Genetics (ACMG).[1] The incidences reported below are from the full report, though the rates may vary in different populations.[2]

Blood cell disorders

- Sickle cell anemia (Hb SS) > 1 in 5,000; among African-Americans 1 in 400
- Sickle-cell disease (Hb S/C) > 1 in 25,000
- Hb S/Beta-Thalassemia (Hb S/Th) > 1 in 50,000

Inborn errors of amino acid metabolism

- Tyrosinemia I (TYR I) < 1 in 100,000
- Argininosuccinic aciduria (ASA) < 1 in 100,000
- Citrullinemia (CIT) < 1 in 100,000
- Phenylketonuria (PKU) > 1 in 25,000
- Maple syrup urine disease (MSUD) < 1 in 100,000
- Homocystinuria (HCY) < 1 in 100,000

Inborn errors of organic acid metabolism

- Glutaric acidemia type I (GA I) > 1 in 75,000
- Hydroxymethylglutaryl lyase deficiency (HMG) < 1 in 100,000
- Isovaleric acidemia (IVA) < 1 in 100,000
- 3-Methylcrotonyl-CoA carboxylase deficiency (3MCC) > 1 in 75,000
- Methylmalonyl-CoA mutase deficiency (MUT) > 1 in 75,000
- Methylmalonic aciduria, cblA and cblB forms (MMA, Cbl A, B) < 1 in 100,000
- Beta-ketothiolase deficiency (BKT) < 1 in 100,000
- Propionic acidemia (PROP) > 1 in 75,000
- Multiple-CoA carboxylase deficiency (MCD) < 1 in 100,000

Inborn errors of fatty acid metabolism

- Long-chain hydroxyacyl-CoA dehydrogenase deficiency (LCHAD) > 1 in 75,000
- Medium-chain acyl-CoA dehydrogenase deficiency (MCAD) > 1 in 25,000
- Very-long-chain acyl-CoA dehydrogenase deficiency (VLCAD) > 1 in 75,000
- Trifunctional protein deficiency (TFP) < 1 in 100,000
- Carnitine uptake defect (CUD) < 1 in 100,000

Miscellaneous multisystem diseases

- Cystic fibrosis (CF) > 1 in 5,000
- Congenital hypothyroidism (CH) > 1 in 5,000
- Biotinidase deficiency (BIOT) > 1 in 75,000
- Congenital adrenal hyperplasia (CAH) > 1 in 25,000
- Classical galactosemia (GALT) > 1 in 50,000
- Severe combined immune deficiency (SCID)

Newborn screening by other methods than blood testing

- Congenital deafness (HEAR) > 1 in 5,000
- Critical congenital heart defects (Screened using pulse oximetry)

Secondary targets

The following disorders are additional conditions that may be detected by screening. Many are listed as "secondary targets" by the 2005 ACMG report.[1] Some states are now screening for more than 50 congenital conditions. Many of these are rare and unfamiliar to pediatricians and other primary health care professionals.[1]

Blood cell disorders

- Variant hemoglobinopathies (including Hb E)[1]
- Glucose-6-phosphate dehydrogenase deficiency (G6PD)

Inborn errors of amino acid metabolism

- Tyrosinemia II[1]
- Argininemia[1]
- Benign hyperphenylalaninemia
- Defects of biopterin cofactor biosynthesis[1]
- Defects of biopterin cofactor regeneration[1]
- Tyrosinemia III[1]
- Hypermethioninemia[1]
- Citrullinemia type II[1]

Inborn errors of organic acid metabolism

- Methylmalonic acidemia (Cbl C, D)[1]
- Malonic acidemia[1]
- 2-Methyl 3-hydroxy butyric aciduria[1]
- Isobutyryl-CoA dehydrogenase deficiency[1]
- 2-Methylbutyryl-CoA dehydrogenase deficiency[1]
- 3-Methylglutaconyl-CoA hydratase deficiency[1]
- Glutaric acidemia type II
- HHH syndrome (Hyperammonemia, hyperornithinemia, homocitrullinuria syndrome)
- Beta-methyl crotonyl carboxylase deficiency
- Adenosylcobalamin synthesis defects

Inborn errors of fatty acid metabolism

- Medium/short-chain L-3-hydroxy acyl-CoA dehydrogenase deficiency[1]
- Medium-chain ketoacyl-CoA thiolase deficiency[1]
- Dienoyl-CoA reductase deficiency[1]
- Glutaric acidemia type II[1]
- Carnitine palmityl transferase deficiency type 1[1]
- Carnitine palmityl transferase deficiency type 2[1]
- Short-chain acyl-CoA dehydrogenase deficiency (SCAD)[1]
- Carnitine/acylcarnitine Translocase Deficiency (Translocase)[1]
- Short-chain hydroxy Acyl-CoA dehydrogenase deficiency (SCHAD)

- Long-chain acyl-CoA dehydrogenase deficiency (LCAD)
- [Glutaric acidemia type II|Multiple acyl-CoA dehydrogenase deficiency]] (MADD)

Miscellaneous multisystem diseases

- Galactokinase deficiency[1]
- Galactose epimerase deficiency[1]
- Maternal vitamin B12 deficiency

References

1. ^ Jump up to:[a b c d e f g h i j k l m n o p q r s t u v w x y z aa] Newborn Screening Authoring Committee (2008). "Newborn Screening Expands: Recommendations for Pediatricians and Medical Homes—Implications for the System". *Pediatrics* **121** (1): 192–217. doi:10.1542/peds.2007-3021. **Jump up^** "Newborn Screening: Toward a Uniform Screening Panel and System: Main Report". *Genetics in Medicine* Amcerican College of Medical Genetics

Prenatal Vitamins available on most State Medicaid Formularies (Oklahoma Formulary)

Example below from http://www.okhca.org/providers.aspx?id=658&menu=74&parts=7719_7723_7725

SoonerCare Preferred Prenatal Vitamins

	Description Details
O-CAL PRENATAL	PRENATAL VIT/IRON FUMARATE/FA ORAL 15-1MG TABLET
O-CAL FA	PRENATAL VIT/IRON FUMARATE/FA ORAL 66-1MG TABLET
PRENATAL PLUS	PNV WITH CA, NO.72/IRON/FA ORAL 27 MG-1 MG TABLET
PRENATAL LOW IRON	PNV WITH CA, NO.74/IRON/FA ORAL 27 MG-1 MG TABLET
PRENATAL LOW IRON	PNV WITH CA, NO.74/IRON/FA ORAL 27 MG-1 MG TABLET

TRINATAL RX 1	PRENATAL VIT27&CALCIUM/IRON/FA ORAL 60 MG-1 MG TABLET
COMPLETENATE	PNV #14/FERROUS FUM/FOLIC ACID ORAL 29 MG-1 MG TAB CHEW
COMPLETE NATAL DHA	PNV2/IRON B-G SUC-P/FA/OMEGA-3 ORAL 29-1-250MG COMBO. PKG
VOL-NATE	PRENATAL VIT NO.73/IRON/FA ORAL 28 MG-1 MG TABLET
VOL-TAB RX	PRENATAL VIT #76/IRON, CARB/FA ORAL 29 MG-1 MG TABLET
VOL-PLUS	PNV WITH CA, NO.71/IRON/FA ORAL 27 MG-1 MG TABLET
VOL-PLUS	PNV WITH CA, NO.71/IRON/FA ORAL 27 MG-1 MG TABLET
VOL-PLUS	PNV WITH CA, NO.71/IRON/FA ORAL 27 MG-1 MG TABLET
TRIADVANCE	PRENATAL VIT 15/IRON CB/FA/DSS ORAL 90-1-50 MG TABLET
FOLIVANE-OB	PNV NO.15/IRON FUM & PS CMP/FA ORAL 85 MG-1 MG CAPSULE
TARON-C DHA	PNV#16/IRON FUM & PS/FA/OM-3 ORAL 35-1-200MG CAPSULE
TRIVEEN-U	PNV W-O CA NO5/FE FUMARATE/FA ORAL 106.5-1MG CAPSULE
TRINATAL GT	PRENATAL VIT 16/IRON CB/FA/DSS ORAL 90-1-50 MG TABLET
TRINATAL ULTRA	PRENATAL VIT 18/IRON CB/FA/DSS ORAL 90-1-50 MG TABLET
SE-NATAL 19	PRENATAL VIT/FE FUM/DOSS/FA ORAL 29 MG-1 MG TABLET
SE-NATAL 19	PRENATAL VIT/FE FUMARATE/FA ORAL 29 MG-1 MG TAB CHEW
MULTINATAL PLUS	PV W-O VIT A/FE FUMARATE/FA ORAL 40-1MG TAB CHEW
PRENATA	PRENATAL VIT37/IRON/FOLIC ACID ORAL 29 MG-1 TABCHEW
PNV FOLIC ACID PLUS IRON	PRENATAL VIT COMBO NO.60/FERROUS FUMARATE/FOLIC ACID

PNV FOLIC ACID PLUS IRON	PRENATAL VIT COMBO NO.60/FERROUS FUMARATE/FOLIC ACID
PNV FOLIC ACID PLUS IRON	PRENATAL VIT COMBO NO.60/FERROUS FUMARATE/FOLIC ACID
VINATE GT	PRENATAL VIT 16/IRON CB/FA/DSS ORAL 90-1-50 MG TABLET
VINATE II	PRENATAL VITAMINS/FE BISGLY/FA ORAL 29 MG-1 MG TABLET
CONCEPT OB	PNV NO.15/IRON FUM & PS CMP/FA ORAL 85 MG-1 MG CAPSULE
CONCEPT DHA	PNV#16/IRON FUM & PS/FA/OM-3 ORAL 35-1-200MG CAPSULE

What should parents know to protect the safety and security of their Baby?

1. If possible, prior to the birth of your child, visit the hospital where you intend to deliver and inquire about their security procedures.

2. After admission to the hospital ask about hospital protocols covering routine nursery procedures, feeding, visitation hours and security measures.

3. Your infant, the father or significant other and you will be banded with identical identification bands. Do not remove these bands: they are used for your and your baby's identification. Only persons with the ID bands may take baby to and from the nursery.

4. **Never** leave your infant unattended in your room (or anywhere when you leave the hospital. If you leave the room or go to the bathroom, send the baby to the nursery, unless a family member is present to watch your baby.

5. Do not carry your infant in the hallway. Anyone carrying an infant in the hallway will be questioned. Always transport your baby in his/her crib.

6. Always place the infant's crib on the side of your bed, farthest from the door. Never go to sleep with the infant in bed with you. There is always a possibility that the infant could roll off the bed or you could roll over onto your infant.

7. Do not give your infant to anyone without proper hospital identification. Find out what special identification is used to identify hospital personnel. Prior to giving your infant to a person with a Hospital ID, inquire as to the reason why the baby must be taken to the nursery. Always be suspicious in the hospital (as well as after you go home) when someone or other personnel want to take or hold your baby.

8. Question unfamiliar person entering your room or inquiring about your infant—even if they are in hospital attire or seem to have a reason for being there. Alert the nurse's station ASAP.

9. Determine where your infant will be when taken for tests and how long the test will take.

10. For your Records at home you should have the following:

    a. Recent color photograph of full face view
    b. Written description of your infant: hair and eye color, length, weight, date of birth and specific attributes (such as any skin blemish or other birthmarks)

11. After discharge, do not allow any "strangers" or other unfamiliar persons into your home. Home health nurse or other agency personnel will schedule an appointment with you and carry proper identification.

12. The use of outdoor decorations to announce a baby's arrival (balloons, large floral wreaths, wooden storks, etc.) is not recommended. Similarly, be careful when using social media in announcing your baby's birth.

13. Do not allow anyone in your home that you are not expecting or who you do not know.

14. Never leave your infant unattended in the supermarket, your vehicle, your physician's office or any other public place.

15. For patients who have private postpartum rooms, only an adult or significant other may spend the night in the room with the patient. Children are not allowed to spend the night in the room with the patient. Patients with semi-private rooms may have another adult in the room if the other bed is not occupied.

COMMON QUESTIONS ABOUT NEWBORN HEARING SCREENS/TESTS

- **WHY ARE YOU TESTING MY BABY?**

    It is a general doctor's order. The doctors at Southwestern Medical Center and the State of Oklahoma want ALL newborns screened before discharge.

    HOW DO YOU TEST MY BABY?

    We use the Auditory Brainstem Response (ABR) test. For this test, earphones are placed over the baby's ears. A computer sends soft clicking sounds to the ears through the earphones. Little sticky sensors are placed on the back of the neck, shoulder and forehead to pick up the responses to the sounds from his/her brain and sends it to a computer which then analyzes the responses. The computer then automatically gives a PASS or REFERS result.

- **HOW LOUD IS THE SOUND?**

    The sounds are very soft tones like a music box.

- **HOW LONG WILL IT TAKE?**

The test can take about 15 minutes or so. The more settled and quiet the baby is, the quicker the test goes.

- **WHY IS THE BABY CRYING? YOU SAID IT WOULDN'T HURT?**

It doesn't hurt. The baby is crying because I am disturbing him/her, the same way he/she may cry when you change a diaper.

- **WHAT DOES "REFER" MEAN?**

REFER simply means the baby needs more testing.

- **DOES THAT MEAN MY BABY CANNOT HEAR?**

No. A REFER result can happen if there is a little bit of fluid in the baby's ear or if there is too much background noise or if the baby moves too much during testing. However, to be sure, the baby needs further testing. It is common for babies to pass a second screening or to have normal hearing after failing two screenings. The important thing is to follow the recommendations and advice from the physician regarding further testing.

APPENDIX E

VBAC Protocol at Southwestern Medical Center, Lawton, OK

(Reprinted with permission from Southwestern Medical Center, Lawton, OK)

SOUTHWESTERN MEDICAL CENTER

POLICY /PROCEDURE TITLE: Vaginal Birth after Cesarean Section (VBAC)	DEPARTMENT(S): LABOR/DELIVERY	Page 1 of 4
APPROVAL SIGNATURE(S)/ DATE: _____ _____ _____ _____ Effective Date:	REVIEW SIGNATURE(S)/ DATE: _____ _____ _____ _____	Date Originated: December 13, 2006 Date(s) of Revision: August 26, 2009

PURPOSE: **To provide guidance in the management of the Vaginal Birth after previous Cesarean Section. (VBAC)**

SCOPE: **The scope of this policy/procedure is to provide guidelines for care of a patient presenting for a pre-consented Vaginal Birth after previous Cesarean Section for live births. A trial of labor will be monitored and provisions will be taken to provide a safe environment for mother and baby. It applies to any individual involved in the care of the obstetrical patient.**

RESPONSIBILITY: **Nursing Administration, Department of OB/GYN, Department Manager, Clinical Supervisor.**

Responsibilities

A. Obstetrical Surgeon
 1. Screen patients for contraindications to a trial of labor in an attempt to VBAC
 2. The obstetrical surgeon is responsible for providing the following documentation by the time of admission
    ➢ Type of existing uterine scar (i.e., copy of previous operative report)
    ➢ Standard consent form signed in the provider's presence
 3. Decide whether or not sufficient resources are available to support TOLAC, and be certain that all of the appropriate staff have been contacted and are immediately available
 4. Prostaglandins should not be used for cervical ripening
 5. Oxytocin should be ordered only by the obstetrical surgeon
 6. In case of fetal demise where VBAC is considered, the management is at the discretion of the attending physician.

B. Registered Nurse
 1. Admit patient to the Birthing Center
 2. Notify OB, Operating Room crew and anesthesia of TOLAC admission

3. Provide nursing care within the established guidelines of this policy

DEFINITIONS:

1. **Vaginal Birth after Cesarean Section (VBAC)** is the successful delivery of a patient whose obstetric history includes one and or more previous cesarean sections(s) with low transverse uterine incision.

2. **Trial of labor after cesarean section (TOLAC)** is the attempt to achieve VBAC. VBAC and TOLAC are often used interchangeably.

3. **Failed TOL** occurs when a VBAC is not achieved with a TOL and the patient is delivered by repeat cesarean section.

4. **Obstetrical surgeon** is a provider with privileges to perform a cesarean section delivery.

5. **Immediately available** means OB/GYN, anesthesia and OR personnel are in house able to be in Labor and Delivery or Operating Room immediately when needed.

POLICY:

Patients considering a trial of labor must be screened by an OB/GYN physician to determine if the procedure is appropriate given their obstetrical history. They will receive information regarding the potential risks and benefits. They will be required to sign consent for Vaginal Birth after Cesarean Delivery (VBAC) stating that they have received and understand the information given to them by their obstetrical provider. A trial of labor after a cesarean section is considered a high-risk labor. An obstetrical surgeon must be immediately available. The obstetrical surgeon will evaluate each VBAC patient on admission and decide if adequate support is available.

Indication for Vaginal Birth after Cesarean Section:

- **One or two previous Cesarean Section with low-transverse uterine incision**
- **Clinically adequate pelvis**
- **No other uterine scars or previous rupture**
- **Physician immediately available throughout active labor capable of monitoring labor and performing an emergency cesarean delivery**
- **Pre-consent for Vaginal Birth after Cesarean Delivery**
- **Informed consent process and the plan of management should be documented in the prenatal record**

Contraindication for Vaginal Birth after Cesarean Section:

- **Any patient at high risk for uterine rupture**
- **Prior classical or T-shaped incision or other transfundal surgery**
- **Contracted pelvis**
- **Medical or obstetric complication that precludes vaginal delivery**
- **Need for induction if no spontaneous onset of labor**
- **Less than 1 year since previous cesarean section**
- **Previous arrest of descent (relative contraindication)**
- **Inability to perform emergency cesarean delivery because of unavailable surgeon, anesthesia, Sufficient staff, or facility (OR suite)**
- **Pre-consent for Vaginal Birth after Cesarean Section unavailable**
- **Informed consent process and the plan of management documentation is unavailable in Patient's prenatal record**

Procedure:

The Registered Nurse participating in the care of the patient attempting Vaginal Birth after Cesarean Section demonstrates competency in electronic fetal monitoring and uterine monitoring, physiology of normal labor, and potential complications of labor. The Registered Nurse must also be aware of the common signs of uterine rupture to include but not limited to non-reassuring fetal heart rate pattern, uterine or abdominal pain, loss of station of the presenting part, vaginal bleeding, and hypovolemia.

1. **Determine whether or not the hospital can meet the facility and staffing needs for TOLAC. If not, consider cesarean section.** OB/GYN to determine when patient is in active labor and will be in house once that diagnosis is made

2. **If the patient has not consented for VBAC, the obstetrical surgeon will be notified immediately. If the patient refuses to sign consent for VBAC and cesarean section, a refusal of care form will be initiated.**

3. **If the patient has signed standard provider TOLAC/ VBAC consent, have her also sign hospital VBAC consent and, simultaneously, cesarean section consent. If patient indicates that she has not received all the information she wants or needs to make an informed decision, notify provider immediately.**

4. **Have the obstetrical surgeon contact the anesthesia provider to discuss patient risk factor and facility capacity.** Anesthesia and OR personnel must be immediately available (defined as in house) to perform emergency cesarean section. The facility (OR suite) must also be ready immediately for emergency cesarean section.

5. **Current history and physical on chart.**

6. **Maternal physical assessment should be performed to include cervical exam to confirm status of Cervix and fetal presentation.**

7. **Continues fetal monitoring will be used to evaluate uterine activity and fetal well-being during labor. If unable to obtain a good tracing via external monitor, obstetrical surgeon should be notified immediately.**

8. Start IV with #18 gauge catheter, obtain routine lab work to include type and screen.

9. Maternal vital signs, fetal heart rate, and uterine activity will be assessed and documented per labor protocol.

10. Provide pain management support. Choice of analgesia or anesthesia does not differ from non-VBAC laboring patients.

11. *Report immediately to physician*:

    ♦ Non-reassuring fetal heart rate pattern, consistent variable decelerations, late decelerations, prolonged decelerations, fetal tachycardia with no maternal fever
    ♦ Acute onset of abdominal pain
    ♦ Unremitting pain or increased pain through an epidural
    ♦ Abrupt loss of fetal station
    ♦ Vaginal bleeding
    ♦ Hypovolemia
    ♦ Dysfunctional labor pattern, ineffective uterine contractions, or poor to absent progress
    ♦ Irregular shape of maternal abdomen or visualization of fetus under skin

12. *If signs of rupture are present*:

    ♦ Notify obstetrical surgeon STAT
    ♦ Notify surgery crew STAT
    ♦ Provide patient oxygen at 10liters by facemask
    ♦ Bolus IV fluids
    ♦ Move patient to OR
    ♦ Fetal scalp electrode if possible
    ♦ Insert foley if possible

13. Patient should be monitored closely for adequate progress in active phase of labor and for continued descent in second stage.

14. Anesthesia provider to notify the obstetrical surgeon if other cases are to be started in the Operating Room during the VBAC patient labor.

15. Obstetrical surgeon should periodically reevaluate facility and staffing needs throughout labor.

Patient Teaching

1. Teaching patient about the importance of maternal and fetal monitoring.

2. Teach the patient about the equipment.

3. Instruct patient to inform RN of any sharp pain at the incision site or of abdominal pain, vaginal bleeding, or any feeling of something wrong.

Documentation

1. Document VBAC on delivery record and assessment sheet.

2. Document all interventions and assessments.

3. Document all physician notification.

4. Document all patient education.

5. Document uterine activity and response in nurses notes. Include resting tone of uterus per palpations or per IUPC.

If deviation from policy occurs, physician documentation will include:

☐ Explanation by the physician regarding policy.

☐ Patient's response to explanation.

☐ Explanation of reason for deviation.

VBAC CONSENT FORM

CONSENT FOR PATIENTS WITH A PRIOR CESAREAN BIRTH

	Patient's Initials
1. I understand that I have had one or more prior cesarean(s).	_____
2. I understand that I have the option of undergoing an elective repeat cesarean or attempting a vaginal birth after a cesarean (VBAC)—the decision is entirely my own.	_____
3. I understand that the risk of a uterine rupture during a VBAC in someone such as myself, who has had a prior low transverse cesarean section, is around 1 in 100.	_____
4. I understand that uterine rupture may be catastrophic and may not be preceded by any advanced warning.	_____
5. I understand that a catastrophic event is defined as being extremely harmful to mother and baby. Examples of a catastrophic event include but not limited to maternal/fetal anoxia (without oxygen) and/or maternal/fetal death.	_____
6. I understand that despite swift medical action, an injury to the mother or the baby can result.	_____
7. I understand that if uterine rupture occurs I may loose my uterus and future childbirth capability. I understand there is a possibility of death as a result of uterine rupture.	_____
8. I understand that if my uterus ruptures during my VBAC, there may not be sufficient time to operate and to prevent the death of or permanent brain injury to my baby.	_____

9. I understand that if I deliver vaginally, I most likely will have fewer problems after delivery and a shorter hospital stay than if I have a cesarean delivery.   _____

10. I understand that if I choose a VBAC and end up having a cesarean during labor, I have a greater risk of problems than if I had an elective repeat cesarean.   _____

11. I understand that due to the size of Southwestern Medical Center, we cannot guarantee that the facility will have all resources immediately available; therefore, a cesarean section may be necessary.   _____

12. I have read or have had read to me the above information and I understand it.   _____

REFERENCES:

AWHONN, ACOG Practice Bulletin (2008) guidelines for Perinatal Care, 6th Edition for the American

Academy of Pediatrics and the American College of Obstetricians and Gynecologists.

APPENDIX F

References and Sources of Information

Williams's Obstetrics, 23rd edition, by Cunningham et al. McGraw-Hill

Human Labor and Birth, by Oxorn and Foote, McGraw-Hill

Obstetrics and Gynecology by Wiillson and Carrington, 9th

American Baby and Americanbaby.com, Meredith Corporation

Motherly Art of Breastfeeding

Breastfeeding Handbook for Physicians, Second Edition, ACOG (sales.acog.com)

Guidelines for Perinatal Care, Seventh Edition (sales.acog.com)

Wikepedia, the Free Encyclopedia, on line *www.wikepedia.com*

As Your Baby Grows from conception to birth, *Publishing* Group of Meredith Corporation

APPENDIX G

Sample of a Birth Plan

The Birth Plan below is courtesy of

Jameca Price, MD, MPH
Oregon Health & Science University
Department of Obstetrics & Gynecology
Female Pelvic Medicine and Reconstructive Surgery

Jeffrey Kingman Smith

**Birth Plan for
Mary Smith and John Smith**

Name: Mrs. Mary Smith

My coach will be: John Smith (husband)

Obstetrician: Dr. William Jones (xxx) xxx-xxxx

Other support person(s): _____(mother), _____(Mother-in-Law), and _____ (sister)

I do not want:

Medical students, nursing students, interns, or non-essential medical personnel observing or assisting during my labor or during the birth

Comfort measures during labor

I would like to have the following:

Use of clear fluids (broth, juice), jello, ice, lollipops, hard candy.

Walking around, as tolerated and if safe for baby and me.

While in bed, freedom to move and reposition for comfort and well-being.

I will bring a CD player and use music or other recordings for relaxation.

The most helpful things I do when I am uncomfortable are: take warm baths/showers; receive massage, and rock hips.

I would like access to birthing ball.

To relax, I listen to soothing music; rock in rocking chair; take warm showers/baths; use massage and/or aromatherapy.

Pain control for childbirth

I have practiced breathing exercises and relaxation/stress reduction techniques.

I prefer an epidural for pain medication; I understand that continuous fetal monitoring is required for epidural anesthesia.

I would like to avoid other forms IV or IM anesthesia or sedation, and in particular any medications that are likely to affect the baby's level of alertness immediately after birth.

PROCEDURES PRIOR TO OR DURING EARLY LABOR

Shave:
I do not want to be shaved unless needed

Induction/Augmentation of Labor:
I would like for my labor to proceed at its own natural pace, and would therefore like to avoid amniotomy and stripping of membranes unless a specific medical need arises. Pitocin may be used if needed.

Fetal Monitoring:
I understand that intermittent fetal monitoring for assessment of fetal well-being is recommended by the American College of Obstetricians and Gynecologists, and that this usually consists of a 20-30 minute strip upon admission and re-evaluation at intervals depending on labor progress and fetal response. This is definitely okay.

I do not want internal fetal monitoring done without a strong medical justification given, and express permission from me or my mother (Name of mother)

Intravenous Access:
I understand that upon admission blood will be drawn for routine lab work, and that at that time tubing will remain in place and a heparin lock created. This is fine.

PROCEDURES FOR DELIVERY

Vaginal Delivery

Leg Support:
Support of legs by John Smith, (name of sister or other person), and/or nurses, if necessary, but stirrups are preferred.

Environment:
Elimination of excessive bright light and excessive noise at birth.

Episiotomy:
Episiotomy only if indicated, if I tear. But please use this as last resort.

Perineal Massage:
I have done perineal massage at home to promote stretching of perineum.

I would like perineal massage done during the birthing process.

Anesthesia:
I would like local anesthesia for repair of lacerations or episiotomy.

Cesarean Delivery
No one plans to deliver by c/s, but if that becomes an issue, I would like to have epidural or spinal anesthesia.

John Smith and I desire to be together during a cesarean delivery. I am aware that John Smith is there to support me, and that if general anesthesia is used, that support will not be needed. However, even if general anesthesia is used, I would like for him to be present during the delivery so that he may bond immediately with the baby while I am still under anesthesia.

If the baby must be taken to the nursery, I would like John Smith to accompany him/her. If I am alert, and the baby is stable, I wish to hold the baby before it goes to the nursery.

POSTPARTUM

Skin to skin contact on my abdomen as soon as feasible after birth.

Apgar evaluation to be done while baby is on my abdomen if possible.

John Smith does wish to catch the baby or cut the cord.

Postpone eye medication until after initial bonding is established, +/- one after birth.

Breastfeed as soon as baby and I are ready.

Allow parental/newborn bonding for as long as mother and baby are stable.

I would like rooming in 24 hours a day.

I would like sitz baths twice a day after delivery.

We have a newborn picture outfit and would like this to be worn for the hospital newborn pictures

NEWBORN CARE

Pediatric Care and Patient Discharge Preferences

I would like normal discharge (48 hours) after normal vaginal delivery.

Our Pediatrician is:

Dr. Justin Jones
Children's Physician Clinic
(xxx) xxx-xxxx

In Case of Medical Problems with Baby

If baby must be taken from room, I would like myself and/or John Smith to accompany the baby at all times.

If medical procedures must be performed on the baby, I would like for myself and/or John Smith to be present at *all* times.

I plan to exclusively breastfeed our baby, and therefore request that s/he not be given artificial nipples of any kind, including bottles (formula or water) or pacifiers.

Circumcision

We have read the information about circumcision. We do want our newborn son to be circumcised.

Our pediatrician, Dr. Justin Jones, will be conducting the circumcision.

APPENDIX H

Baby Weight and Length for each week of Pregnancy

The following information is sourced from The BabyCenter/Expert Advice at **http://www.babycenter.com/average-fetal-length-weight-chart**

Until about 20 weeks, babies are measured from the crown (or top) of the head to the rump (or bottom). This is because a baby's legs are curled up against his torso during the first half of pregnancy and very hard to measure.

After that, babies are measured from head to toe.

Gestational age	Length (US) (crown to rump)	Weight (US)	Length (cm) (crown to rump)	Mass (g)
8 weeks	0.63 inch	0.04 ounce	1.6 cm	1 gram
9 weeks	0.90 inch	0.07 ounce	2.3 cm	2 grams
10 weeks	1.22 inch	0.14 ounce	3.1 cm	4 grams
11 weeks	1.61 inch	0.25 ounce	4.1 cm	7 grams
12 weeks	2.13 inches	0.49 ounce	5.4 cm	14 grams
13 weeks	2.91 inches	0.81 ounce	7.4 cm	23 grams
14 weeks	3.42 inches	1.52 ounce	8.7 cm	43 grams
15 weeks	3.98 inches	2.47 ounces	10.1 cm	70 grams
16 weeks	4.57 inches	3.53 ounces	11.6 cm	100 grams
17 weeks	5.12 inches	4.94 ounces	13 cm	140 grams
18 weeks	5.59 inches	6.70 ounces	14.2 cm	190 grams

Week	Length	Weight	Length (cm)	Weight (g)
19 weeks	6.02 inches	8.47 ounces	15.3 cm	240 grams
20 weeks	6.46 inches (crown to heel)	10.58 ounces	16.4 cm (crown to heel)	300 grams
20 weeks	10.08 inches	10.58 ounces	25.6 cm	300 grams
21 weeks	10.51 inches	12.70 ounces	26.7 cm	360 grams
22 weeks	10.94 inches	15.17 ounces	27.8 cm	430 grams
23 weeks	11.38 inches	1.10 pound	28.9 cm	501 grams
24 weeks	11.81 inches	1.32 pound	30 cm	600 grams
25 weeks	13.62 inches	1.46 pound	34.6 cm	660 grams
26 weeks	14.02 inches	1.68 pound	35.6 cm	760 grams
27 weeks	14.41 inches	1.93 pound	36.6 cm	875 grams
28 weeks	14.80 inches	2.22 pounds	37.6 cm	1005 grams
29 weeks	15.2 inches	2.54 pounds	38.6 cm	1153 grams
30 weeks	15.71 inches	2.91 pounds	39.9 cm	1319 grams
31 weeks	16.18 inches	3.31 pounds	41.1 cm	1502 grams
32 weeks	16.69 inches	3.75 pounds	42.4 cm	1702 grams
33 weeks	17.20 inches	4.23 pounds	43.7 cm	1918 grams
34 weeks	17.72 inches	4.73 pounds	45 cm	2146 grams
35 weeks	18.19 inches	5.25 pounds	46.2 cm	2383 grams
36 weeks	18.66 inches	5.78 pounds	47.4 cm	2622 grams
37 weeks	19.13 inches	6.30 pounds	48.6 cm	2859 grams
38 weeks	19.61 inches	6.80 pounds	49.8 cm	3083 grams
39 weeks	19.96 inches	7.25 pounds	50.7 cm	3288 grams
40 weeks	20.16 inches	7.63 pounds	51.2 cm	3462 grams
41 weeks	20.35 inches	7.93 pounds	51.7 cm	3597 grams
42 weeks	20.28 inches	8.12 pounds	51.5 cm	3685 grams

So please, do not ask your OB the same question *every* visit, "How much does my baby weighs or how long does he measure?" at your next appointment!

INDEX

Symbols

3D Ultrasound 213
39 Week Rule 105
"Daddy's Hands" 184

A

A.A. Milne, Living to a 100 xx
A. A. Milne Quote, Loving too much xx
Abdominal Pain 92
Acne during pregnancy 104
ACOG 31
Acrocyanosis 266
Adverse OB outcomes 72
    Missing fingers and toes 73
Advice from others 52
Afraid of Needles 276
Allergies, Seasonal and Hay Fever 82
Ambien 298
Amniotic Fluid
    Leakage 248
Amniotic Sac 245
Anatomy of Pregnancy 800
Anemia 80
    Postpartum 540
An Example of some maleEye Candy 735
Antacids 78
Appendix A
    100% Whole wheat bread 424
    Dedication of Book 770
    Dr. Zweig's 2013 Graduation Speech 774
    Jude Lyons' Bran Raisin Recipe 772
    Why author chose OB-GYN 766
    Why Author Wrote this Book 765
Appendix B
    A "Doctors Note" 790
    Forceps Illustration 789
    Harmony NIPS Testing 782
    New Sunscreen Labels 786
Appendix C
    How did I become Pregnant 791
Appendix D
    Newborn Screening Tests 811
    Vaccination Guidelines in Pregnancy 801
Appendix E
    VBAC Consent Form 828
Appointments 19

B

Babies and "the light." 642
Baby already waving to everyone in the OR 527
Baby being weighed after C-section 379
Baby Book 189
Baby Books 189
Baby Brain 88
Baby Bump 119
Baby ID Bracelets 511
Baby in Warmer 160
Baby Moon 185
Baby "mummy-wrapped" 161
Baby on Mother's Abdomen 278
Baby sees the light? 641
Baby's head is crowning on the perineum 159
Baby weight and height 70

Bacterial Vaginosis 108
Balanced Meal. 418
Balanced meal plans 421
Barbiturates 299
Bathing and Showering 60
Bendectin© 13
Biophysical Profile (BPP) 212
Birth Canal 240
Birth Canal maneuvers 143
Birth Certificate
    This RN is making footprints to be official 147
    Typical Hospital with babys footprints 148
Birthing Plans 219
Birth Plan Samples 831
Bishop Score
    Components 247
Blankie of his son's "Blankie" 548
Bottle-feeding 583
Braxton Hicks contractions 114
Breastfeeding 151, 554, 602
    Acual Nursing Process 566
    Advantages 555
    Baby favoring one breast 576
    Breast Pumps 581
    Clogged Milk ducts 574
    Disadvantages 556
    Engorgement 565
    Facilitating Milk Expression 579
    Frequency 578
    How to Express 579
    Initiation 563
    Inverted nipples 575
    Key Points 562
    Lactation Consultant's Advice 569
    Lactation suppression 586
    Let down 575
    Losing weight while nursing 576
    Mastitis (breast infection) 573
    Milk Expression 578
    Milk productin 578
    Milk supply 580
    Nutrition for 576
    Postpartum 538
    Preparations for 557
    Requirements for effective 567
    Sequence in Brief 582
    Stored milk thawing 582
    Storing milk 581
    Sustaining milk supply 564
    Swollen Glands 574
    Techniques 558
    Weight Loss Program while breastfeeding 587
Breech Deliveries 391
    ECV (External Cephalic Version) 392
Breech Presentations 391

C

Caffeine Use during pregnancy 474
Calling your OB office 67
Camper Reproduction 668
Carpal tunnel syndrome 92
Caruthers's Triplets at age 2 202
Castor Oil 703
Caval Syndrome 101
Cerclage of cervix 182
Cervix
    Bishop Score 247
    Dilatation 232
    Effacement or thinning of 232
    Incompetent 181
    Ripeness 246
Cesarean Delivery 354
Cesarean section
    Incision care 527
Cesarean Section
    Anemia 529
    Aspiration 261
    Breastfeeding after 530
    Emergency 261
    FAQs 383
    Indications for 360
    Post-Operative pain control 381
    Risks 364
    Sex after 530
    Stairs after 530
    Steps to 368
    Swimming after 530

Cesarean Sections
   Complications 368
   Legal Indications 360
   Medical History 355
Cesarean Secton
   Incision Types 357
Chantrix 125
Charles Krauthammer Quote xiv
Cheese Choices 416
Chicago Musical Song, "Mama" 57
Chicken Taco Soup 435
Chlamydial infections 108
Circle of Life xliii
Circumcision 610
   Post procedure care and appearance 601
Circumcision Prep and Drape 613
Classes
   Childbirth 188
Classic Cradle Position 559
Clothing 60
Colds and Flu 75
Color Doppler of umbilical cord flow 213
colostrum 92
Comanche County Memorial Hospital Picture 62
Common Questions Newborn Hearing Screens 819
Common Symptoms of Pregnancy 8
Compazine 15
Condylomata 111
Constipation 77, 79
Contraction Stress Test (CST) 211
Cord Blood Banking 217
Cowboy saw God today 291
cravings during pregnancy 86
C-sections and obesity 367
C-section surgical planes 359
Cutting Umbilical Cord 159

D

Delivery
   Description 277
   "Ring of Fire" 274
   Shakes and Shivers afterwards 288

Demerol 295
Dental care during pregnancy 177
Dental Hygiene 173
Diabetes 477
   Treatment 480
Diabetes in Pregnancy
   Testing for 218
Diaper "Cake" 608
Diarrhea 76
Diclegis 13
Diet 12
   Breads and Cereals 424
   Calcium intake 430
   Caloric Requirements 408
   Daily Food Guide 431
   During pregnancy 406
   Fats in Protein foods 415
   Fiber 422
   Fish 406
   Fluid Intake 426
   Folic Acid 428
   Food Additives 466
   Food Preparation 442
   Iron 421, 428
   Mercury in Fish 407
   Milk and Dairy Products 419
   Proteins 410
   Salt intake 427
   Sample menu 300 calories 408
   Sample Menus and Food Groups 432
   Weight Gain during pregnancy 409
   Zinc 429
Dizziness 83
Doctors Note 790
Doppler Study 212
doxylamine 14
Drugs during pregnancy
   References 476
Dr. Zweig's daughter 662
Dr. Zweigs Power Table 114
Due Date 18

E

Eclampsia 47, 194

Egg preparing its own bed (or endometrium) it will "sleep" or grow in 794
Electric Blankets 400
Engagement of Fetal Head 237
Environmental Exposures 450
Epidural and spinal spaces in backbone. 305
Epidural Anesthesia 302
    Indications for 311
    Information Sheet 313
    Risks and Side Effects 312
Epiduralplacement 308
Epidural procedure 309
Episiotomy 520
Example of Balanced Meal 418
Example of Cereal food label 436
Exercise and Physical Activities 17
Exercise in Pregnancy 395
    Cardinal Principles 397
    Cautions 397
    Don'ts 395
    Exercise Do's 396
    Scuba Diving 399
    Water or Snow Skiing 399
    Weight Lifting 399
External Fetal Monitoring belts on patient in early labor 289
Extreme long term variability 344
Eye care in pregnancy 178

F

Fainting 83
Family departing 167
Family members to support you 156
Family& Nursing Students 155
Father cutting cord 279
Father of baby cutting his new borns Cord. 278
Fentanly 296
Fertilization of egg, transport down the tube and implantation 797
Fetal Backbone and Ribs 209
Fetal Heart Monitoring 210
    Long Term Variability 338

Type 1 Head Compression Decelerations 339
Type 2 Late Decelerations 340
Type 3 Variable decelerations 341
Fetal Kick Counts 206
Fetal monitor 156
Fetal Monitoring 332
Fetal Movements 206
Fetal Strip showing no "long term variability 338
Fetal strip showing normal short and long term variability 338
Fetal Surveillance Testing 210
FHT pattern Summary 341
Figure 6-2. Complete Dilatation when putting on a turtle neck 235
Figure 6-12 Placenta Praevia 205
Figure.6-16.NormalNSTstrip 211
Figure 7-9. The typical Delivery Room Audience 257
Figure 24-3. Key Protection from Moon rays 638
Figure 26-22. Photograph of Lake Elizabeth and jogging path 733
Figure 26-27. Women's Favorite Story of the Year 758
FigurHamrell's Line 680
FiguVariable or Type III decelerations 342
Fluoride in pregnancy 175
flu vaccine 45
Focal Point on a Picture 273
folic acid 31
Folic Acid 428
Folic Acid deficiency 81
Food for Your Baby 553
Food Labels 435
    Ingredient List 437
    Nutritional Information 437
    Nutrition per Servings 438
Food Poisoning
    Botulism 444
    Salmonella 444
    Staph Infections 443
Food Poisonings

Clostridium Perfringens 444
Food Safety 448
Food Storage 447
Football 559
Foot prints of Baby on the Father's Scrub shirt 149
Forceps Delivery 327
Friedman's Graph of Cervical Dilatation and Time 139
Full Moon for babies 639

G

gas 78
GBS (Group B streptococcus)
    Testing 218
GBS Testing 207
Gender Reveal Party 115
General Anesthesia 319
George Strait
    I Saw God Today 290
Gestational Diabetes
    3 hour glucose tolerance test 218
Gingivitis 178
Glucose Tolerance Test 479
Gonorrhea 110
Graciela at her 6 week 168

H

Hair
    Permanents, Coloring and Manicures 87
Harmony 39
Harmony Prenatal Testing 783
Harmony™ Prenatal Test Summary 784
Headaches 82
Heartburn 77
Height and Weight of baby by week 836
Hepatitis in pregnancy 498
Herpes Infections 109
Herpes in pregnancy 487
    Diagnosis 497
    Mode of Delivery 497
    treatment 494
HIV in pregnancy 498

Hospital
    Preparations 187
    Pre-Registration 187
Hospital Entrance 153
Hospital-issue panties 513
Hospital Stay 511
HPV virus 107
Hygiene in pregnancy 171
Hyperemesis Gravidarum 199

I

Illustration C-2. Mature "Egg Follicle" unit 793
Illustration of a fetal heart strip 334
Illustration of External Version 393
Illustration of forceps application for delivery 331
Illustration of vacuum application 325
Illustration of Vacuum Delivery 324
Infectious Diseases during pregnancy 501
Insomnia 100
insurance coverage 63
Internal Fetal Heart Electrode and Intrauterine Pressure Catheter 135
Internal Fetal Monitoring
    IUPC (intrauterine pressure catheter 227
Interstate 680 Camper 668

K

Kiwi® type of vacuum cup 324

L

Labor
    1st Stage 268
    3rd Stage of 283
    4 P's 236
    4 Stages of Labor 231
    Acitve Management 271
    Active Phase 269
    Coping with 273
    Doctor Presence 258
    Eating and drinking 131

Eating and Drinking 259
False 232
Friedman Curve 270
How do you know? 228
Induction 347
Induction of 150
Induction techniques 348
Labor "Losers" 281
"Last to Know" Phenomenon 131
Length of time 137
Mechanism of 237
Medical Definition 231
Number of support persons 132
Packing for your stay 130
Positions of the Baby 241
Process of 262
Purpose or Goal 232
Time of onset 227
True Labor Definition 244
Turtle Neck Analogy 233
Turtle Neck Sweater Analogy 138
Typical Scenario 264
Umbilical Cord 260
Video and Photographing 255
What to do after starting 249
When to go to hospital 130

laboratory testing 37
Labor, Head Flexion 239
Labor Induction
    39 Week Rule 128
Labor Journey of Birth- 142
Labor Room
    Number of People allowed 256
    Number of people attending delivery 132
Lactation suppression 539
Lactation Suppression 586
Late Deceleration Pattern, Type II 340
LBD Test of Pregnancy 7
Leg swelling 83
LGV 112
Life, the Secret of viii
Lightly sautéed scallops 413
Linea Alba (Black line) 89
Linea Nigra 645

Lip Blisters on breastfeeding baby on 6th day after birth 604
Love, can you feel it tonight? 117
Low Back Pain 94
Low Forceps Application 330
Lying down position 560

M

Manual Removal of a Retained Placenta. 284
Materni21 Prenatal Testing 784
MaterniT21Plus 39
Medications
    Labor analgesics 292
Medications during pregnancy
    General Principles 462
    Specific Harmful Drugs 466
Medications during Pregnancy
    Commonly used Safe Medications 467
Medications for common symptoms 26
Medications in Labor 144
Milk 420
Miscarriage (Abortion) 503
Modified Straddle hold 560
Moluscum 111
Moments that take your breath away xxi, xxiii
Mom leaving Hospital 167
Mom on her "Babymoon." 186
Mom Song sung by Garth Brooks xlii
Morning Sickness 7
Morphine 295
Mother and baby bonding 591
Mother bonding with her newborn 162
Mother holding her baby for first time 161
Motherhood, "Best Job in Life" iii
Mucus plug 129
Multiple Marker 40
My Body is changing 16
Myths about Pregnancy 650

N

nausea and vomiting 76
Neck of Turtle neck sweater 138
Nesting Instincts 219
Newborn
- Acrocyanosis 596
- Advice to your children 631
- Author's Experiences 627
- Baby's Genitalia 600
- Baby's Skin 597
- Circumcision 610
- Concept of Parenting 591
- Cord care and appearance 599
- Diapers 607
- Digestive system 602
- Getting your baby to sleep 625
- Health Screening and Testing 594
- Home Temperatures 605
- Immediate Care after delivery 283
- Keeping your marriage alive 622
- Molding of head 596
- Monitoring and Surveillance Systems 616
- Naming your baby 592
- Newborn Baby Carriers 620
- Newborn baby's physical exam 596
- Pediatrician Specialist 591
- Prenatal visit with Baby's physician 589
- Preparations at home for baby 595
- Songs and Lyrics for inspiration 633
- Supply Checklist for Baby 545

Newborn baby 147
Newborn Drug Addiction 474
Newborn in Warmer 160
Newborn with her mittens on 190
New Father Sleeping Sickness 517
"New Fathers' Sleeping Sickness" 518
New Parents just about ready to take their newborn home. 543
New Sunscreen Labels 787
NIPS or Non-invasive Prenatal Screening 39
Non-stress Test (NST) 211

Normal short and long term variability 339
Nubain 294

O

Obesity 113
OB Nurses "coaching" 158
Obstetrical Forceps 789
Obstetrical Tragedies 502
- Ectopic Pregnancy 509

OB Suite 154
OB Suite Entry 154
OB Table 158
Occupational Safety 454
- Day Care centers 457
- Known Toxic Agents 454
- Medical and Dental Fields 457
- Other Special Exposures 460
- Principles of 456

Oklahoma Sun Rise 126
Old Husband Tales 651
Old Obstetrician Tales 652
- April Fool's Day 666
- Breech baby and Dr. Gandhi 713
- Breech Births by Dr. Dignam 706
- Carmen, the Pregnant Runner 730
- Castor Oil and labor induction 703
- Dr. Branch and the Chairman 701
- Four Babyies in 26 minutes 662
- I want a Pepsi 723
- Juan Garcia and Alviso, CA 673
- Linda Castro Story 753
- Match.com 741
- Melody, the Hairdresser-Athlete 654
- My Little Patient in San Ramon, CA 697
- Pyrimidalis Muscles 729
- Remembering Rita 669
- Story of Jennifer's Birth 658
- Teenager Birth Control 657
- Teen Pregnancy Baby Issue 725
- Teen Pregnancy Lost and Hurt 708
- The Camper on I-680 668

The City Councilman's Wife 655
The DaSilva Family 652
The Garabaldi Family 653
The Hispanic Newly Wed 674
The Isuzu Baby 664
The Redhead from Santa Maria 676
The Story of Patty 735
The Tennessee Trucker Woman 671
Twins in Koerber Family 715
Ultrasound Probe Protection 680
Zweig's Laws of Obstetrics 656

Old Wives Tales 634
Old Wives' Tales
    abies "seeing the light" 640
    Acne Test 644
    Avoid Taking Baths 635
    Baby's Heart Rate 634
    Baby's heart rate and baby's sex 642
    Body changes and baby sex 635
    Cold Feet Test 646
    Demeanor and Agility 649
    Do you smell garlic? 649
    Drano Test 643
    Facial Changes 649
    Food Cravings 635
    Full moon and babies 639
    Hair Growth Theory 648
    Heartburn and hair 636
    How you "carry" your baby 634
    Hubby's sympathy weight gain 636
    Key around neck 638
    Key Test 643
    Linea Nigra Test 645
    Mayan number game 643
    Mayan Number Variations 646
    More Myths about Pregnancy 650
    Morning Sickness Test 644
    Mucus Plug 637
    Pillow Test 646
    Posterior head position 637
    Raising your hands above head 635
    Ring Test 636, 644
    Shape of Belly Test 648
    Show me your hands 649
    Sleeping position 647

"The Drano test 634
Thirsty and drinking water 636
Urine Color Test 647
Operative Vaginal Delivery 321
Our friendly (and beautiful) OB nurses 510

P

Panorama 39
Panorama Prenatal Testing 785
Pap Smears
    Abnormal 123
Patient in 2nd Stage of Labor 157
Patient in Labor 155
Patient with epidural 157
Pediatrician 150
Pelvic Exam Reflex 121
Pentothal 299
Phenergan 15
Phenobarbital 299
phone number 24
Phone numbers 170
Photograph Senior Graduating OU Family Residents of 2013 and 2014 with Dr. Zweig 775
Photo of a Newborn baby 769
Photo of fetal heart electrode and amniohook 137
Photo Resembling "Carmen" 732
Pica 81
Picture of an Isuzu Trooper SUV 664
Placenta
    Separation after birth 285
Placental Abruption 202
Placenta Previa 204
Placing Fetal Scalp Electrode and Amniohook 352
Position of Baby in Labor
    Posterior or OP 243
Postpartum
    After-pains and cramping 520
    Back pain 525
    Bathing and Showering 512
    Bladder problems 524
    Bleeding after delivery 512

Checkup Appointment after delivery 544
Constipation 522
Contraception 532
Depression 532
Hemorrhage 514
Hemorrhoids 523
Leg Swelling and Pain 524
Losing weight after delivery 551
Medications 540
Nutrition and Diet 525
Perineal Care after delivery 519
Physical Activities 526
Physician Rounds 514
Rubella Vaccination 536
Warning Signs 542
Postpartum Checkup 150
Postpartum Depression 532
Postpartum family asleep 543
Postpartum Floor 164
Postpartum mother completely outfitted for her new arrival 163
Postpartum Nursing Station 164
Postpartum Room 163
Pre-eclampsia 47, 191
Pregnancy
"Bump" 120
Dreams more vivid 88
Pregnancy Portraits 224
Pregnancy Q & As 118
Pregnancy symptoms, early 7
Pregnancy Tests, purchase 6
Pregnancy Weight Gain by Trimester 32
Prenatal Classes 63
Prenatal Vitamin Formulary in OK 815
prescriptions 26
Refills 67
Preterm Labor 196
Preterm Rupture of membranes 198
PYRIMIDALIS MUSCLES 729

Q

Quickening
Fetal movements 61

R

Reference Materials 830
Relationship Changes during pregnancy 54
Relatives and friends in Nursery Window 162
Rh Factor 480
Explanation 482
Rhogam 485
Rhogam postpartum 536
Rhogam use 486
Round Ligament Syndrome 92
Rubella Syndrome 730
Rubella Vaccine 471

S

Safety and Security of your baby 817
Salad 423
Saunas 90
Saunas and Hot Tubs 400
Sciatica 96
Seat Belts in pregnancy 179
Sedatives and Tranquiliers 297
Sex during pregnancy 49
Sex in pregnancy 180
sex of your baby 41
Shoes 61
Sickle cell anemia 81
SIDS (Sudden Infant Death Syndrome 619
Silky bordered Baby Blankets 548
Skin Changes 104
sleeping on your back 100
Smoking 25, 402
Postpartum 536
Smoking Cessation 124
medications 125
Nicotine gum 124
Southwestern Medical 62
Spinal Anesthesia 318
Stadol 294
STD's 107
Stillbirth 509
Stretch marks 90

StretchMarks 91
Strip showing normal to increased "Long term variability" 337
Substance Abuse
  Alcohol 473
  Analgesics 473
  Cocaine 474
  Marijuana 474
  Methamphetamines 474
  Tobacco and smoking 474
Sun at the beach require Sunscreen 786
Suntanning 89
Sun Tanning and Skin Tinting 401
Surgical Pause 373
Swelling of feet at end of day 84
Syphilis 112

T

Tanning 90
Thalassemia 82
The "Birthing Kiss." 281
The Girl in a Red Sundress 791
The Simpson Forceps 329
The Snack Machine 407
The Trip to the Hospital 251
The typical Delivery Room Audience 257
The wonder of a child gazing at his newborn sister 165
Third Trimester Changes 222
Thrombophlebitis 538
Tom Stoppard Quote xiv
Traditional Roses for the new mom. 166
travel during pregnancy 59
Traveling 403
Trichomoniasis 108
Trimesters of pregnancy 35
True Knot in cord 261
Turtle Neck is completely dilated or stretched to fit. 236
Twin Placenta 200
Twin Pregnancy 199
Twins on Ultrasound 199
Type II and Type III decelerations 344
Types of Abdominal incisions 357
Types of Uterine Incisions 358

Typical appearance of a Birthing Room 132
Typical Herpes blisters on the Left Labia 109
Typical low transverse bikini incision 357
Typical "Normal" Fetal monitor tracing 336
Typical OR Scene during C-section 354

U

Ultrasound Images of "Blighted ovum 503
Ultrasound of baby in mid-pregnancy 215
Umbilical Cord
  Delayed clamping 267
Unisom 14
Urinary Incontinence 112
Urinary tract infections 103
Urinary Tract Infections (UTIs) 537
Uterine Subinvolution 514
Uterus
  Atony after birth 287

V

vaccinations 46
Vaccinations during Pregnancy 470
Vacuum Delivery 326
Vacuum Extractor 321
Valium 298
Varicose veins 85
VBAC
  Benefits 389
  Protocol 389
  Risks 386
VBAC Protocol at Southwestern 821
VBAC (Vaginal Birth After C-section 386
Vegetables, fruit and protein sources 414
Versed 297
Vertex Position 208
Vistaril (Hydroxyzine) 297
Vitamin B6 13
Vitamin B6 (Pyridoxine) 14
Vitamin B12 anemia 81
Vitamin C 31